Review of Pathophysiology

REVIEW OF PATHOPHYSIOLOGY

Edited by

Christian E. Kaufman, Jr., M.D.

Associate Professor of Medicine, University of Oklahoma College of
Medicine; Staff Physician, Veterans Administration Medical Center,
Oklahoma City

Solomon Papper, M.D.

Distinguished Professor and Head, Department of Medicine, University of
Oklahoma College of Medicine; Staff Physician, Veterans Administration
Medical Center, Oklahoma City

Little, Brown and Company   Boston/Toronto

Contents

Contributing Authors   vii
Preface   xi

| John A. Mohr | **I** | **Aging** |
| | 1 | Physical Consequences of Aging   3 |

Michael D. Ezekowitz	**II**	**Cardiovascular Disease**
Ralph Lazzara	2	Electrophysiologic Basis of Cardiac Arrhythmias 11
Thasana Nivatpumin	3	Myocardial Contraction and Cardiac Performance 21
Dwight W. Reynolds	4	Common Forms of Volume and Pressure Overload 27
Eliot Schechter	5	Atherosclerosis 33
Udho Thadani	6	Biochemical, Physiologic, and Pathologic Consequences of Ischemia 39
Michael F. Wilson	7	Clinical Manifestations of Coronary Artery Disease 45
	8	Valvular Heart Disease 50
	9	Intracardiac Shunts 58
	10	Congestive Heart Failure 65
	11	Mechanisms of Shock 73

Ronald D. Brown	**III**	**Endocrinology, Metabolism, and Hypertension**
John R. Higgins	12	Hormone Action 81
David C. Kem	13	Anterior and Posterior Pituitary 85
Robert H. Roswell	14	Adrenal-ACTH 90
	15	Thyroid and TSH 96
	16	Hypertension 101
	17	Diabetes Mellitus and Glucose Metabolism 106
	18	Reproductive Endocrinology 111

Robert A. Rankin	**IV**	**Gastroenterology**
Jack D. Welsh	19	The Esophagus 119
	20	Peptic Ulcer Diseases of the Stomach and Duodenum 125
	21	The Pancreas 131
	22	The Gallbladder and Biliary Tract 137
	23	The Liver 141
	24	Maldigestion, Malabsorption, and Diarrhea 149
	25	Gastrointestinal Malignancies 154

Sylvia S. Bottomley	**V**	**Hematology**
Philip C. Comp	26	Introduction to Hematology 159
Dilip L. Solanki	27	Disorders of the Erythron 160
	28	Neutrophil Disorders 169
	29	Platelets 175
	30	Disorders of Blood Coagulation 181

Samuel R. Oleinick	**VI**	**Immunology and Rheumatology**
Morris Reichlin	31	Immediate Hypersensitivity Disease 189
Russell T. Schultz	32	Allergic Respiratory Diseases 194
James H. Wells	33	Immunologically Mediated Disease 200
	34	Inflammatory Rheumatic Diseases (Noninfectious): Mediation by Immunologic Mechanisms 206
	35	Degenerative Joint Diseases and Gout 213
	36	Immunodeficiency 220

Everett R. Rhoades	**VII**	**Infection**
	37	Inflammation 231
	38	Hyperthermia and Fever 238

Anthony W. Czerwinski	**VIII**	**Nephrology**
Arnold J. Felsenfeld	39	Disorders of Sodium and Water Metabolism 247
Christian E. Kaufman, Jr.	40	Potassium Homeostasis 260
Henry F. Krous	41	Hydrogen Ion Homeostasis: Metabolic Acidosis and Alkalosis 268
Francisco Llach	42	Calcium, Phosphate, and Vitamin D 279
James A. Pederson	43	Glomerulonephritis and the Acute Nephritic Syndrome 287
Laura I. Rankin	44	The Nephrotic Syndrome 298
	45	Acute Renal Failure 303
	46	The Uremic State 308
	47	Metabolic Bone Disease 313
	48	Renal Cell Carcinoma: Mechanisms of Clinical Manifestations 322

C. G. Gunn	**IX**	**Neurology and Pain**
John W. Nelson	49	Pain 327
	50	Epilepsy 333
	51	Cerebrovascular Disease 337
	52	The Upper Motor Neuron System and the Motor Unit 340

| Don P. Murray | **X** | **Nutrition** |
| Robert Whang | 53 | Clinical Malnutrition 347 |

E. Randy Eichner	**XI**	**Oncology**
Robert B. Epstein	54	Carcinogenesis, Cell Kinetics, and Tumor Immunology 355
J. Lee Murray	55	Extraneoplastic Manifestations of Malignancies 367
Robert B. Slease	56	Neoplasms of the Immune System 375
	57	Cancer of the Breast 386

Ralph C. Beckett	**XII**	**Pulmonary Disease**
Alfred F. Connors	58	Pulmonary Gas Exchange 395
Ann L. DeHart	59	Pulmonary Mechanics 405
Barry A. Gray	60	Control of Breathing 413
David C. Levin	61	Reversible Obstructive Airways Disease (Asthma) 421
D. Robert McCaffree	62	Chronic Airflow Limitation 430
Thomas L. Murphy	63	Interstitial Lung Disease 434
Sami I. Said	64	Pulmonary Edema 442
	65	Pulmonary Vascular Disease 449
	66	Pulmonary Neoplastic Disease 455

| Jay P. Cannon | **XIII** | **Surgery and Trauma** |
| | 67 | The Metabolic Response to Surgery, Injury, and Trauma 463 |

| James A. Merrill | **XIV** | **Toxemias of Pregnancy** |
| | 68 | Hypertensive Disorders (Toxemia) of Pregnancy 475 |

| | | Questions, Answers, and Analyses 485 |
| | | Index 525 |

Contributing Authors

Ralph C. Beckett, M.D.
Formerly Assistant Professor of Medicine, University of Oklahoma College of Medicine. Currently in private practice, Cedar Rapids, Iowa

Sylvia S. Bottomley, M.D.
Professor of Medicine, University of Oklahoma College of Medicine; Staff Physician, Veterans Administration Medical Center, Oklahoma City

Ronald D. Brown, M.D.
Professor of Medicine, University of Oklahoma College of Medicine; Staff Physician, Veterans Administration Medical Center, Oklahoma City

Jay P. Cannon, M.D.
Associate Professor of Surgery, University of Oklahoma College of Medicine; Staff Physician, Veterans Administration Medical Center, Oklahoma City

Philip C. Comp, M.D., Ph.D.
Associate Professor of Medicine, University of Oklahoma College of Medicine, Oklahoma City

Alfred F. Connors, M.D.
Assistant Professor of Medicine, Pulmonary Division, Case Western Reserve University School of Medicine; Director, Medical Intensive Care Unit, Cleveland Metropolitan General Hospital, Cleveland

Anthony W. Czerwinski, M.D.
Clinical Professor, Department of Medicine, University of Oklahoma College of Medicine, Oklahoma City

Ann L. DeHart, M.D.
Formerly Fellow, Pulmonary Disease Section, Department of Medicine, University of Oklahoma College of Medicine. Currently in private practice, Albuquerque, New Mexico

E. Randy Eichner, M.D.
Professor of Medicine and Chief, Hematology Section, Department of Medicine, University of Oklahoma College of Medicine; Staff Physician, Veterans Administration Medical Center, Oklahoma City

Robert B. Epstein, M.D.
Eason Professor and Chief, Oncology Section, Department of Medicine, University of Oklahoma College of Medicine; Staff Physician, Veterans Administration Medical Center; Director of Clinical Oncology, Oklahoma Memorial Research Foundation, Oklahoma City

Michael D. Ezekowitz, M.D., Ph.D.
Associate Professor, Departments of Medicine and Radiology, Yale University School of Medicine, New Haven, Connecticut

Arnold J. Felsenfeld, M.D.
Assistant Professor of Medicine, University of Oklahoma College of Medicine; Staff Physician, Veterans Administration Medical Center, Oklahoma City

Barry A. Gray, M.D., Ph.D.
Associate Professor of Medicine, University of Oklahoma College of Medicine; Director, Medical Intensive Care Unit, Veterans Administration Medical Center, Oklahoma City

C. G. Gunn, M.D.
Professor of Medicine, University of Oklahoma College of Medicine; Staff Physician, Veterans Administration Medical Center, Oklahoma City

John R. Higgins, M.D.	Associate Professor and Associate Chairman, Department of Medicine, and Chief, Endocrinology and Metabolism Section, Texas Tech University School of Medicine, Lubbock
Christian E. Kaufman, Jr., M.D.	Associate Professor of Medicine, University of Oklahoma College of Medicine; Staff Physician, Veterans Administration Medical Center, Oklahoma City
David C. Kem, M.D.	Professor of Medicine and Chief, Endocrinology, Metabolism, and Hypertension Section, Department of Medicine, University of Oklahoma College of Medicine; Staff Physician, Veterans Administration Medical Center, Oklahoma City
Henry F. Krous, M.D.	Associate Professor of Pathology and Pediatrics, University of Oklahoma College of Medicine, Oklahoma City
Ralph Lazzara, M.D.	Professor of Medicine and Chief, Cardiovascular Section, Department of Medicine, University of Oklahoma College of Medicine; Staff Physician, Veterans Administration Medical Center, Oklahoma City
David C. Levin, M.D.	Associate Professor of Medicine, University of Oklahoma College of Medicine; Staff Physician, Veterans Administration Medical Center, Oklahoma City
Francisco Llach, M.D.	Professor of Medicine and Chief, Nephrology Section, Department of Medicine, University of Oklahoma College of Medicine; Staff Physician, Veterans Administration Medical Center, Oklahoma City
D. Robert McCaffree, M.D.	Associate Professor of Medicine, University of Oklahoma College of Medicine; Medical Director, Intensive Care Unit, Oklahoma Memorial Hospital; Staff Physician, Veterans Administration Medical Center, Oklahoma City
James A. Merrill, M.D.	Professor of Gynecology and Obstetrics and Professor of Pathology, University of Oklahoma College of Medicine, Oklahoma City
John A. Mohr, M.D.	Professor of Medicine, University of Oklahoma College of Medicine; Assistant Chief, Medical Service, Veterans Administration Medical Center; Chief, Medical Service, O'Donoghue Rehabilitation Institute, Oklahoma City
Thomas L. Murphy, M.D.	Director, Respiratory Therapy Department, Gaston Memorial Hospital, Gastonia, North Carolina
Don P. Murray, M.D.	Assistant Professor, Department of Medicine, University of Oklahoma College of Medicine; Staff Physician, Veterans Administration Medical Center, Oklahoma City
J. Lee Murray, M.D.	Faculty Associate, Department of Clinical Immunology and Biological Therapy, M. D. Anderson Hospital and Tumor Institute, Houston, Texas
John W. Nelson, M.D.	Professor and Head, Department of Neurology, University of Oklahoma College of Medicine; Chief, Neurology Service, Veterans Administration Medical Center, Oklahoma City

Thasana Nivatpumin, M.D.	Associate Professor of Medicine, University of California at Los Angeles, School of Medicine; Director, Cardiac Catheterization Laboratory, Cedars-Sinai Medical Center, Los Angeles
Samuel R. Oleinick, M.D., Ph.D.	Professor of Medicine and Adjunct Professor of Microbiology-Immunology, University of Oklahoma College of Medicine; Staff Physician, Veterans Administration Medical Center, Oklahoma City
Solomon Papper, M.D.	Distinguished Professor and Head, Department of Medicine, University of Oklahoma College of Medicine; Staff Physician, Veterans Administration Medical Center, Oklahoma City
James A. Pederson, M.D.	Professor of Medicine, University of Oklahoma College of Medicine; Director, Renal Failure Care Unit, Veterans Administration Medical Center, Oklahoma City
Laura I. Rankin, M.D.	Assistant Professor of Medicine, University of Oklahoma College of Medicine; Staff Physician, Veterans Administration Medical Center, Oklahoma City
Robert A. Rankin, M.D.	Assistant Professor of Medicine, University of Oklahoma College of Medicine; Director, Endoscopy Service, Oklahoma Memorial Hospital and Veterans Administration Medical Center, Oklahoma City
Morris Reichlin, M.D.	Professor of Medicine and Chief, Immunology Section, Department of Medicine, University of Oklahoma College of Medicine; Staff Physician, Veterans Administration Medical Center; Head, Arthritis and Immunology Laboratory, Oklahoma Medical Research Foundation, Oklahoma City
Dwight W. Reynolds, M.D.	Assistant Professor of Medicine, University of Oklahoma College of Medicine; Staff Physician, Veterans Administration Medical Center, Oklahoma City
Everett R. Rhoades, M.D.	Formerly Professor of Medicine and Chief of Infectious Diseases Section, Department of Medicine, University of Oklahoma College of Medicine, Oklahoma City. Currently Assistant Surgeon General and Director, Indian Health Service, Washington, D.C.
Robert H. Roswell, M.D.	Assistant Professor of Medicine, University of Oklahoma College of Medicine; Staff Physician, Veterans Administration Medical Center, Oklahoma City
Sami I. Said, M.D.	Professor of Medicine and Chief, Pulmonary Disease and Critical Care Section, Department of Medicine, University of Oklahoma College of Medicine; Staff Physician, Veterans Administration Medical Center, Oklahoma City
Eliot Schechter, M.D.	Professor of Medicine, University of Oklahoma College of Medicine; Director, Cardiac Catheterization Laboratory, Veterans Administration Medical Center, Oklahoma City
Russell T. Schultz, M.D.	Professor of Medicine, University of Oklahoma College of Medicine; Chief of Rheumatology, Veterans Administration Medical Center, Oklahoma City
Robert B. Slease, M.D.	Associate Professor of Medicine, University of Oklahoma College of Medicine; Staff Physician, Veterans Administration Medical Center, Oklahoma City

Dilip L. Solanki, M.D.	Associate Professor of Medicine, University of Oklahoma College of Medicine; Staff Physician, Veterans Administration Medical Center, Oklahoma City
Udho Thadani, M.B.B.S., M.R.C.P.	Associate Professor of Medicine and Vice-Chief, Cardiovascular Section, University of Oklahoma College of Medicine; Staff Physician, Veterans Administration Medical Center, Oklahoma City
James H. Wells, M.D.	Associate Professor of Medicine, University of Oklahoma College of Medicine; Staff Physician, Veterans Administration Medical Center, Oklahoma City
Jack D. Welsh, M.D.	Professor of Medicine and Chief, Digestive Disease and Nutrition Section, Department of Medicine, University of Oklahoma College of Medicine; Staff Physician, Veterans Administration Medical Center, Oklahoma City
Robert Whang, M.D.	Professor and Vice-Head, Department of Medicine, University of Oklahoma College of Medicine; Chief, Medical Service, Veterans Administration Medical Center, Oklahoma City
Michael F. Wilson, M.D.	Professor of Medicine and Associate Professor of Radiology, University of Oklahoma College of Medicine; Associate Chief of Staff for Research, Veterans Administration Medical Center, Oklahoma City

Preface

Knowledge of the mechanisms of disease is vast and rapidly expanding. The purpose of *Review of Pathophysiology* is to summarize selected information that is clinically relevant or likely to become so in the near future; it is not intended as a comprehensive text for this important field.

The term *pathophysiology* refers to the study of alterations in normal body function (physiology and biochemistry) that result from disease processes. Since a knowledge of physiology is essential to an understanding of pathophysiology, each chapter begins with a brief description of normal function, followed by a succinct review of common or classic disease processes. Our goal is to provide understanding of why and how disordered function occurs. Each chapter is concluded by one or two case studies (clinical examples) and related discussions to reinforce important principles and provide clinical relevance.

Review of Pathophysiology was designed to furnish the second-year medical student with a base of clinical information on which to build during subsequent years. In trying to bridge the gap between the basic sciences and bedside observation, we hope we have created a useful format for students, house staff, and practicing clinicians seeking a discussion of pathophysiology that is less detailed than that available in the standard texts.

We wish to thank each of the contributing authors for sharing knowledge and expertise. We are grateful to Beverly Clarke and Libby Price for editorial assistance and to Susie Rose for secretarial support.

C. E. K.
S. P.

Review of Pathophysiology

I Aging

John A. Mohr

1 Physical Consequences of Aging

I. Introduction. There are many physical changes that occur in people directly associated with, or as a result of, the aging process. Failure to recognize this may lead to unnecessary, expensive, and troublesome diagnostic procedures. Furthermore, older people respond differently than younger ones (often adversely) to disease and to our therapeutic endeavors. These differences must be recognized in order to ensure an optimal outcome.

II. Changes in stature and posture

A. Shrinkage in height is common in the elderly. The long bones do not undergo significant shortening; hence, the loss of stature can be ascribed to shortening of the spinal column as a result of both narrowing of the disks and loss in height of the individual vertebrae. In the middle years, this is due primarily to thinning of the disks, whereas in later years vertebral collapse is the major reason for loss of height. Narrowing osteoporotic vertebrae are almost universal in elderly females, but occur less frequently in males. Thus, the elderly are, in general, characterized by shortened trunks and comparatively long extremities.

B. Other changes caused by bone shortening. The thinning of the intervertebral disk and centrum also affects the neck, and to compensate for the upper thoracic spine kyphosis, the head may be tilted backward. In association with shortening of the neck, the thyroid may descend, making it difficult to palpate the lower poles of the thyroid. With shortening of the spine and lengthening of the aorta, the aortic arch elevates and may bring the right innominate artery into the neck with possible kinking of the artery, thus producing a pulsating and sometimes visible mass behind the clavicular portion of the right sternocleidomastoid muscle. The enlarged, rigid aorta may compress the left innominate vein, resulting in dilatation of the left external jugular vein. This can best be seen with the patient sitting up at a 45-degree angle.

Shoulder width and chest size decrease with age. In elderly women, chest diameter decreases 3.3 cm and in elderly men it decreases 2.3 cm. When narrowing is marked, the apical impulse may be present in the anterior axillary line without significant cardiomegaly. Furthermore, the cervical and thoracic spine may become quite rigid, rendering invalid the usual maneuvers attempted in diagnosing meningitis or subarachnoid bleeding.

III. Body hair. Many elderly people demonstrate hair loss over the body suggestive of *alopecia totalis*. Racial, genetic, and sex-linked factors, as well as the changes that occur with aging, determine the amount of hair an individual possesses. American Indian males have little body and facial hair. Caucasian males tend to have far heavier beards, and the onset of graying is earlier than in other races. Facial hirsutism is extremely rare in Japanese women up to 88 years of age, whereas in aging Caucasian women it is quite common. In general, aging is associated with decreased hair everywhere except the face.

IV. Skin. Skin studies of people over the age of 64 have demonstrated lax skin in 94 percent and seborrheic keratoses and cherry angiomas in 88 percent and 75 percent, respectively. Over 75 percent had dry, scaly skin. Other frequent skin features in the elderly include senile purpura, warts, and papillomas. The purpura appear to be a result of the loss of subcutaneous tissue supporting the skin capillaries; hence, minor trauma readily results in ecchymotic lesions. These "spontaneous bruises" occur most frequently on the forearms. There is no evidence that vitamin C deficiency plays any role in their etiology. The number of cells present in the skin declines progressively with age. By the fifth decade of life, the total cell count has decreased almost 50 percent.

V. **Eyes**

A. **Arcus senilis.** One of the most common ocular signs of aging is arcus senilis, i.e., a yellowish-white opaque ring around the iris. It does not interfere with vision and is not related to serum cholesterol; it is a result of deposition of fatty substances in Bowman's and Descemet's membranes.

B. **Visual changes.** Although presbyopia (diminished ability of the lens to focus at different distances) is the most common visual change that occurs in aging, cataracts, macular degeneration, and glaucoma are more serious.

1. **Cataracts.** Cataracts result from opacification of the lens. The lens, a protein-rich organ, doubles its weight and volume in a lifetime. The lens is enclosed by a capsule, layers of which degenerate and form a hard nucleus inside as it grows with age. At the same time, the capsule loses elasticity and accommodation becomes more difficult, thereby contributing to presbyopia.

2. **Macular degeneration.** Macular degeneration results from ischemic changes in the retina, and its frequency increases with advancing age. Impaired vascular supply, especially to the periphery, leads to hyaline infiltration, calcification, and fatty degeneration. Similar changes in the fovea result in impairment of visual acuity.

3. **Glaucoma.** As the lens size increases, the anterior chamber size decreases, producing a more acute angle between the root of the iris and the posterior corneoscleral surface. This, then, clogs the trabecular system, resulting in an increased pressure in the eye (glaucoma).

VI. **Ears.** The age-related changes in the ears are similar to those in the eyes: a slow, progressive loss of acuity known as presbycusis. There is evidence that the noise levels of modern living predispose to lower the age at which hearing begins to deteriorate.

The auditory system consists of four major parts: (1) the middle ear (sound conduction); (2) the inner ear (analysis of mechanical frequency and stimulus transformation); (3) the peripheral neuron (conduction and acoustic selectivity); and (4) the central auditory pathway (integration and interpretation). The latter three are affected by age. The sensory cells of the cochlea appear to be affected first; as a result, high-frequency tones are lost. Impairment of the inner ear results in disturbed intelligibility of speech. With a steady loss of ganglion cells in the auditory nerve, the elderly person loses the ability to discriminate or select individual conversations.

VII. **Body mass**

A. **Muscles.** Muscles are composed of nonmitotic cells and achieve their optimum size and strength when an individual reaches maturity in the middle 20s. Athletic individuals and manual workers who stay in training maintain their muscle mass and strength well into the sixth decade, but then there is a steady atrophy. In general, lean body mass (mus-

Figure 1-1

Influence of age on organ systems. (Modified from graph and text of F. Bourliere, Aging in the individual. Report of the Canadian Conference on Aging, Toronto, 1966, pp. 23–36. In R. Cape, Aging: Its Complex Management. New York: Harper & Row, 1978, pp. 13–38. By permission of Harper & Row.)

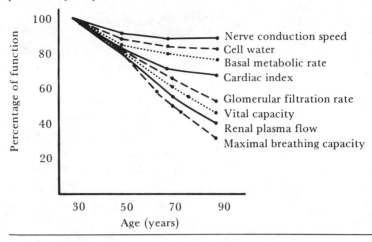

cles, liver, brain, and kidneys) decreases 20 to 50 percent by the age of 70 or 80. A decrease in intracellular water occurs, reflecting changes in cell mass, but there is no associated change in extracellular volume. The clinical implications are real: (1) the need for energy-providing food is reduced; and (2) the target organ mass on which drugs act is reduced. It follows that less food and smaller doses of drugs are required in old people.

B. **Other organ systems.** Most organ systems are similarly affected by age (Fig. 1-1). Particularly prominent changes are described under subsequent headings.

VIII. **Nervous system**

A. **Nerve cell loss.** Nerve cells are postmiotic and, when they are lost, are not replaced. In some cortical areas the loss of cells may be 45 percent. Cerebellar loss may be as high as 25 percent. Even when cells are not lost, they may undergo changes that alter function. For instance, the pyramidal cells in the third layer of the cerebral cortex show a progressive decrease in the number of interconnections between dendrites, thus implying loss of function.

B. **Cellular changes.** At the cellular level the most widely studied change is the intracellular accumulation of lipofuscin pigment, which is highly proportionate to age. Despite the previously mentioned changes, intellectual function is usually well maintained. There are, however, several anatomic changes that do correlate with dementia. These are senile plaques, neurofibrillary tangles, and granulovascular degeneration. Whether senile dementia is a manifestation of aging or a disease process remains unknown.

C. **Brain blood flow.** Recent studies show that from ages 17 to 80 cerebral blood flow declines from 79 to 46 ml per minute per 100 g of brain tissue. A decline in cerebral oxygen consumption from 3.6 to 2.7 ml per minute per 100 g of brain may be the primary reason for the decreased blood flow.

D. **Nerve conduction.** Nerve conduction velocity is most rapid in myelinated fibers and to some degree is proportional to the diameter of the neuron. Motor conduction velocities of the ulnar nerve in infants is about 30 meters per second, and by the age of 5 years reaches maximum adult values (slightly less than 60 m/sec). After the fifth decade of life, the velocity progressively decreases to about 50 meters per second by the eighth or ninth decade.

IX. Cardiovascular system

A. Heart

1. **Myocardium.** In humans the left ventricular wall is usually 25 percent thicker at age 80 than at age 30. There is an increased collagen content and fibrosis in the aged heart; however, their effects on cardiodynamics are unknown.

2. **Heart rate.** The resting heart rate in humans is unchanged by age. When related to body mass, the resting stroke volume and cardiac output are unchanged. However, during maximal work, both stroke volume and cardiac rate are decreased; thus, cardiac output is reduced. Between the third and the eighth decades, the decrease amounts to slightly less than 1 percent per year. The time required for the heart rate to return to normal after exercise is also prolonged with age.

3. **Oxygen consumption.** Maximal oxygen consumption declines at about the same rate as does cardiac output. Obesity, inactivity, and smoking hasten this decline to some extent. At equal work levels, the oxygen uptake is identical in the young and old; thus, the difference lies in work capacity, not in efficiency of oxygen extraction.

4. **Electrocardiographic changes.** The electrocardiogram pattern shows little change with age. However, small but significant increases in the P–R, QRS, and Q–T intervals are frequent.

B. Blood vessels.
Elastin, which gives arteries their resilience, diminishes with age. These fibers progressively straighten, fray, split, and fragment. This process involves both the media of the elastic arteries and the elastic lamina of the muscular arteries. The vascular distensibility is even further compromised by the increasing amount of collagen in the vessels and the cross-linkage of collagen fibers into bundles of larger size. The decrease in distensibility of vessels is reflected in an increase in the pulse wave velocity of blood vessels. The aortic pulse wave velocity increases from 4.1 meters per second at age 5 to 10.5 meters per second at age 65. The change in pulse wave velocity is independent of atherosclerosis. It has been estimated that the energy lost in pulsatile work doubles in the aged because of this diminished elasticity.

X. Renal function.
At birth, the human kidney contains approximately one million nephrons which increase in size until maturity. After maturity, there is a progressive loss of nephrons, owing to sclerosis or scarring of the glomeruli, followed by atrophy of the tubules. Between the ages of 25 and 85, the total nephron loss is 30 to 40 percent. The glomerular filtration rate decreases as much as 46 percent between the ages of 20 and 90. At the same time, renal plasma flow decreases by 53 percent. The reduction of renal tubular cell mass is reflected by a reduction of maximal tubular function; i.e., reabsorption of glucose, secretion of Diodrast, and para-aminohippuric acid are all decreased by about 45 percent. The ability to concentrate urine also decreases with age. Because of the age-related reduction in renal function, the dosage of those drugs dependent upon renal excretion should be modified. Since the aged patient has a reduced muscle mass, less creatinine is produced, and the serum creatinine does not rise in proportion to the fall in renal function. Hence, creatinine clearance, rather than serum creatinine, should be the criterion for renal function or dosage adjustment in the elderly.

XI. Pulmonary function

A. Lung mechanics. Even though the total lung capacity remains unchanged, residual volume and functional residual capacity increase with age, resulting in a decreased vital capacity. Indexes of flow, including maximum voluntary ventilation (MVV), maximum expiratory flow rate (MEFR), and 1-second forced expiratory volume (FEV_1), are all reduced, although airway resistance is unchanged.

B. Gas exchange. The aging process is also associated with impairment of gas exchange, as illustrated by reduced diffusing capacity for carbon monoxide, lowered arterial oxygen tension, and an increased alveolar-arterial oxygen gradient. These changes in lung mechanics and gas exchange are probably caused by a decline in elastic tissues of the lung, weakening of the respiratory muscles, and stiffness of the thoracic cage.

XII. The immune system

A. The thymus gland. The mass of the thymus gland begins to decrease after sexual maturity; by age 50 it has decreased in size to 15 percent of its maximum. The aged thymus is not merely small but is functionally deficient. In young, thymectomized animals given thymus transplants from donors of different ages, the animals receiving the youngest thymus had the T-lymphocyte population and T-cell function effectively restored, whereas those receiving thymuses from older animals did not. Levels of the thymic hormones, thymopoietin and thymosin, decline with age so that by the age of 60, both are undetectable in human serum.

B. T lymphocytes. Sheep red-blood-cell rosette formation is a test for the presence of mature human T lymphocytes. The number of rosette-forming thymocytes declines steadily with age. About 85 percent of the thymic lymphocytes from 20-year-olds form rosettes, while only 50 percent of the lymphocytes of 80-year-old patients do so. This suggests a marked decline in the ability of the thymus to stimulate T-cell maturation.

C. Hypersensitivity. Delayed hypersensitivity, a phenomenon mediated by the helper T cell, is depressed with age. For instance, tuberculin skin reactivity declines after the age of 70, at which time reactivation of tuberculosis is most common. The reaction of T lymphocytes to pokeweed mitogen and phytohemagglutinin is also depressed with age.

D. Antibody response. Antibody response depends upon a complex interaction of different lymphocyte classes and subclasses as well as antigen processing and presentation by macrophages. This interaction has been explored with respect to B and T cells by using an assay system in which plaques of sheep erythrocyte lysis provide a measurable endpoint. When killed staphylococci are used as the antigenic stimulus for isolated human lymphocytes, the number of plaque-forming cells (antibody response) declines with age. Other evidence of decreased humoral immunity includes a decreased antibody response to *Salmonella flagellin* and lower titers of antibodies to AB blood group antigens in older people.

E. Polymorphonuclear leukocytes. The functional properties of the polymorphonuclear leukocytes that can be quantified include migration, chemotaxis, adherence (to nylon fibers), phagocytosis, nitroblue tetrazolium (NBT) dye reduction, and *Candida*-killing activity. Studies in the elderly reveal:

1. Decreased chemotactic activity.
2. Increased adherence.
3. Normal spontaneous migration and phagocytosis.
4. Decreased NBT dye reduction capability.
5. Decreased *Candida*-killing activity.

XIII. **Clinical example of physical consequences of aging**

    A. **Description.** An 84-year-old man was admitted to the hospital because of pneumonia. He also had a history of a progressive loss of recent memory and self-motivation, as well as a progressive inability to carry out his usual daily activities. He was on no medication. Physical examination revealed an elderly, well-nourished, confused man in no distress. The blood pressure was 110/70; the pulse 82 and regular. Arcus senilis and dense cataracts were present bilaterally, and the intraocular pressure was 30 mm Hg (elevated). Rales were noted in the right posterior lung field. His stature was stooped forward with kyphosis of the thorax. The prostate was large but free of nodules. The white count was 10,200 with a shift to immature forms. Urinalysis was within normal limits. The serum creatinine was 1.9 mg per 100 ml, and the BUN 28 mg per 100 ml. An electrocardiogram showed regular sinus rhythm with a rate of 80 and occasional premature ventricular contraction. Chest x-ray showed a tortuous aorta, loss of intervertebral disk space, and an infiltrate in the right lower lobe. Sputum gram stain showed numerous polymorphonuclear leukocytes and gram-positive diplococci.

    B. **Discussion**

       1. Pneumonia is common in the elderly, in part because of the impairment of host defenses and changes in lung mechanics described earlier. *Streptococcus pneumoniae* is probably the offending agent.

       2. Dementia occurring in the elderly is usually of unknown origin. However, metabolic encephalopathy, central nervous system infection, hydrocephalus, and intracranial mass can cause a similar clinical picture and should be excluded by appropriate testing.

       3. The elevated serum creatinine and blood urea nitrogen probably reflected the nephron dropout that occurs with aging. Obstructive uropathy should be excluded and drug dosage modified according to the estimated glomerular filtration rate (creatinine clearance).

       4. The arcus senilis, cataracts, glaucoma, and stooped posture are all common in the aged. The patient's vision and hence his overall function may be improved with proper eye therapy.

Questions

Select the single best answer.

1. Which of the following is not functionally impaired by age?
   a. The middle ear (sound conduction).
   b. The inner ear (analysis of mechanical frequency and stimulus transformation).
   c. The peripheral neuron (conduction and acoustic selectivity).
   d. The central auditory pathway (integration and interpretation).
2. Which of the following is not true concerning skeletal changes related to aging?
   a. The intervertebral disks thin.
   b. The centrum thins.
   c. The long bones shorten.
   d. Shoulder width and chest size decrease.

II Cardiovascular Disease

Michael D. Ezekowitz
Ralph Lazzara
Thasana Nivatpumin
Dwight W. Reynolds
Eliot Schechter
Udho Thadani
Michael F. Wilson

2 Electrophysiologic Basis of Cardiac Arrhythmias

I. **Normal electrophysiology.** Transmembrane potentials of cardiac cells are determined by the differences in concentrations of specific ions in the interior and exterior of the cells and by the relative permeabilities (ease of movement) of the specific ions. In the resting state, the membrane is highly permeable to potassium in comparison with the other major ion species—namely, sodium, calcium, chloride, bicarbonate, and magnesium. The concentration of potassium is much greater inside the cell (150 mM) than outside (5 mM), so this chemical gradient serves to drive potassium out of the cell and generates a counteracting electrical potential gradient to retain potassium in the cell. Since potassium is a positively charged ion, the electrical potential required to retain it in the cell would be a negative potential. Thus, the intracellular compartment has a negative voltage (approximately −90 millivolts [mV]) in comparison with the extracellular compartment—the *resting potential*. When a cell is excited, a marked change in permeability occurs; transiently the membrane becomes relatively much more permeable to sodium than to other ions. Since sodium is in relatively high concentration outside the cell (140 mM) and is a positively charged ion, the increase in sodium permeability results in a transient inward flow of sodium ions (inward current) and a shift in membrane potential toward the positive direction resulting in an *upstroke* and *overshoot* (+30 mV) of the action potential shown in Figure 2-1.

The process of *excitation* occurs when the transmembrane potential in the resting state is shifted to approximately −60 mV, a level called the *threshold potential*. This shift can occur because of the passage of electrical current through the membrane or other stimuli such as mechanical deformation of the membrane. During natural propagation, the shift from resting to threshold potential occurs because of current flow generated by the difference in internal potential between a cell that has been excited to a level of +30 mV and a cell that is in the resting state at a level of −90 mV. Current flows through the interior of the cell and across the membranes because of this potential gradient and because all cardiac cells are connected together in a syncytium by low-resistance junctions. Thus, the process of *propagation* depends on passage of current between the excited cells and the resting cells, and the excitation of the cells in the resting state by this current. The rapidity of propagation (conduction velocity) is strongly dependent on the rate of rise and amplitude of the upstroke, which is the driving force for excitatory current. In turn, the upstroke velocity (V max) is dependent on the level of membrane potential at the time of excitation. At the normal resting potential (−90 mV), excitation results in the maximum upstroke velocity. If cells are excited at lower levels of membrane potential, lesser upstroke velocities are attained and conduction is poor. The relation between upstroke velocity and the level of membrane potential at the time of excitation is shown in Figure 2-2. This relation is called the membrane responsiveness curve and is influenced by a variety of factors including antiarrhythmic agents and the concentrations of certain ions, i.e., Ca^{2+}, as well as by abnormal conditions. Tetrodotoxin (TTX) specifically depresses the sodium channel, causing a downward shift of the curve.

Figure 2-1

Action potential of a normal myocardial fiber.

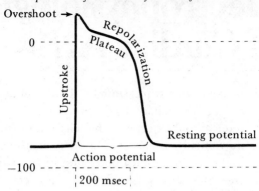

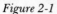

Figure 2-2

Membrane responsiveness curves relating the rate of rise of the upstroke of the action potential to the level of membrane potential at which the cell is excited. TTX = tetrodotoxin; V = membrane potential.

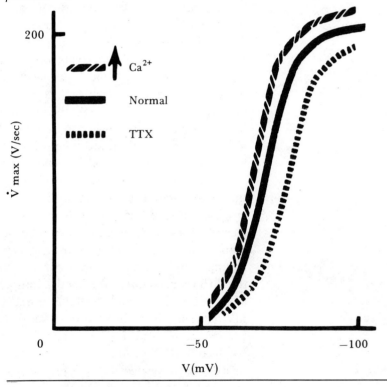

After a cell has been excited, a series of changes in ionic permeabilities occurs. An increase in permeability to calcium results in an inflow of calcium ions because calcium is in higher concentration in the exterior (2.7 mM) than the interior (10^{-7} mM). This inflow of calcium ions is a slower and weaker current than the rapid and transient inflow of sodium ions and is called the *slow inward current* as distinguished from the *rapid inward current* of sodium ions. The inward flow of calcium occurs during the *plateau* of cardiac cells, which is approximately 200 msec in duration. During this time changes occur in permeability to potassium, and as potassium permeability increases during the end of the plateau, the cell repolarizes because potassium again becomes the most permeant ion and because the permeabilities to sodium and calcium have decreased toward the low levels existing in the resting state. In other words, the

Figure 2-3

Refractory periods in relation to action potentials of ordinary myocardial cells (A) and AV nodal cells (B). Double lines on the action potential represent the absolute refractory period; thick lines, the relative refractory period.

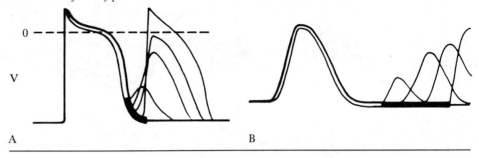

sodium and calcium channels are closed. The sodium channel is open only for a short period of time during the upstroke; the calcium channel is open primarily during the plateau.

The myocardial cells are refractory to excitation for a period after a previous excitation. The *refractory period* generally corresponds approximately to the duration of the action potential. The *absolute refractory period* occurs from the upstroke to the time when the membrane potential has repolarized to the level of the threshold potential; the *relative refractory period* occurs when the membrane potential is repolarizing from the level of the threshold potential to the level of the resting potential. During the absolute refractory period no stimulus will excite the ventricles. During the relative refractory period a larger stimulus is required and the response is poor in the sense that the upstroke velocity and amplitude are reduced, resulting in a poorly conducted action potential. In certain cardiac cells, such as atrioventricular (AV) nodal cells, the refractory period outlasts the action potential duration and the cell is refractory during diastole. It is advantageous for the AV node to have a long refractory period in order to protect the ventricles from excessively rapid firing of the atria. In such a circumstance all the atrial impulses would not traverse the AV node because of refractoriness. The refractory period of ordinary myocardial cells (*A*) and AV nodal cells (*B*) is shown in Figure 2-3.

After its return to the resting state, the ordinary working myocardial cell will remain stable until excitatory current is generated by a cell connected to it. In addition to working myocardial cells in the ventricles and atria, there exist specialized cells which compose a *specialized conducting system* including the *sinoatrial (SA) node*, the *AV node*, the *His bundle, bundle branches,* and *Purkinje network*. The cells in this system have the ability to generate action potentials de novo, that is, to generate action potentials without the stimulus or excitatory current from another cell. This is called the property of *automaticity*. It is based on a slow, gradual depolarization of the membrane potential during diastole. The ionic mechanism for this depolarization is uncertain. When the membrane potential drifts on its own to the threshold potential (−60 mV), excitation occurs. This process of slow diastolic depolarization is influenced by many factors, including adrenergic stimulation, which increases its rate, and vagal stimulation, which decreases its rate. The rate of diastolic depolarization is a primary determinant of the rate of firing of pacemaker cells. Thus, the autonomic modulation of SA nodal firing rate is based primarily on the influence of autonomic mediators on diastolic depolarization. To a certain degree the level of maximum diastolic potential attained after repolarization and the level of threshold potential also influence the rate of firing of pacemakers.

Figure 2-4

Pacemaker action potential illustrating the parameters that determine the firing rate. MDP = maximum diastolic potential; DD = diastolic depolarization; TP = threshold potential; mV = millivolts. Arrow indicates increased calcium.

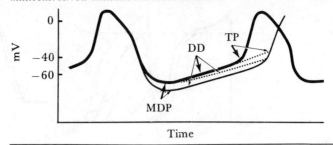

In the normal heart the SA nodal cells have the highest intrinsic firing rate, followed in turn by the AV node, bundle branches, His bundle, and Purkinje network. Pacemaker potentials are shown in Figure 2-4.

In addition to the pacemaker function, the specialized conducting cells have other special properties depending on their location. The AV nodal cells are specialized for slow conduction. Several factors contribute to this property. The upstroke velocities of AV nodal cells are slow. It is probable that AV nodal cells lack rapid sodium channels and generate upstrokes by slow calcium current. The upstrokes are slow and of lesser amplitude; consequently, propagation is slow. Since the excitatory current flows down the interior of the cell, cells that are large in diameter will conduct more rapidly in general. The AV nodal cells are small in diameter. Also they are circuitously arranged. In contrast, the bundle branches and subendocardial Purkinje network are specialized for rapid conduction and dispersal of the impulse throughout the ventricular myocardium. They have this characteristic by virtue of action potentials with rapid upstroke velocities and high overshoots. Also, they have large diameters and are aligned like cables. Between the atria and ventricles normally the only connections are the AV node, His bundle, and bundle branches. The AV node, His bundle, and upper portions of the bundle branches are not connected to adjacent myocardial cells—that is, they are surrounded by a fibrous sheath that does not conduct the impulse. Thus, interruption of these fragile structures at any point will prohibit the impulse from entering the ventricular myocardium. Once the impulse enters the Purkinje network, many connections occur between Purkinje cells and myocardial cells.

The AV node contains two pathways that connect the atria and the His bundle. One pathway conducts relatively more rapidly, but has a longer refractory period, whereas the other pathway conducts relatively more slowly, but has a shorter refractory period. The pathway with the more rapid conduction is the one generally used, but a premature impulse might strike this pathway while it is refractory and utilize the slower pathway with the shorter refractory period.

II. **Abnormalities of electrophysiology.** A common response of cardiac cells to a variety of injuries is a reduction in resting membrane potential, that is, partial depolarization of cells. The reduction in membrane potential results in a diminished sodium current and a diminished upstroke velocity and overshoot. The end result is a slowing or block of conduction. In regions of myocardium where conduction is slow and block occurs, there is a potential for the formation of reentrant pathways. Requirements for a reentrant pathway are: (1) the impulse remains in the pathway for a

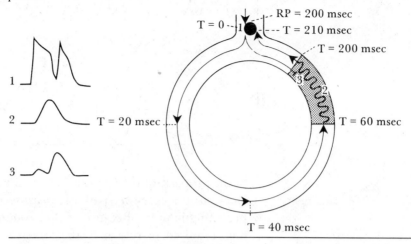

Figure 2-5

Model of reentry with representative action potentials from the input region (1), the region of slow conduction (2), and the region of unidirectional block (3). T = conduction time; RP = refractory period.

period sufficient to allow the surrounding myocardial cells to recover from the previous excitation so that they may be reexcited, and (2) a circuit is formed so that the impulse may return to the adjacent normal myocardium and reexcite the myocardium. The formation of a circuit requires a barrier that the impulse may go around, i.e., a region of complete block of conduction, and a region of unidirectional block where the impulse can proceed in one direction around the circuit but not in the other direction. If the impulse were allowed to proceed in both directions, it would simply enter the circuit, proceed down the entry and exit limbs simultaneously, and extinguish itself by collision somewhere within the circuit. A model of reentry is shown in Figure 2-5. The barrier could be anatomic or functional, i.e., a region of inexcitable myocardium. A number of conditions that lead to slowing of conduction and block can result in reentrant circuits in the intact heart. Ischemia is a common cause of slow conduction and reentry, producing regions of myocardium in which there are barriers, unidirectional block, and slow conduction (see Fig. 2-5).

Another example of a condition that produces reentrant arrhythmias is provided by the Wolff-Parkinson-White syndrome, in which an accessory atrioventricular pathway occurs somewhere along the AV rings. This accessory pathway plus the normal AV conduction pathway (AV node, His bundle, and bundle branches) provides the potential for the formation of a reentry circuit consisting of the atrium, the normal AV pathway, the ventricles, and the accessory AV pathway. Since the AV node is normally a site of slow conduction, all that is required to form this pathway is a site of unidirectional block. The AV rings provide the barrier. For example, a reentrant arrhythmia in Wolff-Parkinson-White syndrome would occur if a premature impulse formed in the atrium and proceeded down the normal AV pathway while it was blocked in the downward (antegrade) direction in a refractory accessory pathway. It could then be conducted through the ventricles back up to and across the accessory pathway, which is no longer refractory in the upward direction (retrograde), to reexcite the atrium. This process might repeat, the circuit thereby generating a continuing tachyarrhythmia. In this example the accessory pathway would form the site of unidirectional block, the AV node the site of slowing of conduction, and the AV rings the barrier. The unidirectional block in the accessory pathway in this example is produced

Figure 2-6

Examples of anomalous automaticity due to early (A) and delayed (B) afterpotentials.

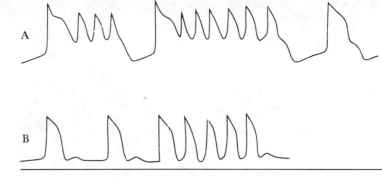

by the property of refractoriness, since the initiating impulse in the atrium blocks in the accessory pathway because it had not recovered from the preceding impulse. Because of slow conduction in the AV node and the time required to return to the accessory pathway retrograde, there is recovery from refractoriness and retrograde conduction. Thus, the basis for unidirectional block might be refractoriness.

It was stated previously that the AV node contains two pathways that connect at the proximal end of the node and again at the distal end of the node. In essence, these pathways form a loop which under appropriate conditions might provide a reentrant circuit. For example, an impulse that strikes one pathway while it is refractory might proceed down the other and then return over the original blocked path at a time when the refractory period of this path had ended, allowing a retrograde propagation. Thus, a circle would be formed by anterograde propagation down one pathway and retrograde propagation up the other. This is probably the mechanism for most supraventricular tachycardias.

Another mechanism for the formation of arrhythmias in the intact heart might be abnormalities of the property of automaticity. For example, the rate of diastolic depolarization of a lower pacemaker might be enhanced by some factor such as increased beta-adrenergic stimulation so that the pacemaker might fire more rapidly than the SA node and usurp control of the heart. Certain types of anomalous automaticity have been observed in cardiac cells and may account for arrhythmias in the intact heart. In one type, cardiac cells after repolarizing show another positive, transient shift of the membrane potential, called a delayed afterpotential; also, the membrane potential during the process of repolarization may shift more positively transiently, called an early afterpotential. If these afterpotentials attain the level of the threshold potential, the cell will fire again. Examples of these types of anomalous automaticity are shown in Figure 2-6. Whether this is a mechanism for arrhythmias remains to be proved in the intact heart.

Bradyarrhythmias may result from failure of pacemakers, especially the upper pacemakers which set the normal heart rate. For example, the SA node if diseased may not fire at the normal rate because of a depression of the rate of diastolic depolarization. Such a situation occurs in patients who have the sick sinus syndrome, owing to pathologic slowing or pauses in the firing of the sinus node. Similarly, if the sinus node impulse is not transmitted into the ventricles because of block of conduction between atrium and ventricles, i.e., heart block, the patient must rely on the automaticity of the His bundle branches and the Purkinje fibers. The intrinsic firing rates of these structures are relatively slow (30–40 beats/

Figure 2-7

Components of the conduction system in the heart with representative action potentials in proper temporal relations to the electrocardiogram. SAN = sinus node; AVN = AV node; HB = His bundle; PF = Purkinje fiber; VM = ventricular myocardium; AM = atrial myocardium.

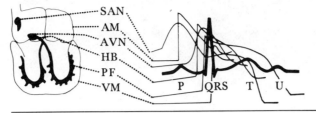

min) and often are not sufficient to sustain the patient in a normal state. Thus, failure of pacemaker firing and failure of AV conduction are common causes of bradyarrhythmias.

The diagnosis of arrhythmias in clinical practice is based on interpretation of the electrocardiogram. The relationship of the electrocardiographic waveforms to electrophysiologic events is shown in Figure 2-7.

The P wave is the potential generated by the process of activation and propagation in atrial myocardial cells. Thus, the sinus node fires just before the beginning of the P wave. The segment between the P wave and the QRS complex is occupied by the conduction of the impulse in the AV node, His bundle, and bundle branches, which, because of their small size, are not reflected in the electrocardiogram. The QRS complex, the largest waveform on the electrocardiogram, reflects activation and propagation in ventricular myocardium. The T wave reflects repolarization of ventricular myocardial cells and is not of great importance in the diagnosis of arrhythmias. The relationship of the P wave and the QRS is very important in the diagnosis of arrhythmias since the normal sequence of atrioventricular activation dictates that a P wave should precede every QRS and the time required for AV conduction dictates that the time (P–R interval) by which the P wave precedes the QRS should fall within certain normal limits. The configuration of the P wave is important. If the impulse begins in the SA node, as it should normally, the shape of the P wave will fall within certain normal limits. Similarly, the shape and duration of the QRS complex are important. If the impulse proceeds down the normal conduction pathway, the QRS is narrow because ventricular activation is facilitated by the Purkinje network. If the ventricles are activated from any other source—for example, an ectopic focus in the ventricles (reentrant or automatic) or an accessory pathway connecting atrium and ventricles—the QRS complex will be widened and distorted because the ventricles are activated by pathways other than normal rapidly conducting Purkinje network. If a tachycardia activates the ventricles by way of the normal conduction system, it arises in the AV junction or atria and is termed a *supraventricular tachycardia*. If a tachycardia activates the ventricles from a site in the ventricles itself, it is called a *ventricular tachycardia*.

III. **Clinical examples of cardiac arrhythmias**
   A. **Ventricular tachycardia and fibrillation**
      1. **Description.** A 48-year-old man had experienced chest pain radiating into the left arm with exertion or excitement for 2 years. This pain had become progressively worse but never lasted more than 15 or 20 minutes at a time. While watching television on the night before admission, he had severe chest pain which lasted several hours and was accompanied by sweating and nausea. He was ad-

Figure 2-8

Examples of ventricular ectopic firing, including a single ectopic beat (A), a run of ventricular tachycardia (B), and ventricular tachycardia leading to ventricular fibrillation (C).

A

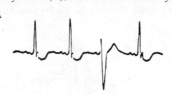

B

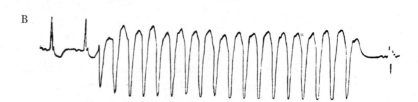

C

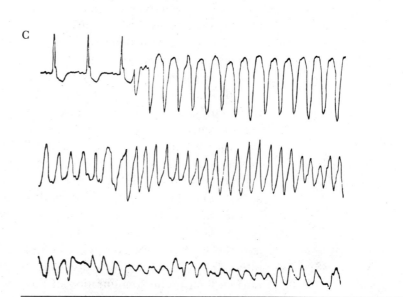

mitted to the hospital where the electrocardiogram indicated an acute myocardial infarction. The electrocardiograms in Figure 2-8 were recorded at different intervals during the first 10 hours after admission.

2. **Discussion.** In Figure 2-8A, the third beat represents an ectopic ventricular beat or premature ventricular beat. Note that the QRS is widened, that is, the duration of it is increased, and it is different from the normal QRS complex. In Figure 2-8B, the ectopic QRS initiates a series of abnormal QRSs which constitute a ventricular tachycardia. In Figure 2-8C, the ectopic QRS initiates a ventricular tachycardia, followed by disorganized chaotic potentials representing ventricular fibrillation. Fibrillation probably represents the formation of multiple and varying reentry pathways, i.e., a disorganization of propagation. It results in loss of pumping action by the heart. Note that the ectopic ventricular beat at the beginning of the abnormal rhythm in C occurs during the T wave, e.g., during repolarization. This has been shown to be a particularly dangerous time (the vulnerable period) for the occurrence of ventricular ectopic beats. Ventricular tachyarrhythmias are common in acute my-

Figure 2-9

Initiation of supraventricular tachycardia by a premature atrial beat (X) in a patient with Wolff-Parkinson-White syndrome. Electrocardiographic leads I, II, and III are shown.

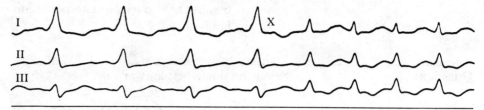

Figure 2-10

Electrocardiogram showing complete heart block.

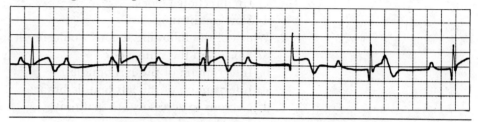

ocardial infarction, and ventricular fibrillation is a common mode of death.

B. Wolff-Parkinson-White syndrome. A 28-year-old man had complained of palpitations since his teens. These occurred unpredictably and consisted of an abrupt onset of a sensation of his heart beating very rapidly for a period of time followed by an abrupt return to normal. He had learned that straining as at stool or coughing might terminate the attacks more quickly. He was hospitalized to determine the cause of the attacks and was found to have Wolff-Parkinson-White syndrome. During the recording of the electrocardiogram an attack of tachycardia began spontaneously, as shown in Figure 2-9. Note that the first few beats show a widened QRS complex and shortened P–R interval, characteristic of Wolff-Parkinson-White syndrome. Note that a premature atrial beat indicated by an early and abnormal P wave (X) initiates a run of tachycardia with a different QRS complex. Usually in Wolff-Parkinson-White syndrome the tachycardia occurs when a premature atrial beat blocks in the accessory pathway and conducts down the AV node, thereby producing a normal QRS complex.

C. Heart block. An 83-year-old white male had felt well until 3 months before admission, when he fainted while walking home from the grocery store. He had been unconscious for only a few minutes when he awoke. Since that time he had several dizzy spells which lasted up to 2 or 3 minutes but had no warning signs. On the day before admission while watching television, his wife noticed that he lost consciousness and turned pale and then blue. She shook him and called the ambulance. As the ambulance was coming he awoke and then his color became better. He was admitted to the hospital where an electrocardiogram was recorded (see Fig. 2-10). This electrocardiogram shows no relationship between the P waves and the QRS complexes. The QRS complexes are much slower in rate than the P waves. The indications are that the atria are under the control of one pacemaker, the sinus node, whereas the ventricles are under the control of another pacemaker firing at a much slower rate. Apparently the impulse is not conducting from atria to ventricles, i.e., there is heart block. Hence, the intrinsic firing rate of ventricular pacemakers is slow and often unstable. Patients with heart block are prone to loss of consciousness because of the inadequate perfusion of the brain during periods of bradycardia.

Questions

Select the single best answer.

1. In the heart the formation of a reentrant circuit generally does not require:
   a. Prolonged refractory period.
   b. Barrier.
   c. Unidirectional block.
   d. Slow conduction.
2. Which of the following lesions would result in complete heart block?
   a. Fibrosis in the sinus node.
   b. Interruption of the His bundle.
   c. Interruption of the left bundle branch.
   d. Necrosis in accessory AV pathway.

3

Myocardial Contraction and Cardiac Performance

I. **The sarcomere and models of myocardial function.** The sarcomere is the fundamental unit of heart muscle and is the active contractile element. It contains both of the major contractile proteins, actin (thin filament) and myosin (thick filament) (Fig. 3-1). During contraction, the actin filaments are "pulled" by the myosin toward the center of the sarcomere, resulting in sarcomere shortening. This is the basic mechanism of myocardial contraction. Since the properties of heart muscle cannot be entirely explained by the contractile proteins (which can be thought of as the "power"), two additional components—the series elastic element and the parallel elastic element—are proposed (Fig. 3-2). These elastic elements are concepts, not anatomical structures. Their role in the pathophysiology of contraction will be pointed out in the following discussion, as will that of the contractile proteins.

II. **Definitions**
   A. **Preload** is the tension exerted on the muscle in the resting state. Preload can be expressed or thought of as either the resting muscle length or the resting tension. The relation between resting length and resting tension is determined by the characteristics of the parallel elastic element.
   B. **Afterload** is the resistance to shortening that the muscle must overcome during contraction.
   C. **Isometric contraction** is contraction without shortening; energy is transferred totally to tension by stretch of the series elastic element.
   D. **Isotonic contraction** is muscle contraction without change in tension. Contraction energy is transformed totally to shortening of the muscle.
   E. **Velocity of shortening** (dl/dt) is the rate of change of muscle fiber length, that is, the change in length in any unit of time. In more familiar terms, for an automobile this could be miles (dl) per hour (dt).

III. **Muscle contraction.** Our review of muscle mechanics begins with analysis of a strip of heart muscle. The application of basic muscle mechanics to the intact heart and to the evaluation of the cardiac function in humans will then be discussed.

   The contraction of muscle can best be understood using a simple "muscle bridge" (Fig. 3-3). The muscle is attached to one side of a pivoting arm and a weight (afterload) to the other. A stop allows a controlled amount of initial stretch (preload). A strain gauge attached to the muscle records the tension, and the movement of the arm indicates the shortening.

   Figure 3-4 shows the changes in force and length during a typical contraction using a muscle bridge. When the muscle fibers are stretched (preload) to any resting muscle length (Fig. 3-4A, lower panel) the force measured is the resting tension (point r to point s). This is due to stretching of the parallel elastic element. When the muscle fibers are stimulated (Fig. 3-4, point s), contraction begins. Muscle tension rises, but there is no muscle shortening. This is due to stretching of the series elastic element of the muscle. When muscle tension exceeds afterload (Fig. 3-4, point a), muscle shortening begins while the tension remains constant and equal to the afterload. The velocity of muscle shortening (dl/dt) is the tangent of

Figure 3-1

The contractile proteins.

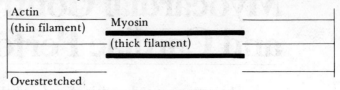

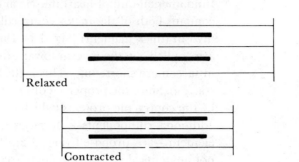

Actin
(thin filament)

Myosin
(thick filament)

Overstretched

Relaxed

Contracted

Figure 3-2

Model of the sarcomere.

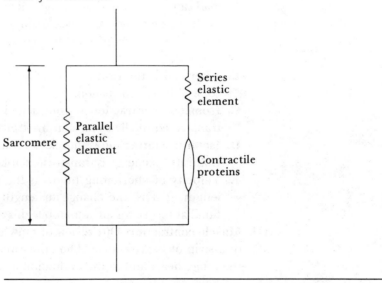

Sarcomere

Parallel
elastic
element

Series
elastic
element

Contractile
proteins

Figure 3-3

The muscle bridge.

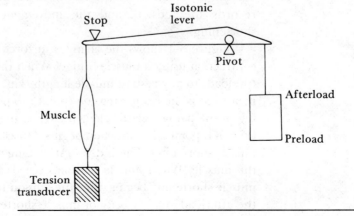

Stop

Isotonic
lever

Pivot

Muscle

Afterload

Preload

Tension
transducer

Figure 3-4

Changes in tension and length of an isolated muscle during contraction. A = low afterload; B = high afterload; r = resting state (preload); s = start of contraction; a = afterload.

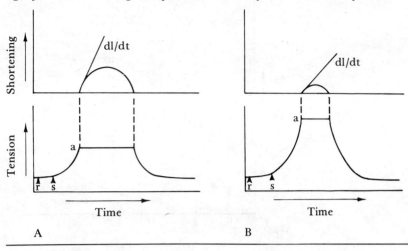

Figure 3-5

The force-velocity curve of isolated muscle. A = force-velocity curve; B = effect of changing preload on the force-velocity curve; C = effect of changing contractility on the force-velocity curve.

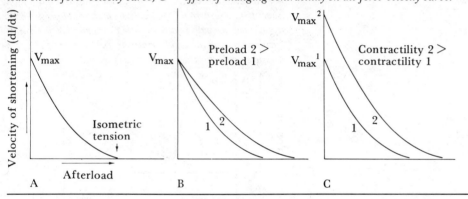

the length-time curve (Fig. 3-4A, upper panel). Muscle shortening velocity is not constant throughout the course of contraction; the initial dl/dt is fastest. If the afterload is increased (Fig. 3-4B), the tension developed is increased, and the velocity and magnitude of shortening is decreased.

A. The force-velocity relationship. Figure 3-5A represents the velocity of muscle shortening (dl/dt) plotted against afterload, expressing the relationship described in Figure 3-4 somewhat differently. At the maximum developed tension (afterload) the shortening velocity is zero; maximum shortening velocity (V max) occurs when the tension developed is zero. In Figure 3-5B the effect of different preloads is illustrated. Preload for curve *2* is higher than preload for curve *1*. In both curves, as afterload increases, the dl/dt decreases. As shown in Figure 3-5B, isometric tension (vertical arrow) is greater with greater preload, while for any given afterload dl/dt *2* is greater than dl/dt *1*. This indicates that preload affects both the force and the velocity of muscle shortening. However, when each of the force curves (*1* and *2*) is extrapolated to zero load, upper left corner, they approach the same point on the velocity axis. Thus, V max is independent of preload and afterload and is a measure of muscle contractility. Figure 3-5C shows that changes in contractility shift the force velocity curve up and to the

Figure 3-6   *The length-tension relationship of isolated muscle.*

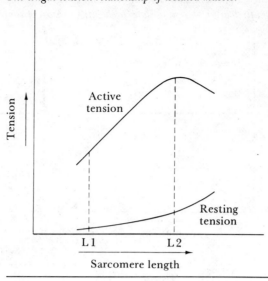

Figure 3-7

The pressure-volume relationship of a cardiac chamber. A = end-diastolic volume and pressure; B = onset of ejection; C = end-systolic pressure and volume; D = early diastole; AB = isovolumic contraction (fixed volume with rapid pressure rise); BC = ventricular ejection (decreasing LV volume with relatively little change in LV pressure); CD = isovolumic relaxation (ventricular pressure falls with relatively fixed volume); DA = ventricular fillings (small change in pressure, with marked increase in ventricular volume).

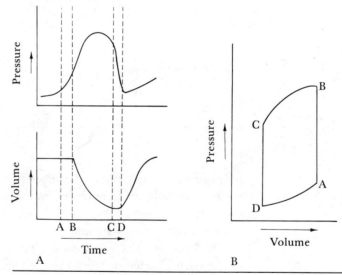

right. Increased contractility will increase the velocity at any afterload; hence V max is increased, reflecting the increased contractility.

B. **Tension-length relationship (Frank-Starling curve).** When a muscle contracts isometrically from varying resting lengths, varying tension is developed. Increases in resting length result in increased tension. This is called the "preload reserve" or the Frank-Starling law of the heart (Fig. 3-6). At some resting length (*L2*) maximum tension (*T2*) is developed. Further increases in length produce no change or a fall in tension.

IV. **Ventricular pressure–volume relationship: The intact heart.**

A. Figure 3-7A shows the plot of ventricular pressure and volume against time during a cardiac contraction. If one plots the ventricular pressure

Figure 3-8

Three diagrams showing relation of stroke volume to afterload (A), preload (B), and contractility (C) with determinants of stroke volume. SV1 and SV2 = different stroke volumes; V1 and V2 = corresponding end-diastolic volumes; P1 and P2 = the respective aortic pressures.

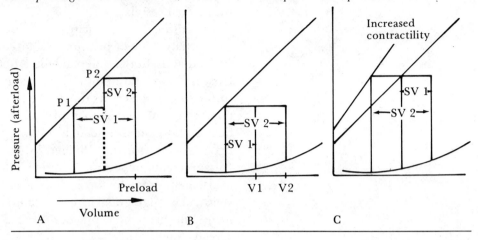

and volume against each other (Fig. 3-7B), a ventricular pressure volume loop is obtained. In the ventricle with a stable contractile state the ratio of ventricular pressure to ventricular volume at end systole (Fig. 3-7, point C) is relatively unaffected by changing preload or afterload. The line joining the end-systolic pressure-volume points at different preloads and afterloads is linear. The slope of this line represents the contractile state of the ventricle; increased ventricular contractility is associated with a steeper slope. Since this line is unaffected by changing preload and afterload and is sensitive to ventricular contractility changes, it has been proposed as a measure of myocardial contractility in humans.

B. Effect of preload, afterload, and contractility on stroke volume. It can be seen from Figure 3-8A that as the afterload (aortic pressure) increases from P_1 to P_2, stroke volume decreases. Thus, ventricular afterload is a major determinant of ventricular ejection. For a given afterload (Fig. 3-8B), increased preload, from V_1 to V_2, results in increased stroke volume. This is "preload reserve" or the Frank-Starling law. When ventricular afterload and preload are constant, increased stroke volume can be achieved by increased cardiac contractility, which shifts the end-systolic pressure-volume line upward and to the left (Figure 3-8C). Thus, stroke volume is determined by preload, afterload, and myocardial contractility. Since ejection fraction is the ratio of stroke volume to end-diastolic volume (EF = SV/EDV), it is a measure of ventricular performance and is also a function of preload, afterload, and myocardial contractile state.

V. Intact cardiovascular system. Since preload and afterload are important determinants of myocardial performance, we shall define them in the intact cardiovascular system. We shall use the ventricle for illustration because it is the more important chamber, but the same analysis applies to the atrium.

A. Preload. In the intact heart, ventricular end-diastolic volume (EDV), ventricular end-diastolic pressure (EDP), or mean atrial pressure can be taken to represent preload.

B. Afterload. The forces resisting ejection of ventricular blood constitute afterload. Because of the complex geometry of the heart and the changing muscle fiber orientation, ventricular wall stress (force/unit muscle mass) is difficult to obtain. For practical purposes, arterial pressure, usually peak systolic or mean pressure, is taken as the afterload of the ventricle. This is closely related to the resistance to flow through the arterial vessels.

C. Contractility. No satisfactory method exists in humans to measure contractility. Rate of pressure rise (dp/dt) has been used, but it is both preload and afterload dependent. Attempts to extrapolate to V max from pressure and dp/dt measurements during isometric contraction suffer from large errors due to the few points available for extrapolation. Since the end-systolic pressure-volume line is independent of both preload and afterload, it could be a useful measure of contractility. It is, unfortunately, limited by the practical problem of making measurements in several different states (e.g., with different afterloads) in order to plot the line (see Figs. 3-7 and 3-8) and of requiring a ventricular angiogram in each state to make the volume measurements. Both of these practical limitations have precluded its widespread clinical use.

Since the heart is a pump, measuring pressure and volume alone does not adequately describe cardiovascular function. Cardiac output increases with increased heart rate and with increased stroke volume. At extremes of heart rate output may fall, since at very rapid rates filling time is reduced and stroke volume falls; at slow rates diastolic compliance limits the degree to which stroke volume can increase to compensate.

Questions

Select the single best answer.

1. In a normal heart, increased cardiac output (CO) can be achieved by:
   a. Reduction of ventricular afterload—arterial blood pressure or arterial resistance.
   b. Increase in ventricular preload—ventricular end-diastolic pressure (EDP) or volume (EDV).
   c. Increased myocardial contractility.
   d. Increased heart rate.
   e. All of the above.
2. Ventricular preload can be estimated by:
   a. Arterial pressure.
   b. End-diastolic pressure.
   c. Ventricular contractility.
   d. Ventricular end-systolic pressure and volume.
   e. Velocity of fiber shortening.

4 Common Forms of Volume and Pressure Overload

I. **Physiology of cardiac pump function**
   A. **Diastolic function of the ventricle (volume).** The diastolic properties of the ventricle are defined by its compliance curve. Compliance is the amount of pressure required to distend the ventricle to any given volume. A less compliant (stiffer) ventricle requires more pressure, and a more compliant ventricle less pressure at any given volume. The compliance curve is not linear but rises more and more steeply as the ventricle is stretched (see Fig. 4-1). The normal left ventricle (curve A) has a volume of about 135 cc at a distending pressure of 12 mm Hg. A less compliant ventricle (curve B) will require a greater pressure to be distended to the same volume (curve shifted upward and left), while a more compliant ventricle (curve C) will have a greater volume at the same pressure (curve shifted downward and right). This diastolic volume of the ventricle is its *preload*. Physiologically preload is the stretch of the myocardial fibers, but clinically it is approximated by the end-diastolic volume or end-diastolic pressure.

   The Frank-Starling curve relates the diastolic or filling status of the ventricle (preload) to its work output (see Fig. 4-2). Up to a point, increased preload (increased volume loading) is associated with an increased output. Beyond that point the output plateaus (or may fall). The heart thus has a mechanism that causes input and output to keep pace (more input = more output) on a beat-to-beat basis over the physiologic range.

   B. **Systolic function of the ventricle (pressure).** During systole the ventricle must develop sufficient pressure to exceed the pressure in the great vessels (aorta or pulmonary artery) so that flow may begin. This pressure development phase (isometric contraction) is determined by the contractile state of the myocardium. This state is impossible to measure accurately clinically, but can be approximated by the rate of rise of ventricular pressure (dp/dt—change in pressure per unit of time).

   Afterload is the resistance (or more properly, impedance) against which the ventricle must empty. A higher afterload (higher resistance) requires the ventricle to develop more pressure in order to empty at the same rate or causes slower emptying at any given pressure. These changes during the ejection phase can be measured clinically by the mean systolic ejection rate, the ventricular ejection time, or, perhaps most accurately, the end-systolic pressure-volume relationship. Figure 4-3 shows the changes in the systolic pressure-volume curve as a measure of ventricular contractile function. Point A in Figure 4-3 demonstrates the normal relationship: at an end-systolic pressure of about 100 mm Hg the ventricle has emptied to about 55 cc. With impaired function the ventricle develops the same pressure, but empties less well (has a higher end-systolic volume) (see Fig. 4-3, point B). With augmented contractility the ventricle can develop higher pressure and yet empty normally (see Fig. 4-3, point C).

   By relating the systolic and diastolic pressure-volume properties of the ventricle, a work curve can be obtained (see Fig. 4-4). During

Figure 4-1

Ventricular compliance curves. A = curve of normal left ventricle; B = curve of less compliant ventricle; C = curve of more compliant ventricle.

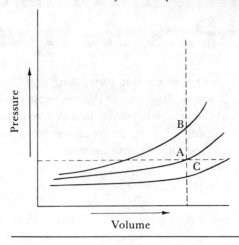

Figure 4-2

The Frank-Starling curve.

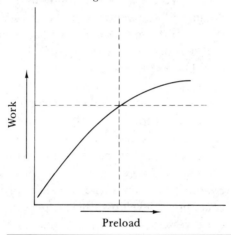

diastole the ventricle fills along its diastolic compliance curve (see Fig. 4-4, points *A–B*). With the onset of systole, pressure builds up (isovolumic phase) until it reaches the level where ejection begins (see Fig. 4-4, points *B–C*), and volume then decreases until the end of systole (see Fig. 4-4, points *C–D*). With the onset of diastole (isometric relaxation) pressure falls abruptly (see Fig. 4-4, points *D–A*) to the level determined by diastolic compliance. The area inside these curves, the pressure-volume loop, represents the work of the ventricle.

II. Pathophysiology of volume and pressure overload
A. Volume overload
1. Volume overload affects the diastolic function of the ventricle. Acute volume load increases the preload by increasing end-diastolic volume. Because of the shape of the diastolic compliance curve (see Fig. 4-1) this is accompanied by an increase in end-diastolic pressure. Increased diastolic stretch, utilizing the Frank-Starling mechanism, results in increased stroke output and maintains a normal end-systolic and early diastolic volume. The stroke volume and ejection fraction increase. Because of the increase in the size of the pressure-volume loop (see Fig. 4-4, move points *B* and *C* to the right), there is an increase in cardiac work. Further, because of

Figure 4-3

The systolic pressure-volume relation. A = normal end-systolic pressure and volume; B = end-systolic pressure and volume with reduced contractility (less emptying; therefore, higher volume at the same pressure); C = end-systolic pressure and volume with increased contractility in response to increased afterload (ventricle generates higher pressure but empties to same volume).

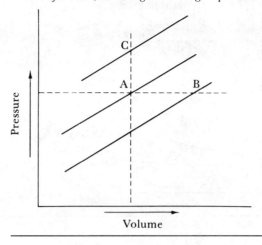

Figure 4-4

The pressure-volume loop. A = beginning of diastole; B = end-diastole; C = beginning of ejection; D = end of systole.

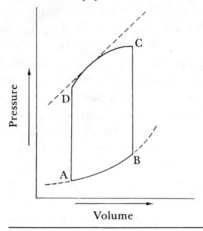

the Laplace relationship (in a sphere wall tension varies directly with the radius) there is an increase in wall tension at the same intraventricular pressure, further increasing myocardial work. If marked, this stretching exhausts the capability of the Frank-Starling mechanism to provide cardiac reserve.

2. **Chronic volume load.** If the volume load is maintained, cardiac dilatation—that is, rearrangement of the myocardial fibers—occurs. In this way the myocardial fiber length returns to normal but the enclosed volume is increased (see Fig. 4-1, lower curve). This response adapts the ventricle to handle the volume load. The thinning of the wall increases its compliance so the pressure within the ventricle drops. The return of end-diastolic fiber length to normal means that the Frank-Starling mechanism can again be used effectively to provide cardiac reserve. However, the increased radius of the ventricle results in an increased wall tension and an increased oxygen demand. If dilatation persists, this increased wall tension leads to some hypertrophy (an increase in the number of myofibrils per cell) along with the dilatation.

Figure 4-5

The effect of hypertrophy on the pressure-volume relationships of the ventricle. The upper two curves represent systole and the lower curves represent diastole. A = normal pressure load; B = increased pressure load; C = the combination of increased pressure load and hypertrophy.

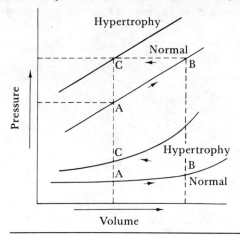

B. Pressure overload. Pressure overload (increased afterload) impairs systolic functioning of the ventricle. Faced with increased resistance to outflow the ventricle empties less completely, resulting in a higher end-systolic and, therefore, early diastolic ventricular volume. The result is increased diastolic stretch of the ventricle (increased preload, dilatation) since it starts filling from a higher volume which then allows for generation of a greater pressure. The initial compensation for a pressure load therefore utilizes the Frank-Starling mechanism.

This initial dilatation is soon replaced by concentric hypertrophy. This shifts the ventricular end-systolic pressure-volume curve upward and left (Fig. 4-5). The ventricle is now able to develop more pressure from the same end-diastolic volume and to empty to a normal end-systolic volume. However, the hypertrophied ventricle becomes less compliant or stiffer. The pressure required to distend it to a normal diastolic volume increases.

III. Clinical examples of volume and pressure overload

Normal Values

Right atrial mean pressure	3–6 mm Hg
Left atrial (pulmonary wedge) mean pressure	6–12 mm Hg
Stroke volume	50–80 cc/beat
Heart rate	60–100 beats/min
Cardiac output	4–6 L/min
Left ventricular end-diastolic volume	60–100 cc/m² body surface
Ejection fraction	55–65%

A. Volume overload after surgery
1. **Description.** A 58-year-old woman developed acute renal failure following surgery for an abdominal aortic aneurysm. She had no history of cardiac disease but received 5 L of saline during the first postoperative night in an effort to increase urine output. The morning following surgery she complained of severe dyspnea and was unable to lie flat. Examination revealed jugular venous distension of 12 cm with the patient at 45 degrees. The apex impulse was

hyperdynamic with a palpable early diastolic filling wave. The first sound was normal; the aortic and pulmonic components of the second sound were accentuated. An S3 gallop was heard at the apex. A short systolic ejection murmur was heard at the base of the heart. There were rales two-thirds of the way up both lung fields. T-wave changes on the ECG suggested a possible myocardial infarction; hence, a Swan-Ganz catheter was inserted and the following data were recorded:

Right atrial mean pressure	12 mm Hg
Pulmonary wedge mean pressure (equivalent to left atrial mean pressure)	20 mm Hg
Cardiac output	9 L/min

Echocardiogram showed a dilated left ventricle. Nuclear ventriculogram revealed an ejection fraction of 75 percent.

2. **Discussion.** This patient's data showed high filling pressures, indicative of either stiff ventricles with a normal end-diastolic volume or an increased diastolic volume in a normally compliant ventricle as a result of volume overload. The high cardiac output, increased left ventricular volume, and high ejection fraction are consistent with the later diagnosis, since the normal heart responds to volume overload by increasing its forward output.

Fluid restriction and dialysis therapy produced a prompt return to normal of the patient's physical findings and hemodynamic measurements, and her symptoms subsided.

B. **Chronic left ventricular pressure overload**

1. **Description.** The patient, a 55-year-old man, had a 20-year history of hypertension. Because of noncompliance with treatment, control of his pressure had been poor. He came to the emergency room with acute pulmonary edema. The patient's pulse was 92 and regular, his blood pressure 210/130. Jugular and carotid pulses were normal. A sustained left ventricular impulse was palpable. The first sound was normal, the aortic component of the second sound was accentuated, and a fourth sound was heard at the apex. Moist rales were heard over the entire extent of both lung fields. The following measurements were obtained after a Swan-Ganz catheter was inserted:

Right atrial mean pressure	6 mm Hg
Pulmonary wedge (left atrial) mean pressure	30 mm Hg
Cardiac output	3.0 L/min

Echocardiogram showed thick ventricular walls (concentric hypertrophy) and normal chamber size. Nuclear ventriculogram showed a reduced ejection fraction of 30 percent.

2. **Discussion.** This patient with hypertension has developed severe left ventricular hypertrophy. In the face of continuing afterload, compensatory mechanisms in the ventricle have failed, and at the present time, despite a high filling pressure, the ejection fraction and cardiac output have fallen, representing loss of compensation. Increasing cardiac output by the Frank-Starling mechanism is impossible because the high filling pressure is already producing pulmonary symptoms. The stiff ventricle and high diastolic pressure

results in the generation of a fourth sound at the apex. The filling pressure on the right side is normal since the left ventricular failure is relatively acute.

Following vigorous therapy of his hypertension with furosemide and sodium nitroprusside, the patient's symptoms cleared. His hemodynamic measurements were then:

Right atrial mean pressure	5 mm Hg
Pulmonary wedge (left atrial) mean pressure	15 mm Hg
Cardiac output	4 L/min
Nuclear ejection fraction	50%

3. **Further comments.** Reduction of ventricular afterload has now allowed a return to more normal function. The severe hypertrophy, however, will not regress completely and still results in some decreased compliance (elevated left ventricular filling pressure) and reduced function (somewhat reduced ejection fraction and cardiac output).

Questions

Select the single best answer.

1. The normal response to an acute volume load is:
   a. Elevated diastolic pressure.
   b. Elevated diastolic volume.
   c. Elevated stroke volume.
   d. None of the above.
   e. All of the above.
2. Chronic pressure loading produces:
   a. Ventricular hypertrophy.
   b. Elevated end-diastolic pressure.
   c. Both.
   d. Neither.

5 Atherosclerosis

I. **Introduction**
  A. **Disease process**
    1. **Atherosclerosis, or hardening of arteries,** is a progressive disorder that causes a gradual and uneven narrowing of medium- and large-sized arteries through the development of atheromatous or fatty plaques within the arterial walls.
    2. **Vascular sequelae** are due either to obstruction of blood flow or to dilatation of the vessel wall. Atherosclerosis is the basic cause of most myocardial infarctions, ischemic heart disease, and peripheral vascular disease, including most aneurysms of the thoracic and abdominal aorta.
  B. **Distribution**
    1. **The clinical disease** is unevenly distributed in the world's population. It occurs primarily in the industrialized countries of North America, Western Europe, and the European portion of the Soviet Union. Atherosclerotic cardiovascular disease is uncommon in Asia, including China, Japan, and India, and in the Near East, Africa, and Latin America.
    2. **The economic and health care burden** of atherosclerosis on the population in the United States is enormous. In the year 1980, the cost was over $40 billion and 700,000 deaths. Atherosclerosis is the leading cause of death in Western countries. It constitutes a twentieth-century epidemic with a medical, social, and economic impact of major proportions.
  C. **Etiology**
    1. **The cellular biological substrate** of atherogenesis is an expression of the normal vascular wall remodeling that occurs throughout life. While the disease process is multifactorial, risk factors have been identified that tend to modify the cellular remodeling into a pathological process of plaque formation.
    2. **Major risk factors** include smoking, high blood pressure, elevated serum lipids, and emotional or environmental stress. The atherogenic process is clearly aggravated by Western dietary habits. The amount and kind of lipoproteins circulating in the blood and interacting with the cellular surface of the vessel wall are important. Diabetes mellitus, particularly when first manifested in childhood, the dyslipidemias, and family history are also important factors that correlate closely with coronary artery disease.
    3. **Cellular mechanisms of atherogenic risk factors.** Probable mechanisms of atherosclerotic plaque formation and the corresponding controllable risk factors are listed in Table 5-1.
    4. **Protection** to some degree is afforded by estrogen in women of child-bearing potential, according to epidemiologic evidence. There is also evidence that regular, moderate exercise may delay the progression of atherogenesis.

II. **Anatomy and physiology.** Knowledge of the structure and function of the walls of large- and medium-sized arteries is important to an understanding of the pathophysiologic process. Microscopic examination of a transverse section of the arterial wall shows three major layers: intima, media, and adventitia.

Table 5-1   *Proposed Cellular Mechanisms of Atherogenic Risk Factors*

Risk Factor	Cellular Mechanism
Elevated serum cholesterol	Increases LDL, which damages endothelium
	Increases passage of cholesterol carried by LDL, especially when HDL is low, leading to increased proliferation of smooth muscle cells
Hypertension	Increases endothelial permeability through
	1. Increased artery wall tension
	2. Endothelial damage from angiotensin
	3. Platelet adherence with release of vasoactive agents
	4. Hemodynamic stress
Cigarette smoking	Damages arterial cell membrane through
	1. Circulating carbon monoxide
	2. Platelet adherence (vasopressin)
	3. Lipid mobilization (catecholamines)

HDL = high-density lipoprotein; LDL = low-density lipoprotein.

A. Intima. The inner layer is composed of the flattened endothelial cells, a basement membrane, and occasional smooth muscle or myointimal cells. There are scattered collagen and elastin fibers as well as mononuclear leukocytes in this inner layer. Within the intimal layer of coronary arteries and some others there can be found multilayered cushions of myointimal cells, even in the young. It is not known whether these cushions are normal or pathologic, or whether they predispose to atherosclerosis. It has been shown that in areas of hemodynamic stress, a fibrous thickening of the intima will develop; when there are elevated serum lipids, this thickening may progress to an atheromatous lesion.

    Low-density lipoproteins (LDL) and fibrinogen penetrate the endothelium to the extent that their concentration in the arterial wall is about one-tenth that in blood. Endothelial permeability is partly controlled by a carbohydrate coating on the luminal side of the endothelial cell. Thinning of the luminal coating has been seen at sites of plaque formation in experimental animals. Passage of macromolecules across the endothelial cell appears to be accomplished through the well-known process of vesicular transport by invaginations and separation of portions of the cell membrane; this is called pinocytosis.

B. Media. The middle portion consists mostly of smooth muscle cells (SMC) and well-defined elastic membranes in alternating layers to form lamellar units; each unit is a SMC with an elastic membrane on either side. The number of units appears to relate to the amount of hemodynamic stress to which a particular artery is subjected. In vitro studies show that the SMC can synthesize collagen, elastin, and other substances. The SMC and platelets are thought to be prominent in the development and regression of the atherosclerotic plaque.

    The metabolic secretory activity of the SMC, particularly collagen and elastin secretion, seems to be influenced by a variety of physical and chemical stimuli; this yields a highly dynamic vessel wall that adapts to different physiologic and pathophysiologic conditions.

C. Adventitia. The outer layer, composed mostly of collagenous substances, provides mechanical strength to support the other layers of the arterial wall. The most common cell is the fibroblast. The vasa vasorum course through this layer to bring nutrients, as do lymphatic channels and the innervation of the arterial wall. Penetrating branches of the vasa vasorum provide nutrient blood supply to the outer layers of the media in large arteries and the thoracic aorta. The lower abdominal aorta in humans lacks these penetrating vasa vasorum. It has been suggested that the high predilection for atherosclerotic plaque formation and aneurysm in the distal aorta may be partly related to this lesser nutrient blood supply.

III. **Clinical importance of atherosclerosis.** The clinically important consequences of atherosclerosis are obstruction to blood flow and therefore to oxygen and metabolic supply to the tissues that the arterial blood flow subserves, the destruction and weakening of large arterial walls with aneurysm formation, and the potential for rupture. Aneurysm formation is particularly likely to occur in the lower abdominal aorta.

The principal sites for clinically important atherosclerosis are listed in order of their incidence: (1) lower aorta and iliacs; (2) proximal coronaries; (3) femorals, popliteals, and thoracic aorta; (4) internal carotids; and (5) cerebral vessels, especially the vertebral, basilar system, and the circle of Willis.

IV. **Mechanisms of plaque formation**

A. **Theories of pathogenesis.** Two principal theories of the pathogenesis of the atherosclerotic plaque are: the *insudation theory* believed to have begun with Virchow and the *encrustation theory* associated with Rokitansky. Insudation implies that there is a form of localized low-grade inflammatory edema causing an increased permeability and therefore the passage and accumulation of constituents from the plasma into the intimal layer of the arterial wall. Encrustation means the deposition of formed elements of the blood (platelets, fibrin, and leukocytes) into mural thrombi at sites of injury to the intimal layer of the artery, as well as the organization of these thrombi by the SMC. Both theories imply that atherosclerotic plaque formation and regression make up a dynamic process. The theory of encrustation relates more strongly to environmental factors that might result in arterial endothelial injury to trigger formation of the "white" thrombi. The theory of insudation relates more closely to the concepts of elevated lipoproteins carrying cholesterol into the arterial wall.

B. **Serum cholesterol.** A sustained elevation of serum cholesterol is closely associated with progressive atherosclerosis. More than 93 percent of the body's cholesterol is contained within cells, where it participates in essential structural and metabolic functions. *Only 7 percent circulates in plasma,* where it can predispose to atherosclerosis. Two-thirds of the cholesterol circulating in plasma is in the low-density lipoprotein (LDL) fraction, which has been implicated as a major cause of atherosclerosis. Elevated serum cholesterol may be of exogenous origin, produced by a high-fat, high-cholesterol diet. However, the hypercholesterolemia may also be of endogenous origin due to genetic factors, such as the 1 in 500 individuals who have familial hypercholesterolemia (FH). Patients with FH have high plasma LDL levels due to a genetic defect in the gene for the LDL receptor.

In hyperlipidemic serum it is the cholesterol carried in the LDL fraction that is important to atherogenesis and plaque formation. With elevated serum cholesterol and endothelial injury from hypertension and cigarette smoking, there may be an accelerated atherogenesis.

Injury to the arterial luminal cell membrane releases peptides from cell fragments, which stimulate the exposed SMC to cellular proliferation.

Hypercholesterolemia alone can cause endothelial injury and increased permeability by an as yet unexplained mechanism. It appears that high levels of LDL are important to the progressive development of an atherosclerotic lesion and plaque formation. High levels of serum LDL in experimental animals are capable of producing endothelial injury, platelet adherence, stimulation of SMC, and accelerated atherogenesis. The combination of prolonged, severe endothelial injury and low- to medium-LDL levels will also produce atherosclerotic lesions. If the endothelial injury is mild or intermittent and LDL levels are low, the lesion will usually regress; if LDL levels are moderately elevated, the lesion may progress.

C. **Cellular components**

1. **Smooth muscle cell.** Immunohistochemical staining shows that most plaque cells resemble the arterial medial SMCs in their staining characteristics. A few cells have morphologic features similar to blood-derived leukocytes. It remains unknown whether the lipid-filled "foam" cells are mostly monocytes derived from the blood or mostly SMCs modified through imbibing large quantities of lipid.

2. **Platelets.** The adherence of platelets to injured or denuded vessel wall surfaces appears to be enhanced by a portion of the factor VIII molecule (von Willebrand's factor). Reduction of von Willebrand's factor leads to defective platelet aggregation and thrombus formation. Vasopressin has been shown to increase factor VIII to induce primary platelet aggregation and to increase plasminogen activator; therefore, it may enhance the role of platelet in both thrombosis and atherogenesis. The prostaglandins are also involved in platelet function; prostacyclin is a vasodilator and inhibitor of platelet aggregation.

3. **The endothelial cell** furnishes a surface to which platelets cannot adhere and also functions as a permeability barrier.

D. **Lipoproteins.** Content of the three major lipoproteins is shown in Figure 5-1.

1. **Low-density lipoprotein (LDL)** or very low-density lipoprotein (VLDL) has been established as the chief macromolecule that carries cholesterol and cholesterol esters in their passage through the intima and the inner media. This is true in all stages of the human atherogenic plaque from the very early "fatty streak" to the most advanced lesions, which have large, necrotic, cholesterol-rich interiors surrounded by foam cells and covered with fibrous tissue.

2. **High-density lipoprotein (HDL)** appears to be a protective molecule that transports cholesterol from the tissue to the liver. The HDL fraction is relatively poor in cholesterol and rich in phospholipid. There is a positive correlation between regular physical exercise of the kind designed to improve cardiorespiratory function, and an increased HDL/LDL ratio. This interesting finding has not been sufficiently explored at the cellular and basic biochemical level. However, it has obvious implications for therapy or preventive medicine. In cell culture preparations, the mitosis-stimulating effect of LDL from hyperlipidemic serum on the SMC can be completely blocked by HDL from normal serum or by estrogen. It is thought that HDL blocks the entrance into the SMC of LDL by

Figure 5-1

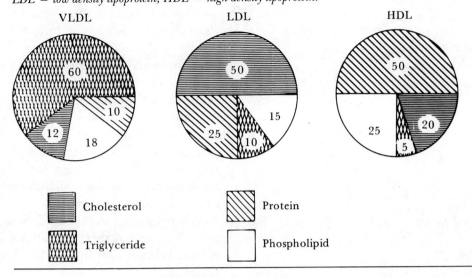

Content of the three major lipoproteins in percentages. VLDL = very low density lipoprotein; LDL = low density lipoprotein; HDL = high density lipoprotein.

interfering in the binding to cell surface receptors. The stimulation of SMC proliferation by hyperlipidemic LDL apparently requires entrance into the cell.

3. **Lipid disorders, dyslipidemias,** are more than a matter of high-serum lipids; they relate to an imbalance of lipid-carrier proteins. High levels of LDL and VLDL and low levels of HDL are correlated with atherogenesis and coronary atherosclerosis; high levels of HDL are correlated with low risk. HDL levels can be elevated by diet, exercise, and specific drug therapy. Therefore, it is now generally recognized that HDL determination should be added to the laboratory measurement of total serum cholesterol and triglyceride values. For example, a cholesterol value between 200 and 250 mg/dl is considered within normal limits for an American; however, with an HDL value below 45 mg/dl, a definite risk of coronary heart disease is present.

V. **Therapeutic considerations.** Treatment of patients with atherosclerosis should consist of: (1) management of the important clinical manifestations, such as ischemic heart disease, peripheral vascular disease, strokes, and aneurysms; (2) efforts to control the various risk factors including lowering serum cholesterol, high blood pressure, and smoking; and (3) programs to promote changes in life style and regular physical exercise.

In experimental animal models the cholesterol-rich atherosclerotic plaque will regress simply by lowering serum cholesterol to less than 150 mg/dl. However, effective and simple therapy to accomplish this and interrupt the disease process at the molecular and cellular level has not been achieved in man.

VI. **Clinical example of atherosclerotic coronary artery disease**

A. **Description.** A 52-year-old salesman gave a history of chest pain described as pressure, heaviness, or a squeezing sensation in the retrosternal location with frequent radiation into the neck. The symptoms developed in association with anxiety, after eating, and in association with effort. The retrosternal distress usually lasted 5 to 10 minutes but occasionally lasted longer.

The patient weighed 235 pounds and was 70 inches in height. The resting electrocardiogram was normal. Serum cholesterol was 270 mg/dl. There was no history of hypertension, diabetes mellitus, or gout. Family history revealed that his father and two uncles died of myocardial infarction in their fifties. The patient smoked one to two packs of cigarettes per day and was a social drinker; he had sedentary habits. Physical examination was noncontributory other than identifying an obese man with normal blood pressure who appeared anxious.

During a treadmill exercise tolerance test, the patient's chest pain was reproduced and the electrocardiogram showed ischemic ST segment depression. Coronary artery disease was diagnosed.

B. Discussion

1. This case history illustrates the multifactorial nature of atherosclerotic coronary artery disease. Risk factors included elevated cholesterol, obesity, cigarette smoking, emotional factors, and family history of coronary disease.

2. Additional studies showed that the serum triglycerides were markedly elevated and there was an abnormal glucose tolerance. The chemical abnormality fit into the category of type IV hyperlipoproteinemia.

3. There are at least five major categories of abnormal lipoprotein patterns. The type IV hyperlipoproteinemia is probably the most common and is associated with increased serum levels of VLDL. Factors commonly associated with increased VLDL levels are obesity, stress, and glucose intolerance. Treatment should include weight reduction and restriction of food precursors of VLDL triglyceride, namely, carbohydrates and alcohol. Cholesterol intake should be reduced to 300 to 400 mg per day. Attention to the major risk factor of cigarette smoking and to the amelioration of emotional stress is also important. Specific therapy to control angina is indicated, and an exercise program should be encouraged.

Questions

More than one answer may be correct.

1. Atherosclerosis with the development of coronary disease is often associated with which of the following?
   a. Cigarette smoking.
   b. High blood pressure.
   c. Elevated LDL cholesterol levels.
   d. Elevated serum high-density lipoprotein (HDL) levels.
   e. All of the above.

2. Select the true statements regarding the relationship between regular aerobic exercise and the progression of coronary atherosclerosis (CAD):
   a. Long-distance runners never experience coronary disease.
   b. Long-distance runners may have coronary disease but do not die from myocardial infarctions.
   c. Epidemiologic studies demonstrate an inverse relationship between regular exercise and CAD.
   d. Physical exercise to improve cardiorespiratory function will increase the HDL/LDL ratio.
   e. None of the above.

6 Biochemical, Physiologic, and Pathologic Consequences of Ischemia

I. **Normal physiology.** The heart is an aerobic organ and can develop only a small oxygen debt without undergoing irreversible damage. Under physiologic conditions myocardial oxygen supply equals myocardial oxygen consumption. In a steady state, determination of the heart's oxygen consumption provides an accurate measure of its metabolism. Factors determining myocardial oxygen consumption are: (1) the tension time index (the area under the left ventricular pressure curve), tension being directly related to the radius and the intraventricular pressure and inversely related to ventricular wall thickness; (2) contractile state of the myocardium (contractility); and (3) heart rate. Acceleration of heart rate increases the frequency of tension development per unit time and also augments myocardial contractility. Oxygen supply is determined by the coronary blood flow. The heart is supplied by the left and right coronary arteries, which course across the epicardial surface of the heart and then give rise to arteries which turn at right angles and penetrate the myocardium. Myocardial blood flow is determined by the driving pressure and resistance offered to flow at the level of precapillary sphincters. Resistance in the vessels is variable due to the compressive effect of the contractile myocardium and is also influenced by neural, metabolic, myogenic, and humoral factors. Effective driving or perfusion pressure is the pressure gradient between the coronary arteries and the coronary sinus. During systole coronary ostia are partly occluded by the open aortic valve leaflets. However, during diastole when the aortic valve is closed, aortic diastolic pressure is transmitted directly to the coronary ostia. Coronary arteries are compressed during systole in the contracting thick left ventricle. Coronary blood flow in the left coronary artery occurs primarily during diastole, while right coronary flow occurs during both systole and diastole. Subendocardial zones are more vulnerable to diminished blood flow than are the subepicardial zones. Normal coronary blood flow is 60 to 90 ml per minute per 100 gm of myocardium but can increase substantially during exercise. Coronary collateral vessels (connections between coronary arteries) are abundant in the canine heart but are highly variable in human hearts. Under physiologic conditions, they are of little consequence but play an important role when coronary blood flow is compromised by obstruction of a major vessel.

II. **Myocardial ischemia** is defined as a state of myocardial oxygen deprivation accompanied by inadequate removal of metabolites secondary to decreased perfusion. Myocardial ischemia results when myocardial oxygen demand outstrips supply; this is brought about either by the reduction or cessation of coronary blood flow or by an increase in oxygen demand during stress that cannot be met by an increase in coronary blood flow. The cross-sectional area of the coronary artery may be reduced by 70 to 80 percent without inducing ischemia at rest. However, with this degree of narrowing in the proximal position of a coronary artery, ischemia can often be induced by any stimulus—i.e., exercise, atrial pacing, or psychologic stress—that augments myocardial oxygen demand.

Myocardial ischemia is most commonly caused by organic narrowing or obstruction of coronary arteries, but it may result from coronary artery spasm or from increased oxygen demand in the presence of normal coronary arteries, as in aortic stenosis and subaortic muscular stenosis. Relative roles of atherosclerosis, arterial occlusion, platelet aggregation, coronary artery spasm, and increased myocardial oxygen demand in the causation of myocardial ischemia are discussed below.

A. **Atherosclerosis** is by far the commonest pathologic process for organic narrowing of the coronary arteries. Invariably atherosclerotic plaques develop in the proximal segments of coronary arteries. However, in some patients there is diffuse involvement of coronary arteries with atherosclerosis. When the lumen diameter decreases to 50 percent or lower (cross-sectional area narrowing of 75% or more), manifestations of myocardial ischemia invariably occur during stress, but as the narrowing progresses, manifestations of ischemia may occur during rest because of a marked reduction in the coronary blood flow. The severity and extent of ischemia varies with the number of vessels involved in the atherosclerotic process and the severity of the lesions.

B. **Nonatherosclerotic coronary disease.** Coronary arteries may be narrowed due to inflammatory and autoimmune processes. The vessels involved are usually small branches of coronary arteries, in contrast to the main or larger coronary arteries affected by atherosclerosis. Small-vessel coronary disease is often seen in polyarteritis nodosa, systemic lupus erythematosus, rheumatoid arthritis, scleroderma, and diabetes; it may be an important cause of myocardial ischemia in this group of patients.

C. **Coronary thrombosis and platelet aggregation.** Recent studies suggest that thrombotic occlusion of an atherosclerotic vessel is an important cause of prolonged myocardial ischemia and is found in as many as 50 to 85 percent of cases following an acute myocardial infarction. What initiates the thrombotic process, however, remains speculative, and both coronary spasm and platelet aggregation have been implicated. In animal experiments, platelet aggregation has been shown to decrease myocardial blood flow. Whether such a process occurs spontaneously in man remains unproved at the present time. Increased platelet aggregation remains a plausible explanation for initiating the thrombotic process in a diseased coronary artery.

Extent of myocardial injury from sudden disruption of coronary blood flow is determined by the presence or absence of collateral circulation in the ischemic area, the site of occlusion, and the status of the remaining coronary arteries. In the absence of collateral blood flow, ischemic myocardium invariably becomes necrotic, but the severity and extent of necrosis varies with the site of occlusion and the size and number of vessels involved.

D. **Coronary artery spasm.** Spasm of a normal coronary artery or a previously diseased coronary artery is an important cause of myocardial ischemia. The exact mechanism by which the coronary artery goes into spasm, however, remains speculative. Current evidence suggests that coronary spasm is in all probability due to an increase in vasomotor tone and reactivity of the coronary arteries and is mediated through the alpha-adrenergic innervation. Furthermore, coronary artery spasm and platelet aggregation may be interrelated. Platelet aggregation releases thromboxane A_2, which is a potent vasoconstrictor and which may be the mechanism of spasm, especially in coronary arteries with obstructive organic narrowing because platelets often adhere to these lesions and under appropriate stimuli might release thromboxane A_2. The end result of coronary arterial spasm is a profound reduction in myocardial blood flow with resultant deprivation or reduction of oxygen supply to the myocardium. Although coronary artery spasm is not a common cause of myocardial infarction, it is nevertheless an important cause of prolonged myocardial ischemia and serious, often fatal arrhythmias.

E. **Coronary embolism.** This is a rare cause of a sudden reduction in coronary blood flow but can produce severe myocardial ischemia and even myocardial necrosis. The source of emboli is usually thrombi in the left atrium or left ventricle. Atrial fibrillation, valvular heart disease, cardiomyopathy, and endocarditis predispose to coronary embolism.

F. **Augmentation of myocardial oxygen demand.** The important determinants of myocardial oxygen demand are heart rate, contractile state of the ventricle, and the tension time index. In the presence of moderate to severe organic narrowing of coronary arteries, any stimulus that increases any or all of the determinants of myocardial oxygen demand will often induce myocardial ischemia. The stress may be exercise, which increases heart rate, myocardial contractility, and tension time index, or anxiety, which augments heart rate and blood pressure. Anemia, thyrotoxicosis, and infection also increase myocardial oxygen demand and may induce myocardial ischemia in a patient who has obstructive narrowing of one or more coronary arteries. However, these conditions rarely precipitate myocardial ischemia in the presence of normal coronary arteries. Increased myocardial oxygen demand in the presence of normal coronary arteries is rarely a cause of myocardial ischemia but can occur in patients with severe aortic stenosis and in those with subaortic muscular stenosis. In these two conditions, myocardial oxygen demand is greatly augmented due to a thickened, hypertrophied ventricle and due to a marked elevation of intraventricular pressure.

III. **Biochemical consequences of ischemia.** Under aerobic conditions the myocardium derives its energy from oxidative phosphorylation. It utilizes primarily free fatty acids (FFA). This preferential utilization of FFA depends on the high activity of several enzyme systems including the acyl-CoA-carnitine transferase systems that facilitate oxidation of FFA, inhibition of glucose uptake, glycolytic flux, and glycogenolysis.

By reducing oxygen availability, ischemia limits the rate of adenosine triphosphate (ATP) synthesis, with subsequent decline in high-energy phosphate stores. Activity of enzymes involved in the intermediate metabolism is altered. Glycolytic flux increases because of enhanced phosphorylation and uptake of glucose. Glycogenolysis accelerates. Augmentation of glycolytic flux may maintain viability by providing ATP. However, this mechanism cannot maintain myocardial ATP stores adequately even in the nonworking heart. Oxygen deprivation inhibits Krebs cycle activity and the metabolism of glucose occurs through the anaerobic pathway. Due to diminished blood flow, lactate accumulates in the cells with resultant decline in pH and accumulation of other metabolites which inhibit glycolytic flux at the phosphofructokinase and glyceraldehyde-3-phosphate dehydrogenase steps. Ischemia increases the intracellular concentration of acyl CoA esters, which in turn inhibit the effective exchange of adenosine diphosphate (ADP) and ATP between the cytoplasm of the cell and the mitochondria by suppressing the activity of adenine nucleotide translocase. Ischemia leads to reduction in synthesis of myocardial proteins and increase in analine release.

Complete oxidation of 1 mole of glucose gives rise to the net production of 36 moles of ATP. However, only 2 moles of ATP are produced during anaerobic metabolism of 1 mole of glucose. The failure of energy production during ischemia results in decline in the concentration of creatine phosphate. Mitochondria have high affinity for oxygen, and cell death varies with duration and extent of ischemia. If ischemia is prolonged, cell death occurs and lysosomal hydrolase activity increases in response to irreversible injury.

During ischemia there is inward influx of calcium across the sarcolemma. Accumulation of calcium in the cell augments hydrolysis of ATP, inhibits ATP synthesis through oxidative phosphorylation, and impairs the mechanical performance of the myocardium. Loss of functional integrity of the sarcolemma allows the liberation of cytoplasm constituents into the circulation (transaminases, lactic dehydrogenase, and creatine kinase).

Ischemia also depresses the energy-dependent membrane sodium-potassium pumping system, which leads to loss of intracellular potassium in the vicinity of the sarcolemma.

IV. **Physiologic consequences.** In animal experiments, ligation of the coronary artery leads to paradoxical motion in the center ischemic zone, reduced contractility in the adjacent area, and increased contractility of the uninvolved normal myocardium through the Frank-Starling mechanism. This situation is simulated in humans during coronary occlusion by a thrombus or spasm. In the absence of myocardial infarction, patients with coronary artery disease usually do not show impaired myocardial function at rest, but increase in myocardial oxygen demand during stress often precipitates myocardial dysfunction. Regional areas of impaired myocardial contractility, whether sustained or transient, may depress overall left ventricular function, producing reductions of left ventricular systolic function (cardiac output, stroke volume, ejection fraction, and stroke work). Myocardial ischemia also affects diastolic pressure–volume relation. Impaired relaxation leads to increased resistance to ventricular filling. Through its direct effect on contractility, ischemia causes incomplete ventricular emptying and elevation of left ventricular end-diastolic pressure, which may lead to left ventricular failure. Cardiogenic shock may ensue when myocardial damage is extensive ($\geq$40%). Within 30 to 60 seconds of coronary artery occlusion, S–T segment elevation occurs (more marked in the central zone) and is probably related to altered ionic transport across the myocardial cell membrane due to reduced intramyocardial oxygen tension. S–T changes during transient ischemia are due to subendocardial injury. During prolonged ischemia, there is increased susceptibility to ventricular arrhythmias due to inhomogenous spread of activation in the ischemic zones and due to altered membrane properties. In general, S–T segment elevation is a reasonable index of the extent of myocardial ischemia. However, it should be recognized that changes in temperature, drugs, and pericardial injury also influence S–T segments.

V. **Pathologic consequences.** When myocardial ischemia is transient, biochemical and physiologic changes are often reversible, and near complete functional recovery occurs. However, during prolonged ischemia, irreversible myocardial damage or myocardial infarction occurs. Site and location of the infarction depends on a number of factors: (1) location and severity of coronary arterial narrowing, (2) the extent of collateral circulation to the ischemic area, (3) the size of the vascular bed perfused by the narrowed vessel, and (4) the oxygen needs of the jeopardized myocardium.

Both during transient and prolonged ischemia, the patient often experiences chest pain and there is electrocardiographic evidence of ischemia (S–T wave changes). If the myocardial damage is irreversible, the affected region appears pale, bluish, and slightly swollen; 18 to 36 hours later the myocardium appears tan or reddish purple. These changes persist for 48 hours, when the infarct turns gray. By 8 to 10 days following infarction, the infarcted muscle is removed by mononuclear cells. Over the next 2 or 3 months, the infarcted area is converted to a shrunken, thin scar, which whitens and firms with time. The endocardium below the infarct becomes thickened and opaque. In man, myocardial infarction may occur after narrowing in one or more arteries. However, it may occur due to coronary arterial spasm without occlusive coronary artery disease. If the coronary artery becomes completely occluded and there is poor collateral blood flow to the ischemic area, the infarct is often transmural (whole thickness of myocardium). Occlusion of the left anterior descending coronary artery results in involvement of the areas supplied by this artery (septum, apical area, and anterior wall). Occlusion of the left circumflex artery may lead to infarction of the lateral and inferoposterior wall of the left ventricle. Occlusion of the right coronary artery results in infarction of the inferoposterior wall of the left ventricle, the inferior portions of the septum, and the posteromedial papillary muscle.

Nontransmural myocardial infarction often occurs in the presence of severely narrowed coronary arteries which are not completely occluded. Myocardial infarction often involves the left ventricle, but right ventricular infarction occurs in some 20 to 30 percent of cases of inferior myocardial infarction.

Myocardial infarction may be complicated by myocardial rupture, which leads to hemopericardium and immediate death from cardiac tamponade. Rupture of the infarcted septum may lead to a communication between the two ventricles (ventricular septal defect). Rupture of the papillary muscle may lead to severe mitral regurgitation and acute pulmonary edema. Many patients die suddenly due to ventricular arrhythmias following an acute myocardial infarction. Of those who survive the first few hours and are hospitalized, 10 to 25 percent die due to various complications (pump failure, arrhythmias, cardiac rupture, mitral regurgitation).

Pericarditis is a frequent complication of myocardial infarction but is usually transient and is secondary to the involvement of the epicardial layer of the myocardium. A late complication of myocardial infarction is left ventricular aneurysm, which develops in 12 to 15 percent of patients who survive. The aneurysm predisposes to clot formation, with resultant increased risk of systemic embolization.

VI. Clinical examples of myocardial ischemia
A. Myocardial infarction
   1. **Description.** A 50-year-old man came to the hospital with severe chest pain of 4 hours' duration. On examination he was in sinus rhythm with a heart rate of 120 per minute and blood pressure of 70/50 mm Hg. He was mentally confused and acutely dyspneic.

   Electrocardiogram showed evidence of a recent anterior myocardial infarction (S–T segment elevation in anterior chest leads V_1–V_6). Chest x-ray showed gross pulmonary edema.

2. Discussion

a. Chest pain is secondary to severe myocardial ischemia. The mechanism by which pain occurs during myocardial ischemia is poorly understood.

b. Mental confusion and severe hypotension indicate severe myocardial impairment and poor ventricular function secondary to extensive myocardial damage.

c. Dyspnea is secondary to marked elevation of left ventricular end-diastolic pressure due to failing left ventricular performance, with resultant increase in end-diastolic pressure. Radiologic evidence of pulmonary edema indicates marked elevation of pulmonary capillary pressure as a consequence of raised left ventricular end-diastolic pressure.

B. Transient myocardial ischemia

1. **Description.** A 54-year-old patient reported having recurrent episodes of chest pain during exertion for the past 3 years. Clinical examination did not reveal any abnormality. A resting electrocardiogram was normal. During exercise, the patient complained of breathlessness and developed S–T segment depression in the anterior chest leads. His heart rate increased from 60 beats per minute to 120 per minute and blood pressure increased from 110/80 mm Hg to 170/90 mm Hg. Electrocardiogram returned to normal within 5 minutes of stopping exercise.

2. **Discussion**

a. Myocardial ischemia was precipitated during exercise, which increases myocardial oxygen demand due to increases in heart rate, systolic blood pressure, and myocardial contractility.

b. Breathlessness was due to a transient increase in left ventricular end-diastolic pressure secondary to myocardial ischemia.

c. Electrocardiographic S–T depression represents subendocardial ischemia.

d. With the cessation of exercise, myocardial oxygen demand decreased and manifestations of myocardial ischemia (S–T changes, chest pain, breathlessness) subsided.

Questions

More than one answer may be correct.

1. A 45-year-old man was admitted to the hospital with severe chest pain. The cardiac rhythm was regular at 90 beats per minute and blood pressure was 150/80 mm Hg. Bilateral basal rales were audible, and chest x-ray showed cardiomegaly and pulmonary edema. Which of the following statements is false?
   a. History is compatible with acute myocardial ischemia.
   b. Basal rales and pulmonary edema indicate severe left ventricular failure.
   c. Pulmonary capillary wedge pressure will be low.
   d. Left ventricular end-diastolic pressure will be elevated.

2. Which situations are associated with an increase in myocardial oxygen demand (MVO_2)?
   a. Tachycardia.
   b. Bradycardia.
   c. Elevated systolic blood pressure.
   d. Reduced myocardial contractility.
   e. Cardiomegaly.

7 Clinical Manifestations of Coronary Artery Disease

I. General considerations

A. **Magnitude of the problem.** Coronary artery disease constitutes the most important health problem facing the United States. By estimates of the American Heart Association, over 4 million Americans have had either a heart attack or angina pectoris. Given current statistics, one in five Americans can expect coronary artery disease to become clinically manifest by the age of 60. The clinical manifestations of ischemic heart disease are, generally speaking, results of an inexorably progressive atherosclerotic process involving the coronary arteries. In some studies of large American populations, coronary artery disease accounts for over 30 percent of deaths from all causes for all ages. There does seem to be a gradual reduction in death rates from coronary artery disease, beginning in the late 1960s. The reason for this decline is actively debated.

B. **Pathology.** Coronary artery disease is best viewed pathologically and clinically as a continuum of progressively severe atherosclerotic lesions roughly (though not uniformly) paralleling a clinical progression from asymptomatic to symptomatic to death.

The symptoms and signs of coronary artery disease are largely due to abnormal functioning of the left ventricular myocardium. The myocardial changes, in turn, are consequences of narrowing of the lumens of the major coronary arteries.

In order for flow to be decreased through a blood vessel, at least 75 percent of the *cross-sectional area* of the lumen must be obliterated. In coronary angiography, lumen size is usually expressed as the diameter reduction. For example, a 30 percent angiographic stenosis (diameter reduction) represents approximately a 50 percent cross-sectional area reduction, a 50 percent stenosis represents a 75 percent cross-sectional area reduction, a 70 percent stenosis represents approximately a 90 percent cross-sectional area reduction, and so on. The mathematical relationship, of course, is cross-sectional area (of remaining lumen) equals πr^2 (where r represents the radius of the remaining lumen).

Some important facts about the pathology of coronary artery disease are: (1) All portions of the extramural (the portions of the coronary arteries on the surface of the heart) coronary arteries tend to be involved in the atherosclerotic process, though some segments are narrowed more severely than others. (2) The atherosclerotic process is limited to the epicardial coronary arteries and does not involve the intramyocardial vessels. (3) Of the three types of atherosclerotic plaques—lipid, fibrous, and complicated—only the last is responsible for causing significant (>75%) reduction in luminal size. (4) Lipid and fibrous plaques have a worldwide distribution, but complicated plaques are generally found in populations that develop symptomatic coronary artery disease.

The role of thrombosis in the development of acute myocardial infarction, sudden death, or even angina pectoris is debated. It appears that the superimposition of thrombus on complicated atherosclerotic plaques is, at least in many situations, a component of acute myocardial infarction.

II. Clinical syndromes. Symptoms and signs of coronary disease are the result of myocardial dysfunction, and they can take the form of angina pectoris, acute myocardial infarction, or sudden coronary death. Cardiac arrhythmias, conduction abnormalities, and congestive heart failure as *isolated* manifestations of coronary disease are uncommon. Exactly what produces which of the major coronary events (angina pectoris, acute myocardial infarction, or sudden coronary death) as the clinical manifestation of coronary disease in a given patient is uncertain. Any of these events may be the first, or the last, manifestation of coronary disease. Sudden coronary death or acute myocardial infarction can occur without preexisting angina, and patients with angina may never have an acute myocardial infarction. About half of patients with sudden coronary death have pathologic evidence of a prior myocardial infarction.

A. Angina pectoris. The original description of angina pectoris is attributed to Dr. William Heberden, who wrote over two centuries ago:

> There is a disorder of the breast, marked with strong and peculiar symptoms, considerable for the kind of danger belonging to it, and not extremely rare. . . . The seat of it, and sense of strangling and anxiety with which it is attended, may make it not improperly be called Angina pectoris.
>
> Those who are afflicted with it are seized, while they are walking, and more particularly when they walk soon after eating, with a painful and most disagreeable sensation in the breast, which seems as if it would take their life away, if it were to increase or to continue: the moment they stand still, all this uneasiness vanishes. In all other respects, the patients are, at the beginning of this order, perfectly well, and in particular have no shortness of breath, from which it is totally different . . . and it will come on, not only when the persons are walking, but when they are lying down, and oblige them to rise up out of their beds every night for many months together: and in one or two very inveterate cases it has been brought on . . . even by swallowing, coughing, going to stool, or speaking, or by any disturbance of mind . . . this complaint was greatest in winter: another, that it was aggravated by warm weather. . . .

This description still applies to a large number of patients with angina pectoris but what we've come to appreciate is that there are many atypical clinical presentations of patients with angina pectoris. Many different patterns of discomfort involving the chest, arms, epigastrium, neck, jaw, or teeth are compatible with angina. Patients whose discomfort manifests as earache have been seen.

There are classical precipitating features of angina pectoris such as effort (physical), eating, cold weather exposure, and emotional stress, though angina can occur at rest, nocturnally, or with arrhythmias of a variety of types.

Effort produces an increase in the work of the heart and, associated with this increase in work, an increase in myocardial oxygen consumption. There typically is a hemodynamic threshold for angina that may be expressed as a product of the heart rate and systolic blood pressure. Regardless of the type of stress, this threshold tends to be reproducible; this threshold is the point at which myocardial oxygen needs exceed the myocardial oxygen delivery, with ischemia being the result. Some patients with coronary disease have an unpredictable response to effort for reasons that are not clear. Occasionally, a patient will have what is referred to as walk-through angina, in which pain appears and then subsides on continuing effort. The mechanism for this phenomenon is also unclear, though it may be related to delayed onset of vasodilatation of collateral vessels in response to metabolic factors that accrue with time.

Excitement, anxiety, anger, and fear can provoke autonomic discharges that also result in angina. Frequently, if heart rate and blood pressure are monitored during those periods of emotional stress associated with angina, the importance of the sympathetic nervous system can be appreciated.

The mechanism of ischemia and resulting pain associated with eating are not well understood. This usually occurs only with severe coronary disease.

As in Dr. Heberden's description, the role of cold weather in provoking ischemia and pain with coronary disease has long been recognized. It has been suggested that the cold produces reflex vasoconstriction that could involve the coronary arteries as well as the peripheral vascular system. The peripheral vascular constriction could elevate the arterial blood pressure, thus increasing the impedance to left ventricular ejection, thus increasing cardiac work.

Frequently in angina that occurs at rest (angina decubitus) there is evidence of sympathetic overactivity manifest by increases in heart rate and blood pressure. Nocturnal angina may have a similar mechanism related to dream activity or other cause of increased sympathetic tone. Angina at rest and angina nocturnally usually indicate severe coronary disease and are two of the criteria for the unstable pattern of angina.

Tachycardia, by reducing diastolic filling time of the coronary arteries and by increasing myocardial oxygen consumption, can precipitate anginal attacks.

B. **Acute myocardial infarction.** Acute myocardial infarction (MI) is a clinical and pathologic event characterized by chest pain that is similar to angina but tends to be more severe and longer lasting and is characterized pathologically by irreversible ischemia-injury-death of myocardial tissue. As previously mentioned, the role of coronary thombosis superimposed on a complicated atherosclerotic plaque in precipitating an acute MI is debated. Coronary spasm may also play a part in some MIs and in angina pectoris as well. The classical time course of an acute MI—described as polymorphonuclear leucocyte invasion within 24 hours, dissolution of necrotic muscle by 4 to 10 days, and the laying down of collagen and total healing by scar formation by 2 months—is probably an oversimplification, since the myocardial necrosis tends to be an ongoing process over a period of hours to days.

Epidemiologic studies suggest that around 25 percent of acute MIs are unrecognized clinically.

Arrhythmias originating in or near the infarcted myocardium, heart failure, and shock (the latter two due to extensive myocardial death) are the most compromising and deadly results of acute myocardial infarction.

C. **Sudden coronary death.** Although proof that sudden coronary death is due to atherosclerosis requires necropsy examination, available statistics suggest that around 90 percent of sudden deaths are caused by coronary atherosclerosis.

The definition of *sudden coronary death* is debated, especially with respect to time following onset of symptoms. Some authors suggest that death must occur within 6 hours of onset of symptoms. Others allow 24 hours to pass. The coronary arteries of patients dying suddenly are remarkably similar to those of patients dying from acute MI. The mechanism of death in virtually all of these patients is ventricular fibrillation. It is much less common to find histologic evidence of sinus or AV node or bundle branch abnormalities in patients dying suddenly.

III. **Clinical examples of coronary artery disease**

A. **Angina pectoris**

1. **Description.** A 62-year-old man with a history of smoking two packs of cigarettes per day for 45 years and a 10-year history of intermittently treated hypertension came to the cardiology clinic with a 2-year history of episodic retrosternal aching discomforts brought on by exertion and by emotional stress. These episodes were occurring with increasing frequency, currently about three times a day and occasionally at night. The pain typically lasted 10 to 15 minutes and was usually relieved by rest. The patient frequently experienced dyspnea with the pain. On examination no cardiac abnormalities were noted. Electrocardiogram (ECG) was normal, though performed while he was having no chest pain. Chest x-ray was normal. Laboratory testing was normal except for a cholesterol level (total) of 279 mg/100 ml. Exercise testing was performed. The patient developed his typical chest pain at a heart rate of 96 beats per minute and a blood pressure of 140/90 mm Hg only 2 minutes after beginning the test (speed 1.7 mph, grade 10%). Upon onset of pain, 4 mm of S–T segment depression was noted in several leads. Coronary angiography was performed and revealed greater than 75 percent narrowing in the left main coronary artery. Left ventricular angiography revealed a normal-sized and contracting chamber. The patient subsequently underwent coronary artery bypass surgery and was pain free when last seen a year later.

2. **Discussion**

a. The patient had multiple risk factors for coronary artery disease: smoking, hypertension, and an elevated serum cholesterol level.

b. The patient was experiencing a worsening in the anginal pattern marked by rest and nocturnal episodes, increasing frequency, and decreasing amounts of exertion to produce angina. This is referred to as unstable angina.

c. The normal ECG at rest and normal chest x-ray are common in even severe disease. The relatively low heart rate and blood pressure at the onset of pain as well as the dramatic depression in S–T segments all suggest severe coronary disease.

B. **Sudden coronary death**

1. **Description.** A 47-year-old woman was attending a horse race in a neighboring state. She had no history of cardiac problems but was a smoker and a diabetic with a history of coronary disease in her family. At the race, she suddenly stood up, clutched her chest, and passed out. Resuscitative efforts were unsuccessful. Postmortem examination revealed severe diffuse coronary artery disease with evidence of a fresh thrombus in her proximal left anterior descending coronary artery. There was no pathologic evidence of acute MI.

2. **Discussion.** Almost certainly this patient died of ventricular fibrillation precipitated by occlusion of her left anterior descending coronary artery. Had she survived, evolution of an anterior myocardial infarction could be expected.

Questions

Select the single best answer.

1. Which of the following is not considered a major isolated manifestation of coronary artery disease?
   a. Sudden death.
   b. Acute myocardial infarction.
   c. Hypotension.
   d. Angina pectoris.
   e. None of the above.
2. Which of the following is the most common cause of sudden coronary death?
   a. Complete (third-degree) heart block.
   b. Cardiogenic shock.
   c. Ventricular fibrillation.
   d. Sinus node arrest.
   e. Ruptured left ventricle.

I. Physiology
   A. Explanation of terms
      1. **Jugular venous pulsation.** The *a* wave is produced with atrial contraction. The *v* wave is due to pressure buildup in the venous reservoir while the tricuspid valves are closed. The x descent occurs between the *a* and *v* waves and is associated with atrial relaxation. The x descent is partly interrupted by a small *c* wave, which is produced by tricuspid valve closure. The y descent occurs between the *v* wave and the succeeding *a* wave of the next cardiac cycle and is produced by emptying of the venous reservoir into the right ventricle.
      2. **The normal heart sounds.** The closure of the atrioventricular (AV) and semilunar valves produces the first and second heart sounds. Because right-sided pressures are far lower than those found on the left side, the sounds produced by the tricuspid and pulmonary valves are softer than those produced by the mitral and aortic. The pulmonary valve closure sound is best heard in the left second intercostal space (the pulmonary area). The tricuspid valve closure is best heard at the fourth left intercostal space (the tricuspid area). The mitral and aortic sounds are heard at all areas; the former better at the apex (the mitral area) and the latter better at the base of the heart. Closure of the AV and semilunar valves on the right side of the heart are not synchronous with the closure of the corresponding valves on the left. Asynchronous closure, therefore, normally gives rise to splitting of the first and second heart sounds. From a diagnostic standpoint, this is more important in relation to the second heart sound. With inspiration, the right ventricle is distended by the augmented venous return. This produces prolonged right ventricular contraction and delayed pulmonary valve closure. Thus, P_2 moves away from A_2. As a result, the second heart sound is more widely split on inspiration. This is a normal finding. With expiration, right ventricular filling is diminished, and P_2 moves closer to A_2. On expiration, the second heart sound is single. Thus, the effect of respiration on the second heart sound is to produce a constant variation in the degree of splitting which is quite characteristic of good health. The third heart sound is generally present in children and young adults, especially with tachycardia and lying on the left side and is considered to be a normal finding in people under age 35. This sound is thought to be produced by vibration of the ventricular walls or tension of the AV valves. The sound, as can be seen in Figure 8-1, occurs during the rapid phase of ventricular filling and is low pitched and best heard at the apex. It may originate from either or both ventricles. All other sounds produced by the heart are abnormal.
II. **Pathophysiology.** There are three functional disturbances that may occur with the mitral, tricuspid, aortic, and pulmonary valves. These are: (a) stenosis, (b) regurgitation, and (c) a combination of stenosis and regurgitation.
   A. **Mitral stenosis**
      1. **Hemodynamic changes.** Until a critical degree of narrowing oc-

Figure 8-1

The cardiac cycle, showing the pressure curves of the great vessels and cardiac chambers, valvular events, heart sounds, left ventricular volume curves, jugular pulse waves, and the apex cardiogram. The electrocardiogram is shown below. The dark line above the right atrium represents the left atrium. MC = mitral component of first heart sound; MO = mitral valve opening; TC = tricuspid component of first heart sound; TO = tricuspid valve opening; AC = aortic component of second heart sound; AO = aortic valve opening; PC = pulmonic valve component of second heart sound; PO = pulmonic valve opening; OS = opening snap of AV valves; IC = isovolumic or isovolumetric contraction wave; IR = isovolumic or isovolumetric relaxation wave; O = opening of mitral valve; RFW = rapid-filling wave; SFW = slow-filling wave. The a, c, and v waves and x and y descents are explained in the text. (From J. Willis Hurst [Ed.], The Heart [4th ed.]. New York: McGraw-Hill, 1978, with permission of the author and the publisher.)

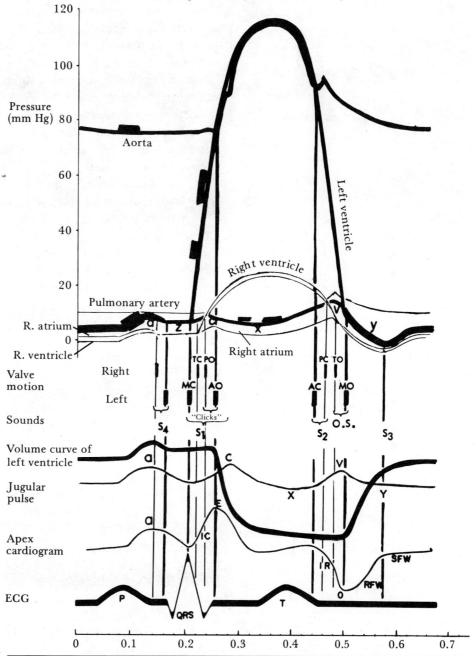

curs, no disturbance of hemodynamic function results from stenosis of the mitral valve. The reserve is so great that the valve orifice has to be at least halved before the obstruction requires any compensatory pressure changes. Even if the obstruction is not hemodynamically important, the increased rate of flow across the narrowed area produces murmurs facilitating early diagnosis, often long before symptoms are felt. With progressive narrowing of the valve orifice, a pressure gradient develops between the left atrium and the left ventricle (see Fig. 8-1). The left atrium hypertrophies and the pressure generated by the left atrial muscle is increased. This pressure is reflected back into the pulmonary veins, capillaries, and arteries with resultant pulmonary hypertension, right ventricular hypertrophy, and even right atrial hypertrophy. With increasing pressure of the left atrium, the pulmonary capillary pressure becomes elevated approaching the blood osmotic pressure so that pulmonary edema can readily occur. Since atrial systole is crucially important as a booster pump to the filling of the ventricle, the onset of atrial fibrillation (the commonest disturbance of rhythm seen in patients with mitral stenosis) is often a milestone in the natural history of this condition. Patients deteriorate rapidly because the rapid heart rate results in a decreased filling time and, therefore, there is a buildup in pressure and volume in the left atrium which is transmitted to the lungs.

2. **Clinical picture.** The symptom complex is usually dyspnea on effort progressing to orthopnea or the inability to lie flat and finally advancing to paroxysmal nocturnal dyspnea, which is a condition where the patient wakes at night short of breath and gets relief by sitting up or getting out of bed and seeking fresh air from an opened window. Hemoptysis is relatively common and can vary from massive amounts to sputum streaking. The patient may also complain of chest pain, which may be typically anginal in quality. Other symptoms include those associated with congestive cardiac failure and cyanosis, which is usually peripheral due to a low cardiac output. Palpitations are common, particularly due to paroxysmal tachycardias and atrial fibrillation. Emboli occur secondary to thrombi forming within an enlarged left atrium or on the valve. These patients are susceptible to recurrent pulmonary infection. They may complain of hoarseness due to paralysis of the left recurrent laryngeal nerve by the enlarged left atrium. Syncope is an occasional symptom. Subacute bacterial endocarditis is uncommon in the patient with pure mitral stenosis.

3. **Signs.** In the presence of heart failure, jugular veins may be distended. A large *a* wave is found in patients with pulmonary hypertension, but in atrial fibrillation, the *a* wave is absent. Patients with secondary tricuspid incompetence usually have a large *c–v* wave and systolic expansion of the liver. The peripheral pulse may be normal, but with significant mitral stenosis, it is reduced in volume. Precordial examination usually reveals the apex to be normal in position; it is often described as tapping. There may be an associated parasternal lift. The second sound is often palpable in the pulmonic area, reflecting pulmonary hypertension. In the mitral area, a palpable first heart sound with a diastolic thrill may be perceived. On auscultation, the most striking features are found at the apex, where the first sound is accentuated. It is associated with

an opening snap, which occurs closely after the second heart sound, and a mid-diastolic rumble. In patients that are in sinus rhythm, the first heart sound may be preceded by a presystolic murmur. In some patients, the opening snap is best heard along the left sternal border, and in others the mid-diastolic murmur is heard only when the patient is rotated on the left side. The loud first heart sound and the opening snap are usually absent in patients with calcific mitral stenosis.

B. Mitral regurgitation

1. **Hemodynamic changes.** The volume of blood regurgitated into the left atrium determines the clinical picture. Significant regurgitation produces left atrial distension. The increased volume of blood must return to the ventricle through the mitral valve. In the absence of obstruction at the mitral valve level, the left ventricle is rapidly filled and a loud third sound results. Torrential flow across the valve produces a diastolic murmur, although no anatomical stenosis may be present. The left ventricle dilates to accommodate the increased volume.

2. **Clinical picture.** When the degree of regurgitation is mild, the patient may be asymptomatic. The major hazard is the development of bacterial endocarditis, which may convert mild mitral regurgitation to a severe lesion. The left ventricle can tolerate mitral regurgitation for many years without impairment of function, but when failure develops it usually progresses steadily and relentlessly, resulting in congestive failure, which can be halted only temporarily by conventional medical management. Symptoms, therefore, are predominantly effort dyspnea progressing to orthopnea and paroxysmal cardiac dyspnea. Acute pulmonary edema, hemoptysis, angina pectoris, and embolism are less frequent than in mitral stenosis. Patients may complain of palpitations (due to the overactive hyperdynamic left ventricle) and the development of atrial fibrillation. Fatigue and loss of energy are common complaints.

3. **Signs.** The pulse is usually normal, but occasionally can be collapsing. Atrial fibrillation is frequent. The jugular venous pressure is usually normal in the absence of heart failure. In the late stages, tricuspid regurgitation, jugular venous distension, and a pulsatile liver are present. Examination of the precordium usually reveals an enlarged left ventricle with an overfilled thrusting apex beat. Right ventricular enlargement as evidenced by a parasternal heave usually occurs late. On auscultation there is invariably a loud apical pansystolic regurgitant murmur. The murmur commences with the first heart sound, which it may obscure, and runs through to A_2. It is maximum at the apex, high pitched, blowing in quality, and usually radiates to the axilla. Less commonly, the jet is directed medially and may not occupy the whole of systole. This usually occurs in association with papillary muscle dysfunction or a ruptured cordi. The severity of the incompetence cannot be assessed from the intensity of the murmur, although generally speaking the loudest murmurs are associated with the greatest degree of incompetence. A third heart sound is usually present at the apex and this may be followed by a mid-diastolic flow murmur.

C. Aortic stenosis

1. **Hemodynamic changes.** Aortic stenosis results in obstruction of flow from the left ventricle to the aorta. As narrowing of the valve

occurs, the left ventricular pressure in systole increases to achieve an adequate cardiac output. This results in a pressure gradient between the left ventricle and the aorta. The increased pressure load in the ventricle results in concentric hypertrophy of the left ventricle. When heart failure occurs, cardiac output drops and the gradient falls. The jet of blood through the narrow orifice may produce post-stenotic dilatation of the aorta. Inadequate coronary filling of the hypertrophied muscle may occur, producing myocardial ischemia.

2. **Clinical picture.** The characteristic picture in aortic stenosis is a long asymptomatic period. Symptoms of dyspnea, angina pectoris, and syncope are evidence of severe disease and associated with a poor prognosis unless valvular replacement is undertaken. The pulse is characteristically slow rising. In the elderly, the pulse contour may be deceptive, since the atherosclerotic vessels tend to produce a brisker upstroke than one would anticipate for the degree of stenosis. Thus, the diagnosis may be missed. The jugular venous pressure is usually normal unless there is heart failure. A prominent *a* wave is a sign of an advanced disease and is usually associated with hypertrophy of the septum, causing obstruction to the outflow of the right ventricle. The precordium is characterized by an apex that is displaced downward and outward. It is usually localized and has the character of a pressure overload ventricle. An aortic ejection murmur is characteristic. It is usually loudest at the base of the heart and may radiate to the neck as well as to the apex. Occasionally, it is loudest at the apex, and even more rarely, it may be totally confined to the apex. The first sound is often inaudible or replaced by an ejection click. Frequently, a harsh, loud systolic murmur is all that is heard. The aortic sound is often soft. Paradoxical splitting of S_2 may occur. Usually, the degree of stenosis can be clinically assessed by the slowness of the upstroke of the carotid and peaking of the aortic systolic murmur. The longer the ejection period, the later the peaking, the more severe the lesion. This is true only if left ventricular function is good.

D. **Aortic regurgitation (chronic)**
   1. **Hemodynamic findings.** Aortic regurgitation produces reflux of blood from the aorta to the left ventricle during diastole. Most of the leak occurs during early diastole and the increased volume of blood is accommodated by ventricular dilatation and later hypertrophy.
   2. **Clinical picture.** The natural history of this disease includes a prolonged asymptomatic period followed by the onset of symptoms of shortness of breath, orthopnea, paroxysmal cardiac dyspnea, or pulmonary edema, which present as late signs and reflect an ominous prognosis unless the valve is replaced. Palpitations and awareness of arterial throbbing in the neck are sometimes troublesome.
   3. **Signs.** Characteristically, the pulse is collapsing and full. Examination of the precordium usually reveals an apex that is displaced laterally and downward. On auscultation, the most characteristic finding is an early diastolic murmur, which commences with A_2 and is usually high pitched and soft. With increasing degrees of incompetence, the murmur becomes louder and longer and radiates more widely.

E. **Tricuspid regurgitation** most commonly occurs secondary to right heart failure and is due to disturbance of the architecture of the tricuspid valve apparatus. The hemodynamic picture is similar to mitral regurgitation except that it occurs on the right side of the heart.

   The patient usually presents or has signs of right heart failure. The physical examination is characterized by a large *v* wave in the neck and systolic expansion of the liver. Auscultation reveals a systolic murmur that increases with inspiration, and is heard best along the left sternal border.

F. **Tricuspid stenosis** rarely occurs as an isolated lesion. Physical examination reveals an increased *a* wave on the jugular venous pulse. The characteristic feature is a mid-diastolic murmur at the tricuspid area with presystolic accentuation intensifying remarkably on inspiration with an opening snap.

G. **Pulmonary stenosis and regurgitation**

   1. **Pulmonary stenosis.** The etiology of this condition is usually congenital; it may be mild and nonprogressive, attention being drawn to the heart by the detection of a systolic murmur. The murmur varies widely in intensity and is usually present along the left sternal border, increasing markedly with inspiration. Wide splitting of the second heart sound on expiration is characteristic, with the pulmonary component delayed and soft.

   2. **Pulmonic regurgitation** is extremely rare as an isolated lesion. It occurs postoperatively following correction of a tetralogy of Fallot and is usually of little clinical importance. It is characterized by an early to mid-diastolic murmur occurring along the left sternal border. The murmur increases with inspiration.

III. **Clinical examples of valvular heart disease**

A. **Mitral stenosis with pulmonary hypertension**

   Description. A 38-year-old white woman gave a history of a constitutional illness with joint pains at the age of 15. The doctor told her that she had a heart murmur. She recovered uneventfully and remained totally asymptomatic until after her first pregnancy 7 years later, when she noticed that she had become short of breath when she exerted herself. She successfully delivered a second child 5 years later and again noticed some deterioration in her effort tolerance. However, she performed her housework adequately and denied symptoms of orthopnea and paroxysmal nocturnal dyspnea. She had pneumonia, requiring hospitalization and treatment with antibiotics, 6 years later. She was told that she had a heart murmur but the lesion was not characterized further. Following discharge from the hospital, she noted that her effort tolerance had diminished even further, and she began for the first time to have some difficulty doing her housework. She also complained of being tired and at times coughed up blood-stained sputum. About 4 years after that, she noticed some irregularity of her heart beat and consulted her doctor. On physical examination, there was no evidence of heart failure. Her blood pressure was 105/80. Her pulses were all present, but the rhythm was totally irregular. On examination of her precordium the cardiac apex was located in the midclavicular line, fifth intercostal space. She had a parasternal heave, indicating right ventricular hypertrophy, and the first heart sound was palpable. On auscultation in the mitral area, the first heart sound was accentuated, the second heart sound was normal. She had an opening snap, which followed closely upon the second heart sound and preceded a long diastolic rumble. The pulmonary component of her second heart sound was increased. Chest x-ray showed an enlarged left atrium and a straight left heart border. The lung fields showed some cephalization of blood flow. ECG showed P mitral, indicating left atrial enlargement and right ventricular hypertrophy. M-mode echocardiogram showed an enlarged left atrium. The mitral valve showed a reduced E to F slope; the valve was thickened and the posterior leaflet moved anteriorly. The clinical diagnosis of mitral stenosis with pulmonary hypertension was made.

B. Acute mitral regurgitation

Description. A 42-year-old white man who was previously perfectly well came to the emergency room with a prolonged episode of chest pain with shortness of breath and sweating. The pain radiated to the neck and down the left arm. On physical examination, there was no evidence of heart failure. Pulse rate was 72 and regular. Examination of the precordium was normal. ECG showed S–T segment elevation in leads V_2 through V_6 and chest x-ray showed some redistribution of blood flow to the upper lobes. The heart size was normal. The patient was admitted to the coronary care unit with the diagnosis of acute myocardial infarction and did well until the fourth hospital day, when he had a second episode of chest pain followed by significant shortness of breath. On physical examination, a new murmur was heard. The murmur was pansystolic, heard maximally at the mitral area, and radiated to the axilla and to the left sternal border. A loud third heart sound was audible. The diagnosis of acute mitral regurgitation due to infarction of one of the papillary muscles of the mitral valve apparatus was suspected and later confirmed by cardiac catheterization and surgery.

C. Symptomatic aortic stenosis

Description. A 72-year-old white woman was active and asymptomatic until 6 months before seeing her physician. She complained of chest pain only on exercise. She had no other symptoms. On physical examination, there was no evidence of heart failure. Her carotid pulse had a slow upstroke and was not easily palpated. The blood pressure was 110/70. Examination of the precordium revealed an apex beat well localized, normally situated, and thrusting in nature. On auscultation, an ejection systolic murmur was heard at the base of the heart. It radiated to the apex and was associated with a very soft A_2 component to the second heart sound. The first sound was also inaudible and an ejection click preceded the murmur. The murmur was late peaking. An ECG showed left ventricular hypertrophy. Chest x-ray showed a normal-sized heart with normal lung fields. Echocardiogram showed a heavy calcified aortic valve with evidence of left ventricular hypertrophy without dilatation of the left ventricle. Left ventricular function was normal. The diagnosis of symptomatic aortic stenosis was made.

Questions   Select the single best answer.

1. Which statement does not apply to the left ventricular pressure curve?
   a. At the time of mitral valve closure, the left atrial pressure equals the pressure in the left ventricle.

b. At the time of aortic valve closure, the aortic pressure equals the pressure in the left ventricle.
c. In a normal heart during systole there is always a measurable difference in pressure between the left ventricle and aorta.
d. In the normal heart during diastole the left atrial pressure never measurably exceeds the pressure in the left ventricle.
e. All of the above.

2. Which of the following is false concerning the jugular venous pulsation?
a. The *a* wave is produced by atrial contraction.
b. The X descent occurs between the *a* and *v* waves and is associated with atrial relaxation.
c. In pulmonary hypertension, the *a* wave is accentuated.
d. In pulmonary stenosis, the *a* wave is accentuated.
e. In atrial fibrillation, the *a* wave is always present and well seen but diminished in size.

9   Intracardiac Shunts

I. Normal physiology

A. **Fetal circulation.** To understand the pathophysiology of intracardiac shunts, one must have basic knowledge of the fetal circulation (Fig. 9-1). Much of the available data on this subject has been taken from the various works of Heymann and Rudolph and their co-workers in their experience with fetal lambs.

In the fetus, systemic (nonpulmonary) blood returns to the heart through the vena cavae and coronary sinus into the right atrium. Venous drainage from the upper part of the body and the heart returns to the right atrium through the superior vena cava and the coronary sinus and is then directed into the right ventricle through the tricuspid valve. Venous drainage from the lower part of the body (including the placenta) returns to the right atrium through the inferior vena cava. This inferior vena cava drainage is made up of venous blood from the lower body of the fetus and from the umbilical veins (the umbilical venous blood either courses directly into the inferior vena cava through the ductus venosus or is directed through the hepatic circulation into the inferior vena cava). About half of the inferior vena caval blood is directed through the right atrium, across the foramen ovale, and into the left atrium; the other half joins the superior vena cava and coronary sinus blood in crossing the tricuspid valve into the right ventricle. Almost 90 percent of the blood ejected by the right ventricle (the right ventricle ejects about twice as much blood as the left in the fetus) is shunted through the ductus arteriosus into the thoracic aorta; only the remaining fraction is carried through the pulmonary vascular bed and into the left atrium through the pulmonary veins. The blood which is ejected from the left ventricle is comprised mostly (approximately 80%) of the inferior vena caval blood that is shunted through the right atrium across the patent foramen ovale and into the left atrium and, to a lesser extent (approximately 20%), of the pulmonary venous blood that escaped being shunted from the pulmonary artery into the thoracic aorta through the ductus arteriosus. Of the blood in the descending thoracic aorta, a large proportion is directed into the placenta because of low resistance in that circulation.

In the fetus, oxygenation of blood takes place in the placenta. The umbilical vein has a PO_2 of approximately 30 torr and thus, the inferior vena caval blood, which includes umbilical venous blood, has a higher PO_2 than does the superior vena caval blood. The blood in the ascending aorta has a PO_2 of approximately 25 torr because the inferior vena cava provides most of the blood to the left atrium and left ventricle. On the other hand, blood entering and leaving the right ventricle, being an admixture of superior and inferior caval blood, has a lower PO_2 of approximately 18 torr. The blood in the descending aorta, distal to the ductus arteriosus, is derived primarily from the pulmonary artery with only a small contribution from the aortic arch; thus, the PO_2 is lower (approximately 22 torr) than in the ascending aorta.

There is equalization of pressures in the aorta and pulmonary artery, and the left ventricular and right ventricular systolic pressures

Fetal circulation. (Reproduced with slight modification from S. Kaplan, Congenital heart disease. In V. C. Vaughan and R. J. McKay (Eds.), Nelson Textbook of Pediatrics (10th ed.). Philadelphia: Saunders, 1975, p. 1019. By permission of the author and W. B. Saunders Co.)

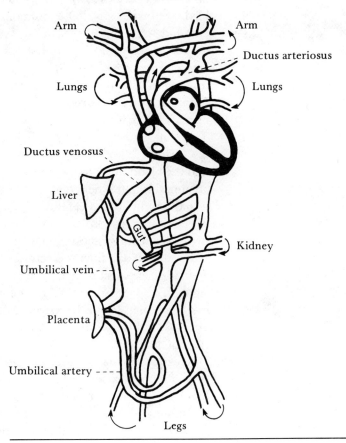

are essentially equal. The equalization is due to the patency of the ductus arteriosus between the right and left heart circulations.

B. Postnatal circulatory events. A number of important changes in circulation occur at birth. In general, the two most significant are ventilation of the lungs and elimination of the placental circulation. At birth, the lungs are filled with air, resulting in a marked fall in pulmonary vascular resistance. At approximately the same time, clamping of the umbilical vessels eliminates the low resistance placental circulation from the systemic circulation, thus markedly increasing systemic vascular resistance (as opposed to pulmonary vascular resistance, which decreases with pulmonary ventilation).

1. Pulmonary circulatory events. The pulmonary vascular (or arteriolar) resistance in the fetus is high. This is due primarily to pulmonary vascular smooth muscle vasoconstriction in response to the marked hypoxemia in the pulmonary arteries (~18 torr), though, in addition, lack of lung expansion by air contributes to this high resistance. At birth, with ventilation of the lungs, there is significant increase in pulmonary arterial PO_2 and a marked vasodilatation associated with a decrease in pulmonary vascular resistance (augmented by expansion of the lungs with air) and a marked increase in flow of blood through the lungs. Thus, within several minutes of birth, there is as much as a tenfold increase in pulmonary blood flow owing to this reversal of pulmonary vasoconstriction. In view of the above discussion and in the context of understanding shunts, recollection of the hemodynamic application of Ohm's law is appropriate: Resistance = Pressure/Blood flow. While vasodilatation of pulmonary smooth muscle occurs at birth with rise in PO_2, pulmonary arterial pressure remains elevated for 6 to 10 weeks post delivery and the large amount of muscle regresses to its adult status, at which time the pulmonary arterial pressures attain their normal adult levels (systolic about 24 mm Hg or less, diastolic about 12 mm Hg or less).

2. **Foramen ovale closure.** The cleft-like interatrial opening, the foramen ovale, is located in the lower part of the interatrial septum. This cleft is covered by a flap-like structure that protrudes into the left atrium. With the slightly higher pressures in the right atrium and the blood flow from the inferior vena cava directed into the left atrium, this flap is held open in the fetus. At birth, the flow of blood into the right atrium is reduced due to elimination of the umbilical circulation. This also reduces the right atrial pressure. Left atrial pressure increases at essentially the same time due to the increase in pulmonary blood flow and return of blood to the left atrium associated with expansion of the lungs. These two events, decrease in right atrial pressure and increase in left atrial pressure, combine to cause the flap-like valve covering the foramen ovale on the left atrial side of the septum to be pressed against the septum, closing the opening.

3. **Ductus arteriosus closure.** As noted above, the smooth muscle in the pulmonary arterioles relaxes with increased PO_2; on the other hand, smooth muscle in the ductus arteriosus, which is considerable in amount, constricts. This vasoconstriction is important because the prenatal size of the ductus arteriosus is similar to that of the aorta. In a mature infant, the ductus arteriosus is effectively closed by vasoconstriction within 24 hours of birth. Thrombosis and fibrosis of the wall continue the closure process, occurring over the next 2 weeks or so.

II. **Determination of intracardiac shunting**

A. **Principles.** Intracardiac shunting is defined by the direction and the magnitude of the shunt. There are a number of factors that influence these, but the following three predominate and are interrelated: (1) the size of the communication between the chambers or the vessels involved, (2) the pressure differences between the chambers or the vessels connected by the shunt, and (3) the outflow resistances of the chambers on either side of the shunt (Fig. 9-2). If the communication is small, the direction and magnitude of the shunt will be determined largely by the difference in pressures in the communicating chambers or vessels, with outflow resistances having little effect on the magnitude of the shunt except by influencing the amount of pressure in the chambers or vessels. For example, a small communication with a higher pressure in the chamber on the left side of the communication than on the right and a lower resistance on the right than on the left (as in Fig. 9-2A) will produce a left-to-right shunt.

If the communication is large, there may be a resulting equalization of pressures and the shunt will depend on the outflow resistances. For example, large communication with equal pressures in both chambers and a lower outflow resistance on the right than the left will produce a left-to-right shunt (seen in Fig. 9-2B). On the other hand, if

Figure 9-2

Diagram of interrelations among size of communication, pressure (P) differences between chambers or vessels, and outflow resistances (R) of the chambers. A shows left-to-right shunt: small communication, higher pressure and resistance on left (L) than right (R). B shows left-to-right shunt: large communication, equal pressures, lower resistance on R than L. C shows bi-directional or nonshunting: large communication, equal pressures, equal outflow resistance. (From A. M. Rudolph and M. A. Heymann, Neonatal circulation and pathophysiology of shunts. In H. J. Levine [Ed.], Clinical Cardiovascular Physiology. New York: Grune & Stratton, 1978, p. 603. By permission of the author and Grune & Stratton, Inc.)

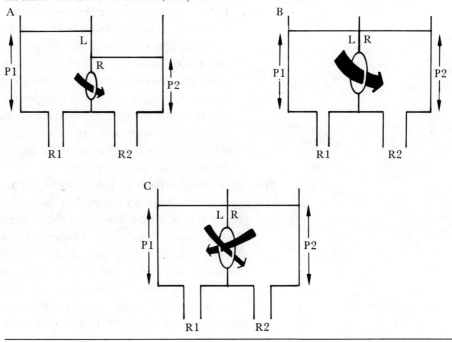

the communication is large, with equalization of pressures and equal outflow resistances, either there will be no shunt or there will be bi-directional shunting (see Fig. 9-2C).

B. Fetal circulation. Normally, before birth there is an extremely low resistance in the placental circulation (in the systemic circuit) and high resistance in the nonexpanded pulmonary vascular bed. Additionally, the large ductus arteriosus produces equalization of pressures in the pulmonary artery and the aorta. These factors combine to produce a large shunt from the pulmonary artery into the aorta.

C. Postnatal circulation. After birth, with the drop in pulmonary resistance and the increase in the systemic resistance, there is reversal of the shunt, with blood flowing from the aorta into the pulmonary artery. This continues in a decreasing manner until ductal closure by vasoconstriction.

D. Congenital heart disease. Several types of congenital cardiac defects involve abnormal communications between the pulmonary and systemic circulations and associated shunting of blood between the two circulations. A shunting of blood from the pulmonary to the systemic circulation is usually referred to as a right-to-left shunt and a shunting of blood from the systemic to the pulmonary circulation is called a left-to-right shunt. In a right-to-left shunt, de-oxygenated blood is shunted into the systemic circulation from the pulmonary circulation. In a left-to-right shunt, oxygenated blood is shunted into the pulmonary circulation from the systemic circulation. In the normal child or adult, the left ventricular systolic pressure (aortic systolic pressure) is about five times the right ventricular systolic pressure (pulmonary artery systolic pressure). Also, the left ventricular outflow resistance (systemic vascular resistance) is about 10 times the right ventricular outflow resistance (pulmonary vascular resistance). Thus, in a small communication between the left and right circulation, the higher pressures on the left produce shunting from left to right. With large communications between the left and right circulations, while there is frequently equalization of pressures, the much lower resistances in the pulmonary circulation favor shunting from left to right.

After birth, almost all cardiac shunts occur initially in a left-to-right direction. These include defects such as atrial septal defects, ventricular septal defects, patent ductus arteriosus, aorticopulmonary windows, truncus arteriosus, single atria, single ventricles, shunts from left ventricle to right atrium, shunts from sinus of Valsalva in aorta to the right atrium, and (as an example of noncongenital cause of intracardiac shunting) rupture of the interventricular septum with an acute myocardial infarction.

III. **Myocardial effects of left-to-right shunts.** In left-to-right shunts at the aorticopulmonary artery level or the ventricular level, a portion of the left ventricular output is lost from the systemic circulation and directed into the pulmonary circulation. The left ventricle attempts to compensate for this by increasing its output. This is facilitated by increases in circulating catecholamine levels and adrenergic neural stimulation of the myocardium, both of which produce increased left ventricular output (and work). If the sympathetic-adrenal system is not functioning properly, the lack of myocardial stimulation can contribute to a failing myocardium. The myocardium also responds to the volume load that occurs with shunting by dilatation and hypertrophy. The increase in work load on the ventricle in the above situation also increases the oxygen demands of the myocardium. However, oxygen supply to the myocardium can be compromised by (1) a lowering of aortic diastolic pressures (in aorticopulmonary communication due to a siphoning-off of blood by the pulmonary circulation) since a majority of coronary blood flow occurs during diastole, (2) an increase in heart rate that encroaches significantly on diastole, and (3) by an increase in diastolic ventricular pressure which could impede coronary filling and flow.

IV. **Pulmonary circulatory effects of left-to-right shunts.** Regardless of the type of left-to-right shunt, high pulmonary blood flows or pressures produced by the shunting can create a progressive increase in pulmonary vascular resistance by thickening the pulmonary arteriolar smooth muscle and intima with eventual obliteration of the vessels by thrombosis and fibrosis. At some point, this process becomes irreversible even with correction of the shunt. With increase in pulmonary vascular resistance to greater than systemic levels, there will be a reversal in the shunt to right to left. (This creates the so-called Eisenmenger physiology.)

V. **Clinical examples of intracardiac shunting**

    A. **Ventricular septal defect with left-to-right shunting**

        1. **Description.** A 6-year-old boy was evaluated for a heart murmur. The child had experienced normal growth and development and could easily keep up with his peers, participating actively in soccer and gymnastics. On examination there was a prominent left parasternal lift, a slightly loud pulmonic component of the second heart sound, a palpable systolic thrill associated with a grade 5/6 holosys-

Figure 9-3

Oxygen saturations and pressures in a patient with a ventricular septal defect and left-to-right shunting. Ao = aorta; IVC = inferior vena cava; LA = left atrium; LV = left ventricle; PA = pulmonary artery; RA = right atrium; RV = right ventricle; SVC = superior vena cava.

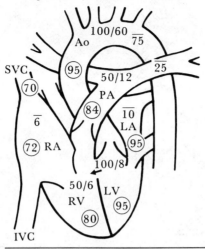

tolic murmur at the lower left sternal border with wide radiation of the murmur. No cyanosis or clubbing was detected, and the boy appeared normal otherwise. Cardiac catheterization was subsequently performed (Fig. 9-3).

2. **Results of cardiac catheterization**
   a. Stepup of O_2 saturation from right atrium (RA) to right ventricle (RV) indicated a left-to-right shunt at the ventricular level.
   b. Shunt quantification revealed 2.2 times more pulmonary blood flow than systemic blood flow.
   c. Resistance quantification revealed essentially normal pulmonary vascular resistance and systemic vascular resistance.

3. **Discussion**
   a. This was a moderate-sized ventricular septal defect (VSD) and left-to-right shunt. The normal left ventricle (LV) diastolic pressure (12 mm Hg) implied no LV failure. The normal pulmonary vascular resistance implied no irreversible changes in the pulmonary arterioles.
   b. In this situation there is typically no impairment in physical abilities.
   c. The loud murmur was secondary to turbulent flow across the VSD.
   d. The loud pulmonic component of S_2 was related to a mild elevation in pulmonary artery pressure due to increased flow.
   e. The parasternal lift was related to increased right ventricular size from the increased volume.

B. **Patent ductus arteriosus with right-to-left shunting**
   1. **Description.** A 21-year-old woman was evaluated for the recent onset of cyanosis of the lower extremities. She had been told she had a loud murmur as a child. In the past 10 years she had had some difficulty in physically keeping up with her peers. On exam, the patient had lower extremity cyanosis and clubbing, and a very loud and palpable pulmonic component of S_2, a large apical impulse, and no audible murmur. A cardiac catheterization was performed (Fig. 9-4).

Figure 9-4

Oxygen saturations and pressures in a patient with a patent ductus arteriosus and right-to-left shunting. Ao = aorta; IVC = inferior vena cava; LA = left atrium; LV = left ventricle; PA = pulmonary artery; RA = right atrium; RV = right ventricle; SVC = superior vena cava.

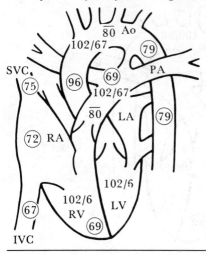

2. **Results of cardiac catheterization**
   a. A drop in O_2 saturation was found at the aortic arch suggesting patent ductus arteriosus (PDA) with right-to-left shunting.
   b. Shunt quantification revealed three times as much systemic blood flow as pulmonary blood flow.
   c. Resistance calculations revealed a markedly elevated pulmonary vascular resistance and a mildly reduced systemic vascular resistance with pulmonary vascular resistance being three times the systemic vascular resistance.

3. **Discussion**
   a. This was a large PDA with severe and irreversible pulmonary hypertension related to irreversible elevation in pulmonary vascular resistance secondary to obliteration of the pulmonary arterioles.
   b. The lower extremity cyanosis was related to nonoxygenated blood being delivered to the systemic circulation through the patent ductus arteriosus at a point distal to the departure of the arteries to the upper extremities and head.
   c. There was no murmur audible because there was no pressure gradient across the PDA (the flow from right to left occurs in this situation because of lower systemic vascular resistance).

Questions

Select the single best answer.

1. Which of the following is not a *direct* determinant of the direction and magnitude of an intracardiac shunt?
   a. Difference in pressure between the communicating chambers.
   b. The difference in oxygenation of the right- and left-sided blood.
   c. The size of the communications.
   d. The outflow resistance from the communication chambers.
2. After birth, most intracardiac shunts are initially which of these?
   a. Right-to-left shunts.
   b. Left-to-right shunts.
   c. Bi-directional shunts.
   d. None of the above.

10 Congestive Heart Failure

I. **General description.** Congestive cardiac failure is the pathophysiologic state in which an abnormality of cardiac function is responsible for the failure of the heart to pump blood at a rate adequate for the metabolic demand of peripheral tissues (organs). Clinical presentations result from the combination of depressed ventricular performance and inadequate peripheral organ function. It is usually, but not always, associated with exhaustion of the cardiac compensatory mechanism. The degree of congestive cardiac failure is dependent on the rate, duration, and magnitude of the development of the pathophysiologic state. In acute heart failure attributable either to sudden increase in afterload to the heart (for example, acute hypertensive crisis) or to a sudden volume overload (for example, mitral regurgitation secondary to papillary muscle rupture), the heart does not have adequate time to develop compensatory mechanisms. Therefore, heart failure is abrupt and more severe. Regardless of whether it is acute or chronic, heart failure leads to further heart failure—it is a vicious cycle.

II. **Compensatory mechanisms**

A. **Three principal compensatory mechanisms** are needed to maintain adequate cardiac output in the early stages of heart failure:

1. **The Frank-Starling law of the heart (preload reserve)** is achieved by increasing ventricular end-diastolic volume (increasing preload), which leads to cardiac dilatation with resultant increase in cardiac output.

2. **Increased catecholamine release** from adrenergic nerves and adrenal medulla results in increased heart rate and myocardial contractility.

3. **Cardiac hypertrophy** leads to augmentation of the heart pump function due to an increased myocardial muscle mass. However, myocardial contractility per unit muscle mass may be normal or depressed.

All these compensatory mechanisms are of limited and finite potential and at the expense of increasing myocardial metabolic demand-oxygen consumption. Heart rate, myocardial contractility, and myocardial tension developments are the major determinants of myocardial oxygen consumption. Myocardial tension (T) is directly related to the ventricular pressure (P) and the radius (R) of the ventricular cavity ($T = PR$), thus myocardial dilatation leads to increased R and results in increased myocardial oxygen consumption. In early stages of heart failure, cardiac compensatory mechanisms may be adequate to maintain ventricular performance but ultimately ventricular function deteriorates and clinical heart failure becomes manifest. In severe heart failure, there is a marked increase in circulating catecholamines and depletion of myocardial catecholamines, resulting in decreased myocardial contractility and increased afterload. Cardiac dilatation may increase until the heart exhausts the preload reserve and functions on the plateau limb of the Frank-Starling curve; thus, stroke volume does not increase with further increases of end-diastolic volume (Fig. 10-1).

B. **Systemic adaptation to heart failure**

1. Sodium (Na^+) and water retention occur secondary to decreased

65

Figure 10-1

Frank-Starling function curves in normal and in mild and severe heart failure. SV = stroke volume; CO = cardiac output; LVEDP = left ventricular end-diastolic pressure; LVEDV = left ventricular end-diastolic volume.

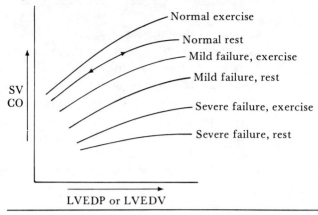

renal blood flow and glomerular filtration rate and other mechanisms that enhance reabsorption of sodium in both proximal and distal nephron segments. The resulting expansion of the blood volume further enhances ventricular filling pressures and end-diastolic volumes (preload).

2. Low cardiac output and reduced tissue perfusion lead to an increase in red blood cell 2,3-diphosphoglycerate (2,3-DPG) level, which facilitates the release of oxygen from the red blood cells. Thus, oxygen supply to the tissues is augmented at any given partial pressure of oxygen.

III. **Classification of heart failure (according to pathogenesis)**
   A. **Increased tissue metabolic demand (high output failure).** This type of heart failure occurs in states such as hyperthyroidism, beriberi, anemia, arteriovenous shunt, and Paget's disease. In all these conditions, the heart is called upon to pump an abnormally large volume of blood in order to deliver enough oxygen to meet the increased metabolic demands of the tissues. In addition, myocardial metabolism in beriberi and thyrotoxicosis may be impaired. In this form of heart failure the resting cardiac output may be in the upper limits of normal value or increased similarly to the mild exercise state. Myocardial contractility may be normal or increased.

   B. **Mechanical constraint of ventricular filling: External constraint (constructive pericarditis, cardiac tamponade); internal constraint (mitral valve stenosis).** In constrictive pericarditis or cardiac tamponade, diastolic ventricular filling is impaired by the external pressure and physical limitations exerted on the heart such that the heart (right and left ventricles) cannot dilate adequately, with resultant decrease in end-diastolic volume and preload. Paradoxically, end-diastolic pressure, which is transmitted from pericardial pressure, increases markedly.

   In mitral valvular stenosis, ventricular diastolic filling is decreased because of the obstruction across the mitral valve. Myocardial contractility and left ventricular systolic functions are usually not impaired. The left ventricular stroke volume decreases because of decreased left ventricular end-diastolic volume. The heart responds to these conditions by increasing heart rate in order to maintain cardiac output. However, increased heart rate has a deleterious effect by further shortening the left ventricular filling period and thus diminishing diastolic ventricular filling and ventricular diastolic volume, with resultant decrease in cardiac output.

C. **Mechanical obstruction of ventricular systolic ejection (increased afterload, pressure load).** Hypertension, aortic valvular stenosis, and coarctation of aorta (constriction of aorta) are the examples of increased left ventricular afterload. The resting cardiac output may be normal; however, the heart cannot increase cardiac output adequately during exercise. The primary cardiac compensatory mechanism in these conditions is cardiac hypertrophy. Because of the thickened, hypertrophic ventricle, ventricular diastolic compliance decreases—i.e., the ratio of the rate of ventricular diastolic volume (v) change per unit ventricular pressure (P) change (v/P) decreases. Decreased ventricular compliance is characterized by ventricular stiffness. The left ventricular end-diastolic pressure is usually increased, resulting in increased left atrial and pulmonary capillary wedge and pulmonary arterial pressures.

D. **Increased ventricular volume (volume load).** In mitral valvular regurgitation or aortic valvular regurgitation, ventricular diastolic volume is increased in order to accommodate the regurgitant blood volume in addition to the normal blood return from the left atrium. Subsequently, the heart dilates. Because myocardial oxygen consumption from diastolic tension is less than systolic ventricular tension, the heart tolerates volume load conditions better than pressure load.

E. **Myocardial disease.** Characteristically, myocardial contractility is depressed in myocardial disease. Decreased myocardial contractility could happen at a regional level or involve the whole heart. This condition occurs in ischemic heart disease (that is, inadequate coronary blood supply to the heart secondary to coronary occlusive disease); in cardiac anoxia, inadequate oxygen supply to the heart secondary to hypoxemia (the coronary arterial system is normal); or in infiltrative and inflammatory myocardial disease. The heart compensates by increasing heart rate and by dilatation. Because myocardial contractility is impaired, myocardial shortening is decreased, which leads to increased end-systolic volume. Stroke volume and cardiac output at rest may be normal, but during exercise, cardiac performance is invariably depressed.

IV. **Physiologic consequences of heart failure**

A. **Four characteristic features.** Regardless of the mechanism, cardiac failure is often associated with four characteristic features:

1. **A depressed ventricular function curve (Frank-Starling curve).** In the normal heart, the ventricle functions on the ascending limb of the ventricular function curve (see Fig. 10-1). Stroke volume and cardiac output vary physiologically with the end-diastolic ventricular volume (preload). During exercise, cardiac output may increase five- to tenfold over the resting level. This is brought about by increased myocardial contractility and heart rate and decreased peripheral resistance. The ventricular function curve shifts upward and to the left. In severe heart failure, the heart usually exhausts the compensatory mechanisms. The ventricular function curve is flat and markedly depressed and shifted downward and to the right of the normal curve. The heart usually functions at the plateau part of the ventricular function curve (maximum preload reserve). Thus, for a given heart at the same level of end-diastolic volume,

stroke volume is markedly depressed in severe heart failure. During exercise the heart responds poorly, with minimal increase in stroke volume, or the heart may fail further by moving to the descending limb of the ventricular function curve.

2. **Increased arteriovenous oxygen content difference.** Normally, total body oxygen consumption is rather constant. The amount of oxygen delivered to the tissues in the arterial blood is the product of blood flow (CO) and arterial oxygen concentration, which is expressed as ml of O_2 per liter of whole blood (CaO_2 = ml O_2 per liter). The amount of oxygen returning to the heart and lungs in the central venous blood is the product of CO and oxygen content of mixed venous blood (CvO_2 = ml O_2 per liter). The difference between these two quantities is the amount of oxygen consumed by the tissues (total body oxygen consumption per unit time, $\dot{V}O_2$). These relationships can be expressed mathematically.

$$\dot{V}O_2 = CO(CaO_2 - CvO_2)$$
$$\dot{V}O_2/CO = CaO_2 - CvO_2$$
$$CO = \dot{V}O_2/CaO_2 - CvO_2$$
$$CO \sim 1/CaO_2 - CvO_2$$

CO = cardiac output (L/min)
CaO_2 = arterial O_2 content (ml/L)
CvO_2 = mixed venous O_2 content (ml/L)
$\dot{V}O_2$ = total body oxygen consumption (ml/min)

$CO \sim 1/CaO_2 - CvO_2$ implies that the cardiac output varies inversely with the arteriovenous oxygen difference (normally 30–50 ml/L). For a given metabolic state, widening of the arteriovenous O_2 difference signifies decreased cardiac output and narrow arteriovenous O_2 difference represents high cardiac output state. However, this relationship applies only if $\dot{V}O_2$ is constant and there is no blood shunting at the peripheral tissue level.

3. **Elevation of left atrial pressure (LA)** with resultant pulmonary congestion.

4. **Elevation of right atrial pressure (RA)** or central venous pressure (CVP) with resultant systemic congestion.

B. **Closed circuit system.** The cardiovascular system is a closed circuit system (Fig. 10-2). At any point in this closed circuit system, if there is an increase in pressure it will be reflected forward or backward within the circuit as long as there is no mechanical obstruction to the pressure transmission, e.g., vascular obstruction or valvular stenosis within the circuit. For example, increased left ventricular pressure is transmitted to left atrium and pulmonary veins, with resultant increase in left atrial and pulmonary venous and pulmonary capillary pressures. Eventually there is an increase in pulmonary arterial pressure, which leads to elevation of right ventricular and right atrial pressures.

It is important to remember that the pressure measured in any cardiac chamber is dependent on the pressure volume characteristic of that particular chamber. For example, increased left ventricular end-diastolic pressure, which is transmitted to the left atrium, leads to a lesser degree of increase in left atrial pressure when the left atrium is enlarged than when this chamber is small. This is because a large atrium is more compliant than a small one. In clinical situations, a marked increase in left atrial pressure with resultant pulmonary

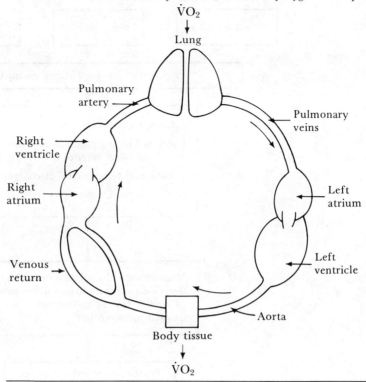

edema is observed following rupture of a papillary muscle leading to acute mitral regurgitation. In this situation, the left atrium is invariably of normal size. In contrast, in chronic mitral regurgitation, the left atrium is greatly enlarged, the increase in left atrial pressure is less pronounced, and pulmonary congestion and edema occur late in the disease process.

The pathophysiologic consequences of heart failure discussed above may occur simultaneously in any sequence, or in some instances, only one or two of them may be evident. All these changes usually are present in the most severe form of heart failure. Figure 10-3 summarizes the sequence of the pathophysiologic state of heart failure.

V. **Hemodynamic alterations and correlation with physical signs and symptoms in heart failure.** Various signs and symptoms of heart failure can be explained easily on the basis of hemodynamic alterations that occur following myocardial failure. The raised left ventricular pressure is transmitted to the left atrium, pulmonary veins, and capillaries and results in pulmonary congestion and pulmonary edema. The latter becomes clinically manifest as dyspnea (shortness of breath) during exertion and at rest, orthopnea, and bilateral pulmonary crepitations.

The fourth heart sound is often audible and is due to the forceful contraction of the atrium in order to boost the ventricular filling. However, this is not pathognomic of heart failure and may be audible in patients without heart failure, especially in the elderly with underlying coronary artery disease and stiff left ventricle. The third heart sound is more pathognomic of heart failure and is usually audible in moderate and severe heart failure.

Increased right atrial pressure is eventually transmitted to the systemic veins and leads to systemic congestion. Engorgement of neck veins; congestion of liver, which is often tender due to stretching of the liver

Figure 10-3   *The pathophysiology of heart failure.*

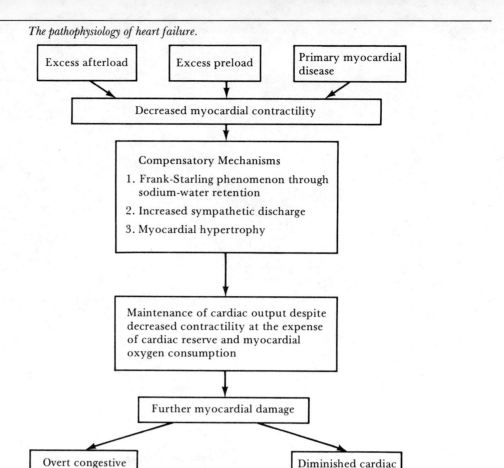

capsule; accumulation of fluid in tissues (pitting ankle and leg edema); and increase in body weight are manifested clinically.

Diminished cardiac output results in diminished renal blood flow, glomerular filtration rate, and urine flow; increased blood urea nitrogen and creatinine levels; and increased arteriovenous oxygen difference.

It is well recognized that right heart failure is usually secondary to left heart failure, in which instance signs and symptoms of right heart failure develop quite late in the disease process. However, patients with severe pulmonary parenchymal or occlusive pulmonary vascular disease may present primarily with signs and symptoms of right heart failure. In these patients symptoms of low cardiac output are secondary to low right ventricular output with resultant decrease in pulmonary blood flow and left ventricular output.

The relation among various pathologic states accounting for heart failure and their physiologic consequences are summarized in Table 10-1.

VI. **Clinical examples**
  A. **High output failure**
    1. **Description.** A 65-year-old woman came to the hospital with a 6-month history of palpitations, heat intolerance, and breathlessness on exertion. During the last 2 months she had noticed ankle swelling and had noted episodic breathlessness at night. Examination revealed sinus tachycardia (heart rate 130 beats/min), jugular venous distension, bounding high volume pulses, blood pressure of 160/80 mm Hg, cardiomegaly, prominent eyes, and an enlarged thyroid gland.

Pathologic State	HR	SV	CO	LVEDV	LVEDP	LAP	RAP	Cardiac Contractility	Heart Size
Increased tissue demand (high output failure)	↑	↑↑	↑↑	↑↑	↑ or NL	↑ or NL	↑	↑ or →	↑ all chambers
Diminished LV filling									
Mitral stenosis	↑	↓	↓	NL or ↓	↓	↑	↑ or NL	NL	NL or ↑ (LA ↑)
Pericardial constriction	↑↑	↓↓	↓	NL or ↓	↑↑↑	↑↑↑	↑↑↑	↓ or NL	↑ or NL
Increased volume load (aortic and mitral regurgitation)	↑	NL or ↑	NL or ↓	↑↑↑	↑	↑	↑	↓	↑↑
Increased pressure load (aortic stenosis)	↑	NL or ↓	NL or ↓	NL or ↑	↑↑	↑↑	↑	NL, ↑ or ↓	NL or ↑
Myocardial disease	↑	↓	↓	↑↑	↑↑	↑↑	↑	↓↓	↑
Complete heart block	↓↓	↑↑	↓	↑	↑	↑	↑	NL	↑

HR = heart rate; SV = stroke volume; CO = cardiac output; LVEDV = left ventricular end-diastolic volume; LVEDP = left ventricular end-diastolic pressure; LAP = left atrial pressure; RAP = right atrial pressure; NL = normal; LV = left ventricular; ↑ = increased; ↓ = decreased; → = no change.

2. **Discussion.** This patient has thyrotoxicosis (overactive thyroid gland). Thyrotoxicosis leads initially to a hyperdynamic state and in some patients, as in this case, subsequently to high-output cardiac failure. Tachycardia, high bounding pulse, and an elevated blood pressure indicate a hyperdynamic state. Jugular venous distension, cardiomegaly, and ankle edema are due to heart failure.

B. **Low output failure**

1. **Description.** A 60-year-old man had sustained an extensive acute myocardial infarction 4 years before his recent admission. Since that time he had become progressively breathless on exertion and during the past 6 months had developed swelling of his abdomen and feet despite vigorous diuretic and digoxin therapy. Examination revealed an emaciated man who was breathless even at rest. Cardiac rhythm was regular and blood pressure was 90/60 mm Hg. Jugular venous pressure was elevated, and there was ankle edema, hepatomegaly, and ascites. Heart sounds were faint but a loud fourth sound was audible. Chest x-ray revealed marked cardiac enlargement, bilateral pleural effusions, and pulmonary venous congestion. Cardiac catheterization revealed severe inoperable three-vessel coronary artery disease, poor left ventricular function with marked elevation of left ventricular end-diastolic pressure, and low cardiac output.

2. **Discussion.** In this patient myocardial infarction was responsible for extensive damage to the left ventricular muscle, which resulted in chronic elevation of left ventricular end-diastolic pressure. This accounted initially for breathlessness on exertion and, with time, exudation of fluid into the alveoli (pulmonary edema). Subsequently, the right heart also started to fail, manifested by venous congestion (elevated jugular venous pressure, ascites, ankle edema, and liver enlargement).

    The final outcome in this kind of patient remains grave. Afterload-reducing agents such as hydralazine often lead to some improvement in left ventricular performance by reducing the impedance to left ventricular outflow. The nitrate group of drugs are also useful; their venodilator effects reduce venous return to the heart, which leads in turn to a reduction in ventricular volumes and end-diastolic pressures.

Select the single best answer.

1. Which statement does not apply to congestive heart failure secondary to mitral valvular stenosis?
   a. The left atrial pressure is elevated.
   b. The pulmonary arterial pressure is elevated.
   c. The heart failure is due to left ventricular failure.
   d. All of the above.

2. When pulmonary edema results from chronic aortic valvular regurgitation, all but one of the following statements should apply. Select the *one* incorrect statement.
   a. The left atrial pressure, pulmonary arterial pressure, and right atrial pressure are elevated.
   b. Enlarged left ventricular and left atrial volume is present.
   c. Ventricular hypertrophy is the primary compensatory mechanism of this type of heart failure.
   d. Decreased aortic blood pressure (left ventricular afterload) will increase forward aortic blood flow, decrease regurgitation of blood to the left ventricle, and decrease left ventricular volume.

11   Mechanisms of Shock

I. **Introduction.** In normal circulatory physiology the circulation is designed to supply oxygen and nutrients to the tissues of the body for maintenance of cellular metabolism. Cardiac output, expressed as the systemic or pulmonary capillary blood flow, increases or decreases in response to the body's oxygen demands. The equation that expresses this relationship is: oxygen consumption (ml/min) = cardiac output (L/min) × difference in arterial minus venous O_2 content (ml/L). The principal components of the circulatory system—the cardiac pump, the arterial and venous conduits, and the capillary exchange vessels—function together in order to maintain constancy in the body's internal environment and to support cellular integrity. The cardiac pump, through conversion of metabolic to mechanical energy, produces the necessary hydrostatic pressure in the arterial system to account for blood flow. The process involves a change from hydrostatic to kinetic energy plus heat due to blood viscosity and peripheral vascular resistance. Systemic and pulmonary blood flow are equal, since the two circulations are in a series configuration. However, systemic arterial pressure is much (about six times) higher than pulmonary arterial pressure, which reflects the differences in overall vascular resistance between the two circulations. Cardiovascular regulation is brought about through a complex and interactive control system with many stabilizing or negative feedback loops—including the responses to cellular metabolites, local and baroreceptor reflexes, sympathetic and vagal reflexes, and other neuroendocrine controls and also including cardiorespiratory and cardiorenal responses to protect the organism and keep its internal environment constant.

II. **Pathophysiology of shock**

A. **The clinical syndrome of shock** is characterized by inadequate tissue perfusion and the signs and symptoms resulting from the poor perfusion of vital organs. The patient is usually anxious and may be pale and cold due to reflex vasoconstriction and poor perfusion to the skin and mucous membranes; the skin is often clammy due to stimulation of sweat glands; there is tachypnea and tachycardia; oliguria occurs because of reduced renal perfusion; and in severe shock with hypotension the patient will have altered sensorium secondary to inadequate cerebral perfusion.

B. **Classification.** Circulatory shock states have been classified into four main categories for purposes of understanding the pathophysiology: (1) hypovolemic shock, which may result from hemorrhage, trauma, burns, or severe diarrhea; (2) cardiogenic shock, secondary to myocardial infarction, severe heart failure, or cardiac arrhythmia; (3) distributive shock, seen with severe sepsis, barbiturate intoxication, ganglionic blockade, and transection of the spinal cord; and (4) obstructive shock, commonly due to cardiac tamponade, but also seen with dissecting aneurysm, embolism, a ball-valve thrombus, vena caval obstruction, and other causes.

1. **Hypovolemic shock** such as that due to hemorrhage is caused by a loss of central blood volume resulting in a decreased central venous pressure, cardiac output, the low-flow state, and hypotension. Compensatory responses include increased heart rate, vasoconstriction, and increased myocardial contractility. Redistribution of blood

volume occurs, with greater fractions of the cardiac output being delivered to the liver, heart, and brain and lesser fractions in differing proportions to the kidney, splanchnic, and cutaneous tissues. Greater tissue extraction of oxygen per unit of blood occurs as a compensatory mechanism. Metabolic acidosis (lactic) results from the low-tissue-flow state but the initial compensatory response is hyperpnea and tachypnea, resulting in a respiratory alkalosis. Trauma produces a generalized increase in autonomic and neuroendocrine activity. This stimulation of cardiac, respiratory, and hypothalamic centers increases heart rate, myocardial contractility, and ventilation. It also causes vasoconstriction, reduction of urinary excretion, and preservation of central venous volume. If the blood volume deficit is minimal or absent, stroke volume and cardiac output will be increased. Important therapeutic measures include replacement of circulating volume and correction of metabolic and electrolyte imbalances.

2. **Cardiogenic shock** is caused by a marked decrease of cardiac function, otherwise known as pump failure. If, in the course of an acute myocardial infarction, there is sufficient myocardium destroyed or malfunctioning, cardiac output will decline despite the compensatory elevation of left ventricular end-diastolic pressure. The resultant fall of arterial pressure will activate arterial baroreceptors that cause a reflex tachycardia, positive inotropic stimulation of the myocardium, and increased systemic vascular resistance, which will minimize the fall of arterial pressure. In patients with a profound decrease in cardiac function and cardiac output, the shock syndrome will develop in the face of intense vasoconstriction. However, it has been shown that many patients who have an acute myocardial infarction and a moderately decreased cardiac output will have a normal systemic vascular resistance despite a fall of arterial blood pressure. Experiments have shown that systolic expansion of the freshly infarcted region can activate myocardial stretch receptors whose afferent inputs to central coordinating centers cause inhibition of sympathetic outflow. Thus, during severe myocardial ischemia and infarction, the vasomotor coordinating centers in the brain may receive conflicting signals. It is not surprising, therefore, that patients with acute myocardial infarction exhibit variation in their peripheral vascular response to their illness.

Therapy is directed toward preservation of functioning myocardium, maintenance or restoration of ventricular performance, and the establishment of adequate systemic tissue perfusion. The important hemodynamic parameters essential to management are: left ventricular filling pressure, obtained by a venous Swan-Ganz catheter as pulmonary artery wedge pressure (PAWP), and systemic arterial pressure, which should be measured by an intraarterial line. Cardiac output is obtained by the thermodilution technique using the Swan-Ganz catheter. To obtain maximum intrinsic myocardial performance and yet avoid pulmonary edema the PAWP should be maintained between 20 and 24 mm Hg. This is accomplished by judicious use of intravenous fluids, diuretics, and vasodilators. The latter are also useful to improve tissue perfusion and lower output impedance to improve cardiac output. Support of systemic arterial pressure is accomplished, if necessary, by use of cardiac inotropic agents such as dopamine. If pressure and flow cannot be maintained, then the intraaortic balloon pump (IABP)

Figure 11-1

Development of septic shock may follow either of two major pathways through a hyperdynamic (high cardiac output) or a hypodynamic (low cardiac output) state. (From L. Hinshaw, Overview of endotoxin shock. In R. A. Cowley and B. F. Trump [Eds.], Pathophysiology of Shock, Anoxia and Ischemia. Baltimore: Williams & Wilkins, 1982, p. 223. Copyright © 1982, The Williams & Wilkins Co., Baltimore. Reproduced with permission from the author and publisher.

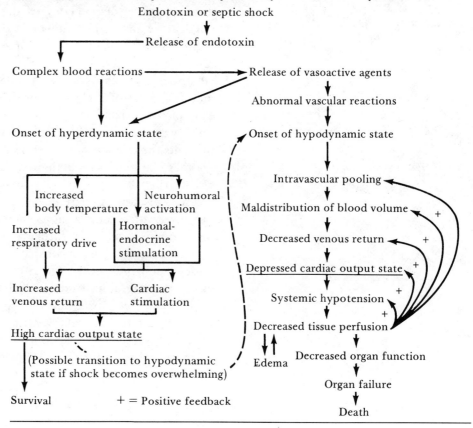

can be instituted to stabilize the hemodynamics while a cardiac catheterization procedure is performed to evaluate for a surgically correctable lesion; these include aneurysm, septal rupture and shunt, and papillary muscle rupture with flail mitral leaflet and significant mitral regurgitation. The IABP device lowers systolic pressure, thereby assisting cardiac output, and raises diastolic pressure, which improves coronary perfusion, thereby tending to preserve the myocardium and restore ventricular performance.

3. **Distributive shock** with normal or elevated peripheral vascular resistance commonly occurs with severe sepsis due to gram-negative bacillary organisms, especially *Escherichia coli;* this shock state is due in part to release of endotoxin and appears to be a primary disorder of venous capacitance with a maldistribution of blood flow and volume (Fig. 11-1). Regional vascular resistance alterations, myocardial dysfunction, intravascular coagulopathy, and capillary leakage also contribute to the maldistribution. The defect may not be reversed by infusion of large volumes of fluid. However, the early use of massive doses of corticosteroids, appropriate antibiotics, and general circulatory support therapy may be lifesaving. This contrasts to the conditions of barbiturate intoxication, central nervous system injury, and ganglionic blockade, in which secondary venous capacitance changes due to altered neuromotor controls respond readily to fluid distension.

A low-resistance type of shock is also recognized, which more often occurs with gram-positive infection or with mixed gram-positive and gram-negative organisms, as in peritonitis, pneumonia, and abscess formation. Vascular resistance is decreased, and cardiac output is usually increased. Despite the high-output state a critical tissue perfusion deficit may exist, which is characterized by an increase in blood lactate concentration. Management and therapy must be directed toward identifying and treating the bacterial agent with specific antibiotics, toward surgical drainage when indicated, and toward rational correction of the hemodynamic derangements.

4. **Obstructive shock** is due to an inadequate cardiac output commonly because of a blockage of diastolic filling of the heart. For example, in cardiac tamponade due to pericardial effusion and rapid accumulation of fluid, the increased intrapericardial pressure prevents the dilation of the ventricles that normally occurs during diastolic filling. As a result there is impaired filling and a disproportionate rise of intraventricular diastolic pressures compared with volume, resulting in a reduced stroke volume and narrow pulse pressure, with a compensatory increase in heart rate that may not be adequate to maintain cardiac output. Venous distension in the neck and arms is often a conspicuous feature, and an absent apex impulse may indicate a large effusion. This may be demonstrated by echocardiographic studies, which may demonstrate a large, "relatively echo-free" space not only posterior to the left ventricle but also anterior to the right ventricle. Pulsus paradoxus, resulting from a lowered arterial pressure during inspiration, is often present, but in the most severe cases with a significantly reduced arterial blood pressure this exaggerated respiratory variation may be absent. In shock due to cardiac tamponade, hemodynamic studies will show equalization of atrial, ventricular diastolic, and pulmonary artery diastolic pressures. When the compensatory mechanisms of tachycardia, increased venous pressure, an augmented inotropic myocardial state, and peripheral vasoconstriction fail to correct the problem, profound reduction in cardiac output and death will ensue. An emergency pericardiocentesis will usually give dramatic relief by drawing off the fluid to relieve the acute obstruction.

III. **Clinical example of distributive shock**

A. **Description.** A 42-year-old man whose wife said he had been unusually depressed recently was brought to the emergency room after taking an overdose of sleeping pills. The patient was unconscious; he had a pale and cold skin indicating obvious vasoconstriction. Respiration was shallow and the pulse was rapid and weak. Systolic blood pressure was 60 mm Hg. The neck veins were flat; there was no edema. Stomach contents were emptied by tube, ventilation was supported, and lines placed for measurement of cardiac output and venous and arterial pressures. Loading of intravascular compartment with intravenous saline was instituted; subsequently the patient had a diuresis and returned to normal hemodynamics.

B. **Measurements**

	Initial	Final
Cardiac output (L/min)	3.0	6.0
Mean arterial pressure (mm Hg)	45	90
Systemic vascular resistance (dynes sec cm^{-5})	1,200	1,200

C. Discussion

1. The findings are typical of the circulatory generalized distributive defect seen in shock due to barbiturate intoxication.
2. Plasma volume expansion and ventilatory support have proved to be successful in patients such as this one with potentially fatal blood levels of barbiturates.

Questions

More than one answer may be correct.

1. Which statement or statements do not apply to the pathophysiology of circulatory shock?
   a. Compensatory responses to hypovolemia include tachycardia, tachypnea, vasoconstriction, and reduced urine excretion.
   b. Maldistribution of cardiac output, coagulopathy, and capillary leakage are features of severe sepsis due to gram-negative organisms.
   c. In the course of shock due to acute myocardial infarction, ventricular filling pressure will always be elevated; therefore intravenous fluids are contraindicated.
   d. Cardiogenic shock is rarely due to acute myocardial infarction.
   e. All of the above.
2. Select the correct statement or statements regarding the pathophysiology of shock.
   a. Circulatory shock and a new cardiac murmur developing after myocardial infarction suggest a ruptured septum or papillary muscle.
   b. The intraaortic balloon pump (IABP) assists both cardiac output and coronary blood flow.
   c. In shock due to barbiturate overdose plasma volume expansion is an important part of the treatment.
   d. In a septic patient with a normal cardiac output we can safely assume that critical tissue perfusion is preserved.

III Endocrinology, Metabolism, and Hypertension

Ronald D. Brown
John R. Higgins
David C. Kem
Robert H. Roswell

12 Hormone Action

I. **Introduction.** Hormones are unique secretory products of the endocrine glands, which are released directly into the circulation and interact with specific target tissues to regulate their metabolic activity. This regulatory effect is mediated through highly specific receptors within the target tissues that must first bind the hormone before a change in metabolic activity can occur. Thus, an alteration of either the hormone concentration or the receptor can lead to a pathologic condition characterized by either an increase or a decrease in the regulated activity. Hormones can be chemically classified into three groups: polypeptide hormones, steroid hormones, and amine hormones, which include catecholamines that tend to behave like peptide hormones and iodothyronines or thyroid hormones that are more like steroid hormones in their behavior. The different classes of hormones vary in their characteristics and receptors; they are discussed below.

II. **Peptide and catecholamine hormones**

A. **Hormone production and secretion.** The peptide hormones are proteins that vary in size from a few to well over a hundred amino acids. While these hormones are too numerous to list individually, some of the more important peptide hormones include insulin, parathyroid hormone, and all of the pituitary hormones. The catecholamines, which are amino acid analogues, are discussed with the peptide hormones because of their close similarities in both physical-chemical characteristics and receptors. Generally speaking, peptide hormones are synthesized on the ribosomes in the endocrine gland cells as prohormones, large peptide molecules that are cleaved to yield active hormones. These hormones are then packaged by the Golgi apparatus in secretory granules, which remain in the cytoplasm until needed. The hormones reach the circulation by exocytosis of the secretory granule in response to a specific stimulus, such as an elevation of blood glucose in the case of insulin.

B. **Mechanism of action.** Several steps are involved before an actual alteration of cellular metabolism occurs, once the peptide hormone has been secreted. First, the hormone binds to a specific receptor on the target tissue cell membrane. Here adenylate cyclase is activated by the hormone-receptor complex and adenosine triphosphate (ATP) is converted to cyclic adenosine monophosphate (cAMP), which acts as a second messenger. Some of the peptide hormone may act through a second messenger other than cAMP, such as cyclic guanosine monophosphate (cGMP) or calcium. In either case, the second messenger activates a protein kinase, which in turn phosphorylates a protein substrate, yielding an activated enzyme. This activated enzyme then carries out the regulatory function of the hormone. Catecholamines act in a similar manner, binding first to a membrane receptor and stimulating the formation of a second messenger.

C. **Characteristics of peptide and catecholamine hormones.** The peptide hormones and catecholamines have a number of physicochemical properties that distinguish them from steroid hormones. These properties include a high molecular weight, water solubility, a short plasma half-life due in part to the absence of a plasma carrier protein, membrane receptors, and a rapid onset of action, mediated by a second messenger, which is usually cAMP.

III. Steroid hormones

A. Hormone production and secretion. The steroid hormones are all derived from cholesterol and as a result are all structurally quite similar. The major steroid hormones include the adrenal steroids, cortisol and aldosterone; the gonadal steroids, testosterone in the male and estradiol and progesterone in the female; and the active vitamin D metabolite 1,25-dihydroxyvitamin D. The thyroid hormones, which are iodinated amino-acid analogues, are discussed with the steroid hormones because of their close similarities in both physicochemical properties and receptors. Generally speaking, the steroid hormones are synthesized by multiple enzymatic steps in response to a specific stimulus, which is often a peptide hormone such as adrenocorticotropic hormone (ACTH) in the case of cortisol synthesis. Unlike peptide hormones, the steroid hormones are not stored to any appreciable degree, and hormone release due to a specific stimulus is a result of increased biosynthesis rather than release of preformed hormone.

B. Mechanism of action. As for peptide hormones, several steps are involved before steroid hormones exert their metabolic effects. Following release into the circulation, the steroid hormone is largely bound to a plasma-carrier protein, leaving only a small fraction of unbound or free hormone. This free hormone diffuses into the cytoplasm of the target tissue cell, where binding to a specific cytoplasmic receptor occurs. The hormone-receptor complex is then translocated to the nucleus, where binding at specific nuclear chromatin sites occurs. Thyroid hormones differ slightly from the steroid hormones in that they bind directly to their nuclear receptors. Once the hormone is bound to the chromatin acceptor site, synthesis of specific messenger ribonucleic acids occurs, which in turn leads to the synthesis of specific proteins. It is this final protein synthesis step that is responsible for the metabolic effects of the steroid or thyroid hormone.

C. Characteristics of steroid and thyroid hormones. The steroid and thyroid hormones have a number of properties that distinguish them from peptide hormones. These characteristics include a low molecular weight, fat solubility (which allows the hormone to diffuse intracellularly to bind to a cytoplasmic receptor), a long plasma half-life due in part to binding to a plasma-carrier protein, and a slow onset of action mediated by protein synthesis.

IV. Endocrine disease due to disorders of hormone-receptor systems

A. Increased hormonal activity. The overproduction of a given hormone can result from hyperplasia of the endocrine gland, due to known or unknown stimuli, or from an autonomously functioning neoplasm within the endocrine gland, such as a pituitary adenoma-producing growth hormone. Additionally, the hormone may be produced ectopically, usually by a malignancy such as an oat cell carcinoma of the lung, producing ACTH. Increased hormone-mediated metabolic activity due to increased receptor sensitivity or concentration has not been well documented, but has been speculated to be partly responsible for certain hyperadrenergic states.

B. Decreased hormonal activity. A decrease in various hormonally mediated metabolic activities may occur due to a number of abnormalities of the hormone-receptor system. First, the congenital absence or subsequent destruction of an endocrine gland due to trauma, neoplasm, or autoimmune phenomena will result in decreased or absent hormonogenesis. Decreased hormone production may also occur as a result of a specific enzyme deficiency leading to impaired production of certain steroid hormones. An example here would be impaired cortisol biosynthesis in patients with congenital adrenal hyperplasia due to 21-hydroxylase deficiency. Additionally, in certain rare instances, an endocrine gland may produce a biologically inactive hormone, such as an abnormal insulin resulting in diabetes mellitus. Decreased hormone-mediated activity may also result from a decrease or absence of the hormone receptors or a competing hormone antagonist that occupies the receptor but does not activate it. The most common clinical example of a receptor deficiency is the insulin resistance and hyperglycemia often seen in obesity as a consequence of decreased insulin-receptor concentration. Finally, a post-receptor defect within the target cell has been postulated to be responsible for decreased hormone-mediated activity in some instances.

V. **Clinical example of hormone action—testicular feminization**

A. **Description.** A 17-year-old female referred for evaluation of primary amenorrhea gave a history of normal breast development beginning at age 12, but she had not yet had a menstrual period. Physical examination revealed a normal female body habitus but no axillary or pubic hair. Pelvic examination demonstrated an atrophic vagina ending in a blind pouch without palpable internal genitalia. Closer examination revealed small bilateral inguinal masses.

The serum testosterone was 960 ng/dl (normal: males 400–1,000, females 20–80), and a chromosome analysis demonstrated a normal male 46-XY karyotype.

B. **Discussion**

1. This patient demonstrated the classic features of the rare disorder of testicular feminization.
2. The disease is characterized by end-organ resistance to testosterone and thus a female phenotype despite a male genotype.
3. The defect lies in the cytoplasmic receptor for the steroid hormone testosterone.
4. Since testosterone does not bind to its cytoplasmic receptor, nuclear translocation of the hormone-receptor complex cannot occur.
5. The result is a complete lack of androgen effects, or virilization, even though testosterone levels may be normal or elevated.
6. Because the defect is congenital, embryonic sexual development is phenotypically female and patients are reared as females.
7. Treatment consists of removing the small inguinal testes to prevent malignant degeneration and the administration of estrogens to maintain normal secondary female sexual characteristics.

Questions

Select the single best answer.

1. The following statements concerning peptide hormones are all true except:
   a. The peptide hormones include insulin, parathyroid hormone, and all of the pituitary hormones.
   b. Catecholamine hormones are similar to peptide hormones with regard to physicochemical characteristics and receptors.
   c. Peptide hormones act by binding initially to a cytoplasmic receptor, which is then translocated to a nuclear receptor site.
   d. In general, peptide hormones work through activation of a protein kinase, which in turn phosphorylates a protein substrate, yielding an activated enzyme.

2. Endocrine disease may result from which of the following disturbances of a hormone-receptor system?

a. Increased hormone-mediated activity due to autonomous production of the hormone by an adenoma.

b. Increased hormone-mediated activity due to ectopic production of the hormone by a malignancy.

c. Decreased hormone-mediated activity due to production of an abnormal, biologically inactive hormone.

d. Decreased hormone-mediated activity due to a defect or absence of the hormone receptor.

e. All of the above mechanisms may result in endocrine disease.

13 Anterior and Posterior Pituitary

I. **Review of normal physiology of the anterior pituitary**
   A. **Anterior pituitary hormones**
      1. **Adrenocorticotropic hormone (ACTH)** stimulates the adrenal glands to produce and secrete cortisol.
      2. **Beta-lipotropin** is a complex molecule that contains beta-melanocyte-stimulating hormone (MSH) and endorphins. While this hormone has lipolytic activity, its clinical importance is not yet established.
      3. **Thyroid-stimulating hormone (TSH)** controls production and release of L-thyroxine and L-triiodothyronine.
      4. **Follicle-stimulating hormone (FSH) and luteinizing hormone (LH)** control ovarian and testicular function.
      5. **Growth hormone (GH)** affects growth of skeletal structures, as well as controlling cellular function through nutrient production and availability.
      6. **Prolactin** acts as a mediator of milk secretion in the female and may have other activity in modulating secretion and end-organ responsiveness to gonadotropins.
   B. **Control of secretion.** Releasing factors and release-inhibitory factors originate in the hypothalamus and reach the pituitary through a dense capillary network. Except for prolactin, the anterior pituitary hormones are primarily controlled by releasing factors; that is, if the hypothalamus is destroyed or if the pituitary stalk is severed, prolactin secretion increases while the secretion of ACTH, beta-lipotropin, TSH, LH, FSH, and GH decreases. When target organ hormones (cortisol, thyroid hormone, estrogen, or testosterone) are stimulated to appropriate levels, they inhibit further release of their corresponding pituitary hormone in a homeostatic fashion, primarily by appropriate changes in these releasing factors.

   Some of the hypothalamic factors identified include the following:
      1. **Corticotropin releasing factor (CRF)** stimulates ACTH release; this factor has recently been isolated and purified.
      2. **Thyrotropin releasing hormone (TRH)** stimulates the release of both TSH and prolactin.
      3. **Somatostatin** inhibits growth hormone release.
      4. **GH secretion** is inhibited by increases in blood glucose and free fatty acids.
      5. **Dopamine** inhibits prolactin release.

II. **Pathophysiology—general principles**
   A. **Alterations in pituitary hormone secretion** can result from disease processes involving either the hypothalamus-pituitary unit or the target gland.
      1. Tumors of the pituitary can hypersecrete ACTH, GH, prolactin, and (rarely) TSH.
      2. Hypothalamic or pituitary destruction (tumor, trauma, infection, etc.) may result in partial or complete hypopituitarism.
      3. Target organ deficiencies (e.g., hypothyroidism, Addison's disease,

or hypogonadism) release the pituitary from negative feedback inhibition and lead to a rise in the appropriate pituitary hormone.

4. Autonomous hormone production by target glands (e.g., Graves' disease or Cushing's syndrome through an adrenal adenoma) suppresses the corresponding pituitary hormone.

5. Neoplasia (e.g., carcinoma of the lung) may produce pituitary hormones ectopically.

6. Drugs may alter pituitary hormone secretion (e.g., phenothiazines frequently elevate plasma prolactin).

B. **The clinical picture** associated with a pituitary hormone alteration is often a manifestation of the effect on the target gland. Common examples of this include hypothyroidism due to TSH deficiency and Cushing's disease due to ACTH overproduction.

III. **Disorders of anterior pituitary**

A. **Acromegaly**

1. **Etiology.** Acromegaly is usually due to excessive GH production by a pituitary tumor. Overproduction of GH-releasing factor by the hypothalamus may also occur, but this is an uncommon event.

2. **Clinical finding.** Gigantism occurs if onset is before epiphyseal closure at puberty. Enlargement of acral parts of body, such as jaw, hands, and feet, and of internal organs continues despite closure of the growth centers in the long bones. Patients may complain of headaches and may have visual disturbances from compression of the tumor on the anterior commissure of the optic nerve. Hypogonadism is frequently observed due to concurrent damage to LH- and FSH-producing cells.

3. **Diagnosis.** This rests on finding high blood levels of GH that do not subside 1 hour after an oral glucose load.

4. **Treatment** generally involves removal of the tumors. Recent studies suggest that a dopamine agonist, bromocriptine, partially inhibits GH secretion and may be useful in suppressing some tumor growth.

B. **Hyperprolactinemia**

1. **Etiology.** Drugs which inhibit the effect of dopamine, including phenothiazines, methyldopa, and buterophenones, may be potent causes of prolactin release. Estrogen directly stimulates the pituitary cells, which secrete prolactin, leading occasionally to hyperprolactinemia when patients take birth control pills or estrogen supplements. Other causes include prolactin-secreting tumors (e.g., chromophobe adenoma) and hypothalamic disease, which may increase release of prolactin by decreasing dopamine-mediated inhibition of prolactin secretion.

2. **Clinical findings.** Patients with a prolactin-secreting tumor frequently present with galactorrhea and hypogonadism. Amenorrhea or oligomenorrhea is frequent in women, while impotence and loss of libido are most frequent in men; infertility is found in both sexes.

3. **Diagnosis** is confirmed by finding a high blood level of prolactin and by the result of a search for underlying causes, such as a drug or pituitary tumor.

4. **Treatment.** If an estrogen or other medication is suspected, one should withdraw the offending drug. If a microadenoma or larger tumor is observed, surgical removal of tumor is generally recommended. There is now evidence that some of these tumors will

recede in size and reduce the secretion of prolactin during suppressive therapy with bromocriptine.

IV. **Review of normal physiology of the posterior pituitary (neurohypophysis)**

A. **The neurosecretory unit.** Vasopressin is synthesized in the paraventricular and supraoptic nuclei of the hypothalamus. The axons of these neurons, which make up the supraopticohypophyseal tract, terminate in the median eminence of the pituitary stalk and in the posterior pituitary. Vasopressin is stored in the nerve terminals bound to a carrier protein, neurophysin. In response to physiologic stimuli, vasopressin is split from neurophysin and released into adjacent capillaries.

B. **Control of vasopressin secretion**

1. **Osmotic factors** are the principal regulators of vasopressin release under physiologic conditions. The supraoptic and paraventricular nuclei are osmoreceptors. *Increased* osmolality (hypernatremia) of extracellular fluids activates the neuroendocrine cells in these nuclei. Impulses are carried down their axons and elicit vasopressin release. *Decreased* osmolality inhibits activation of the cells, and vasopressin release is decreased.

2. **Blood volume** also regulates vasopressin release. A decreased effective blood volume stimulates baroreceptors in the left atrium and pulmonary veins. Neural afferents from the baroreceptors activate the hypothalamus and stimulate vasopressin release. With severe hypovolemia, osmoregulation can be overridden and can result in water retention in the face of hypo-osmolality. Factors which increase the effective blood volume will inhibit vasopressin release.

3. **Pain, stress, sleep, and exercise** also stimulate vasopressin release through neural pathways.

4. **Pharmacologic agents** such as nicotine, morphine, and barbiturates stimulate vasopressin secretion through different receptors, while alcohol, phenytoin, and glucocorticoids inhibit vasopressin release.

C. **Mechanism of action of vasopressin**

1. **Vasopressin** binds to a specific receptor on the renal tubular cell membrane and stimulates the production of cyclic adenosine monophosphate (cAMP). This acts in an undetermined manner in the distal tubules and collecting ducts to make them more permeable to water.

2. As the collecting duct passes through the renal medulla, water passively enters the hypertonic interstitial tissues and the remaining urine becomes more concentrated.

V. **Disorders of posterior pituitary function**

A. **Diabetes insipidus**

1. **Pathogenesis.** Diabetes insipidus (DI) results from a lack of vasopressin release or a resistance to its action. Central DI can result from any process (surgery, trauma, tumors, infiltrative diseases) that damages the hypothalamus or severs the pituitary stalk. Up to 50 percent of cases of central DI, however, are idiopathic and 2 to 4 percent are familial.

   Hereditary nephrogenic DI is a rare sex-linked condition of males in which the kidneys do not respond to vasopressin. Acquired nephrogenic DI can result from chronic hypokalemia or hypercalcemia, lithium, demeclocycline, and methoxyflurane. Patients with sickle cell anemia also have an impaired response of the kidney to vasopressin but the reasons for this are not entirely known.

2. **Clinical aspects**
   a. Symptoms of polyuria and polydipsia are due to excretion of large quantities of dilute urine.
   b. Plasma osmolality is only mildly elevated as long as the thirst mechanism is intact and the patient has free access to water.
   c. The presence of a relatively low urinary osmolality (<250 mOsm/kg water) with an elevated plasma osmolality after a period of dehydration is usually sufficient for diagnosis of this condition.
   d. The concentrating defect is improved markedly by administration of exogenous vasopressin.

B. **Syndrome of inappropriate ADH (SIADH)**
   1. **Pathogenesis.** SIADH may result from either pituitary or ectopic production of vasopressin. Causes include:
      a. Central nervous system disease—i.e., head trauma, meningitis, brain tumor.
      b. Lung conditions—i.e., oat cell carcinoma, tuberculosis, pneumonia.
      c. Secretion of vasopressin from certain neoplasms, including those of the mediastinum and gastrointestinal tract.
   2. **Clinical aspects**
      a. Patients may have central nervous system symptoms (headache, nausea and vomiting, encephalopathy) if the resulting hypo-osmolality is acute or severe.
      b. The diagnosis depends on finding hypo-osmolality and a concentrated urine that is otherwise unexplained (see Chap. 39, Disorders of Sodium and Water Metabolism).

VI. **Clinical example of galactorrhea and amenorrhea**
   A. **Description.** A 25-year-old woman sought medical attention after failing to menstruate for 4 months. She was not pregnant, and her physical examination was entirely normal except that a small amount of milky fluid could be pressed from both breasts.
   B. **Discussion**
   1. Perhaps the most important issue for treating this young woman was deciding whether or not she had a prolactin-producing pituitary tumor.
   2. She was carefully questioned regarding the possibility that she might be taking a medicine that elevates prolactin production. The phenothiazine tranquilizers block the dopamine receptor in the pituitary and cause hyperprolactinemia by releasing the prolactin-producing cells of the pituitary from the inhibitory effect of dopamine coming from the hypothalamus. Methyldopa and reserpine, two commonly used antihypertensives, deplete dopamine from the hypothalamus and allow prolactin to increase. Estrogens, such as those found in oral contraceptives, directly stimulate prolactin-producing cells in the pituitary.
   3. Her blood level of prolactin was measured. A greatly elevated level would indicate a pituitary tumor. Moderate elevation suggests a pituitary tumor, but other causes of hyperprolactinemia are more likely. Included among these other causes could be primary hypothyroidism, a history of chest wall injury or chest surgery, and

chronic renal disease. Each of these possibilities can be ruled out by a careful history, physical examination, and simple laboratory studies. High prolactin levels do not have a recognizable cause in a significant percentage of people; this condition is referred to as idiopathic hyperprolactinemia.

4. Special radiographic studies (sellar tomography) were done to search for enlargement of her sella turcica or erosion of the floor of the sella.

5. When radiographic studies indicated the likelihood of a pituitary tumor, she was given a formal visual field examination to determine if the tumor extended above the sella to involve the optic chiasm.

6. When a pituitary tumor was found, trans-sphenoidal surgery made it feasible to remove the tumor while leaving behind normal pituitary tissue.

7. If no specific cause for her galactorrhea and amenorrhea had been found and if she desired to become fertile, medical treatment with bromocriptine would have been considered. Bromocriptine binds to the dopamine receptors in the pituitary and inhibits the secretion of prolactin.

Questions

Select the single best answer.

1. If the connection between the hypothalamus and pituitary is destroyed, which one of the following will occur?
   a. Increase in prolactin.
   b. Increase in prolactin and growth hormone secretion.
   c. Increase in the secretion of all anterior pituitary hormones.
   d. Decrease in the secretion of all anterior pituitary hormones.
   e. Increase in ACTH secretion if the adrenals are intact.

2. Which is the incorrect statement regarding control of vasopressin secretion?
   a. A rise in serum osmolality, such as that caused by hypernatremia, stimulates vasopressin release.
   b. Osmotic factors are the principal regulators of vasopressin release under physiologic conditions.
   c. Decreased effective blood volume stimulates vasopressin release.
   d. Severe hypovolemia can override osmoregulation and result in vasopressin release in a patient with hyponatremia.
   e. Pain and stress inhibit vasopressin release.

I. **Normal physiology.** The functions of the adrenal cortex and the presence of the adrenocortical hormones, cortisol and aldosterone, are essential to life.

A. **Functional anatomy**

1. **The adrenal glands** consist of an outer cortex, which secretes steroid hormones, and an inner medulla, which secretes catecholamines. The cortex and medulla are separate endocrine glands; they are essentially independent in their hormone production and distinct in their function. The adrenal medulla is discussed in Chapter 16, Hypertension.

2. **The arterial blood supply** to the adrenal glands is from small branches of the aorta, renal arteries, and the inferior phrenic artery. Venous drainage is collected from sinusoids that run through the gland, terminating in the medulla. The left adrenal vein empties into the left renal vein and the right drains into the inferior vena cava.

3. **The adrenal cortex** is composed of three zones:

   a. **Zona glomerulosa.** This zone consists of a thin layer of cells subjacent to the capsule; it secretes aldosterone.

   b. **Zona fasciculata.** This zone, the widest, is made up of cells located in the mid-portion of the cortex that secrete cortisol.

   c. **Zona reticularis.** This zone consists of the innermost cells. They secrete small amounts of sex steroids, testosterone and estradiol, and relatively large amounts of their precursors.

B. **Steroid secretion**

1. **All hormones** secreted by the adrenal cortex are *steroids*. The two principal hormones, cortisol and aldosterone (Fig. 14-1), are secreted at rates of approximately 25 mg per 24 hours and 100 μg per 24 hours, respectively. Other steroids secreted in quantitatively significant amounts are dehydroepiandrosterone and Δ_4-androstenediol. They are measured as 17-ketosteroids in the urine.

2. **Adrenocortical hormones** are derived from cholesterol. Most of the cholesterol (85%) is derived from the cholesterol of the blood perfusing the adrenal gland. The remainder (15%) is synthesized within the adrenal gland.

C. **Regulation of cortisol secretion.** There are three major secretory control mechanisms for ACTH and hence cortisol:

1. **Negative feedback inhibition of ACTH**

   a. Decreased free plasma cortisol concentration leads to increased release of ACTH by the pituitary; conversely, increased cortisol concentration leads to decreased ACTH release.

   b. This push-pull relationship acts predominantly at the level of the hypothalamus, which has a sensitive sensor for plasma cortisol concentration. Low cortisol levels trigger the release of corticotropin-releasing hormone (CRH), a 41-amino acid peptide, into the portal blood vessels, by which it is transported to the anterior pituitary and stimulates the release of ACTH. There appears to be a secondary and less sensitive sensing mechanism in the pituitary gland itself.

Figure 14-1

Chemical structures of cortisol and aldosterone.

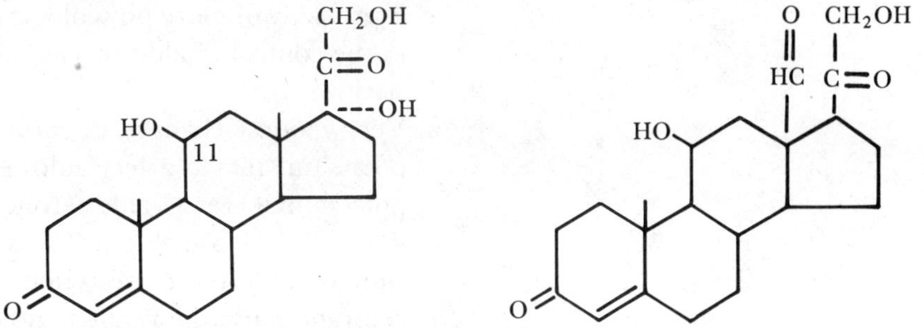

Cortisol
(hydrocortisone)

Aldosterone

2. Circadian variation

   a. There is a systematically varying set point for the minimum plasma-free cortisol concentration to suppress ACTH secretion during the course of the day. This variation is synchronized by the daily environmental shift from darkness to light and from sleep to wakefulness. Day workers have their highest ACTH levels during the morning and their lowest levels late in the evening.

   b. The stimulus for the continual variation of the set point is not dependent on the plasma cortisol concentration.

3. Stress

   a. During episodes of severe physical or emotional stress, ACTH is secreted independently of the set-point mechanism. In severe stress, there is no level of plasma cortisol high enough to inhibit the release of ACTH.

   b. The response to stress is mediated through higher centers of the central nervous system to release CRH or to bypass the negative feedback system.

D. Regulation of aldosterone secretion. There are three mechanisms that regulate the secretion of aldosterone:

   1. Renin-angiotensin system

   a. Under most physiologic circumstances, the renin-angiotensin system is the major regulator of aldosterone secretion. Changes in effective blood volume (renal perfusion pressure) are monitored by the juxtaglomerular apparatus of the afferent arteriole, and changes in sodium concentration (or flux) in the distal tubule are monitored by the macula densa of the tubule. A decrease in renal perfusion pressure or a decrease in sodium concentration in the fluid of the distal tubule causes the juxtaglomerular cells to release renin.

   b. Stimulation of renal sympathetic nerves also releases renin.

   c. Renin is a proteolytic enzyme that acts on a circulating α_2-globulin made in the liver (renin substrate) to split off angiotensin I. Angiotensin I, a decapeptide, is converted to angiotensin II by an enzyme (converting enzyme) located predominantly in the lung.

   d. Angiotensin II, an octapeptide, is a potent vasoconstrictor of arterioles. It is also a potent stimulator of aldosterone secretion and can be converted to angiotensin III (a heptapeptide), which also stimulates aldosterone secretion. Angiotensin II, however, is probably of more physiologic importance than angiotensin III in the control of aldosterone secretion.

2. **Potassium**
   a. Very modest changes in serum potassium concentration and potassium intake affect aldosterone secretion. An increase in potassium increases aldosterone secretion, and potassium depletion will decrease aldosterone secretion. These effects of potassium on aldosterone secretion are independent of sodium concentration and the renin-angiotensin system.
   b. It is not known whether an alteration in the intracellular or extracellular potassium is responsible for potassium-induced alterations of aldosterone secretion.

3. **ACTH**
   a. Under normal circumstances, ACTH plays a minor role in aldosterone regulation. ACTH accounts for part of the circadian rhythm of aldosterone.
   b. Large amounts of ACTH stimulate aldosterone secretion, but this effect is only temporary since aldosterone secretion returns to pre-ACTH levels in 2 to 3 days, even though ACTH administration continues.
   c. Under conditions of sodium depletion or potassium loading, the adrenal glomerulosa becomes more sensitive to the steroidogenic effects of ACTH and angiotensin II.

II. **Abnormalities of cortisol secretion**
   A. **Hypercortisolism—effects on the pituitary adrenal axis**
      1. Increased glucocorticoid levels, above the set point, suppress ACTH and, consequently, cortisol secretion. Induced increases in cortisol concentration may be achieved by exogenous ACTH or cortisol administration. This phenomenon is used diagnostically when graded doses of exogenous glucocorticoids are given to determine at what level ACTH secretion ceases. This bioassay system, designed to evaluate the set point, is the basis for the dexamethasone suppression test used clinically to evaluate patients with hypercortisolism (Cushing's syndrome).
      2. Prolonged ACTH stimulation results in adrenal hyperplasia, increased steroid output, and greater adrenal sensitivity to ACTH. On the other hand, prolonged exogenous cortisol administration results in adrenal atrophy, decreased steroid output, and decreased adrenal sensitivity to ACTH. In both situations, ACTH secretion is suppressed.
      3. After withdrawal of exogenous ACTH or cortisol, the hypothalamic-pituitary mechanism and the adrenal glands may take up to a year to recover and interact normally. During the recovery period, ACTH secretion resumes first, and as the adrenal glands become responsive to ACTH, cortisol increases toward normal.
   B. **Mechanisms of Cushing's syndrome.** Prolonged excessive circulating cortisol leads to the clinical state of Cushing's syndrome. There are several etiologies:
      1. **Excess pituitary secretion of ACTH (Cushing's disease).** In this form of Cushing's syndrome, the ACTH set point is abnormally high; ACTH will be hypersecreted until endogenous hypercortisolism results.
      2. **Adrenocortical tumor.** An adrenal tumor produces excess cortisol, independent of ACTH. The chronically elevated cortisol levels

suppress ACTH secretion, just as the chronic administration of cortisol inhibits ACTH secretion.

    3. Ectopic ACTH. A non-pituitary tumor produces excess ACTH, independent of circulating cortisol levels and the physiologic needs of the body. The resulting chronically elevated cortisol suppresses pituitary secretion of ACTH.

C. Metabolic effects of glucocorticoids. Glucocorticoids affect virtually all tissues in the body. The response to glucocorticoids of a tissue may be catabolic or anabolic.

    1. Liver. There is an increase in glycogen. Glucose production from protein increases (gluconeogenesis). RNA synthesis and protein synthesis also increase.

    2. Adipose tissue. There is an increase in free fatty acid and glycerol release, and a decrease in glucose utilization and lipogenesis.

    3. Muscle. There is a decrease in glucose utilization and protein synthesis, and an increase in protein breakdown.

    4. Connective tissue. There is a decrease in protein synthesis and collagen formation.

    5. Sodium. There is an increase in sodium resorption by the distal tubule and collecting duct, accompanied by an increase in the excretion of potassium. These effects reflect the mineralocorticoid activity of cortisol.

D. Hypercortisolism—clinical manifestations. The clinical manifestations of Cushing's syndrome are the result of the metabolic effects of cortisol on various body tissues.

    1. Adipose tissue. Obesity with centripetal fat distribution is evident. Supraclavicular fat pads increase, and a buffalo hump appears due to deposition of fat over the upper thoracic spine.

    2. Protein. There is thinning of the skin with purple striae over the abdomen, thighs, and upper arms. The skin bruises easily and wounds heal poorly. Muscle wasting and weakness develop. Loss of bone (osteoporosis) with compression fractures of the vertebrae, dorsal curvature of the spine, and rib fractures occur. The hypercalcuria from the destruction of bone and release of calcium may cause renal stones.

    3. Carbohydrate metabolism. Diabetes mellitus, overt and latent, commonly occurs.

    4. Mineral metabolism. Hypertension and hypokalemic alkalosis may appear. Some patients become edematous.

    5. Menstrual dysfunction, hirsutism, and acne commonly occur due to the increased secretion of androgens.

E. Hypocortisolism—clinical manifestations. The clinical manifestations of hypocortisolism, whether the condition results from inadequate pituitary secretion of ACTH, primary adrenal disease (Addison's disease), or an enzymatic defect (congenital adrenal hyperplasia), reflect the effect of a lack of cortisol on various tissues in the body.

    1. Gastrointestinal. The patient may have anorexia, nausea, vomiting, abdominal pain, and weight loss.

    2. Central nervous system. Decreased vigor, lethargy, apathy, and confusion may appear.

    3. Energy metabolism. Impaired gluconeogenesis, impaired fat mobilization, and liver glycogen depletion may cause fasting hypoglycemia.

    4. Cardiovascular-renal. Impaired free-water excretion, excessive losses of sodium in the urine, and retention of potassium and hydrogen ions, may cause hyponatremia, pre-renal azotemia, and hyperkalemic metabolic acidoses, respectively. Eventually, hypotension and shock may ensue.

5. **Pituitary.** In primary adrenal insufficiency, the unrestrained secretion of ACTH results in hyperpigmentation of the skin and the mucosa of the mouth. In secondary adrenal insufficiency, the lack of ACTH may result in hypopigmentation.

III. Clinical example of Cushing's disease

A. Description. A 36-year-old woman noted a gradual increase in weight, fatigue, weakness, oligomenorrhea, facial hair growth, and easy bruising. Examination revealed a plethoric, hirsute woman with central obesity, purple striae, ecchymoses, and marked proximal muscle weakness. Her blood pressure was 164/102 mm Hg.

Laboratory values: hemoglobin 16.2 gm/dl, serum sodium 140 mEq/L, potassium 3.5 mEq/L, fasting glucose 180 mg/dl, morning plasma cortisol 32 μg/dl (normal, 8–26), and late evening plasma cortisol 28 μg/dl (normal, <8). Her urinary 17-hydroxycorticosteroids (17-OHCs) were 15 mg/gm creatinine (normal, <7.5). After dexamethasone, 2.0 mg (low dose) daily for 2 days, plasma cortisol was 30 μg/dl and urinary 17-OHCs were 13 mg/gm creatinine. After dexamethasone, 8.0 mg (high dose) daily for 2 days, an 8 A.M. plasma cortisol was 12 μg/dl and urinary 17-OHCs were 4 mg/gm creatinine.

A pituitary adenoma was removed; 4 days postoperatively, while she was receiving 0.75 mg of dexamethasone daily, a morning plasma cortisol was 1.5 μg/dl. Six months later a morning plasma cortisol was 16.0 μg/dl, and after a low-dose dexamethasone test, the plasma cortisol was 3.0 μg/dl.

B. Discussion

1. This woman had the classic physical findings of a patient with Cushing's syndrome. They can be explained by the known effects of excess cortisol on protein, carbohydrate, fat, and sodium metabolism.

   a. Muscle weakness, striae, and ecchymoses reflect protein catabolism.

   b. Elevated blood glucose is caused by increased gluconeogenesis and decreased glucose utilization.

   c. The central obesity reflects the effect of cortisol on lipogenesis in selected fat cells.

   d. The hypertension and decreased serum potassium reflect the mineralocorticoid action of cortisol.

2. The oligomenorrhea is due to excess sex-steroid secretion and suppression of FSH and LH secretion from the pituitary gland.

3. The lack of a diurnal or circadian rhythm of plasma cortisol is typical of patients with Cushing's syndrome.

4. The resistance of plasma cortisol and urinary 17-OHCs to low-dose dexamethasone and its partial suppression with high-dose dexamethasone indicates that the set point of ACTH release is abnormally high and tells us the patient has pituitary Cushing's syndrome (i.e., Cushing's disease), rather than an adrenal tumor or the ectopic ACTH syndrome.

5. The abnormally low plasma cortisol 4 days postoperatively indicates that the remaining nontumorous ACTH-secreting cells in the pituitary have been suppressed by the prolonged elevation of circulating cortisol.

6. The normal cortisol levels and the normal response to dexamethasone several months later indicate that the patient has been cured, that the previously suppressed ACTH-secreting cells are functioning, and that the set point for ACTH secretion is now normal.

Questions

Select the single best answer.

1. Adrenal insufficiency is usually associated with:
   a. Hyperglycemia.
   b. Decreased serum sodium and potassium.
   c. Normal or low aldosterone.
   d. Need for catecholamine replacement therapy.
   e. All of the above.
2. Patients with Cushing's disease (hypercortisolism due to excess pituitary ACTH) usually have:
   a. Resistance to the ACTH-suppressive effects of exogenous glucocorticoids.
   b. Loss of the diurnal rhythm of ACTH secretion.
   c. A failure of ACTH secretion to respond to hypoglycemic stress.
   d. Normal plasma aldosterone.
   e. All of the above.

I. General aspects of thyroid function

A. **Embryology and anatomy.** The human thyroid originates from the fourth and fifth branchial pouches, forming a discrete organ by the twelfth week of fetal life. In the adult, the thyroid normally weighs from 20 to 30 g and lies over the second and third tracheal rings in the anterior neck. Histologically, the thyroid consists of numerous follicles composed of cuboidal epithelial cells and filled with a colloid substance that consists largely of thyroglobulin.

B. **Thyroid hormones**

   1. **T_4 (tetraiodothyronine or thyroxine)** is made exclusively in the thyroid and is the major product of thyroid hormone synthesis. T_4 present in the circulation is almost all (99.97%) bound to thyroid-binding globulin, thyroxine-binding prealbumin, and albumin.

   2. **T_3 (3,5,3'-triiodothyronine)** is produced primarily from peripheral monodeiodonation of T_4, although about 20 percent of T_3 is secreted directly from the thyroid. T_3 is much less tightly bound to proteins in the circulation and appears to be the metabolically active form of the hormone. Decreased conversion of T_4 to T_3 occurs during stress, illness, starvation, or with the administration of a number of drugs including glucocorticoids, propranolol, and propylthiouracil. This may be a protective mechanism to decrease metabolic activity in adverse situations.

   3. **rT_3 (3,3'5'-triiodothyronine or reverse T_3)** is produced almost exclusively from peripheral monodeiodonation of T_4. Production of rT_3 is enhanced during those situations that inhibit T_4 conversion to T_3, listed above. With no known physiologic role, rT_3 appears to be an inactive product.

C. **TSH regulation of thyroid function.** Thyroid-stimulating hormone (TSH) is a glycoprotein made in the anterior pituitary; it is secreted in response to thyrotropin-releasing hormone (TRH), a tripeptide produced in the hypothalamus and transported to the pituitary through the hypothalamic hypophyseal portal system. TSH stimulates the thyroid production of T_4 and T_3 by binding to membrane receptors on the follicular cells, which in turn activate adenylate cyclase-producing cyclic adenosine monophosphate (cAMP), resulting in increased thyroid hormone synthesis. T_3 and possibly T_4 as well feed back directly to the anterior pituitary to inhibit the production of TSH.

II. Hyperthyroidism

A. **General.** Hyperthyroidism is a condition resulting from the overproduction of thyroid hormones and is characterized by an elevation of both T_3 and T_4, although rarely only T_3 is elevated (T_3 toxicosis). Hyperthyroidism may also occur with the administration of an excessive amount of exogenous thyroid hormone. The clinical manifestations of hyperthyroidism are due to the effects of increased metabolic and sympathetic activity.

B. **Pathogenesis of hyperthyroidism.** The elevations of T_4 and T_3 seen in hyperthyroidism may result from a number of different mechanisms.

   1. **Graves' disease.** The pathogenesis of Graves' disease, the most common cause of hyperthyroidism, is still not completely understood. It appears, however, that abnormal IgG antibodies are pro-

Metabolic effects of increased thyroid hormones
   Weight loss
   Muscular weakness
   Hair loss
   Thin skin
   Onycholysis
   Menstrual irregularities
Hyperadrenergic effects of increased thyroid hormones
   Tachycardia
   Tremor
   Increased perspiration
   Heat intolerance
   Nervousness
   Palpitations

duced that occupy the TSH receptors, stimulating T_3 and T_4 production. The resulting elevation of T_4 and T_3 feedback inhibits pituitary production of TSH but has no effect on these abnormal thyroid-stimulating immunoglobulins (TSI), so thyroid hormone overproduction continues. The TSIs probably arise from a random mutation in B lymphocytes, but only those patients with a genetic defect in suppressor T lymphocytes, who are unable to suppress the production of these immunoglobulins, develop the disease. These abnormal immunoglobulins are probably responsible for the other manifestations of Graves' disease that are not seen with other types of hyperthyroidism; they include ophthalmopathy and, rarely, pretibial myxedema and thyroid acropachy.

2. **Nodular hyperthyroidism.** Occasionally a thyroid nodule or adenoma becomes autonomous in its production of thyroid hormone, resulting in hyperthyroidism. TSH is suppressed, and thyroid hormone production ceases in the surrounding normal thyroid tissue. This type of hyperthyroidism may also develop in a multinodular goiter; it is more commonly seen in the elderly.

3. **Subacute thyroiditis** is a viral disease that affects the thyroid, resulting in a painful, slightly enlarged gland. The associated inflammation causes a release of stored T_3 and T_4, and hyperthyroidism ensues. Unlike other forms of hyperthyroidism, the condition is transient, lasting only a few weeks.

4. **Chronic thyroiditis.** Hashimoto's thyroiditis, or chronic lymphocytic thyroiditis, is an autoimmune thyroid disease characterized by the presence of antithyroid antibodies and lymphocytic infiltration of the gland. Occasionally, patients with this disorder may develop transient hyperthyroidism.

5. **Exogenous or factitious hyperthyroidism.** The administration of exogenous thyroid hormones by the physician (iatrogenic) or surreptitiously by the patient (factitious) may result in hyperthyroidism. In this instance, TSH is suppressed and the gland is not enlarged or tender.

C. **Clinical aspects of hyperthyroidism.** The elevation in T_3 and T_4 seen in hyperthyroidism is due to an exaggeration of normal thyroid hormone action, leading to increased metabolic and adrenergic activity. Although the etiology of the elevation varies, the clinical manifestations do not (Table 15-1).

D. Treatment of hyperthyroidism should be individualized and may be either symptomatic or definitive. For example, only symptomatic therapy is indicated in the self-limited hyperthyroidism associated with subacute thyroiditis.

1. **Symptomatic treatment** usually consists of a blocking agent. Propranolol is the adrenergic blocking agent of choice and has the additional advantage of blocking the peripheral conversion of T_4 to the more metabolically active T_3 form of the hormone.

2. **Definitive therapy** is indicated in hyperthyroidism that is not spontaneously reversible. Three basic modalities are utilized according to specific needs: surgery, drugs, or radioactive iodine.

   Radioactive iodine is the treatment of choice for most cases of hyperthyroidism, but has the disadvantage of a high incidence of hypothyroidism following treatment. It is also contraindicated during pregnancy due to its ability to destroy the developing fetal thyroid.

III. Hypothyroidism

A. General. Hypothyroidism results from the underproduction of thyroid hormones and is characterized by a reduction in both T_4 and T_3, with an associated rise in TSH due to loss of feedback inhibition at the pituitary. However, TSH may be low in cases of secondary hypothyroidism (see the following). The clinical manifestations of hypothyroidism are due to the effects of decreased T_3 and T_4 on metabolic activity.

B. Pathogenesis of hypothyroidism. The reduction in T_4 and T_3 seen in hypothyroidism may be due to a number of different mechanisms.

1. **Autoimmune destruction of the thyroid.** Autoimmune thyroid disease is the most common cause of hypothyroidism and is responsible for most cases of idiopathic hypothyroidism. Hypothyroidism may also occur in other autoimmune thyroid disease, including Graves' disease and chronic (Hashimoto's) thyroiditis. Early in the course of the disease, increased TSH secretion may compensate for the decreased ability to produce thyroid hormones, but as thyroid destruction by antithyroid antibodies continues, the gland can no longer compensate and T_4 and T_3 levels fall despite high TSH levels.

2. **Results of therapy for hyperthyroidism.** Radioactive iodine or surgery occasionally results in excessive loss or destruction of thyroid tissue, and hypothyroidism ensues. The onset of symptoms following therapy may be rapid or gradual, occurring several years after treatment. This therapeutic outcome is the second most common cause of hypothyroidism seen in the United States today.

3. **Secondary hypothyroidism.** Surgical removal or damage to the pituitary by infection, tumor, or infiltrative diseases leads to hypothyroidism, due to the inability to produce TSH. Thus, unlike other forms of hypothyroidism, this condition is characterized by a low TSH. Often there are associated deficiencies of other pituitary trophic hormones, but occasionally isolated TSH deficiency occurs. The degree of thyroid hormone deficiency seen in this condition is usually less severe than other types of hypothyroidism.

4. **Drug-induced hypothyroidism.** A number of drugs have the ability to inhibit thyroid hormone synthesis or release. These include iodine, propylthiouracil, methimazole, lithium carbonate, oral hypoglycemic agents, and 6-mercaptopurine.

Table 15-2   *Clinical Features Common in Hypothyroidism*

Lethargy
Easy fatigability
Dry skin
Cold intolerance
Peripheral edema
Constipation
Hair loss
Menstrual irregularities
Coarsening of the voice
Memory impairment
Weight gain

C. **Clinical aspects of hypothyroidism.** The reduction in T_4 and T_3 seen in hypothyroidism results in a dramatic decrease in both metabolic rate and a number of cellular processes that give rise to characteristic changes listed in Table 15-2.

D. **Treatment of hypothyroidism.** When a reversible cause of hypothyroidism is detected, such as drug-induced hypothyroidism, specific therapy or elimination of the offending agent is indicated. When replacement of thyroid hormone is necessary, the drug of choice is levothyroxine or synthetic T_4. This hormone is converted to T_3 in the body in a manner similar to endogenously produced T_4; thus, T_3 replacement is not necessary. Hormone replacement should be started cautiously and gradually increased until the patient is euthyroid, in order to avoid angina or other cardiac complications produced by a sudden increase in metabolic demands. When thyroid replacement is adequate, the TSH level returns to normal.

IV. **Clinical example of Graves' disease**

A. **Description.** A 26-year-old woman presented with a 3-month history of palpatations, nervousness, increased perspiration, scant irregular menses, and a 15-pound weight loss, despite a noticeable increase in appetite. Physical examination revealed a resting pulse of 140. The skin was smooth, warm, and moist. Eye examination revealed bilateral exophthalmus with a lid lag. The thyroid was approximately three times the normal size and was smooth and firm. A fine resting tremor was present. The remainder of the exam was unremarkable.

B. **Laboratory evaluation** revealed a serum T_4 of 22.8 μg/100 ml (normal, 4.5–11.5) and a T_3 of 310 μg/100 ml (normal, 70–210). The 24-hour ^{131}I uptake was 68 percent (normal 10–30%) and the thyroid scan revealed homogenous uptake of the isotope throughout both lobes.

C. **Discussion**

1. The history and physical findings in this patient strongly suggested the diagnosis of hyperthyroidism.

2. The elevation of serum T_3 and T_4 confirmed the diagnosis of hyperthyroidism.

3. The increased ^{131}I uptake by the thyroid indicated the thyroid was the source of thyroid hormone excess and eliminated the diagnostic possibilities of exogenously administered thyroid hormone or subacute thyroiditis.

4. The homogenous uptake on thyroid scan excluded the possibility of nodular hyperthyroidism or chronic thyroiditis.

5. The correct diagnosis, Graves' disease, is made by a process of elimination of other etiologies of hyperthyroidism.
6. Symptomatic therapy should be instituted and would normally consist of an adrenergic blocking agent, such as propranolol.
7. Definitive therapy could then be instituted and would consist of radioactive iodine, antithyroid drugs, or surgery depending on individual circumstances.
8. Symptomatic treatment should continue until the patient is made euthyroid by definitive means.
9. The patient will require long-term follow-up for the possible development of hypothyroidism regardless of the means of initial treatment.

Questions

Select the single best answer.

1. Hyperthyroidism may be characterized by all of the following except:
   a. Weight loss.
   b. Cold intolerance.
   c. Tremor.
   d. Tachycardia.
2. The most common cause of hypothyroidism is:
   a. Pituitary destruction.
   b. A congenital defect in thyroid hormone synthesis.
   c. Autoimmune thyroid disease.
   d. Ingestion of thyroid-inhibiting drugs.

16 Hypertension

I. Background. Hypertension, defined as a blood pressure of 140/90 mm Hg or greater, is a major health problem in most societies. Numerous studies have documented that the higher the blood pressure, the greater the risk for a variety of cardiovascular events including stroke, myocardial infarction, and congestive heart failure. The cause of most hypertension, i.e., essential hypertension, is unknown. Hypertension may be secondary to a variety of specific diseases. In these cases we have a better understanding of the pathogenesis than of essential hypertension.

II. Hemodynamics

    A. There are two fundamental hemodynamic variables that determine the magnitude of arterial pressure. They are:

        1. Cardiac output (CO) = total systemic blood flow.

        2. Total peripheral resistance (TPR) = resistance offered by the blood vessels to forward flow.

    B. Mean arterial blood pressure (MAP) can be related mathematically to CO and TPR as follows: $MAP = CO \times TPR$.

    C. Hypertension is a dynamic disease that can result from any factor which alters the relationship between CO and TPR. CO, for example, is dependent on two basic variables, stroke volume and heart rate. Stroke volume, in turn, is influenced by factors affecting the left ventricular preload, afterload, and myocardial contractility. These, in turn, may be influenced by such factors as blood volume and adrenergic tone. Heart rate, the other determinate of cardiac output, is determined primarily by vagal tone and adrenergic factors. Total peripheral resistance is a function of several variables, including viscosity of the blood and the length of the blood vessels. However, the most important determinant of peripheral resistance is the radius of the blood vessels, as is evident from the resistance equation: $TPR = (k \times viscosity \times length)/radius^4$. Approximately 70 percent of total peripheral resistance is offered by the small-diameter vessels, mostly the muscular-walled arterioles. There are multiple neural and humoral factors that can influence peripheral vascular resistance (Table 16-1). However, the exact role of these factors in the pathogenesis of hypertension is largely unknown.

III. Major humoral regulators of blood pressure. There are several humoral factors that are often incriminated in some well-defined hypertensive diseases. A deficiency of any one of these hormones usually causes hypotension and a primary excess frequently causes hypertension.

    A. Norepinephrine is a catecholamine that increases blood pressure by stimulating the alpha-adrenoreceptors of arteriolar smooth muscle.

    B. Angiotensin II is a small peptide (8 amino acids) that increases blood pressure directly by stimulating receptors of arteriolar smooth muscle, thereby causing vasoconstriction, and indirectly by stimulating the secretion of aldosterone, thereby causing sodium retention.

    C. Aldosterone is an adrenal steroid (mineralocorticoid) that increases blood pressure by stimulating mineralocorticoid receptors in the distal and collecting tubules of the kidney, which causes the kidneys to reabsorb sodium and excrete potassium. Sodium retention, in turn, causes expansion of the extracellular fluid volume and an increase in effective blood volume.

Arteriolar Constrictors (↑ TPR)
   Adrenergic neurons
   Circulating catecholamines
   Angiotensin II
   Vasopressin (not important in man)
   Calcium
Arteriolar Dilators (↓ TPR)
   Stimulation of beta-adrenergic receptors
   Cholinergic and histaminergic nerves
   Dopamine
   Bradykinin
   Prostaglandin E_2

↑ = increased; ↓ = decreased.

D. Cortisol is an adrenal steroid (glucocorticoid) that increases blood pressure through several mechanisms:

1. Sensitizes arteriolar smooth muscle to vasopressor agents.
2. Increases renin substrate, thereby increasing angiotensin II formation.
3. Increases sodium reabsorption by the kidney due to its mineralocorticoid activity.

IV. **Endocrine models of hypertension.** It is presumed that the blood pressure elevation in patients afflicted with these syndromes is causally related to the hormonal excess, since correction of the excess ameliorates the hypertension. These types of hypertension are rare, but we understand the etiology and pathogenesis of the hypertension far better than we do the pathogenesis of essential hypertension. Therefore, the clinical picture and hemodynamic status of these endocrine models will be detailed. Analysis of the hemodynamic status of patients with these models of hypertension has led to a better understanding of the alterations in cardiac output and total peripheral resistance that are caused by the major humoral regulators of blood pressure. Secondary adjustments of the neurocirculatory system and the kidney, however, may modify the primary effect of these humoral substances.

A. **Pheochromocytoma**

1. **Mechanisms of hypertension.** Pheochromocytoma is a catecholamine-secreting tumor, usually in one of the adrenal glands, but it may be bilateral or extra-adrenal in location. The hemodynamic features are a direct result of adrenergic stimulation of cardiac and vascular receptors. Typically, total peripheral resistance is markedly increased secondary to the alpha-adrenergic stimulation of arterioles from the high circulating norepinephrine levels. Cardiac output may be elevated primarily from the beta-adrenergic effects of epinephrine, which increase heart rate and myocardial contractile force. However, in most cases cardiac output is normal, probably due to several factors, including a decrease in plasma volume and the effects of hypertension per se, which by increasing impedance to left ventricular emptying tends to decrease stroke volume.

2. **Clinical picture.** The palpitations, excess sweating, pallor, headache, hypermetabolism, and glucose intolerance reflect the effects of epinephrine and norepinephrine on the heart, sweat glands, arterioles, liver, and pancreas.

B. Renal vascular hypertension

1. **Mechanisms of hypertension.** Renal ischemia due to diseases of the major renal vessels may cause hypertension by several mechanisms. When one kidney is involved, inappropriately high levels of circulating angiotensin II result in an increase in total peripheral resistance. This is the major mechanism of the hypertension. Cardiac output is typically normal but may be somewhat high or low, depending on the state of extracellular volume. When both major renal arteries are stenotic, hypertension results primarily from expansion of extracellular volume and is similar to that seen with renal parenchymal disease (discussed below).

2. **Clinical picture.** There are usually no specific symptoms, but the patient may have pain and hematuria if there are renal infarcts. There is an abdominal bruit in about 50 percent of patients. The bruit results from turbulent flow through the narrowed artery. The diagnosis is made by the demonstration on angiogram of a narrowing of a renal artery and the functional significance of the stenosis is confirmed by the demonstration of increased renin concentration in the venous effluent of the kidney involved.

C. Primary aldosteronism

1. **Mechanisms of hypertension.** Primary aldosteronism is caused by an adrenal adenoma or bilateral adrenal hyperplasia, resulting in autonomous secretion of excessive amounts of aldosterone. The aldosterone excess, in turn, causes sodium retention, resulting in expansion of extracellular fluid volume. Consequently, cardiac output increases, although some patients with longstanding primary aldosteronism have a normal cardiac output. There is also typically an increase in total peripheral resistance. The mechanism is not clear, but it probably reflects a secondary neurogenic adjustment to the elevated cardiac output.

2. **Clinical picture.** There are usually no symptoms but some patients may have muscle weakness, paresthesias, and urinary frequency due to urinary potassium wastage and resultant hypokalemia.

V. Renal hypertension.

Renal hypertension is the most common form of secondary hypertension, but unlike the other secondary forms outlined above, it is usually not curable.

A. **Mechanisms of hypertension.** In most patients (90%) with renal parenchymal disease, hypertension is caused by an increase in extracellular fluid volume due to impairment of renal sodium excretion. An increased cardiac output results, and this may lead to a secondary increase in total peripheral resistance. Control of extracellular fluid volume by diuretic or dialysis therapy usually controls the hypertension, demonstrating the importance of "volume." However, about 10 percent of patients have a renin-dependent hypertension. Here, the extracellular fluid volume and cardiac output are normal or low. Renin-inhibiting drugs and vasodilators, or in some cases bilateral nephrectomy, may be needed to control the hypertension. There is some evidence to support a deficiency of vasodilators (prostaglandins or neutral lipids), and as a consequence, an increase in TPR unrelated to angiotensin II may play a role in renal hypertension.

B. **Clinical picture.** Uremia commonly dominates the clinical picture. The diagnosis is established by a markedly elevated serum creatinine and a greatly reduced glomerular filtration rate (GFR) (usually less than 15 ml/min). The urinary sediment is usually abnormal. Some

Table 16-2   *Typical Hemodynamic Features of Essential Hypertension*

Early hypertension
  Normal TPR
  Increased CO
Established hypertension
  Increased TPR
  Normal CO
Advanced hypertension
  Increased TPR
  Low CO

CO = cardiac output; TPR = total peripheral resistance.

patients with early polycystic kidney disease and some types of glomerulonephritis become hypertensive before they develop a marked impairment of renal function.

VI. Essential ("idiopathic") hypertension. We do not know the cause of the most common type of hypertension in man and understand far less of its pathophysiology than that of endocrine or renal hypertension. Steroids, catecholamines, renin, and subtle renal abnormalities have been implicated at various times but never proved to be causes. Excess sodium intake is probably a contributing factor in most cases, but it is not the basic cause of essential hypertension.

  A. Mechanisms of essential hypertension. The current major theories (all of which are speculative) of the mechanisms of essential hypertension include: (1) an abnormality of the renal-body fluid pressure control mechanism that normally regulates the amount of sodium excreted as a function of arterial pressure, (2) increased vascular reactivity, (3) increased central nervous system sympathetic outflow, (4) increased or inappropriate activity of the adrenal cortex, and (5) decreased activity of vasodepressor systems.

  The hemodynamic features of essential hypertension are variable, depending on the stage of the hypertensive disorder (Table 16-2).

  The mechanism of evolution of these hemodynamic changes is unknown. Many investigators believe that increased cardiac output, which occurs early in the course of essential hypertension, is the abnormality that triggers the increase in TPR. The cause of the increased cardiac output is unknown.

  B. Clinical features. There are usually no symptoms. It has been called the silent disease. Symptoms do not appear until damage to the kidney, heart, or brain (target organs) is sufficiently extensive to cause renal failure, congestive heart failure, or a stroke.

VII. Clinical example of hypertension

  A. Description. A 52-year-old woman had mild essential hypertension for 20 years. Until 12 months ago, her elevated blood pressure responded well to sodium restriction and diuretics; but since then, her blood pressure has been difficult to control and rather large doses of clonidine and hydralazine are now required. She had been treated for menopausal symptoms (flushing, sweating, anxiety) with Premarin (conjugated estrogens) for 1½ years. At examination, her blood pressure was 180/110 mm Hg recumbent and 160/90 mm Hg standing. Funduscopic exam revealed marked arteriolar narrowing. A systolic bruit was heard in the epigastrium. She had an elevated serum creatinine (3.4 mg/dl) and 1+ proteinuria. An intravenous pyelogram revealed that the pole-to-pole length of the right kidney was 3 cm less than the left.

B. Discussion

1. The patient's blood pressure was readily controlled for several years but then became resistant to therapy. This clinical course suggests that a secondary form of hypertension has developed.

2. Premarin (a type of estrogen preparation) was begun 6 months before the increase in the patient's blood pressure. Estrogens can cause or worsen hypertension, in part, by increasing the activity of the renin-angiotensin system. When the Premarin was discontinued, the patient's blood pressure control improved, but she still required multiple drugs.

3. Some menopausal symptoms are similar to those caused by a pheochromocytoma. A marked postural fall in blood pressure is frequently seen in patients with a pheochromocytoma. Therefore, plasma catecholamine levels were measured, but they were normal. The postural change in blood pressure was, therefore, probably due to clonidine.

4. The epigastric bruit and difference in kidney size suggested the patient had renal artery stenosis. A renal arteriogram did reveal a marked narrowing of the right renal artery near its origin.

5. The rather high serum creatinine suggested that there was an abnormality in the function of both kidneys. Indeed, the renal arteriogram showed narrowing of the smaller arteries of both kidneys, suggesting nephrosclerosis from her longstanding hypertension.

6. The right renal venous renin content was three times higher than the left, which indicated that the stenosis of the right renal artery was functionally significant.

7. The stenosis was surgically bypassed and within a week her blood pressure was 146/94; since then, only a diuretic has been required to maintain her blood pressure below 140/90.

8. Her serum creatinine decreased to 1.6 mg/dl following the bypass and has remained stable with better control of her blood pressure and improved perfusion of the right kidney.

Questions

Select the single best answer.

1. Which of the following cause exacerbation of previously well-controlled longstanding essential hypertension?
   a. Damage to the renal vasculature.
   b. Increased sodium intake.
   c. Acceleration of atherosclerosis.
   d. Superimposed secondary forms of hypertension.
   e. All of the above.

2. Select the correct statement concerning essential hypertension.
   a. The etiology and pathophysiology are known.
   b. Sodium intake of patients with essential hypertension exceeds that of normotensive patients and is the cause of essential hypertension.
   c. The sympathetic nervous system is overactive in all patients with essential hypertension.
   d. Total peripheral resistance may be normal or increased.
   e. None of the above is correct.

17 Diabetes Mellitus and Glucose Metabolism

I. **Review of normal physiology**
   A. **Actions of insulin.** The effects of insulin on cellular metabolism are manifested by changes in carbohydrate, protein, and fat metabolism. Insulin stimulates glucose transport across cell membranes, increases hepatic glycogen synthesis, and inhibits glucose formation from glycogen (glycogenolysis) and from amino acid precursors (gluconeogenesis). The result of all these actions is a decrease in blood glucose. It also promotes the transfer of amino acids across plasma membranes, stimulates protein synthesis, and inhibits proteolysis.

   It markedly increases the incorporation of fatty acids into adipose triglyceride, stimulates lipid synthesis, and inhibits lipolysis. The net result of these actions is to increase the availability of substrate and nutrients for cellular metabolism.

   B. **Secretion of insulin.** Insulin is formed in the beta cells of the pancreas from its precursor, proinsulin. Proinsulin consists of three connected peptide chains designated as alpha, beta, and the connecting peptide (C-peptide). Prior to release, the connecting peptide is split off from the alpha and beta chains and is secreted concurrently with the insulin molecule as a discrete peptide. Because commercial insulin preparations consist of only the alpha and beta chains and contain little if any C-peptide, the presence of connecting peptide in the circulation can be used as an index of endogenous insulin secretion.

   C. **Mechanism of action.** Insulin initiates its action by binding to a specific receptor located on the plasma membrane of responsive tissues. These receptors normally exist in great numbers on responsive cells, and insulin effects are produced when a relatively small number are occupied.

   Acting through unidentified second messengers, the insulin-receptor complex causes glucose to be transported across the cell membrane and to be metabolized to $CO_2 + H_2O$, yielding energy in the process. The effects on lipolysis are mediated by inhibition of adenyl cyclase. Those effects on amino acid transfer are less well understood and may involve a post-membrane intracellular effect of the insulin molecule.

   D. **Other hormones involved in glucose homeostasis.** By various mechanisms the counter-regulatory hormones, including glucagon, growth hormone, cortisol, and epinephrine, all antagonize the effect of insulin. These include changes in hepatic glucose production and glycogen storage, as well as changes in end-organ sensitivity to insulin action.

   Gastrointestinal hormones may stimulate insulin release after a meal. Gut glucagon appears to be particularly important in enhancing insulin release. Somatostatin inhibits both insulin and glucagon production. In patients with absent insulin production, the inhibition of glucagon may result in the lowering of the blood sugar. It has potentially important pathophysiologic and therapeutic implications.

II. **Pathophysiology of diabetes mellitus**
   A. **Insulin dependent diabetes mellitus (type I diabetes, IDDM).** This

ketosis-prone diabetes was formerly known as juvenile diabetes, a term which has been abandoned because older individuals may also develop diabetes due to deficient insulin production and because some individuals develop insulin-resistant diabetes during childhood or teenage years. The basic defect in this type of diabetes is inadequate insulin production by the pancreatic cells. The genetics of IDDM are complex, but there is an increased incidence in those with HLA 8 and HLA BW 15 loci. Because the concordance rate of this type of diabetes is relatively low in twins, however, environmental factors are also at play; they may include exposure to certain viral infections, such as mumps, measles, and Coxsackie viruses. One hypothesis suggests that a viral infection or the sequelae of such an infection may produce insulin deficiency in a patient whose pancreatic islet cells are genetically more susceptible to such damage.

B. **Non–insulin-dependent diabetes mellitus (type II diabetes, NIDDM).** This type of diabetes was formerly called adult-onset diabetes, but can occur at any age. The basic defect in this type of diabetes is resistance to the action of insulin. Many patients have normal or even elevated insulin levels, although some exhibit a delay in the release of insulin after meals. Individuals seem to inherit a susceptibility for this type of diabetes; the disease is expressed in mid-life, especially if a susceptible subject becomes obese. Both obese individuals with mild impairment of carbohydrate tolerance and patients with NIDDM have decreased numbers of available insulin receptors; this plays some role in their insulin resistance. There are also postreceptor defects, characterized by inadequate transport of glucose across cell membranes and inadequate metabolism of glucose within cells. The nature of these postreceptor defects has not been fully elucidated.

III. **Clinical picture**
  A. **Signs and symptoms**
    1. Patients with IDDM (type I) often present in ketoacidosis, generally following a brief period of symptoms as in NIDDM.
    2. Patients with NIDDM (type II) experience polydipsia, polyuria, fatigue, and weight loss.
  B. **The diagnosis** is established by finding consistent elevations in either fasting (>140 mg/dl) or postprandial blood glucose (>210 mg/dl).
    1. Formal glucose tolerance tests are rarely indicated.
    2. Although not an established approach, some favor the use of hemoglobin A_{1c} as a screening test (see Treatment).
  C. **Treatment (general principles)**
    1. In IDDM (type I), insulin therapy is indicated and may require more than one injection daily to achieve optimal control of blood sugar.
    2. In NIDDM (type II), diet is the cornerstone of therapy. If dietary measures fail, oral hypoglycemic agents or insulin may be employed to keep blood sugars in a manageable range.
  D. **Complications.** Most of the complications of diabetes are mediated through changes in small blood vessels supplying the eyes, kidneys, and nerves. The pathophysiology of these lesions is still being debated, but may involve glycosylation of proteins on a mass action basis, which alters the structure and metabolic function of the proteins. Hemoglobin A_{1c} is an example of this phenomenon. Clinically, the complications of diabetes are expressed as retinopathy and decreased vision, peripheral vascular disease, proteinuria, hypertension, neuropathy,

and peripheral vascular disease. Evidence is accumulating that in IDDM complications may be prevented or retarded by good control of blood sugar. Similar data are not yet available for NIDDM.

IV. Diabetic ketoacidosis

A. Pathophysiology.
Insulin deficiency leads to increased lipolysis, causing an increase in the free fatty acid concentration in plasma. As a result, the liver increases ketogenesis.

Glucagon excess contributes to ketosis by activating acyl carnitine transferase. This enzyme is important in the transfer of fatty acids into the mitochondria, where ketones are formed. Ketones are important, since during starvation they may provide energy for all the body, including the brain. The ketones that are formed are beta-hydroxybutyric acid (BHB), acetoacetic acid (AAA), and acetone. Acetone is volatile and results in the characteristic fruity smell of the breath during ketoacidosis and occasionally during starvation. It is not acid and therefore does not contribute to the acidosis.

In ketoacidosis there is a change in the redox state of the body. The redox pairs are reduced, favoring production of BHB over AAA. However, the test to determine the amount of ketones in the plasma, the nitroprusside reaction, responds only to AAA. Therefore, since BHB is more abundant than AAA, the amount of ketones shown by the nitroprusside reaction can be low, even in severe ketoacidosis. Upon successful treatment of ketoacidosis, the redox state returns to normal; BHB is converted back into AAA and then metabolized. Hence, the nitroprusside reaction may increase before decreasing, even though the ketoacidosis is steadily improving.

The hyperglycemic state of ketoacidosis causes an osmotic diuresis by the kidneys. There is loss not only of water but also of electrolytes. The hyperglycemia and the water loss cause the blood to be hyperosmotic, the degree of which can be estimated by using the equation:

$$\text{Blood osmolarity} = \frac{\text{Blood sugar}}{18} + 2\,(\text{Na}^+) + \frac{\text{BUN}}{2.8}$$

B. Treatment.
Treatment of diabetic ketoacidosis is based on knowledge of the pathophysiology; hence, the basic principles of therapy will be outlined.

1. **Sodium and water replacement.** Isotonic saline is needed rapidly to correct the extracellular fluid depletion and to maintain blood pressure. Total deficits of 5 to 8 L of H_2O and 350 to 500 mEq of sodium are frequently encountered.

2. **Insulin replacement.** Small doses should be administered continually or every hour so as to maintain serum insulin levels of 100 μU/ml. Adipocyte release of free fatty acids is inhibited, thus removing the substrate for ketone production.

3. **Potassium replacement.** Due to the ketoacidosis, there is an intracellular K^+ depletion which may exceed 120 to 400 mEq. Upon insulin administration, glucose and K^+ migrate into the intracellular compartment. K^+ must be replaced to prevent arrhythmias and other consequences of the resulting hypokalemia. This phenomenon may occur within 2 to 3 hr after insulin therapy.

4. **Phosphate replacement.** Phosphate depletion is common and results from the osmotic diuresis that usually occurs. Phosphate de-

pletion leads to a decrease in red cell 2,3-diphosphoglycerate (2,3-DPG). This decrease in 2,3-DPG causes hemoglobin to have a greater affinity for oxygen. During ketoacidosis this is not a problem because acidosis allows for oxygen to go into the tissues (Bohr effect), while a decrease in 2,3-DPG does the opposite. However, when the ketoacidosis is treated successfully, the 2,3-DPG deficiency tends to decrease the availability of O_2 to the tissue. Phosphate can be given in the potassium phosphate form to correct the problem.

5. **Glucose administration.** When the blood sugar falls below 250 to 300 mg/dl, glucose should be added to the intravenous fluids, since there is relatively little stored glucose in the body to provide substrate for cellular function.

6. **Further treatment.** Any underlying infection or disease that may precipitate or worsen the ketoacidosis should be sought and treated.

V. **Clinical example of impaired carbohydrate tolerance**

A. **Description.** A 54-year-old man had a 2-day history of fever and a productive cough. On physical examination, he was found to have rales in his right lower lung field, and a chest x-ray confirmed the presence of pneumonia. Some routine laboratory tests were ordered, and the patient was admitted to the hospital for treatment.

During more detailed questioning, the patient admitted to a mild decrease in energy for the past several months and stated that he had been getting up two or three times a night to urinate. Both his mother and his paternal grandfather had developed diabetes during middle age. The patient was 5 ft 10 in. tall and weighed 195 pounds.

B. **Laboratory values** were blood urea nitrogen (BUN), 25; sodium, 132; potassium, 4.5; chloride, 97; bicarbonate, 30; and glucose, 585.

C. **Discussion**

1. The patient probably inherited a susceptibility to non–insulin-dependent diabetes.

2. Because of his obesity, he probably has a decrease in the number of available insulin receptors.

3. The stress associated with his pneumonia has been accompanied by a rise in counter-regulatory hormones such as cortisol epinephrine and has increased his insulin resistance.

4. Until his pneumonia improves, it may be necessary to administer insulin to prevent the development of dangerously high levels of blood glucose or of ketoacidosis.

5. After his pneumonia has resolved, his blood glucose may fall dramatically, perhaps even to normal values.

6. Weight reduction will be of crucial importance either to treat his diabetes if his blood sugar remains high after the resolution of this pneumonia or to prevent the future development of overt diabetes if his blood sugar falls to normal after the resolution of pneumonia.

7. While his mildly elevated BUN might be due to diabetic nephropathy, it was probably caused by volume depletion secondary to heavy glycosuria and resulting osmotic diuresis.

8. The low serum sodium concentration is the result of the high level of blood sugar, which has drawn water into the extracellular space and diluted the sodium, lowering its concentration.

9. The fact that this patient has a rather severe elevation of blood

sugar but was not in ketoacidosis underscores the fact that patients with non–insulin-dependent diabetes are resistant to the development of ketoacidosis.

Questions

Select the single best answer.

1. Choose the *least* appropriate statement regarding the pathophysiology of non–insulin-dependent mellitus.
   a. A decrease in the number of insulin receptors contributes to the insulin resistance seen in this type of diabetes.
   b. Patients will have no measurable blood levels on connecting peptide.
   c. Patients inherit a susceptibility for this type of diabetes even though the disease may not be manifested until after the age of 40.
   d. Basal insulin secretion may be normal or increased, but there is often a subnormal or delayed rise in insulin after meals.
   e. This type of diabetes can occur at any age.
2. Which one of the following is *not* a part of the pathophysiology of diabetic ketoacidosis?
   a. Lipolysis with liberation of free fatty acids into the circulation.
   b. Oxidation of glucose to ketone bodies in the liver.
   c. Osmotic diuresis resulting in sodium and water depletion.
   d. Enhanced gluconeogenesis.
   e. Failure of glucose to be transported inside cells.

Reproductive Endocrinology

I. Introduction. The gonads, the testes in the male or the ovaries in the female, are paired organs that possess two primary functions. The first function is gametogenesis, which involves production of spermatozoa in the testis or release of an ovum from the ovary. The second function of the gonads is the production of sex hormones necessary for normal secondary sexual characteristics. Although the testes and ovaries will be considered separately, it is important to realize the parallel function of the gonads in the two sexes.

II. The testes

A. Normal testicular function

1. **Spermatogenesis** occurs within the seminiferous tubules of the testes in response to follicle-stimulating hormone (FSH) secreted by the pituitary, although the local production of testosterone is also necessary for both initiation and maintenance of the process. FSH binds to the Sertoli cells, which along with the germinal epithelium or spermatogonia line the seminiferous tubules. The spermatogonia then undergo a number of transformations, from spermatocytes to spermatids and finally to spermatozoa, a process that takes approximately 70 days to complete. The Sertoli cells not only act as a receptor for FSH, but also nourish the developing spermatozoa and produce a protein known as inhibin, which feeds back to the pituitary to inhibit FSH production.

2. **Testosterone** is a steroid hormone necessary for maintenance of normal male secondary sexual characteristics. Testosterone production occurs in the Leydig cells, located between the seminiferous tubules within the testes, in response to luteinizing hormone (LH) produced by the anterior pituitary. The biosynthetic process begins with cholesterol, which undergoes a number of metabolic conversions to yield testosterone and smaller amounts of the weak androgens, dehydroepiandrosterone (DHEA), and androstenedione. LH secretion by the pituitary is regulated through feedback inhibition by circulating testosterone.

B. Testicular dysfunction.

1. **General.** Testicular dysfunction results in hypogonadism, which may be either primary or secondary. In primary hypogonadism, the defect lies in the Leydig cell, the seminiferous tubules, or both; it is associated with elevated gonadotropins (FSH and LH). In secondary hypogonadism, the Leydig cells and seminiferous tubules are normal, but fail to function normally, due to low levels of FSH, LH, or both. Some of the more common causes of hypogonadism are discussed in the following paragraphs.

2. **Primary hypogonadism.** Klinefelter's syndrome is an extremely common cause of primary hypogonadism affecting approximately 1 in 500 males. Klinefelter's syndrome results from a 47 XXY karyotype and is characterized by a eunuchoidal body habitus, gynecomastia, and small firm testes. Both spermatogenesis and testosterone production are impaired due to the testicular involvement.

Reifenstein's syndrome is an X-linked recessive disorder characterized by a normal 46 XY karyotype, but with clinical features similar to those of Klinefelter's syndrome, with hypospadias and incomplete virilization. Laboratory studies usually reveal an elevated LH level with normal or even elevated levels of testosterone. The syndrome is due to a defect in testosterone receptors leading to partial androgen insensitivity.

Viral orchitis, usually due to mumps, is a relatively common cause of testicular failure. Involvement may be bilateral or unilateral and usually affects the seminiferous tubules, leading to decreased spermatogenesis, although in severe cases testosterone production may be impaired as well. Clinical evidence of hypogonadism may require several years to develop following the viral infection.

Sertoli-cell-only syndrome is an unusual disease characterized by complete absence of the germinal epithelium within the seminiferous tubules, resulting in completely absent spermatogenesis and elevated FSH levels. The Leydig cells are not involved, and serum testosterone and LH are usually normal.

3. **Secondary hypogonadism.** Kallman's syndrome is characterized by a eunuchoidal body habitus, gynecomastia, and small testes, in association with anosmia (inability to smell) and low levels of FSH and LH. The syndrome is usually familial, with an autosomal dominant inheritance pattern, and appears to be the result of absent gonadotropin-releasing hormone production by the hypothalamus.

Hypopituitarism—which may result from a number of conditions including pituitary tumors, surgery, radiation, or trauma—leads to secondary hypogonadism due to the absence of FSH and LH production. In rare instances, an isolated deficiency of LH or FSH has been demonstrated.

C. **Therapy for testicular dysfunction**

1. **Testosterone production.** When testosterone production is subnormal, therapy with either oral or intramuscular testosterone will result in maintenance of normal libido and secondary sexual characteristics.

2. **Fertility.** When subnormal spermatogenesis is the result of primary hypogonadism, little can be done to enhance fertility. However, when decreased spermatogenesis is due to secondary hypogonadism, the administration of exogenous gonadotropins, gonadotropin-releasing hormone, or clomiphene, which causes an increase in endogenous gonadotropin, often results in improved spermatogenesis and fertility.

III. **Ovaries**

A. **Normal ovarian function**

1. **The two major functions** of the ovaries, like those of the testes, are reproduction and sex hormone production. Normally, ovulation occurs at approximately day 14 of the 28-day menstrual cycle. During the early part of the cycle, an ovarian follicle enlarges and produces estrogen, which triggers the midcycle surge in LH and FSH that is responsible for rupture of the follicle and release of the ovum. During the latter half of the cycle, the ruptured follicle develops into a corpus luteum, producing large amounts of progesterone and leading to development of a secretory endometrium that will allow implantation to occur if the ovum is fertilized. If fertilization and implantation occur, human chorionic gonadotropin (HCG) produced by the trophoblastic tissue maintains the corpus luteum. However, if fertilization does not occur, the corpus luteum

involutes, progesterone production ceases, and the endometrium is shed, thereby initiating a new cycle.

2. **Estrogen** is the hormone responsible for maintenance of normal secondary sexual characteristics in the female; it is produced primarily by the granulosa and theca cells of the ovarian follicles in response to LH. Estrogen production follows the same biosynthetic pathway as testosterone in the male, but an additional step in the female converts testosterone and other weak androgens into the potent estrogen, estradiol, and the weaker estrogen, estrone.

B. **Ovarian dysfunction**

1. **General.** Ovarian dysfunction may lead to several clinical syndromes in the female. If estrogen production is subnormal due to an ovarian lesion or pituitary disease with low FSH and LH, the result is a loss of normal secondary sexual characteristics. Like testosterone underproduction in the male, this situation is referred to as primary or secondary hypogonadism or ovarian failure, depending on the site of involvement. Another common syndrome in the female is excessive production of the estrogen precursors, testosterone and androstenedione, which because of their androgenic properties may lead to excessive hair growth or virilization. Infertility in the female may be due to an anatomic defect such as obstruction of the fallopian tubes; however, it is often the result of anovulation, which may be due to either estrogen deficiency or androgen excess, resulting in a disturbance of cyclic ovarian function. The loss of cyclic ovarian function may also be associated with absent menses (amenorrhea). These common syndromes of ovarian dysfunction are discussed in more detail in the following paragraphs.

2. **Estrogen deficiency.** Primary ovarian failure is associated with subnormal estrogen production and elevated gonadotropins. This clinical picture is normally seen at the time of the menopause, when ovarian function decreases, but earlier it is an abnormal occurrence. Primary ovarian failure may be the result of a congenital defect in gonadal development, such as in Turner's syndrome, characterized by a 45 XO karyotype, short stature, and gonadal dysgenesis, or an acquired defect of the ovaries, such as surgical removal, radiation damage, or idiopathic ovarian failure due to autoimmune disease.

   Secondary ovarian failure is associated with normal ovaries; however, there is loss of cyclic function and estrogen production, due to low or absent gonadotropins. Secondary ovarian failure may be due to any destructive lesion of the pituitary or hypothalamus, such as pituitary tumor, surgery, or infiltrative disease. A unique cause of secondary hypogonadism in the female is Sheehan's syndrome, or postpartum pituitary necrosis resulting from infarction of the pituitary during delivery. An elevation of serum prolactin—due to drug ingestion, a pituitary lesion, or idiopathic causes—may also result in secondary ovarian failure due to the interference of gonadotropin secretion and action by the elevated prolactin.

3. **Androgen excess.** Androgen excess in the female is usually associated with hirsutism and menstrual disturbances, but when severe may cause actual virilization of the female patient. The large majority of cases of androgen excess in the female are due to ovarian androgen overproduction, but some cases are the result of adrenal androgen excess. Women who show signs of ovarian androgen ex-

cess without enlargement of the ovaries are said to have idiopathic hirsutism. This is an extremely common disorder, which in most cases probably represents a mild form of the polycystic ovary syndrome. Polycystic ovary syndrome is characterized by enlarged cystic ovaries, androgen excess, infertility, and menstrual disturbances. Although the exact etiology of polycystic ovary syndrome is not well understood, it is associated with increased pituitary LH production, which stimulates the ovarian overproduction of testosterone and androstenedione. FSH release is suppressed by these androgens, leading to follicular atresia and anovulation. Androstenedione is peripherally converted to the weak estrogen, estrone; by a positive feedback mechanism, this results in further pituitary LH production, leading to continuation of the syndrome. In rare cases, androgen excess may be the result of an ovarian tumor.

4. **Infertility.** Infertility due to absence of the normal cyclic ovarian release of a mature ovum (anovulation) is a common clinical problem in the female; it may result from any of the previously discussed abnormalities of ovarian function—either primary or secondary ovarian failure with decreased estrogen production, idiopathic hirsutism, or polycystic ovary syndrome with increased androgen production. Usually anovulation is associated with irregular or absent menses. Clinically, the determination of ovulation is made by demonstration of the biologic effects of progesterone produced by the corpus luteum after ovulation has occurred. These effects of progesterone include a rise in basal body temperature, development of a secretory endometrium, and an alteration of the cervical mucus.

C. **Therapy for ovarian dysfunction**

1. **Estrogen production.** When estrogen production is subnormal, therapy with estrogens administered orally, intramuscularly, or even topically will result in maintenance of the normal female secondary sexual characteristics.

2. **Androgen excess.** Treatment of ovarian androgen overproduction involves suppression of pituitary LH by oral contraceptives, resulting in decreased ovarian androgen production, or the use of direct androgen antagonists such as spironolactone. When androgen excess is the result of an ovarian tumor, treatment is obviously surgical.

3. **Infertility.** When anovulation is the result of a destructive lesion of the ovaries, little can be done to return fertility to the female patient. However, when anovulation is the result of a hypothalamic-pituitary disturbance or ovarian androgen overproduction associated with increased LH, ovulation can often be induced by the administration of clomiphene, which triggers a rise in both FSH and LH, leading to follicular maturation and ovulation. In patients who do not respond to clomiphene, the administration of human FSH and LH may be utilized to stimulate ovulation.

Finally, when anovulation is associated with elevated prolactin levels, the use of bromocriptine to reduce prolactin levels may result in the return of normal ovulatory cycles.

IV. **Clinical example of Klinefelter's syndrome**

A. **Description.** A 19-year-old white male complained of bilateral, painless breast enlargement. There was no past history of drug ingestion, marijuana use, or testicular trauma. Physical examination revealed a tall, thin white male in apparent good health. Facial hair was sparse, and bilateral subareolar breast tissue was palpable. Examination of the genitalia revealed normal penile development with small firm testes measuring 2.0 cm in their greatest dimension.

B. Laboratory evaluation revealed a serum testosterone of 320 ng/dl (normal, 400–1,000) with an FSH of 48 (normal, 5–30) and LH of 36 (normal, 5–20).

C. Discussion

1. This patient demonstrated the classic manifestations of Klinefelter's syndrome. Additionally, semen analysis usually reveals absent spermatozoa (azoospermia).

2. Histologically, the syndrome is characterized by dysgenesis of the seminiferous tubules, leading to tubular hyalinization and fibrosis with clumping of the Leydig cells.

3. The fundamental defect is the presence of an extra X chromosome in a male, resulting in a 47 XXY karyotype. This is usually due to chromosomal nondisjunction during meiosis, producing a gamete containing a 24-chromosome complement.

4. The diagnosis is based on the demonstration of the extra X chromosome. Usually a chromatin-positive buccal smear is adequate, but confirmation can be made by conventional karyotyping.

5. Treatment consists of testosterone replacement in patients who demonstrate evidence of androgen deficiency. If gynecomastia is severe or psychologically disturbing, surgical reduction may be indicated.

Questions

Select the single best answer.

1. Infertility in the female due to anovulation may be the result of which of the following?
   a. Decreased pituitary production of FSH and LH.
   b. Increased pituitary production of prolactin.
   c. Decreased ovarian production of estrogens.
   d. Increased ovarian production of androgens.
   e. All of the above.

2. Androgen deficiency in the male results in a loss of normal secondary sexual characteristics and may be due to all of the following except:
   a. Decreased pituitary production of LH.
   b. A destructive lesion of the Leydig cells.
   c. Congenital absence of spermatogonia (Sertoli-cell-only syndrome).
   d. A defect in testosterone receptors (partial androgen insensitivity).

IV Gastroenterology

Robert A. Rankin
Jack D. Welsh

19 The Esophagus

I. **Functional anatomy.** The cricopharyngeus (upper esophageal sphincter), which is the lowermost segment of the inferior pharyngeal constrictor, denotes the beginning of the esophagus. The body of the esophagus is a cylindrical, distensible tube that extends from the cricopharyngeus through the posterior mediastinum to the stomach. The aortic arch, the left main stem bronchus, and the left atrium are all in close proximity to the esophagus.

   The lumen of the esophagus is lined with squamous epithelium throughout its course. The upper one-fourth is striated muscle and the lower one-third is smooth muscle, with variations, but no intermixing, in between. No serosa is present; thus, there is no containment mechanism for the spread of cancer. The lower esophageal sphincter (LES) is poorly defined histologically, but is well defined functionally and pharmacologically. It consists of a specialized segment of circular, smooth muscle in the terminal 2 to 4 cm of the esophagus. It is located at the gastroesophageal junction, where squamous epithelium of the esophagus changes to columnar epithelium of the stomach.

II. **Physiology**

   A. **Normal swallowing.** There are three major components of swallowing. The oropharyngeal component begins with a well-coordinated sequence of events, including pushing the bolus of food to the back of the throat with the tongue, coupled with cricopharyngeal relaxation. The cricopharyngeal muscle has a normal resting pressure of 50 to 100 mm Hg, which decreases to less than 5 mm Hg during the swallowing process. The body of the esophagus has a normal resting pressure that is subatmospheric, a reflection of the intrathoracic pressure. Three patterns of pressure changes can be seen within the body of the esophagus: (1) a primary wave is a peristaltic stripping wave initiated by swallowing; (2) a secondary wave is a peristaltic wave initiated by distension of the esophagus and not preceded by a swallow; and (3) a tertiary wave is a nonpropulsive contraction of most of the esophagus at the same time. Tertiary waves can be seen in normals and are not considered abnormal unless they occur frequently.

   The LES has a normal resting pressure of 15 to 30 mm Hg. It appears to be mediated by inhibitory influences carried in undefined extravagal pathways. It relaxes as the cricopharyngeus opens and remains open until the peristaltic wave has reached the lower esophageal sphincter. Esophageal distension, by causing a secondary wave, will also cause relaxation of the LES.

   B. **Mechanisms for maintenance of normal LES resting pressure.** There are numerous mechanisms for maintenance of the LES resting pressure that limit reflux of gastric contents into the esophagus. Both mechanical and structural factors are important. The phrenoesophageal ligaments help hold the LES in position. The diaphragmatic opening normally limits just how far the LES can open. The acute angle of entry of the esophagus into the stomach results in a mucosal flap valve that helps prevent reflux of gastric material. The intraabdominal pressure, a positive pressure, surrounds the subdiaphragmatic portion of the LES. Since the thoracic pressure is negative, this pressure difference helps to keep the LES closed.

Table 19-1   *Agents That Alter Basal LES Pressure*

Increase Pressure	Decrease Pressure
Autonomic Agents	
Cholinergic (muscarinic) agents (bethanechol)	Cholinergic (nicotinic) agent (nicotine)
Alpha-adrenergic agonists (phenylephrine, norepinephrine)	Beta-adrenergic agonists (epinephrine, isoproterenol)
Anticholinesterase (edrophonium)	Alpha-adrenergic antagonists (phentolamine)
	Anticholinergics (atropine)
	Dopamine
*Hormones**	
Gastrin and pentagastrin	Secretin
Motilin	Cholecystokinin
Bombesin	Glucagon
Prostaglandin F_2	GIP and VIP
	Prostaglandins E_1, E_2, A_2
	Progesterone and estrogen
Others	
Histamine (through H1 receptor)	Histamine (through H2 receptor)
Gastric alkalinization	Nitrites and nitrates
Metoclopramide	Caffeine
Protein meal	Fatty meal
	Theophylline
	Chocolate
	Ethanol (high dose)
	Sedatives
	Peppermint

*These hormones have been shown to affect the LES in pharmacologic doses, not in physiologic doses.

GIP = gastric inhibitory peptide; LES = lower esophageal sphincter; VIP = vasoactive intestinal peptide.

Source: Reproduced with permission from J. R. Meadows, *Sophomore Introduction to Medicine*, Gastroenterology Section, Department of Medicine, Indiana University School of Medicine, 1978, p. 105.

Intrinsic myogenic activity of the sphincteric smooth muscle is probably the most important factor in maintenance of LES pressure. Control of myogenic activity is poorly understood and probably represents the interplay between hormones and neural mechanisms. Agents, including medications and some foods, that affect the LES do so primarily by influencing myogenic tone (Table 19-1).

III. Signs and symptoms of esophageal problems

A. Dysphagia (difficulty in swallowing)

1. **Oropharyngeal dysphagia** can occur secondary to a pharyngeal motor problem (such as a neurological or muscular disease) or from a hypopharyngeal mass. If incoordination of cricopharyngeal relaxation occurs, a hypopharyngeal outpouching (called Zenker's diverticulum) can be caused by the effects of swallowing pressure on the left hypopharyngeal wall. In patients with oropharyngeal dysphagia, liquids often cause as many problems as solid foods do, if not more. Tracheal aspiration as well as regurgitation through the nose may result.

2. **Esophageal dysphagia** may be due to motor abnormalities, masses, or strictures of the body of the esophagus or of the LES area.

Figure 19-1

Possible mechanism for symptoms in reflux esophagitis.

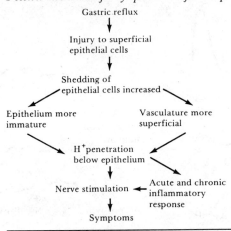

Failure of the LES to relax during the swallowing process often results in the sensation of dysphagia. Solids, especially meats, usually cause the most difficulty. When chest pain is associated with difficulty in swallowing, it is called odynophagia.

3. **Globus hystericus** is a condition in which the patient feels as though there were a lump in the lower pharynx or at the base of the tongue. It is thought to be a psychogenic problem since no motor abnormalities are noted on testing. The mechanism is unknown.

B. **Pain.** Heartburn (pyrosis) is a substernal burning sensation usually associated with reflux of acid contents from the stomach into the esophagus. The same symptoms can be caused by reflux of bile into the esophagus, but this is much less common. The exact mechanism of pain is not completely understood, but a reasonable possibility is shown in Figure 19-1.

Chest pain not related to reflux esophagitis may also arise from either esophageal spasm or acute distension of the esophagus. It can be unusually severe and may mimic angina pectoris or myocardial infarction.

IV. **Tools available for the study of the esophagus.** Although the history and the physical examination are basic, more specific tests can directly document the pathophysiology of the esophagus. Barium contrast radiography and esophagoscopy can be done to look for specific pathology in the esophagus. In addition, esophageal manometry, intraesophageal pH monitoring, and acid perfusion studies of the esophagus can demonstrate disturbances of function. Esophageal manometry utilizes pressure transducers to show whether or not the swallows progress in an orderly manner down the esophagus, what the pressure is in the lower esophageal sphincter, and whether or not the LES relaxes appropriately with swallowing. Intraesophageal pH monitoring can be done to check for frequency of acid reflux into the esophagus. The acid perfusion study (Bernstein study) is performed by dripping normal saline, alternating with 0.1 N hydrochloric acid, into the esophagus. Reproduction of the patient's symptoms with acid suggests that they are due to acid reflux.

V. **Some common diseases of the esophagus**

A. **Motor disorders (Fig. 19-2)**

1. **Achalasia** is characterized by low-amplitude tertiary waves without peristaltic activity, increased LES pressure, and failure of the LES to relax with swallowing. Its exact etiology is unknown, but the mechanism is thought to involve vagal denervation of the esopha-

Figure 19-2 *Some common motor disorders of the esophagus.*

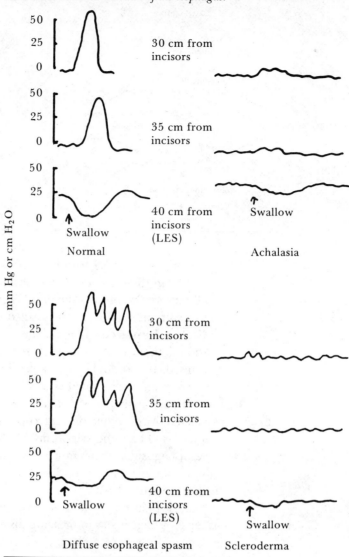

gus. As a result, there is marked dilatation of the esophagus with chronic stasis changes of the mucosa (which may include apparent thickening and a dull gray appearance). Symptoms are mainly related to the inability of the lower esophageal sphincter to relax with swallowing. Dysphagia occurs because it is difficult for food to get into the stomach, and weight loss occurs for the same reason. Spontaneous regurgitation of food retained in the esophagus is a fairly common symptom and sometimes results in pulmonary aspiration. The diagnosis is made by a combination of barium studies, esophagoscopy, and manometry, the last being of major importance.

2. **Diffuse esophageal spasm** is a disease characterized by repetitive, vigorous, tertiary contractions with variable LES relaxation. The etiology is unknown. Symptoms induced by the vigorous contractions include chest pain, dysphagia as the progress of the food is interrupted, or odynophagia. The diagnosis is made primarily with manometric measurements.

3. **Systemic diseases.** Diseases that affect the striated or smooth muscle of the esophagus can also cause esophageal symptoms. Scleroderma is a systemic disease in which the smooth muscle por-

tion of the esophagus is often involved. Replacement of the smooth muscle by fibrosis results in loss of LES competence and loss of primary waves of the lower esophagus. Reflux of acid back into the esophagus is common and often associated with stricture formation. Diseases that affect the striated muscle portion of the esophagus, such as polymyositis, often cause symptoms of oropharyngeal dysphagia as well as loss of peristaltic activity in the upper portion of the esophagus.

B. **Reflux esophagitis.** The most common disease of the esophagus, reflux esophagitis, is due to reflux of gastric acid (or less commonly, alkaline bile) through the lower esophageal sphincter and into the esophagus. The etiology of the LES incompetence is usually unclear, but it certainly does not require an associated hiatal hernia. A hiatal hernia (herniation of the stomach into the thoracic cavity) may contribute to LES incompetence, but by itself does not necessarily cause incompetence.

The severity of resultant esophagitis appears to be dependent on four factors. (1) The frequency and duration of reflux constitute probably the most important factors, in that the longer the retention of acid within the esophagus, the more apt there are to be symptoms. A patient with symptomatic reflux esophagitis would typically have acid present in the lower esophagus for about 10 percent of a 24-hour period. (2) The effectiveness of the esophageal clearing mechanism is also of great importance. With reflux of material out of the stomach and back into the esophagus, a secondary wave should be generated. If this does not occur, or occurs inadequately, acid will stay within the esophagus for a longer period of time. (3) The nature of the reflux material is also of importance. Commonly, acid from the stomach is refluxed into the esophagus, but bile can cause the same symptoms. (4) Mucosal defense factors are also important. There appears to be some patient-to-patient variation both in the mucosal lesions that can develop and in the symptoms. Some patients with severe mucosal disease will have few if any symptoms, whereas other patients with minor mucosal abnormalities will have severe symptoms.

There appear to be three types of reflux patients. Upright refluxers are those whose reflux episodes occur only in an upright position, usually following a meal. Supine refluxers are patients in whom reflux episodes almost always occur while they are lying down, especially following a meal or when going to bed at night. The third and most common type consists of patients with severe symptoms of reflux esophagitis who will reflux in either the supine or the upright position.

The most common complications of severe erosive esophagitis include ulcerations, stricture formation secondary to inflammation and fibrosis, and bleeding when erosions or ulcerations involve vessels.

Symptoms are variable from patient to patient, but the most common symptom is heartburn. As described earlier, this is a substernal burning sensation associated with acid in the esophagus. Chest pain of a more continuous nature can occur and is usually associated with more severe forms of reflux esophagitis in which ulcerations are present. Dysphagia is usually seen with stricture formation, but can occur during periods when severe inflammation is present. Bleeding that can be seen with erosions or ulcerations can present either as hematemesis, melena, or an iron deficiency anemia due to chronic occult blood loss. Aspiration pneumonitis can occur; it appears to be more common in the elderly patient. Patients may often have symptoms of water brash (a bitter taste in the back of the mouth), which can occur when acid refluxes up the entire esophagus and into the hypopharynx. Some patients complain only of regurgitation in which they spontaneously find food in the back of their mouths.

Beyond the history and physical exam, combined pH monitoring and esophageal biopsy appear to be the most sensitive and accurate diagnostic tests.

VI. Clinical example of esophageal disease
  A. **Description.** A 35-year-old male patient reported having had difficulty swallowing for 5 years. It had been worse during the past 2 years, and recently he had trouble at each meal. Soft foods and liquids went down more easily than solids. During meals, he typically got a full feeling behind his sternum. On some occasions he induced vomiting and then could go back to finish his meal. He had not noticed any bile in the vomitus, only food he had just eaten. He had some trouble with regurgitation of food at night when he lay down, but denied any heartburn. The patient had lost 15 pounds over the past 6 months.

  Physical examination revealed a somewhat thin man, in no acute distress. His vital signs were normal, and his general physical examination revealed no abnormalities. Routine laboratory studies were all normal.

  An esophagram showed a dilated esophagus containing food and a bird-beak narrowing of the lower esophageal sphincter area. Esophagoscopy revealed some stasis changes in his esophagus and a tight LES area. No cancer was apparent. Esophageal manometry demonstrated low-pressure tertiary waves and a high LES pressure that did not relax with swallowing.

  After balloon dilatation of the esophagus, the patient's symptoms improved markedly.
  B. **Discussion**
    1. The combination of difficulty in swallowing solid foods and of nocturnal regurgitation suggests esophageal disease.
    2. The x-ray and esophagoscopy findings suggest achalasia.
    3. The manometric findings of a high-pressure zone in the area of the LES, without relaxation during swallowing, and low-pressure tertiary waves in the body of the esophagus help confirm the diagnosis.
    4. Dilatation of the tight LES area was associated with relief of symptoms.

Questions

Select the single best answer.

1. Dysphagia noted in achalasia patients is probably caused by:
   a. Inability of the esophagus to contract.
   b. Inability of the LES to relax.
   c. Inflammation within the esophagus.
   d. Cricopharyngeal incoordination.
2. Which of the following can be symptoms of reflux esophagitis?
   a. Waterbrash.
   b. Coughing.
   c. Odynophagia.
   d. All of the above.

Peptic Ulcer Diseases of the Stomach and Duodenum

I. **Anatomy.** The radiologic divisions of the stomach and duodenum are useful in understanding both anatomy and physiology.

The cardia of the stomach lies around the esophageal opening on the lesser curvature and contains a narrow zone of junctional epithelium made up of mostly mucous-producing cells. The fundus of the stomach is above a line from the cardia to the greater curvature. The antrum is the distal-most portion of the stomach. It lies beyond the angulus and extends to the pylorus, where the stomach empties into the first portion of the duodenum, the duodenal bulb. The body of the stomach is located between the fundus and the antrum.

II. **Gastric physiology**

A. **Secretion**

1. **Cell type and function.** There are four major cell types found within the stomach: (1) The gastrin-producing cells (G cells) are found in the antrum and, with stimulation, release gastrin into the blood stream. (2) Mucous-producing cells are located throughout the stomach. Their major function is to produce lubricating mucus. (3) Parietal cells, found in the stomach body and fundus, secrete hydrochloric acid (HCl), an intrinsic factor. (4) The chief cell is also found in the body and fundus of the stomach. It produces pepsinogen, which is cleaved by acid to pepsin, a proteolytic enzyme. Secretion from chief cells is stimulated by protein and also by factors that stimulate HCl secretion.

The three known in-vivo agonists of hydrochloric acid secretion are acetylcholine, gastrin, and histamine. (Of the two types of histamine receptors, I and II, only type II receptors are found in the stomach.) These three agonists seem to work through a final common pathway to cause HCl secretion: maximum hydrochloric acid secretion by the parietal cell can be accomplished by maximum stimulation of acetylcholine release, maximum histamine receptor stimulation, or infusion of large amounts of gastrin. Blockage of any one of these three agonists will decrease hydrochloric acid secretion, even if maximum stimulation by one of the other agonists is maintained.

2. **Normal control of secretion.** During periods of time when there is no stimulation of acid production (i.e., without sight, smell, or taste of food), the stomach secretes HCl at approximately 2 mEq per hour. Maximum secretion approximates 8 to 10 mEq per hour and is mediated by a cephalic phase, a gastric phase, and an intestinal phase of agonism/antagonism.

The cephalic phase is mediated by the vagus nerve and triggered not only by smell or taste of food but also by hypoglycemia. All this results in direct cholinergic stimulation of parietal cells to secrete hydrochloric acid and of the G cells in the antrum to secrete gastrin.

The gastric phase is mediated by the long vagal and short intramural reflexes. It is apparently triggered by gastric distension as well as by products of protein digestion, alcohol, and caffeine.

Alkalinization of the antrum also stimulates the gastric phase. Antral acidification below a pH of 2 causes a feedback inhibition, especially of gastrin release. These also result in cholinergic stimulation of parietal cells and release of gastrin from G cells.

The intestinal phase is triggered by food entering the duodenum, is probably hormonally mediated, and is mostly inhibitory in nature.

B. Motility. Motility within the stomach is under neurohormonal control, with the vagal nerve being of major importance. As a motor unit, the stomach is considered to have two functional areas: a proximal receptacle that includes the fundus and the body of the stomach, and a distal pump that includes the antrum. Motility waves begin in about the midbody of the stomach as shallow contractions and move to the pylorus with increasing rate and vigor. The body and fundus of the stomach also function as an area for storage, volume adaptation, and regulation of osmolarity. The antrum mixes gastric contents and propels these contents into the duodenum.

The stomach therefore releases into the duodenum food that is nearly isosmotic and is of small particle size. In a normal stomach, food is released into the duodenum at a fairly constant rate of kilocalories per minute. In general, liquids move faster than solids, since the osmolarity and particle size are more easily regulated. Foods higher in caloric content (such as fat) empty at a slower rate than carbohydrates. This means that a large meal containing many calories will take much longer to empty out of the stomach than a small meal of fewer calories.

III. The common diseases

A. Acute erosive gastritis (stress erosions). The stress erosions that are demonstrated in acute erosive gastritis are superficial ulcerations involving only the mucosa of the stomach. Important factors in their formation include aspirin, alcohol, and bile, as well as stress. Hydrochloric acid must be present for their formation, but not necessarily in large quantities. With the intake of aspirin or alcohol, there is a change in the potential difference of the gastric mucosa. This allows backdiffusion of the hydrogen ion and is, therefore, a possible means of cellular damage. In areas where erosion occurs, the first thing seen is an area of hyperemia surrounding a blanched portion of mucosa. For this reason, it is also postulated that some change in blood flow may be important in the pathogenesis of erosions. Because the erosion does not involve an area where nerves are typically found, pain is usually not a feature. Hemorrhage is the main clinical problem. With involvement of the mucosa, hemorrhage is typically from small vessels and does not pose a life-threatening problem. (If the mucosal erosion extends below the muscularis mucosae, it is considered an ulcer, and major hemorrhage can occur.) With therapy, the lesions are able to heal quickly because of the fast cell turnover time in the stomach of 4 to 6 days.

B. Chronic atrophic gastritis is associated with little or no secretion of acid, enzymes, or intrinsic factor. It is typically seen with advancing age. If there is a complete lack of intrinsic factor secretion, pernicious anemia results. It is also a predisposing factor in carcinoma of the stomach.

C. Gastric ulcer. By definition, an ulcer is a lesion that extends through the mucosa and beyond the muscularis mucosae into the submucosa. It is more commonly seen in people from 40 to 60 years of age. Hydrochloric acid hypersecretion is not a primary factor since most of these older patients have normal, or even less than normal, rates of maximum stimulation of hydrochloric acid secretion. Acid does need to be present for the formation of a benign (peptic) ulcer. The possible mechanisms of mucosal injury and increased permeability to hydrogen ion include: (1) Reflux of bile salts and lysolecithin into the stomach from the duodenum can cause direct damage to the cell membrane. (2) Ingestion of aspirin or alcohol can cause a change in the potential difference across the cell membrane, allowing hydrogen ion back-diffusion to occur and cause cellular damage. (3) Stress, as mentioned earlier, can lead to gastric erosions that can go on to form ulcerations. (4) Gastric outlet obstruction may occur and keep the gastric mucosa bathed in acid.

The mucosal defensive barrier may be defective in patients who develop gastric ulcers. As a result, the back-diffusion of hydrogen ion can cause pepsin activation (and therefore protein digestion) and histamine release (and therefore further stimulation for hydrogen ion production). Mucous protection or secretion of a protective substance by the parietal cells may be impaired. There appears to be a very thin mucous barrier probably containing a bicarbonate gradient (regulated by prostaglandins) that is an important first line of defense against the hydrogen ion. If epithelial renewal is slowed from its normal 4- to 6-day turnover time to a longer period, the regenerative capacity of the stomach will be impaired. This may become important in patients who are malnourished.

Given the preceding discussions, it is not surprising that gastric ulcers are common in patients with gastric outlet obstruction due to pyloric channel or duodenal bulb disease, in patients taking aspirin or alcohol on a regular basis, in patients suffering from stress (whether neurosurgical or psychic, from burns or septicemia), and in those patients with chronic diseases such as rheumatoid arthritis, chronic lung disease, and renal failure.

Patients with a gastric ulcer may experience pain in the epigastric area, nausea and vomiting, bleeding with or without pain, and anorexia or early satiety. The pain is not as classic as in duodenal ulcers and can occur during a meal, after a meal, or between meals. It does not always respond to food intake. The area of the stomach involved with the ulcer has decreased motility because of inflammation and scarring. The most common location for a gastric ulcer is at the division of the body and the antrum (between parietal cell and gastrin-producing cell territories), an area where considerable motility normally occurs. For this reason poor gastric emptying is common, and nausea and vomiting may result. Prepyloric ulcers with surrounding inflammation can block the pylorus, causing gastric outlet obstruction with resulting nausea and vomiting. Hemorrhage occurs when the ulceration extends through a blood vessel, and can be massive when an artery of some size is disrupted.

Penetration of a gastric ulcer into an adjacent structure may also cause symptoms. For instance, ulcer penetration into the pancreas can cause pancreatitis and pain. Perforation of an ulcer will release air and gastric juice into the abdominal cavity, resulting in signs of peritonitis and free air under the diaphragm. Patients, therefore, demonstrate marked abdominal pain, loss of bowel sounds, and board-like rigidity of the abdomen, all consequences of peritonitis. Gastric ulcers commonly recur, approximating 40 percent at 1 year. The number of recurrences tends to decrease after the second or third sequential ulcer. Gastric ulcers usually heal more slowly than duodenal ulcers, probably because they are typically larger. Gastric ulcers do not lead to gastric cancer.

D. Duodenal ulcer. Approximately 95 percent of duodenal ulcers are found in the duodenal bulb, with most of the rest occurring in the immediate postbulbar area. As with gastric ulcers, acid needs to be present for a duodenal ulcer to occur. On the average, patients with duodenal ulcers secrete more acid in the basal and stimulated states than do normals. However, a large overlap exists between normals and duodenal ulcer patients with respect to both basal and maximal states of gastric acid secretion. The mechanism of duodenal defense against ulcer formation includes rapid mucosal cell turnover, relative impermeability of the mucosal cell to acid, and neutralization of acid as it leaves the stomach with pancreatic and biliary secretions. Ulceration is related to pH and the rate of acid entering the duodenal bulb. Since pancreatic and biliary secretions enter the duodenum beyond the duodenal bulb, the bulb is the only small-bowel segment regularly bathed in acid.

Pain from a duodenal ulcer typically occurs in the right upper quadrant or epigastric area after the stomach has been emptied of a meal (usually 3–4 hr after eating). Pain relief can sometimes be obtained by eating food, which neutralizes acid within the stomach and the duodenum. Pain often awakens a patient at night, usually around 2 A.M., a time of maximum nocturnal gastric acid output.

Recurrences are common, approximately 50 to 60 percent at 1 year, but this decreases with time in most patients. Hemorrhage, perforation, penetration, and gastric outlet obstruction can occur. Hemorrhage of a life-threatening nature occurs when a major vessel is eroded by the ulcer. Perforation of a duodenal ulcer is the most common cause of free air under the diaphragm in an otherwise healthy individual. It accounts for approximately 85 percent of cases in which free air is noted. The pancreas is the most common area of ulcer penetration; the gastrohepatic ligament and the biliary tree are the next most frequent targets. Therefore, signs and symptoms of pancreatitis can occur secondary to a penetrating duodenal ulcer. Occasionally, jaundice or biliary tract fistulae may also occur secondary to a duodenal ulcer.

The Zollinger-Ellison syndrome is caused by a gastrin-secreting tumor (gastrinoma). The gastrinoma is usually found in the pancreas and is almost always malignant, but grows very slowly. With continuous gastrin production by the tumor, the parietal cells of the stomach are in a continuous state of hydrochloric acid secretion. Hence, basal acid secretion is greatly increased, but stimulated acid production (from food, histamine, or vagus stimulation) increases little, since almost maximum stimulation is usually occurring.

A gastrinoma is sometimes found in association with type I multiple endocrine adenomatosis involving the pituitary, parathyroid, and pancreatic glands. In the Zollinger-Ellison syndrome, ulcers are most commonly found in the duodenal bulb, although gastric, postbulbar, or jejunal ulcers may be found. A jejunal ulcer is otherwise rare and should make one suspect a gastrinoma. In these patients a high, fasting plasma gastrin level is usually found. Ulcer recurrence is the rule without specific therapy, and recurrence is also common following the usual surgery for ulcer disease.

IV. Clinical examples

A. Benign gastric ulcer

1. **Description.** A 65-year-old housewife noticed recurrences of epigastric pain, often coming within an hour of eating. She had been awakened at 4 to 5 A.M. with the pain and received only partial relief with antacids. Two days before being seen, she passed several sticky, black stools. She felt faint on one occasion but never passed out.

   Her hemoglobin was 10 gm/dl. A nasogastric tube was placed in her stomach, and some coffee grounds–appearing material was aspirated.

   When the patient was hospitalized, upper gastrointestinal x-rays revealed a 2-cm by 2-cm ulcer at the gastric angulus, and endoscopy with biopsy was performed. The biopsies showed benign gastric tissue. She was treated for 6 weeks with antacids 1 and 3 hr after meals, as well as at bedtime. Symptoms resolved and repeat upper gastrointestinal x-rays at 2 months revealed healing of the ulcer.

2. **Discussion.** This patient presents a typical clinical picture of gastric ulcer disease. The pain was partly relieved by antacids, but often worsened by eating. The passage of black stools (melena) indicated that blood had been in contact with acid, thus implicating an upper gastrointestinal bleeding site.

   Endoscopy was performed to exclude an ulcerating gastric carcinoma, which will occasionally present a similar clinical and radiographic appearance. As is often the case, no clues to the origin of the ulcer were discovered. Fortunately, the ulcer healed without producing major bleeding or other serious complications.

B. Hemorrhagic gastritis

1. **Description.** A 27-year-old male came to the emergency room after vomiting bright red blood. He gave a 1-week history of mild epigastric discomfort starting after a night on the town, during which he fell and hit his head. He had been taking 8 to 10 aspirins a day for his headache and mild abdominal pain. There was no history of previous ulcer disease.

   Physical exam revealed a pulse of 105 and a blood pressure of 120/80 that dropped to 105/60 with standing. His conjunctiva were pale. Abdominal exam revealed mild epigastric tenderness, but no guarding or rebound.

   He was hospitalized, and his stomach was lavaged with iced saline to clean out the blood and help control the bleeding. Gastroscopy was performed, revealing hemorrhagic gastritis (stress erosions). There was no evidence of a gastric or duodenal ulcer. Therapy with antacids was begun and no further bleeding was noted.

2. **Discussion.** It is likely that the combined effects of aspirin and ethanol led to the stress erosions that were the source of the patient's gastric bleeding. Both agents impair the gastric mucosal barrier to the hydrogen ion. Antacids are helpful therapy by reducing H^+ concentration until the mucosa can heal and recover its normal resistance to autodigestion.

More than one answer may be correct.

1. Regarding *gastric* ulcer formation, which of the following are true?
   a. Acid secretion from the stomach is normal or below normal.
   b. Acid is not required for ulcer formation.
   c. Alcohol can increase gastric cell permeability to H^+.
   d. Stress can play some role in ulcer formation.
2. Major determinant(s) of gastric acid secretion include(s):
   a. Gastrin.
   b. Acetylcholine.
   c. Histamine.
   d. All the above.

The Pancreas

I. **Anatomy.** The pancreas is a relatively small organ weighing 60 to 110 g and is retroperitoneal in location. It has no capsule but is located close to several vital structures, including the stomach, duodenum, spleen, portal vein, and distal common bile duct. The pancreas receives efferent nerves from the vagus and splanchnics through the hepatic and celiac plexuses. Sympathetic efferents supply the blood vessels. Afferent nerves traveling through the celiac plexus are responsible for the pain of pancreatic disease but the mechanisms are poorly understood.

   A. **The exocrine pancreas** consists of clusters of microscopic, spherical acini that form lobules. Each acinus consists of a cupped layer of acinar cells that secrete a large variety of proteins into the central lumen. The ductal lumen is partially lined by pale-staining, centroacinar cells that secrete water and sodium bicarbonate.

   B. **The endocrine pancreas** consists of approximately a million islets of Langerhans scattered among the loose tissue between lobules. Their known cell types and secretory products are: beta cells, insulin; alpha cells, glucagon; delta cells, somatostatin; d_1 cells, vasoactive intestinal peptide (VIP); and d_2 cells, pancreatic polypeptide.

II. **Physiology and biochemistry.** The pancreas can secrete up to 4,000 cc of fluid per day and produces more protein per gram of tissue than any other organ in the body. It has a tremendous reserve capacity and requires 80 to 90 percent destruction before maldigestion or malabsorption occurs. The average daily secretion includes:

Water	2,500 ml
Total protein	5–10 g/day
Na^+	145 mEq/L
K^+	5 mEq/L
Ca^{2+}	1.6 mEq/L
Mg^+	0.4 mEq/L
$HCO_3^- + Cl^-$	155 mEq/L

Water and electrolyte secretion is stimulated by secretin released by the duodenal mucosa when acid enters the duodenum.

Pancreatic enzymes are made by the acinar cells and are stored intracellularly until stimulation for release occurs. A large variety of enzymes are found in the pancreatic juice (see Table 21-1). Because the proteins produced in the pancreas could destroy it, protective mechanisms are available to prevent autodigestion from occurring. Many enzymes are produced as inactive proenzymes. Membrane packaging occurs within the cell to protect the cell as it stores the enzyme. Since trypsin is the major activator for most of the proenzymes, trypsin inhibitors are secreted along with the enzymes into the pancreatic duct. With some exceptions (amylase and lipase for instance), enzymes are activated only upon reaching the duodenal lumen where enterokinase (released from the duodenum) converts trypsinogen to trypsin, which in turn activates the proenzyme. The pancreatic enzymes are secreted in response to cholecystokinin, which is released from the duodenal wall in response to fat and amino acids entering the duodenum. When both secretin and cholecystokinin act on the pancreas simultaneously, the effects are addi-

Table 21-1 *Enzymes of Mammalian Pancreatic Secretion*

Zymogen	Enzyme	Activator
Trypsinogen	Trypsin	Enterokinase, Ca^{2+}, trypsin
Chymotrypsinogen	Chymotrypsin	Trypsin
Procarboxypeptidase A	Carboxypeptidase A	Trypsin
Procarboxypeptidase B	Carboxypeptidase B	Trypsin
Proelastase	Elastase	Trypsin
Proelastomucase	Elastomucase	Trypsin
	Amylase	Chloride
	Lipase	Emulsifying agents
	Esterase	Bile salts
Prophospholipase A	Phospholipase A	Bile salts
		Trypsin
	Cholesterol esterase	Bile salts

Source: Reproduced with permission from J. R. Meadows, *Sophomore Introduction to Medicine*, Gastroenterology Section, Department of Medicine, Indiana University School of Medicine, 1978, p. 74.

Figure 21-1

Classification of pancreatitis according to the definition of Marseille. (From R. Ammann, Acute pancreatitis. In H. L. Bockus (Ed.), Gastroenterology (3rd ed.). Philadelphia: Saunders, 1976, vol. 3, p. 1021. Reproduced with permission of the publisher and R. Ammann.)

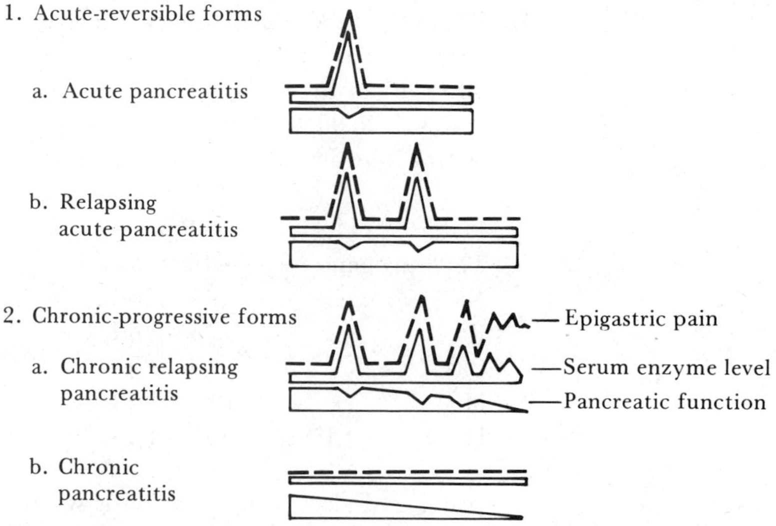

1. Acute-reversible forms
   a. Acute pancreatitis
   b. Relapsing acute pancreatitis
2. Chronic-progressive forms
   a. Chronic relapsing pancreatitis
   b. Chronic pancreatitis

— Epigastric pain
— Serum enzyme level
— Pancreatic function

tive. Consequently, more enzymes are released when secretin is acting upon the pancreas in conjunction with cholecystokinin than with cholecystokinin alone.

III. **The common diseases**

A. **Acute pancreatitis.** Defined, *acute pancreatitis* is acute inflammation with secretory cell damage; complete structural and biological restitution is possible if the cause is eliminated. Two types of acute pancreatitis can occur (see Fig. 21-1): (1) Edematous pancreatitis occurs more frequently and is milder in severity; the pancreas becomes swollen, but no major hemorrhage occurs. (2) Hemorrhagic pancreatitis is a more severe variety often associated with major retroperitoneal bleeding and a relatively high mortality.

Acute pancreatitis is called acute relapsing pancreatitis if more than one episode occurs from the same cause. For instance, this can occur with recurrent passage of gallstones through the common bile duct.

1. **Pathogenesis.** The pathogenesis of acute pancreatitis appears to be autodigestion. Activation of the pancreatic enzymes occurs within the pancreas with subsequent cellular destruction and inflammation. Fat necrosis, which may be intrapancreatic or peripancreatic, can also occur because of lipase activation. Calcium and magnesium soaps can therefore be formed, leading to hypocalcemia and hypomagnesemia. Elastase can break down arterial walls, leading to hemorrhage. Trypsin can cause clotting and bleeding problems, due to activation of circulating procoagulants. Sequestration of extracellular fluid in the pancreatic bed and abdomen may deplete the plasma volume; the release of kinins into the blood also contributes to the hypotension that commonly occurs. Islet cell damage may cause insulin deficiency, but this is usually mild and transient unless major pancreatic destruction occurs.

   In approximately 75 percent of patients acute pancreatitis is associated with gallstones. The mechanism by which gallstones cause pancreatitis is not known, but most of these patients have passed stones through the sphincter of Oddi. Impaction of a stone at the sphincter of Oddi can cause pancreatic duct obstruction that might be associated with backwash of bile into the pancreas, inciting pancreatitis. Lymphatic spread of infection from the gallbladder to the pancreas has been postulated, but there is even less evidence to support this theory.

   Trauma, either accidental or from abdominal surgery near the pancreas, can cause pancreatitis. An infection such as mumps can involve the pancreas; metabolic states such as hypercalcemia and hyperlipidemia (type V) are also associated with acute pancreatitis. Drugs such as thiazide diuretics and corticosteroids, which cause increased pancreatic secretion, or oral contraceptives (possibly by causing increased serum lipids) are occasionally associated with pancreatitis. Alcohol is commonly associated with chronic relapsing pancreatitis but rarely causes the acute variety.

2. **Clinical aspects.** Symptoms, signs, and complications of pancreatitis vary with the severity of pancreatic injury. Pain is the most common symptom and is usually localized to the periumbilical or epigastric area with radiation straight through to the back. Shock can follow hypovolemia or kinin release. Nausea, vomiting, fever, adynamic ileus, peritonitis, and ascites are all possible complicating features of severe inflammation or infection. Tetany may result from rapid calcium or magnesium sequestration following fat necrosis. Jaundice can occur from pancreatic edema around the common bile duct where it traverses the pancreas. Gastric bleeding may occur, usually from gastritis in the area of the stomach adjacent to the inflamed pancreas. Retroperitoneal bleeding from hemorrhagic pancreatitis can cause blood loss, hypovolemia, and shock. If diabetes accompanies acute pancreatitis, it is usually a transient result of inflammation near the islets of Langerhans. Pseudocysts and abscesses are relatively common complications, pancreatic abscesses causing a high mortality.

   Mortality is related to the severity of necrosis, hemorrhage, and so on. The most common causes of death include refractory hypotension, acute tubular necrosis, respiratory failure, and sepsis.

B. Chronic pancreatitis. With chronic pancreatitis, permanent structural and functional damage already exists at the time of presentation. There are two general types of chronic pancreatitis, persistent and relapsing (see Fig. 21-1). In chronic persistent pancreatitis, pain is not a typical feature. Serum amylase and lipase elevations are not commonly seen, and patients usually present because of pancreatic insufficiency with either diabetes or steatorrhea or both. Chronic relapsing pancreatitis is the most typical form found in alcoholic pancreatitis. Recurrent painful episodes are typical, and slowly progressive pancreatic destruction results.

1. **Pathogenesis.** The mechanisms by which chronic pancreatitis develops are unclear, but the etiology of chronic relapsing pancreatitis seems to include alcohol in at least 75 percent of the patients. This may be also true for chronic persistent pancreatitis. In chronic pancreatitis secondary to alcoholism, pathologic changes of fibrosis and acinar destruction occur before symptoms of pain in at least 90 percent of patients. Alcohol appears to increase the protein concentration within the pancreatic secretions. This is thought to cause pancreatitis by the following scheme. Initially, there is precipitation of the protein in the lumen of the ductules, resulting in obstruction and proximal ductular and acinar dilatation. This in turn results in a chronic inflammation or fibrotic reaction around the small ductules that can further compromise the lumen. The acinus eventually becomes atrophic or is totally destroyed and replaced by fibrosis. Progressive inflammation, necrosis, and parenchymal cysts may occur. Eventually, calcifications appear within the pancreas, both in the parenchyma and within the small ductules. Islet cells also can atrophy or be destroyed and replaced by fibrosis. Later the large ducts become involved with periductular inflammation and fibrosis, often resulting in alternating stenosis/dilatation. The pressure in the large duct remains low. Overall, approximately 10 to 15 percent of chronic alcoholics with more than 10 years of alcohol abuse develop chronic pancreatitis.

   Hereditary conditions such as cystic fibrosis, hemochromatosis, or familial pancreatitis may also be associated with chronic persistent pancreatitis.

2. **Clinical aspects.** As in acute pancreatitis, pain is the biggest problem in chronic relapsing pancreatitis. It is again periumbilical in location with radiation through to the back. The classic triad in chronic pancreatitis is calcification of the pancreas (found in approximately 20% of cases), diabetes mellitus secondary to destruction of the islets of Langerhans, and steatorrhea from inadequate lipase secretion.

   Major complications include pseudocyst formation, bile duct obstruction, splenic vein occlusion, and drug addiction. Pseudocyst formation may occur when a duct becomes obstructed with secretion continuing behind the obstruction. Common bile duct obstruction can occur either from fibrosis around the common bile duct as it courses through the head of the pancreas or from inflammation and edema during some of the relapsing, painful episodes. Splenic vein occlusion can occur when the inflammation within the pancreas impinges on the splenic vein. Since many patients have chronic pain, drug addiction may result from efforts to relieve the pain.

IV. Clinical example of chronic pancreatitis

A. **Description.** A 54-year-old man was admitted for evaluation of epigastric pain. He had apparently been well until approximately 18 months prior to admission, when he experienced several episodes of right–upper-quadrant pain. Oral cholecystography at that time revealed gallstones. Six months later he suffered an especially severe episode of right–upper-quadrant pain and epigastric pain with radiation to the back. He underwent cholecystectomy; at surgery the gallbladder was inflamed but was easily removed. The common bile duct was not explored. Gallstones were seen within the gallbladder. Two months later the patient experienced another episode of periumbilical and epigastric pain which radiated through to his back. He required hospitalization because of the pain but rapidly improved with intravenous fluids and pain medications. He was noted to have an elevated urinary amylase, but a normal serum amylase. Between that admission and the present admission he suffered numerous episodes of similar epigastric pain radiating to his back, but treated himself at home with codeine. Although the codeine would relieve his pain temporarily, he often noted pain again after eating or drinking. The present admission was precipitated by an especially severe episode of pain and mild jaundice. He has lost 40 pounds over the past several months.

Review of his past medical history revealed no serious illnesses except as noted. He considered himself a social drinker and had consumed approximately a pint of liquor per day for the last several years.

On physical exam he appeared moderately ill, with a blood pressure of 110/80 and no postural hypotension. General examination was normal except for evidence of muscle wasting and malnutrition. The liver was approximately 15 cm in total span in the right midclavicular line. There was tenderness to palpation throughout the epigastric area that was especially noted in the periumbilical area. Mild scleral icterus was noted. There was a trace of edema in the lower extremities.

During hospitalization he was found to have a normal blood count. Urinalysis revealed 1^+ glucose and some bilirubin. His serum and urine amylase were normal and his alkaline phosphatase was four times the upper limit of normal. His serum bilirubin was slightly elevated. Examination of his stool showed neutral fat globules and meat fibers. His fasting blood glucose was 200 mg/dl. An endoscopic retrograde cholangiopancreatogram showed alternating stenosis and dilatation of the pancreatic duct indicating chronic pancreatitis. The common bile duct was slightly dilated except in its distal portion, where it went through the head of the pancreas. At this point it narrowed in a gradual fashion. No stones were seen.

B. **Discussion.** The patient has chronic relapsing pancreatitis, probably secondary to his alcohol intake. As opposed to acute recurrent pancreatitis, such patients may not have serum amylase elevations late in their disease because much of the pancreas may be destroyed. For this same reason they may develop diabetes (destruction of the islets of Langerhans) and fat, protein, and carbohydrate maldigestion (because of inadequate enzyme production). This patient also developed mild obstructive jaundice because of scarring and inflammation around the common bile duct where it courses through the head of the pancreas.

The diabetes was controlled with insulin and the patient's maldigestion improved with pancreatic enzyme supplementation. He was asked to abstain from alcohol because in some patients abstinence will lessen the painful attacks.

Select the single best answer.

1. Regarding gallstones as a cause of pancreatitis, the only connection known with any certainty is that most patients with pancreatitis and gallstones:
   a. Reflux bile into the pancreatic duct.
   b. Pass gallstones into the duodenum.
   c. Have gallstones impact at the sphincter of Oddi.
   d. Have lymphatic spread of infection from the gallbladder to the pancreas.
2. The first step in alcohol causing chronic relapsing pancreatitis appears to be:
   a. Protein precipitates within the ductules.
   b. Acinar cell destruction.
   c. Increased protein in the pancreatic secretions.
   d. Stenosis of the main pancreatic duct.
   e. Periductular inflammation.

22 The Gallbladder and Biliary Tract

I. Functional anatomy. Small biliary radicals coalesce within the liver to form right and left hepatic ducts, which in turn join to form the common hepatic duct. The cystic duct from the gallbladder joins this to form the common bile duct, which empties into the duodenum through the sphincter of Oddi. The gallbladder is a distensible organ lined by columnar epithelium, which has a capability for salt and water absorption. The nerve supply of the gallbladder is through a branch of the vagus. Arterial blood supply is through a branch of the celiac trunk.

II. Physiology. Normal bile is approximately 80 percent water, 4 percent phospholipids (over 95% of which is lecithin), less than 1 percent cholesterol, and approximately 12 percent bile salts. Normal bile salts are conjugated with either glycine or taurine. Primary bile salts produced in the liver include cholic and chenodeoxycholic acids. Secondary bile salts are formed in the colon by action of the bacteria on the primary bile salts; these include deoxycholic and lithocholic acid. The solubility of cholesterol in the gallbladder bile depends upon the dry weight percentages of bile salts, lecithin, and cholesterol (Fig. 22-1). Of these, bile salts make up approximately 70 percent. When it exceeds 10 percent, cholesterol is taken from an unsaturated to a saturated form. At this point, the metastable zone, cholesterol can go in and out of solution. As the percentage of cholesterol increases, it is much more likely to remain in the crystal phase and therefore be able to form gallstones.

Hepatic synthesis of bile salts approximates 0.3 to 0.6 g per day. The total bile salt pool is usually 2 to 3 g, and it recirculates through the enterohepatic cycle five to ten times daily. The hepatic secretion rate of bile salts thus approximates 15 to 30 g per day. Since the ileum reabsorbs 95 percent of the bile salts, only 0.3 to 0.6 g is excreted in the stool each day.

The main function of the gallbladder is storage of bile and concentration of bile salts, cholesterol, and lecithin. The gallbladder fills because the sphincter of Oddi remains closed while hepatic bile secretion continues. The gallbladder therefore offers a path of least resistance. Concentration and emptying of the gallbladder occur when stimulation by cholecystokinin takes place. Cholecystokinin is released from the duodenum when fat or amino acids enter the duodenum.

III. Gallstone formation. The most common type of gallstone found in humans is the cholesterol gallstone. Formation of cholesterol gallstones can be divided into five stages:

A. Metabolic stage. This involves the genetic, biochemical, or metabolic defect that can lead to the production of bile with excess cholesterol relative to bile salts and lecithin.

B. Chemical stage. The bile contains excess cholesterol, but it is still in a soluble form.

C. Physical stage. This begins when cholesterol crystals form and can be seen within the bile.

D. Growth stage. Stones are present but no symptoms are occurring.

E. Symptomatic stage. During this stage, symptoms occur that are caused by the gallstones.

Figure 22-1

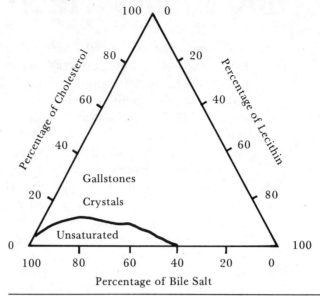

IV. Gallstone disease. The incidence of gallstones is approximately three times as high in females as in males. There are marked variations in gallstone prevalence. In the United States, the prevalence for 40-year-old white females is 10 percent; for American Indians, 70 percent.

Three major types of gallstones occur: (1) Cholesterol gallstones are by far the most common, and contain at least 60 to 70 percent cholesterol. (2) Pigmented stones are composed mainly of bile pigments (bilirubin) and are found in hemolytic diseases such as sickle cell anemia. (3) Mixed gallstones, a combination of pigmented and cholesterol stones, are the least common type. Pigmented gallstones, some of the mixed gallstones, and some cholesterol gallstones with calcium deposits will show up on a regular x-ray. Overall, however, only 15 percent of gallstones are seen on plain films of the abdomen.

Cholelithiasis is usually asymptomatic until stone migration occurs. Migration through or impaction in the cystic duct or at the ampulla of Vater can cause pain without infection. Classic symptoms include right–upper-quadrant pain with radiation to the right scapula area, nausea and vomiting, and relief of pain as the stone is passed. The gallbladder usually functions normally and can be visualized with oral cholecystography.

Acute cholecystitis is almost always associated with cholelithiasis. It occurs with obstruction of the cystic duct and infection in the gallbladder wall behind the gallstone. Chemical inflammation can occur, and vascular congestion is usually seen in the wall of the gallbladder. Symptoms of cholecystitis include right–upper-quadrant pain with radiation to the right subscapular area. Fever and leukocytosis occur because of the infection. Nausea and vomiting may also occur because of the infection, and localized peritonitis may be noted if inflammation extends through the gallbladder wall. Sometimes a slight bilirubin elevation can be noted because of inflammation of the common duct and partial obstruction of bile flow. Empyema (filling of the gallbladder with pus) can sometimes occur;

it would be more common if infection occurred behind a totally obstructed cystic duct. Gangrene and perforation secondary to marked inflammation of the gallbladder wall and vascular congestion can occasionally be seen. If localized inflammation and necrosis in the gallbladder wall occur and penetration through a portion of the duodenum follows, an internal biliary fistula can be formed.

Choledocholithiasis implies gallstones within the common bile duct. Symptoms can occur as the stone passes through the sphincter of Oddi or is impacted above the sphincter of Oddi. They include right–upper-quadrant pain with radiation to the right subscapular area, nausea and vomiting, and possibly jaundice from the obstruction to bile flow. Pancreatitis can occur because of passage of a stone through the sphincter of Oddi. Chills and fever are common if infection occurs. Major complications associated with choledocholithiasis include ascending cholangitis and secondary biliary cirrhosis. Ascending cholangitis develops when infection within the common bile duct progresses into the intrahepatic bile ducts. Secondary biliary cirrhosis can occur if the obstruction persists (usually 3–6 mo).

V. Clinical examples

    A. Description. A 40-year-old, slightly obese, white female with four children reported that she had been in excellent health until 4 months ago when she awakened at 1:00 A.M. with moderately severe, right–upper-quadrant pain. Partial relief was experienced by pressing the right–upper-quadrant area and the pain subsided spontaneously in 2 hours. Two months later she experienced the same sequence of events, this time associated with nausea and vomiting. The episodes of pain then became more frequent and occurred during the day, usually after her largest meal. Two days before admission she again developed pain that subsided somewhat but never completely went away. The next day her urine was dark and she had a slight fever. She began taking penicillin, which had been prescribed for her son's sore throat, but the fever continued until an episode of shaking chills brought her to the physician's office. She had received no relief with antacids or food, and only minor relief with aspirin.

    Physical exam revealed an obese white female appearing to be in moderate distress. Slight scleral icterus was noted and there was tenderness to palpation in the right upper quadrant. With deep inspiration the pain increased enough to make her catch her breath.

    Laboratory studies revealed a hemoglobin of 13 and a white count of 14,000 with a shift to the left. Alkaline phosphatase was five times normal and her bilirubin was 5.0 mg/dl.

    She was admitted to the hospital, given intravenous fluids and antibiotics, and a nasogastric tube was put in place. A sonar study revealed gallbladder stones and mild intrahepatic bile duct dilatation. She was taken to surgery that afternoon; a stone was found impacted above the sphincter of Oddi as well as in the cystic duct. Her recovery was uneventful.

    B. Discussion. This woman is typical of patients with gallstone disease. She first experienced episodes of pain as small stones were being passed (or impacted) in the cystic duct. Later, as a stone became impacted at the sphincter of Oddi, she developed fever and white blood count elevation to secondary infection in the bile ducts. She became jaundiced, since bile could not pass into the duodenum.

Select the single best answer.

1. Which of the following is the most important factor in gallstone formation?
   a. The concentration of cholesterol in the bile.
   b. The concentration of bile salts found in the bile.
   c. The relative percentage of cholesterol in comparison to the percentage of bile salts and lecithin.
   d. The age of the patient.
   e. None of the above.
2. If a gallstone were impacted in the distal common bile duct as opposed to the cystic duct, which statement is correct?
   a. The patient would be more likely to have fever.
   b. The patient would be more likely to have pain.
   c. The patient would be more likely to have nausea and vomiting.
   d. The patient would be more likely to be jaundiced.

23   The Liver

I. **Gross anatomy and vascular supply.** The liver is a two-lobed organ, each lobe having separate afferent and efferent blood vessels. The afferent vessels enter the liver at the hilus and branch within the liver substance; they are accompanied by the branches of the bile ducts. The hepatic artery originates from the celiac and is responsible for 25 to 30 percent of the total afferent blood flow, but provides approximately 50 percent of the available oxygen. The portal vein is made up from the superior mesentery vein after it is joined by the splenic vein and carries approximately 75 percent of the total afferent blood flow to the liver. The portal vein includes all veins that collect blood from the alimentary tract, spleen, pancreas, and gallbladder. The regular branching of the portal vein allows each lobe of the liver to be subdivided into four functional segments. The liver is drained by two or three large hepatic veins, which empty into the inferior vena cava. The hepatic veins run independently from the branches of the hepatic artery, portal vein, and hepatic duct system.

II. **Functional anatomy.** On microscopic examination, the hepatocytes are seen to be arranged as radial cords around the terminal hepatic venules (central veins). The basic anatomic framework of the liver, however, is the microcirculatory unit, which provides functional integration for the hepatic acinus.

   A. The simple hepatic acinus consists of a number of hepatocytes surrounding their terminal hepatic arterioles and portal venules, bile ductules, lymph vessels, and nerves. The portal venules anastomose with sinusoids, which carry blood to the terminal hepatic vein. The hepatic arterioles open into some of the sinusoids.

   B. The periphery of the simple acinus drains into at least two terminal hepatic venules (central veins). Each hepatic venule drains at least three to six simple hepatic acini (Fig. 23-1).

   C. Pressure in the portal venule is low. In the axial sinusoids, which are the site of shunting of hepatic arterial and portal venous blood, the higher arterial pressure ensures a high rate of blood flow.

   D. Each simple acinus is divided into three zones on the basis of their proximity to the axial flow of the blood from the hepatic arteriole. Zone 1 is the closest to the arterial flow, is the most metabolically active, has the highest oxygen supply, is the most resistant to damage, and is the area to regenerate first after damage. Zone 3 is the farthest from the axial flow and closest to the hepatic venules. For these reasons, zone 3 is the first to respond to injury and the last to regenerate. Zone 2 lies between the others (Fig. 23-1). The organelles and enzyme content of the hepatocytes in the three zones are different, although the significance of the differences has not been fully elucidated.

   E. The three zones of the simple acinus are defined by their proximity to their arterial and portal terminal branches, not by their apparent microscopic proximity to the portal space. Hepatocytes seen in a microscopic section of a needle biopsy present a two-dimensional picture of a three-dimensional structure. Hence, the cells located near a portal area may actually be supplied by sinusoidal branches off the axial stream of an adjacent simple acinus and thus function as part of zone 3.

   F. A complex acinus is composed of at least three simple acini and the

141

Figure 23-1

Simple acinus. PA = portal area; THV = terminal hepatic venule (central vein); 1, 2, and 3 = three zones of the simple acinus. (Modified from A. M. Rappaport, Physioanatomic considerations. In L. Schiff (Ed.), Diseases of the Liver *(5th ed.). Philadelphia: Lippincott, 1982, p. 8. Reproduced with permission of the publisher and A. M. Rappaport.)*

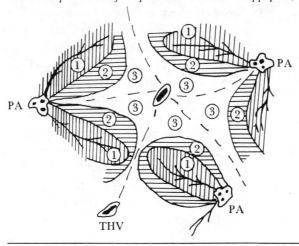

hepatocytes adjacent to the terminal vascular branches. The preterminal arterioles and portal venule divide into three terminal branches, which are the axial vessels for each of the three simple acini.

G. The acinar agglomerates are composed of three or four complex hepatic acini and of the perivascular hepatic parenchyma.

III. Physiologic events that change liver blood flow. In comparison with flow rates at rest, eating a meal markedly increases portal vein and superior mesenteric artery flow without a substantial change in hepatic or splenic artery flow. In contrast, during jogging, portal vein flow is decreased, due to a reduced splenic artery and superior mesentery artery flow, while hepatic artery flow may almost double. The sinusoids play a major role in controlling portal pressure. In the normal liver with usual blood flow, only about 20 percent of sinusoids are utilized. As portal flow increases, more sinusoids are opened to reduce intrahepatic resistance. Portal pressure equals flow times the hepatic resistance; it is the pressure that is required to perfuse the liver.

IV. Cardinal manifestations of liver disease. The liver responds to insult in a limited number of ways. Hence, the pathophysiologic consequences of liver disease usually involve jaundice, portal hypertension, ascites, or portosystemic encephalopathy. The mechanisms of these major manifestations of liver disease will therefore be described.

A. Jaundice

1. Definition. Jaundice is the yellow color of the skin and ocular sclera resulting from increased bilirubin in the blood. In the deeply jaundiced patient, urine and sweat are also colored. The depth of the jaundice depends on bile pigment production, bile excretion, and the amount of conjugated bilirubin present. The conjugated form is water-soluble and penetrates fluids more readily than the unconjugated forms. Since jaundice signals disordered bilirubin metabolism, a brief review of the latter is in order.

2. Bilirubin metabolism. Unconjugated bilirubin is produced from heme, which comes primarily from hemoglobin. Approximately 30 mg of bilirubin is produced each day from 6 g of hemoglobin. The unconjugated bilirubin is transported in plasma bound to albumin.

Hepatic uptake at the sinusoidal membrane involves detachment from the albumin. The bilirubin is transported in the hepatocyte by Y and Z transport proteins to the microsomes, where it is conjugated to a water-soluble polar compound. It is then excreted through the canaliculi and through the bile ducts to the duodenum. After passage to the colon, bacteria hydrolyze the conjugated bilirubin to urobilinogen. Urobilinogen is nonpolar and well absorbed from the small intestine, but only slightly from the colon. The portion that is absorbed is re-excreted by the kidney and liver.

3. **Mechanisms of jaundice.** Jaundice can result from a defect of bilirubin metabolism or excretion, which is either prehepatic, hepatic, or cholestatic in origin.

   a. **Prehepatic.** If red cell destruction (hemolysis) is brisk, even a normal liver may be unable to handle the increased load of unconjugated bilirubin. Under these circumstances, the bilirubin elevation is usually modest unless there is an additional disturbance of bilirubin metabolism or transport.

   b. **Hepatic.** Impairment of bilirubin uptake by the hepatocytes, altered transport within the hepatocytes, or defects in bilirubin conjugation have been described in a variety of liver diseases.

   c. **Cholestatic jaundice.** Here the defect occurs distal to bilirubin conjugation. It may involve impaired transport out of the hepatocyte or along the bile canaliculi through the bile duct system to the duodenum.

   d. **Multiple mechanisms.** Jaundice is usually not due to a single isolated defect. For example, in the condition called familial unconjugated nonhemolytic hyperbilirubinemia, there may be a defect in uptake by the hepatocyte membrane, a defect in conjugation, and also mild hemolysis. In viral hepatitis, both failure of bilirubin conjugation and cholestasis contribute to the jaundice. The duration of the insult is also important. In common duct obstruction, the initial mechanism is cholestasis, but with prolonged obstruction, there is hepatocyte damage that leads to alterations in bilirubin transport and conjugation.

B. **Portal hypertension.** Portal hypertension may be defined as an increased pressure in the portal vein that is above normal physiologic levels. It can broadly be classified into three types, depending on the site of origin.

   1. **Classification**

      a. **Suprahepatic.** Hepatic vein thrombosis (Budd-Chiari syndrome), right-sided heart failure, and constrictive pericarditis can all increase portal pressure, primarily by increasing resistance through the hepatic veins.

      b. **Intrahepatic.** A number of factors are frequently operational in this condition. Portal hypertension is usually the result of increased intrahepatic resistance to blood flow through the liver. Altered architecture due to inflammation, cellular infiltrate, collagen formation, and regenerating nodules may increase hepatic vascular resistance. Sinusoids are destroyed and altered, so that the liver cannot lower resistance by increasing sinusoid flow. Since hepatic arterial flow stays relatively constant, the shunted arterial blood may contribute to the increased pressure on the venous side. With cirrhosis, portal flow is actually reduced, owing to the increased resistance. Flow may even be reversed, so that some hepatic arterial blood leaves by retrograde passage into the portal vein.

   c. Infrahepatic. In this instance, the resistance and pressure in the portal vein segment are increased.

2. **Collateral circulation with portal hypertension.** Portal hypertension leads to the development of a characteristic pattern of collateral venous circulation. However, these collateral channels rarely lower the portal pressure to the normal range. The consequences of this collateral circulation relate to the transmission of the high pressure within the portal venous system to the systemic venous circulation. The collaterals develop in the submucosa of the esophagus and stomach, the azygous system, the submucosa of the rectum, the anterior abdominal wall, and the left renal vein. With portal vein obstruction (infrahepatic), additional collaterals may be formed.

     Hemorrhoids, which may be a source of pain and bleeding, are a result of the collaterals in the rectal submucosa. Multiple intraabdominal collaterals may complicate abdominal surgery. However, the most potentially serious collateral channels are those of the submucosa of the esophagus and the stomach. Bleeding from these varices accounts directly or indirectly for about one-half the deaths in patients with hepatic cirrhosis. Hence, pathophysiology of these varices will be described in some detail.

     Approximately 80 percent of the esophageal varices are supplied by the coronary system, a tributary of the main portal vein that courses the lesser curvature of the stomach. About 50 percent of varices are also supplied by the short gastric vein; in about 15 percent, this is the exclusive supply. The reasons for esophageal variceal bleeding are not clear. A number of factors may account for the susceptibility of these vessels to bleeding, including little supporting tissue, esophagitis, and local erosions. Pressure changes during respiration have been implicated. The height of the portal blood pressure is probably also important. Esophageal varices may be asymptomatic when bleeding occurs, but bleeding is usually a dramatic event that may lead to death or hepatic decompensation, ascites, and hepatic encephalopathy.

C. Ascites

1. **Mechanisms.** Ascites may occur in any edema-forming state as well as numerous intraabdominal conditions. This discussion, however, will be limited to the mechanisms of ascites associated with liver disease. Ascites formation may involve local factors and renal factors.

   a. Local factors

    (1) Portal hypertension with its increased venous pressure favors passage of fluid out of the vessels.

    (2) Lowered plasma colloid osmotic pressure, due to decreased plasma albumin, diminishes the intravascular force for fluid reabsorption.

    (3) Increased hepatic sinusoid pressure causes increased lymph formation, which may then exude from the hepatic surface.

    (4) The relative importance of these local factors varies considerably among patients. For example, with more severe portal hypertension, less depression of the plasma albumin is required for ascites formation. The increased vascular pressure causes loss of fluid from vessels of the mesenteric bed, which, along with increased lymph leakage, favors localization of fluid accumulation to the peritoneal cavity.

    b. Renal factors. For ascites to accumulate, the renal excretion of sodium and water must be less than the amounts ingested. There is still much controversy in this area since it is a dynamic system, but the primary mechanisms thought to be involved are as follows:

        (1) Ascites formation due to local factors decreases the effective blood volume so that there is a reduction in renal perfusion.

        (2) The reduced blood volume also stimulates the renin-angiotensin-aldosterone system.

        (3) Increased plasma renin and aldosterone may result from a number of other factors, including impairment of metabolism and intrarenal redistribution of plasma flow.

2. Major theories of ascites formation. There are two major theories that rely on the above mechanisms to explain ascites formation. Unfortunately, both of these theories are probably too simple, rely too much on renal factors, and do not elucidate the variable and complex factors that occur in the heterogeneous population with liver disease who develop ascites.

    a. In the first theory, sodium retention is secondary to the ascites formation. Because of the loss of fluid into the peritoneal cavity and pooling of splanchnic blood, the effective extracellular fluid and blood volumes are reduced. As a consequence, renal perfusion decreases and the kidney retains sodium, partly from activation of the renin-angiotensin-aldosterone system and also for less well-understood reasons.

    b. In the second theory, the renal retention of sodium and water, due to liver disease, is the primary event. The increased extracellular fluid overflows into the peritoneal cavity if local factors (portal pressure, plasma oncotic pressure, hepatic lymph drainage) favor fluid transudation.

3. Clinical consequences of ascites. Ascites due to liver disease implies a poor prognosis. Among patients with cirrhosis, only 40 percent survive 2 years after ascites develops. Ascites may be precipitated by a high salt intake or any event impairing hepatic function, such as gastrointestinal bleeding. Complications of ascites include patient discomfort, umbilical hernia, and respiratory embarrassment due to elevation of the diaphragm. Spontaneous bacterial peritonitis may occur and should be considered in any patient with cirrhosis and ascites who experiences an acute clinical deterioration.

D. Hepatic encephalopathy (portosystemic encephalopathy)

1. Definition. This is a complex syndrome of neuropsychiatric disturbances occurring in patients with liver disease. It is reflected by various degrees of deterioration in intellectual function, personal behavior, and state of consciousness. There are no liver chemistry or plasma electrolyte disturbances invariably associated with hepatic encephalopathy. Blood ammonia is not always elevated.

2. Pathogenesis. In patients with hepatic encephalopathy, portal blood enters the systemic vascular system and passes to the brain without metabolism of its content. This may result from inade-

Table 23-1   *Clinical Stages of Hepatic Encephalopathy*

Stages	Asterixis*	Mental State
I	+	Intermittent disorientation and confusion
II	+ +	Sleepy, altered behavior
III	+/−	Stuporous, but responds to pain
IV	−	Coma, unresponsiveness

*Asterixis is a coarse, flapping tremor most easily demonstrated in the hands (not specific for hepatic encephalopathy).

quate hepatocellular function and/or from the portal blood bypassing the liver through collaterals and shunts. Alterations in ammonia metabolism are a factor. An amino acid imbalance, mercaptans, and short-chain fatty acids have also been incriminated. As the condition becomes chronic, the patient's brain appears to become more sensitive to a number of insults.

3. **Clinical features.** Hepatic encephalopathy may be due to acute fulminant liver disease or progressive deterioration of chronic liver disease. Gastrointestinal bleeding, with increased blood (protein) in the gastrointestinal tract and associated deterioration of liver function, is often a precipitating event. Increased protein intake, infection, electrolyte imbalance, sedatives, and constipation may all contribute to the pathogenesis. The untreated course typically progresses through several stages of severity (see Table 23-1). However, the prognosis depends on the nature of the associated liver disease. When the onset is acute, such as acute fulminant hepatitis, the prognosis is poor. Intermittent or chronic encephalopathy may be found in stable diseases, such as cirrhosis. In these cases, the prognosis is better.

V. **Clinical examples of liver disease**

A. **Hepatic encephalopathy**

1. **Description.** The family of a 55-year-old man telephoned to say he had been acting strangely for at least the last 6 months. He had become forgetful and irritable; at work he fell asleep during conferences, but was up part of every night. The family wanted to know the name of a psychiatrist.

This patient was followed for 5 years for biopsy-proved, stable cirrhosis. When seen in the physician's office the next morning, the patient was neat, well dressed, and superficially normal. However, he said that he had been forgetting things more easily, he had trouble staying awake during the day, and his secretary had been complaining about his writing. His only other complaint was that he had been more constipated the last few months since he went on a high-protein, low-calorie, and low-fiber reducing diet. There was no history of head trauma or other neurologic symptoms. Physical examination was unchanged except for mild asterixis. When he wrote his name, it was almost illegible, which was a change when compared with his previous signature. Biochemical studies were unchanged.

Bulk was added to his diet, dietary protein was reduced, and a mild laxative was prescribed. He returned with his wife in 10 days at which time he reported that his bowels had been more regular, and his wife said he was himself again.

2. Discussion. This patient illustrated the following points.

    a. Portal systemic encephalopathy (PSE) may vary in its severity throughout the day.

    b. It is frequently confused with primary psychosis. To make the diagnosis, one must consider other neurologic conditions.

    c. Liver chemistries do not help establish the diagnosis; it is basically a clinical diagnosis. Although often elevated, blood ammonia levels frequently do not help in establishing a diagnosis.

    d. Chronic constipation, increased protein intake, and medications may precipitate PSE in the setting of chronic, stable liver disease. Removing these causes may be adequate to help the patient.

B. Portal hypertension

  1. Description. A 65-year-old man was brought to the emergency room with a history of having vomited bright red blood. He had been in good health all of his life and retired as a bank president 10 years ago. He denied any abdominal pain, but on occasion had taken antacids for an upset stomach. He had been a social drinker all of his life, but for the last 6 to 7 years had been drinking up to a fifth of vodka a day. Yearly examinations had been normal, except for some mild abnormality of his liver chemistries last year. On physical examination, he showed muscle wasting of the upper extremities and shoulders. His blood pressure decreased slightly, and his pulse increased when he sat up. The liver and spleen were just palpable. Initial laboratory studies revealed a moderate anemia and slight abnormalities of the liver chemistries. He was hospitalized and stabilized with blood transfusions. When endoscoped, large esophageal varices were seen with a clot adherent to one area. There was no more bleeding. He refused surgery to reduce portal hypertension and was discharged after 4 weeks. It was recommended that he stop drinking.

  2. Discussion. This patient illustrates the following points.

    a. Rather severe liver damage can occur with few symptoms and signs. Chemistries are usually deranged early, but may not be increased in proportion to the degree of liver disease.

    b. Esophageal variceal bleeding may be the first sign of liver disease with portal hypertension, although this is not usually the case.

    c. The patient's ultimate prognosis depends on the degree and extent of liver damage (how reversible it is), if he stops drinking or not, and other factors we have not identified.

Questions

More than one answer may be correct.

1. An alcoholic man with histologically proved cirrhosis had not drunk alcohol in 2 years. He and his wife had an argument and he went to the local bar, where he drank three beers. Along with the beer, he ate three large packages of potato chips, an unspecified number of pretzels, and two salty ham sandwiches. That evening his pants were tight, and the next day he could not button them. On physical examination he had obvious ascites. Which of the following are true?

  a. He had been in a fragile balance of hepatic compensation.

  b. The alcohol in the three beers caused his ascites.

  c. The salt was a bigger load than his kidneys could excrete.

d. He should have a diagnostic paracentesis.

e. The amount of fluid in the three beers caused his ascites.

2. A 24-year-old nurse who had been receiving treatment for chronic active hepatitis for 4 years was referred by her supervisor, who complained that recently the patient had begun confusing medications, writing rambling notes, and napping on duty. When seen in the office, the patient was slightly confused and had asterixis. Which statement(s) are true?

a. The patient probably has hepatic encephalopathy.

b. Her liver chemistries will be more abnormal than before.

c. If a blood ammonia is obtained and it is normal, the diagnosis of hepatic encephalopathy may be ruled out.

d. Recently she had been on a high-carbohydrate diet to increase her weight, and this was probably the cause of her problem.

e. A careful search should be made for all possible causes of her problem.

Maldigestion, Malabsorption, and Diarrhea

I. **Normal physiology**
   A. **Salivary gland amylase** partially hydrolyzes starch and glycogen into maltose and a variety of larger fragments.
   B. **Gastric function.** The stomach mixes ingested materials, reduces particle size, and controls the rate of delivery into the duodenum. Gastric proteases attack many proteins, but produce only slight hydrolysis; they are not essential for protein hydrolysis. The combined effects of proteases and hydrochloric acid release vitamin B_{12} from its dietary sources. Intrinsic factor necessary for intestinal absorption of vitamin B_{12} is secreted by gastric mucosa.
   C. **Pancreas (exocrine).** The pancreas secretes a variety of digestive enzymes, electrolytes, and bicarbonate. The bicarbonate neutralizes acid entering the duodenum, making the intraluminal pH alkaline. Pancreatic secretions are controlled primarily by two hormones: (1) Cholecystokinin-pancreozymin (CCK-PZ) released from the duodenum in response to intraluminal acid, peptones, amino acids, digested fats, and fatty acids. CCK-PZ increases the secretion of all pancreatic enzymes. (2) Secretin, which stimulates water and bicarbonate secretion, is released from the duodenum in response to low intraluminal pH. There are three types of pancreatic enzymes:
      1. **Pancreatic amylase** is virtually identical with salivary amylase. It splits starches and glycogen into their constituent maltose or maltotrios units, at a pH optimum of 6.9.
      2. **Pancreatic proteases** are secreted as inactive zymogens. In the intestine, enterokinase secreted by the intestinal mucosa activates trypsinogen to trypsin. Trypsin, in turn, activates chymotrypsinogen to chymotrypsin and procarboxypeptidase to carboxypeptidase. Although some amino acids are formed by the action of these proteases, the main products are peptides.
      3. **Pancreatic lipase** is secreted as an active enzyme, not a proenzyme. It is secreted in great excess. Its activity is destroyed by a pH less than 3 and is optimal at a pH of about 6 to 7.
   D. **Small intestine**
      1. **Digestive function.** There are digestive enzymes on the border of the surface epithelial cells of the small intestine. Disaccharidases hydrolyze dietary disaccharides to monosaccharides, which can be absorbed. Peptidases hydrolyze peptides to amino acids. Some peptides are absorbed intact and are hydrolyzed by intracellular peptidases.
      2. **Absorptive function.** The proximal small intestine provides a large area for absorption of protein products, fats, carbohydrates, minerals, water, and vitamins. The maximum absorptive capacity for water is approximately 10 to 12 L per 24 hr, and the normal water load is about 7 to 9 L per 24 hr. Water movement is passive, coupled to active solute transport. The terminal ileum is the exclusive site for absorption of bile acids and vitamin B_{12}.

E. Colon. The major function of the large intestine is to absorb water and electrolytes. Maximum absorptive capacity for water is approximately 4 to 6 L per 24 hr, and the normal water load is 2 to 3 L. The only significant nutrients absorbed by the colon are short-chain fatty acids.

II. **Mechanisms of fat digestion and absorption**

A. **Intraluminal digestion.** The mechanisms for intraluminal digestion depend on the form of the ingested lipid and can be divided into three types.

1. **Hydrolysis** followed by micellar dispersion (e.g., triglyceride).

2. **Micellar dispersion** alone (hydrolysis unnecessary) (e.g., cholesterol and fat-soluble vitamins A, D, E, and K).

3. **Hydrolysis alone.** The products of hydrolysis are water soluble, so micellar dispersion is unnecessary (e.g., synthetic medium-chain triglycerides).

B. **Triglyceride digestion and absorption.** Essential steps in triglyceride digestion and absorption are:

1. **Emulsification** of ingested fat in stomach and small intestine.

2. **Release** of cholecystokinin-pancreozymin, which causes pancreatic enzyme and bile secretion into the duodenum.

3. **Hydrolysis** by pancreatic lipase of ingested triglyceride to lipolytic products.

4. **Transfer** of lipolytic products from oil phase to aqueous phase by micellar dispersion with bile acids.

5. **Diffusion** of micelles with uptake of the lipolytic products by the enterocytes.

III. **Maldigestion and malabsorption.** *Maldigestion* is the inability to absorb one or more dietary constituents as a result of inadequate digestion. *Malabsorption* is the failure of the intestinal tract to absorb or reabsorb any substance. Both are usually defined on the basis of the presence of steatorrhea (increased stool fat), but this is an inadequate definition. For example, 10 to 15 percent of patients with gluten-sensitive enteropathy do not have steatorrhea. Some patients may have combined defects; for example, the patient with gluten-sensitive enteropathy has maldigestion because of loss of intestinal digestive enzymes and malabsorption because of loss of absorptive surface.

A. **Maldigestion**

1. **Gastric enzyme/acid deficiency.** Lack of gastric juice proteolytic enzyme activity or acid has no significant effect on protein absorption. Their absence can, however, prevent the release of vitamin B_{12} bound to food sources. Hence, patients who secrete small amounts of intrinsic factor may become B_{12} deficient because they cannot release dietary B_{12}, whereas they can absorb oral crystalline vitamin B_{12} (e.g., postgastric surgery).

2. **Pancreatic insufficiency.** Lack of proteases, lipase, and amylase leads to inadequate digestion of dietary proteins, fats, and complex carbohydrates. There is normally a large excess of lipase; it must be reduced by at least 90 percent to produce steatorrhea.

3. **Intestinal disaccharidase deficiency.** Lack of specific (primary) or all (secondary) disaccharidases produces decreased digestion (hydrolysis) of dietary disaccharides, with subsequent malabsorption.

4. **Intestinal protease deficiency.** May be primary (rare) or secondary, due to mucosal disease (tropical sprue).

5. **Impaired fat digestion.** This can result from a number of defects:

a. Impaired release of CCK-PZ (e.g., duodenal mucosal disease).

b. Delayed release of CCK-PZ with poor mixing of dietary fat and enzymes (e.g., Billroth II—partial gastrectomy with gastrojejunal anastomosis).

c. Pancreatic lipase deficiency (e.g., chronic pancreatitis).

d. Acid inactivation of lipase (e.g., gastrinoma with secretion of large amounts of gastrin that stimulate high acid secretion—the amount of acid is too great to be neutralized, and lipase is inactivated by the acid).

B. Malabsorption. Despite adequate digestion, nutrients may not be absorbed for a variety of reasons.

1. Lack of a secreted carrier, i.e., intrinsic factor. In adults, this is usually related to prior gastric surgery or atrophy of the gastric mucosal cells. The stomach is also unable to secrete acid and proteolytic enzymes, but it is primarily the lack of intrinsic factor that results in the vitamin B_{12} deficiency.

2. Bacterial overgrowth syndromes with increased numbers of bacteria present in various parts of the small intestine may occur as a result of a lack of gastric acid, a blind loop, or altered intestinal motility. Depending on the type and number of bacteria and their metabolic requirements, they may compete for various dietary and intraluminal constituents, with resulting malabsorption.

3. Diseased small intestinal mucosa (gluten-sensitive enteropathy, tropical sprue) may reduce absorptive capacity.

4. Decreased intestinal surface area. Large resections of jejunum and ileum can result in the short bowel syndrome, with malabsorption of multiple nutrients. Disease or surgical resection of the terminal ileum may result in vitamin B_{12} and bile acid malabsorption. Malabsorption of either is rare, however, with a resection of less than 50 to 55 cm of terminal small bowel. When 50 to 100 cm is resected, there may also be fat malabsorption.

IV. Diarrhea

A. Definition. Normal bowel movement frequency in healthy people ranges widely from about three per week to three per day. An increase in stool volume may provide a better definition. A stool weight of greater than 150 to 200 g per 24 hr can be considered diarrhea. A marked decrease in stool consistency is another criterion for diarrhea.

B. Classification of diarrhea. The mechanisms of diarrhea can be categorized as either osmotic or secretory in type.

1. Osmotic. Osmotic diarrhea results from retention in the bowel lumen of nonabsorbable material. Examples include lactose in patients with lactase deficiency and some osmotic laxatives. Osmotic diarrhea is characterized by a stool fluid osmolality significantly greater than twice the concentration of sodium plus potassium (an osmotic gap).

2. Secretory. Most diarrheas fall into the secretory group. Diarrhea will result whenever the rate of intestinal secretion in the small intestine or colon exceeds the rate of fluid reabsorption. Secretory diarrhea is characterized by stool fluid osmolality approximately twice the sum of the sodium and potassium concentrations in the stool. The following are four examples of secretory diarrhea:

a. Diarrhea may be caused by the effect of bacterial toxins on the intestinal mucosa (e.g., cholera).

b. Secretion may be the result of a hormone produced by a tumor (e.g., vasoactive intestinal peptide [VIP]).

  c. Increased colonic secretions may result from the effects of unabsorbed bile acids.

  d. Diarrhea from unabsorbed fats can result from either of two mechanisms. When there is a lipase deficiency, unabsorbed fats reach the colon and are hydrolyzed by bacterial lipase, producing increased fatty acids in the stool contents. The fatty acids stimulate colonic secretion, causing diarrhea. Similarly, when fat has been hydrolyzed by adequate lipase, but is not absorbed due to mucosal disease or bile acid deficiency, the increased amount of fatty acids reaching the colon may stimulate secretion and cause diarrhea.

 3. Mixed osmotic and secretory. In many clinical examples, both mechanisms may be operative.

C. Interrelationships of small intestine and colon. When small intestinal secretion is increased, diarrhea does not necessarily result unless the absorptive capacity of the colon is exceeded. Also, diarrhea may occur when the amount of fluid reaching the ileocecal valve is normal, but either colonic absorption is decreased or there is active colon secretion.

V. Clinical examples

A. Gluten-sensitive enteropathy

 1. Description. A 32-year-old woman reported having diarrhea with three to five stools a day for the last 3 years. Milk made the diarrhea worse. She lost 26 pounds during this period although her appetite was good. A year ago she was noted to have a mild anemia, which did not respond to oral enteric-coated iron tablets.

  On physical examination she was pale and her abdomen slightly distended. The rest of the examination was within normal limits. Barium x-rays of the upper gastrointestinal tract and small intestine revealed an abnormal mucosal pattern. Laboratory studies showed the following: a low total serum protein concentration, mild anemia, an increased stool fat, and evidence of low D-xylose absorption. Biopsy of the jejunal mucosa demonstrated a flat appearance due to loss of villus structures. A gluten-free diet was instituted; within 3 weeks diarrhea had disappeared, and the patient had gained 7 pounds.

 2. Discussion

  a. There was laboratory evidence of malabsorption, intestinal villus atrophy, and a response to a gluten-free diet—sufficient data for a diagnosis of gluten-sensitive enteropathy.

  b. The diseased intestinal mucosa frequently cannot absorb iron from enteric-coated tablets.

  c. Most patients with this disease have an inability to absorb fat and carbohydrates, including D-xylose.

  d. The mucosal damage produces a secondary lactase deficiency, explaining the mild lactose intolerance which contributes to the diarrhea.

B. Pancreatic insufficiency

 1. Description. Over a period of a few months, a 54-year-old alcoholic man's bowel movements increased in amount but not in frequency. He noted a fat ring around the water level in the toilet. His appetite was good, but he lost 20 pounds. Physical examination revealed evidence of caloric-protein malnutrition. A plain x-ray of the abdomen demonstrated flaky calcifications in the area of the pancreas.

Laboratory data showed a mild anemia, slightly elevated fasting blood sugar, and increased stool fat. The D-xylose test was normal.

2. **Discussion**

   a. Patients with malabsorption/maldigestion are starving but may have a good appetite.

   b. The abnormal stool fat was due to a digestive defect (lack of adequate lipase). The carbohydrate, D-xylose, was normally absorbed because it did not need pancreatic enzymes (i.e., hydrolysis not required) for its absorption.

   c. Patients with pancreatic insufficiency frequently have large, bulky stools. There was increased passage of fat into the colon, where it was hydrolyzed by bacterial lipase. The increased concentration of fatty acids produced increased (net) water secretion by the colon.

Questions

More than one answer may be correct.

1. A 72-year-old woman complained of increasing weakness. She had felt tired for the last few years, but during the last 2 months the weakness had worsened. Recently she had also noted shortness of breath and swelling of her ankles. There was no history of other disease or prior surgery. She was sallow and had signs of congestive heart failure. Initial laboratory studies were essentially normal, except for a marked macrocytic anemia (Hgb of 3.1 g/dl) and a very low serum level of vitamin B_{12}. Which of the following are true?

   a. A maximum stimulated gastric analysis for the presence of acid would probably give abnormal results.

   b. Addition of intrinsic factor to oral radioactive vitamin B_{12} would demonstrate normal B_{12} absorption, if the patient has pernicious anemia.

   c. She probably absorbs dietary vitamin B_{12} normally.

   d. A biopsy of her gastric mucosa would be normal.

2. An alcoholic man is diagnosed as having chronic pancreatitis with pancreatic insufficiency, based on findings of calcification of the pancreas and increased stool fat. Studies for other causes for the steatorrhea were negative. Which of the following are probably true?

   a. The patient secretes inadequate amounts of lipase.

   b. This represented a digestive defect.

   c. Pancreatic lipase is a stable enzyme and not influenced by acid.

   d. His diarrhea is due to an osmotic load.

25 Gastrointestinal Malignancies

I. **General.** Malignancies of the gastrointestinal (GI) tract can be considered as involving either hollow organs or solid organs. Cancers of hollow organs (esophagus, stomach, small intestine, and colon) produce gastrointestinal symptoms because of the organs' tubular structure, functions, and communication with the outside of the body. Symptoms from cancers of solid organs (liver and pancreas) stem from the location more than the function of the affected organ, although loss of function may also cause symptoms. Gastrointestinal malignancies may also be associated with the systemic signs and symptoms of cancer described in Chapter 55, Extra-Neoplastic Manifestations of Malignancies.

II. **Malignancies of hollow organs.** Primary cancers of the hollow organs are much more common than metastatic lesions. Histologically, most malignancies of the esophagus are squamous, while those of the rest of the intestinal tract are adenocarcinomas. The cancers may infiltrate the wall of the organ, or they may protrude into the lumen as a mass; occasionally, both manifestations will be seen with the same cancer. The most common symptoms are due to obstruction, bleeding, or pain. The degree of obstruction depends in part on the size of the lumen and the consistency of the intraluminal material at the point of cancer involvement. Dysphagia (difficulty in swallowing) is common in cancer of the esophagus. Marked weight loss from the patient's inability to eat is often the presenting symptom.

Early satiety can be caused by gastric malignancies, as the distensibility of the organ decreases when cancer infiltrates the wall or fills the lumen. Gastric outlet obstruction from a gastric carcinoma may cause nausea and vomiting. Abdominal distress, cramping pain, and a change in bowel habits are frequent signs of small intestine or colon obstruction secondary to a cancer. Obstruction is less common in a right-colon malignancy than in a sigmoid-colon malignancy. In the right colon, the stool is in a liquid form and the lumen of the colon is at its maximum size. Toward the sigmoid colon, the lumen decreases in size and more water is removed from the stool. For this reason, obstruction of the sigmoid colon with formed stool is much more common than obstruction of the right colon with liquid stool.

Bleeding may result from ulceration of the tumor, vascular erosion, or tumor friability. Esophageal or gastric cancers that bleed may lead to hematemesis (vomiting blood), but may also produce melena. On occasion, iron-deficiency anemia may be documented in patients who experience no obvious blood in their stools. Bleeding is frequent in carcinoma of the colon and almost always occurs before the tumor has spread outside the lumen of the colon. Some patients may demonstrate hematochezia, but more often they have no obvious bleeding. For this reason, testing of the stool for blood may lead to an early diagnosis of carcinoma of the colon.

Pain from cancers of hollow organs usually results from contractions related to partial obstruction, but nerve involvement (usually of the serosa or peritoneum) from spread of the cancer can also cause pain. Metastases to the peritoneal surface can cause ascites, which is also a frequent source of discomfort for the patient.

III. **Solid organ malignancies.** Metastatic lesions to the liver are more common than primary hepatic malignancies (although the reverse is true of pancreatic cancer). Frequently, metastatic lesions to the liver are asymptomatic until the liver has been almost replaced by cancer. Pain may result from enlargement of the liver or from location of the tumor on the organ surface so that the peritoneum is irritated. Hepatic encephalopathy may occur as a preterminal event as the liver is destroyed and its ability to detoxify substances in the blood decreases. Jaundice, and rarely portal hypertension, may occur late in the course of the illness.

Pancreatic malignancies typically cause obstructive jaundice and pain. Small, asymptomatic, and therefore potentially curable cancers are infrequently found. Dull, localized epigastric pain is often the first symptom of pancreatic malignancy, although it usually occurs late in the growth of the tumor. The retroperitoneal location of the pancreas causes the pain to radiate to the patient's back.

Obstruction of the common bile duct where it enters the head of the pancreas often occurs with carcinoma located in the pancreatic head. With obstruction of the common bile duct, many changes can occur. Patients develop itching as bile salts are deposited in the skin along with the bilirubin that causes them to be jaundiced. Fat maldigestion secondary to inadequate micelle formation occurs, and steatorrhea may result. Since bile pigments cause the dark color of stool, when they no longer enter the bowel the stools become gray in appearance. Diabetes mellitus from destruction of islet cells or maldigestion from loss of enzyme-producing cells may result when there is far-advanced tumor replacement of the organ.

IV. **Clinical example of gastrointestinal malignancy**

A. **Description.** A 62-year-old male was admitted to the hospital with a 2-month history of dull, epigastric pain radiating to his back and a 10-pound weight loss. Recently, he had noted some itching, followed a few days later by dark urine and light-colored stools.

On physical exam he was thin and mildly jaundiced. Excoriations were noted on his arms and legs. A firm lymph node was found in his left supraclavicular area. The rest of his physical exam was unremarkable. Laboratory examination showed a low serum albumin concentration and elevated serum bilirubin and alkaline phosphatase levels. Sonography of the abdomen revealed a mass in the head of the pancreas and a large gallbladder without stones. Endoscopic retrograde cholangiopancreatography revealed destruction and narrowing of the pancreatic duct, as well as tumor involvement of the distal common bile duct.

He went to surgery, where biopsy of the lymph node revealed adenocarcinoma. Palliative abdominal surgery was done to relieve his jaundice and to protect against duodenal obstruction by the tumor (choledochaljejunostomy and gastrojejunostomy). The celiac ganglion was destroyed to help alleviate his pain.

Following surgery the jaundice and itching went away and his pain was somewhat better. He was able to return home until his death 10 months later, from pneumonia and malnutrition.

B. **Discussion.** This case illustrates many of the signs and symptoms of pancreatic carcinoma. The jaundice and itching (bile salt deposits in the skin) were caused by common bile duct obstruction. The pain location was typical and was apparently mediated by traffic through the celiac ganglion. His course was unfortunately typical for most patients with pancreatic cancer. The malignancy is rarely found at a small, curable stage, and the average life span following the diagnosis is approximately 6 to 8 months.

Questions

More than one answer may be correct.

1. Based on the assumption that the tumor size is the same, symptoms of partial obstruction would occur earliest with carcinoma of the:
   a. Esophagus.
   b. Stomach.
   c. Right colon.
   d. Sigmoid colon.
2. The steatorrhea that can be seen with pancreatic carcinoma can be caused by:
   a. Malabsorption secondary to jejunal abnormalities.
   b. Inadequate micelle formation from obstruction to the flow of bile.
   c. Inadequate amounts of lipase entering the duodenum from the pancreas.
   d. Malnutrition.
   e. Inadequate mixing of food, pancreatic enzymes, and bile salts.

V

Hematology

Sylvia S. Bottomley
Philip C. Comp
Dilip L. Solanki

Introduction to Hematology

The hematologic system is traditionally discussed in terms of its individual cellular components (i.e., the erythrocytes, leukocytes, and platelets) and the blood clotting process. Although each of these has unique physiologic characteristics and derangements in disease, they share other features. For example, the survival of the different blood cell types is variable yet finite, and the source of their replenishment is a common precursor cell, the totipotent stem cell (Fig. 26-1). This stem cell gives rise to: (1) a committed lymphocyte precursor, which initiates the lymphoid cell line, ultimately producing lymphocytes and plasma cells, and (2) a pluripotent myeloid precursor cell, which initiates development of the erythroid, granulocytic, and megakaryocytic cell lines, ultimately producing erythrocytes, granulocytes, monocytes, and platelets. The totipotent and pluripotent stem cells are self-renewing in response to their depletion as they feed to committed stem-cell compartments. The committed stem cells are not self-renewing, but respond to specific regulatory humoral factors that initiate their differentiation. What regulates the transition between the uncommitted and committed stem cells is not yet defined.

Lesions in early precursor cells (i.e., totipotent and pluripotent stem cells) usually affect the quality or quantity of all the various blood cells. An appropriate soil (the hematopoietic microenvironment) comprised of a reticular framework, the vasculature of the marrow tissue and stromal cells, ensures the integrity and potential of the seed (the stem cell population); a disease process affecting the soil can also derange hematopoietic cell development. Abnormalities of the individual cell types reflect (1) developmental defects at the committed stem cell stage and beyond or (2) their undue loss or destruction beyond the normal bone marrow reserve capacity. The physiology and pathophysiology of blood coagulation, while relating to a large extent to fluid phase components of the blood, are importantly integrated with the blood platelets and sometimes with erythrocytes and leukocytes.

Figure 26-1　　　　*Hematopoietic cell differentiation.*

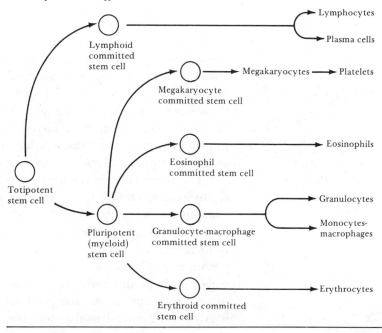

Disorders of the Erythron

I. **Normal physiology**

A. **Erythrocyte production (erythropoiesis) and survival.** The term *erythron* is applied to the entire erythrocytic tissue, comprising the circulating erythrocytes (the red cell mass) and the immature erythroid cell component in the bone marrow. The erythrocyte develops in approximately 5 days (Fig. 27-1): the erythropoietin-responsive cells (ERC), under the influence of the hormone erythropoietin, differentiate and acquire the specific capacities for erythroid development; then each proliferates through four cell divisions (yielding 16 cells), and simultaneously matures as nuclear and cell size decrease and cytoplasmic hemoglobin accumulates. Finally the nucleus is extruded, resulting in a reticulocyte. In a couple of days, the reticulocyte is released into the circulation, where during the ensuing 24 hours it produces the last small percentage of its hemoglobin before the residual hemoglobin-synthesizing organelles are lost. Hence, the reticulocyte content in the peripheral blood reflects the birth rate of new erythrocytes and is a quantitative index of erythroid marrow function.

The erythrocyte remains intravascular for 120 days, during which there is progressive loss of membrane, critical enzymes, and metabolic intermediates necessary for its structural and functional integrity; it is removed by the reticuloendothelial (RE) system. At this point the erythrocyte's membrane and proteins are catabolized, heme is converted to bilirubin, and iron is salvaged and transported to the marrow for reutilization in hemoglobin (Hb) synthesis. To maintain 25×10^{12} circulating erythrocytes (750 g Hb) in an adult man, the marrow must produce 2×10^{11} reticulocytes (6 g Hb) per day. It can increase this production rate six- to eightfold (half a pint of blood per day), so that the red-cell life span has to be reduced to below 15 to 20 days for anemia to ensue.

B. **Regulation of erythrocyte production.** During its 175-mile voyage through the bloodstream, the erythrocyte's principal function is as a vehicle for hemoglobin, the respiratory pigment that accepts oxygen in the lung, then transports and releases it to tissues. While reduction in tissue oxygen supply promptly engages certain general physiologic mechanisms—such as an increase in cardiac output, an increase in active tissue capillaries, or a rightward shift of the oxygen-dissociated curve (to enhance release of oxygen to tissues at lower pressures)—tissue oxygen supply is the fundamental factor regulating red-cell production through the humoral mediator erythropoietin (Fig. 27-1). The principal hypoxia sensor tissue resides in the kidney and in response to oxygen requirements releases erythropoietin.

The three current theories are: (1) the kidney releases a renal erythropoietic factor (REF), an enzyme that activates a precursor globulin (formed by the liver) to produce the active erythropoietin; (2) the kidney releases a proerythropoietin, which is activated by a serum factor; and (3) the kidney releases the active hormone. Some erythropoietin is produced in extrarenal sites (e.g., the liver) because it is detectable in plasma and urine of anephric individuals. Other regulators of erythropoiesis are the hormones from the testes and the pituitary, thyroid, and adrenal glands, since hypofunction of these tissues

Figure 27-1

Regulatory circuits of erythrocyte production. Hb = hemoglobin; TSC = totipotent stem cell; PSC = pluripotent stem cell; ERC = erythropoietin-responsive cell; RBC = red blood cell; Retic = reticulocyte; REF = renal erythropoietic factor.

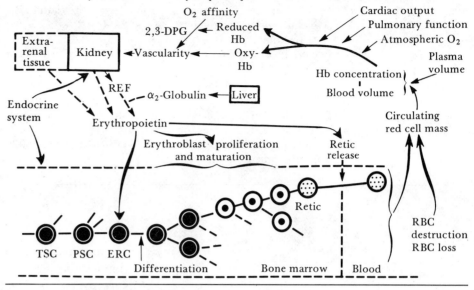

results in diminished rates and hyperfunction in increased rates of erythropoiesis. The precise mechanisms of action of these hormones have not been defined. Oxygen requirements play the major role in thyroidal control of erythropoiesis. Androgens enhance production of erythropoietin by increasing its release by the kidney and appear to enhance erythroid marrow cell differentiation, explaining the higher circulating red cell count in males.

II. Mechanisms of anemia

A. Diminished bone marrow capacity for erythrocyte production

1. **Hypoproliferative anemia.** Loss of stem cells or inhibition of their function reduces or may halt erythroid differentiation and proliferation. The erythroid marrow becomes hypoplastic, and the number of reticulocytes in the peripheral blood approaches zero. While dysfunction of erythroid-committed stem cells results in pure red-cell aplasia, in clinical practice damage to the pluripotent stem cells is more commonly encountered; consequently, leukopenia and thrombocytopenia accompany such anemia (aplastic anemia). Marrow toxins (e.g., drugs, chemicals, and x-rays) cause a variably reparable injury of stem cells. Proliferation of tumor cells and a fibrosis process within the marrow space disrupt the critical stem-cell environment. Stem-cell function can also be inhibited by antibodies or abnormal lymphocytes (suppressor lymphocytes). The effects of a lack of erythropoietin on the erythron are analogous to dysfunctions of erythroid-committed stem cells because they represent the target tissue of the hormone. Erythropoietin production is impaired in diseases of tissues involved in its generation, namely, renal and liver disease (Fig. 27-1). Erythropoietin production is also reduced in chronic infection and inflammation. Finally, antibodies to erythropoietin may arise that inhibit the biologic activity of the hormone.

   The morphologic evidence for these disorders is a hypoplasia or aplasia of the erythroid cell line (and often also the other cell lines)

Table 27-1   *Mechanisms of Vitamin B$_{12}$ and Folic Acid Deficiency*

Deficiency	Cause	Physiologic Basis
Vitamin B$_{12}$ deficiency	Loss of intrinsic factor (e.g., pernicious anemia, infiltrative tumor of gastric fundus, gastrectomy)	Vitamin B$_{12}$ must be complexed with intrinsic factor for absorption in the ileum
	Bacterial colonization of small intestine	Bacteria consume the vitamin B$_{12}$ ingested in the diet
	Diseases of the terminal ileum	Vitamin B$_{12}$ is not absorbed because terminal ileum is its site of absorption
Folic acid deficiency	Dietary lack, or insufficient supply for increased needs (e.g., hemolysis, pregnancy)	Body reserves (stores) of folic acid are limited—sufficient for 5 mo
	Malabsorption diseases of the small intestine	Dietary folic acid is not absorbed
	Folic acid antagonist drugs	Drugs compete for enzymes that transform folate to metabolically active forms

in the marrow. In the case of stem-cell disorders those erythrocytes still produced tend to be macrocytic, presumably because of the great erythropoietin stimulus in response to anemic hypoxia, causing more rapid accumulation of hemoglobin with skipping of precursor cell divisions and thus resulting in larger cells. In disorders associated with decreased erythropoietin production, the erythrocytes are of normal size.

2. **Hyperproliferative anemia.** Disturbances in the orderly subcellular events during maturation of erythroid cells result in faulty erythroblasts, many of which are destroyed by marrow RE cells, a process called intramedullary hemolysis. Because stem-cell function is intact and erythropoietin production in response to the anemia is appropriate, the erythroid marrow is hypercellular, but the peripheral reticulocyte count is low. This constellation of features is termed ineffective erythropoiesis, characteristic of all erythroid maturation defects.

Cell division and nuclear maturation are slowed due to impaired nucleic acid production, specifically deoxyribonucleic acid (DNA), which can result from depletion of certain essential coenzymes or defects of enzymes involved in nucleic acid synthesis or other disturbances of nucleic acid metabolism. Vitamin B$_{12}$ and folic acid represent the principal coenzymes that can be depleted in man, each in certain settings of nutritional or metabolic aberrations (Table 27-1). Drugs, particularly chemotherapeutic and antineoplastic agents, inhibit nucleic acid biosynthesis. Impairment of DNA synthesis prolongs the resting phase of the dividing precursor cells between mitoses while cytoplasmic development proceeds unimpeded. The consequence is a megaloblastic cell, which is larger than normal and has excessive cytoplasm and a disproportionately immature nucleus. Only a proportion of such cells mature into large erythrocytes and are released into the circulation (macrocytic anemia), but have a reduced life span (see section **B** below). Leukocyte and megakaryocyte maturation is similarly affected, so that pancytopenia commonly accompanies megaloblastic anemia. Distinct effects of vitamin B$_{12}$ deficiency are neural deficits (particularly of peripheral sensory nerves and the dorsal and corticospinal tracts) because vitamin B$_{12}$ is also an essential coenzyme for myelin formation.

Defective hemoglobin synthesis interferes with cytoplasmic maturation. Here erythroid cells seem to continue to divide; the resulting erythrocytes are small and poorly hemoglobinized (microcytic-hypochromic anemia) and also have a reduced life span. Iron deficiency (e.g., from chronic blood loss) and the unavailability of iron (e.g., in chronic inflammation/infection where RE iron salvaged from effete erythrocytes is not sufficiently released for reutilization in the normal renewal of red cells) represent the most common mechanisms. With the genetic loss of the ability to form one or more globin chains, as in the thalassemias, there is less hemoglobin produced per cell; in addition, the associated relative cytoplasmic excess of the normally synthesized complementary globin chain interferes with erythroid cell maturation as well as survival of those erythrocytes that reach the circulation (see section **B** below). Incompletely defined defects in heme biosynthesis or iron metabolism in sideroblastic anemias constitute the third mechanism impairing hemoglobin synthesis. In these instances, enormous amounts of iron characteristically accumulate in mitochondria of erythroblasts, impeding their development.

B. **Increased erythrocyte destruction (hemolysis).** The rate of erythrocyte loss (hemorrhage) or destruction (hemolysis) must exceed the production capacity of the normal marrow for anemia to develop; thus, a mild hemolysis will not produce anemia. Signs of increased red-cell regeneration (e.g., reticulocytosis or marrow erythroid hyperplasia) or of increased Hb breakdown (e.g., hyperbilirubinemia) are therefore the only clues for compensated hemolytic disease. Among the numerous causes of hemolysis, erythrocytes succumb to premature destruction through one of three general pathophysiologic mechanisms:

1. **Decreased erythrocyte deformability.** The erythrocyte does not survive beyond 120 days in individuals who have had splenectomy. However, the erythrocyte's survival for 120 days in the presence of the spleen is largely dependent upon its ability to deform, or change from its round, biconcave, 7-micron disk shape into an elongated shape that can traverse from the red pulp of the splenic cords through the 0.5- to 2.5-micron space between endothelial cells lining the venous sinuses of the spleen. A prolonged sojourn of a less deformable erythrocyte in splenic cords, where viscosity is high and pH, glucose concentration, and partial pressure of oxygen are low, reduces its limited metabolic resources and favors premature phagocytosis. A decreased or increased membrane-to-volume ratio, increased cytoplasmic viscosity, and damage to the membrane of the erythrocyte all reduce its normal deformability (Table 27-2).

2. **Enhanced erythrocyte phagocytosis.** Antibody- or complement-coated erythrocytes (e.g., due to incompatible blood transfusion, drugs, or autoantibodies) are removed in part or entirely by splenic or hepatic macrophages through interaction of the Fc fragment receptor or complement receptor on the macrophage and the Fc fragment of the antibody or the complement on the erythrocytes. Partial phagocytosis removes more membrane than cytoplasm, resulting in a spherocyte. These functions of the RE system lead to a work hypertrophy of the organs of erythrocyte destruction (splenomegaly and hepatomegaly). On the other hand, an enlarged spleen from other causes (e.g., congestive or infiltrative splenomegaly) can sequester normal erythrocytes excessively (hypersplenism).

Table 27-2 *Causes of Decreased Erythrocyte Deformability*

1. Decreased membrane-to-volume ratio
   a. Normal aging erythrocyte
   b. Spherocyte (e.g., hereditary spherocytosis, immune hemolysis)
2. Increased membrane-to-volume ratio
   a. Target cell (e.g., hypochromic anemias)
   b. Spur cell (increased membrane cholesterol, e.g., liver cirrhosis)
3. Increased cytoplasmic viscosity and cell rigidity
   a. Sickle cell (hemoglobin aggregation due to hypoxia)
   b. Dehydrated cells (loss of cell water from ATP lack, e.g., pyruvate kinase deficiency)
4. Membrane damage (stretched, distorted, denatured membrane)
   a. Fragmented cell (from shear stress forces in the vasculature, e.g., angiopathic hemolysis)
   b. Heinz bodies (precipitation of denatured hemoglobin on the membrane, e.g., from oxidant drugs, G-6-PD deficiency, excess globin chains in thalassemias)
   c. Oxidant-induced cross-linking of the membrane skeleton

G-6-PD = glucose 6-phosphate dehydrogenase.

Figure 27-2 *The handling of hemoglobin released into plasma.*

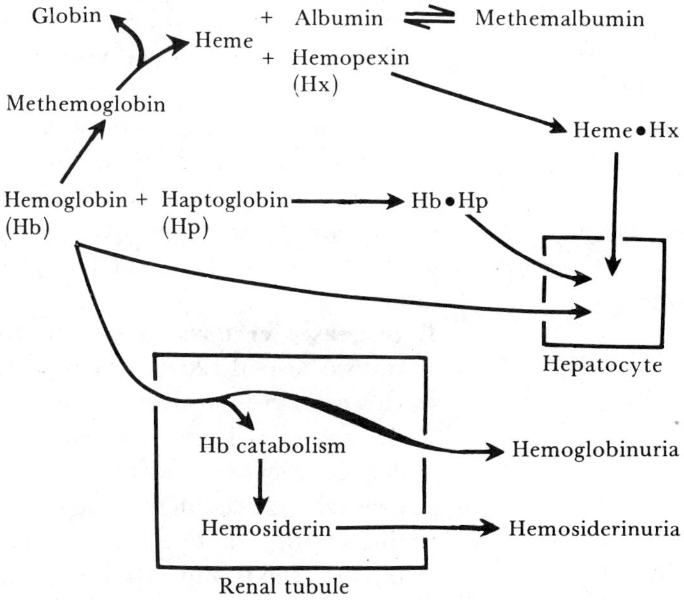

3. **Disruption of the erythrocyte membrane in the vasculature (intravascular hemolysis).** The erythrocyte may be prematurely destroyed by outright lysis within the circulation by: (a) mechanical disruption in angiopathic states mentioned above; (b) antibody-mediated hemolysis when complement is bound to the erythrocyte and becomes fully activated; (c) complement-mediated hemolysis without antibody, unique for the paroxysmal nocturnal hemoglobinuria defect; (d) an oxidant stress sufficiently severe (usually from oxidant drugs) to disrupt the integrity of the membrane; and (e) lysins generated by certain bacteria (e.g., *Clostridium welchii*) or venoms reaching the circulation. Hemoglobin is released into the plasma (hemoglobinemia) and the mechanisms of its subsequent disposal are accompanied by distinct biochemical features useful in recognizing the event of intravascular hemolysis (Fig. 27-2): low serum haptoglobin and hemopexin (these become depleted),

Table 27-3   *Pathophysiologic Classification of Polycythemia*

I. Appropriate
   A. Hypoxemic states (decreased PaO_2)
      1. Pulmonary disorders
      2. Cardiac right-to-left shunt
      3. High altitude
   B. Impaired oxygen delivery (normal PaO_2)
      1. Carboxyhemoglobinemia (smokers)
      2. Hemoglobinopathies with increased oxygen affinity
      3. Congenital methemoglobinemia
      4. Congenital decrease of red cell 2,3-DPG
II. Inappropriate
   A. Excess erythropoietin production
      1. Tumors (kidney, cerebellum, liver, uterus, adrenal)
      2. Renal lesions (renal artery stenosis, cysts, hydronephrosis, nephrotic syndrome)
      3. Familial erythrocytosis
   B. Autonomous erythropoiesis (polycythemia rubra vera)
III. Pseudopolycythemia (relative erythrocytosis)

2,3-DPG = 2,3-diphosphoglycerate.

methemalbuminemia, and hemosiderinuria with or without hemoglobinuria. Prolonged hemosiderinuria can also lead to iron deficiency.

C. Physiologic effects of anemia. The severity of anemia and the rate at which it has developed determine the hypoxic effects on other systems and hence on symptoms. Rapid blood loss (hemorrhagic anemia) may proportionately produce the symptoms of tachycardia, hypotension, and shock. With slow evolution of anemia, remarkable adaptation occurs and few if any symptoms appear in the absence of physical exertion. Once anemia is sufficiently severe, the status of the cardiovascular system, the principal physiologic compensatory mechanism for anemic hypoxia, determines clinical manifestations, e.g., shortness of breath, increased heart rate, palpitations, angina, and in older individuals, heart failure; other symptoms are referable to the muscular and central nervous system, e.g., fatigue, irritability, dizziness, and headache. Cardiac output remains relatively constant until the hemoglobin falls below 7 or 8 g/dl, when less than the normal 6 ml of O_2/dl of circulating blood can be made available to tissues (each gram of Hb carrying 1.36 ml of O_2 when completely saturated). Then cardiac output increases in proportion to the hemoglobin deficit, blood flow is redistributed to the most vital centers, renal blood flow may be reduced by 50 percent, and cutaneous flow is markedly decreased. Liver function is well maintained in severe anemia.

III. Mechanisms of polycythemia

   A. Appropriate increase of erythrocyte production. Polycythemia is most often encountered as a physiologic response to tissue oxygen deficits (Table 27-3). In this case, oxygen delivery is compensated by an erythropoietin-mediated increase in red-cell production, and one finds a direct relation between the red-cell mass and arterial oxygen saturation. The common examples are many pulmonary disorders, cardiac abnormalities accompanied by a right-to-left shunt, and the reduced oxygen saturation of hemoglobin associated with carboxyhemoglobinemia of heavy smokers. Uncommonly, mutations may impart to the hemoglobin molecule an increased affinity for oxygen, impairing its release to tissues. The classic example of a physiologic polycythemia is that which develops in individuals after sojourns at high altitude.

B. Physiologically inappropriate increase of erythrocyte production. Here one finds no direct relation between the red-cell mass and arterial oxygen saturation.

1. **Excessive erythropoietin production.** Large amounts of erythropoietin may be produced and released by several types of tumors (e.g., kidney, cerebellum, liver, uterus, or adrenal) or through local renal ischemia produced by certain benign lesions (e.g., renal artery stenosis, renal cysts, hydronephrosis). Removal of such lesions or repair of a renal artery stenosis corrects the polycythemia.

2. **Autonomous erythropoiesis.** In polycythemia rubra vera, a genetically altered pluripotent stem cell arises whose progeny committed to the erythroid, as well as granulocytic and megakaryocytic cell lines, proliferate independently of the normal humoral controls, the erythroid cell line proliferating most markedly. The stem-cell defect is such that the altered target cell for erythropoietin either is unduly sensitive to low levels of the hormone or proliferates autonomously. The massive red-cell overproduction possible in this disorder may double the circulating red-cell mass, iron supply becomes a rate-limiting factor, and the erythrocytes are often microcytic-hypochromic. It is the continued iron depletion achieved by phlebotomy therapy that serves best as a brake on the excessive erythroid proliferation. After 5 to 10 years or more, this process slows down, may be followed by bone-marrow fibrosis, and may terminate in acute leukemia.

C. Consequences of polycythemia. The physiologically harmful effects of polycythemic states are due mainly to increased blood viscosity that rises sharply with a hematocrit over 60 percent, particularly impairing cardiac hemodynamics and reducing oxygen transport, which in turn can further increase the erythrocytosis. The symptoms are similar to those of anemia. The cardiovascular stress from hypervolemia may be manifested as chest pain or fullness, increased heart rate, shortness of breath, or claudication; the effect on the central nervous system may result in irritability, light-headedness, or fatigue. In polycythemia rubra vera, the high blood viscosity, particularly when coupled with the thrombocytosis and occasionally coexisting atherosclerotic vascular disease, notably promotes arterial and venous thromboses and infarctions. The paradox of simultaneous hemorrhagic manifestations may also accompany this disease because of impaired platelet function as part and parcel of this myeloproliferative disorder (see Chap. 29, Platelets, section C, Platelet function).

D. Relative erythrocytosis. If the venous blood hemoglobin and hematocrit alone are relied upon, an apparent or relative polycythemia, caused by a reduction in plasma volume without a raised red-cell volume, may be overlooked. This combination is a common clinical occurrence, and isotopic measurements of the circulating red-cell and plasma volumes are necessary to establish the presence of true polycythemia. The common settings for a contracted plasma volume are hypertensive and atherosclerotic vascular diseases. The pathophysiologic mechanisms for the reduced plasma volume are not defined but are commonly accentuated by diuretic agents.

IV. Clinical examples

A. Anemia

1. Description. A 35-year-old man had experienced fatigue, intermittent, cramping abdominal pain, and occasional tarry stools for 3 months and had lost 30 pounds in weight. He appeared pale, there was a right–lower-quadrant mass, and the stool was positive for occult blood. With x-ray studies the diagnosis of regional enteritis was made. The Hb was 9 g/dl, and the anemia was corrected with iron therapy. Three years later, the man again complained of fatigue. Laboratory data were:

	3 Yr Ago	Now	Normal
Hemoglobin (g/dl)	9.0	7.5	14–18
Hematocrit (%)	30	20	40–53
Mean corpuscular volume (fl)	75	115	82–100
Reticulocytes (%)	1.0	1.2	0.8–2.5
Leukocytes ($\times\ 10^3/mm^3$)	11	3	4.5–10
Platelets ($\times\ 10^3/mm^3$)	400	90	200–400
Serum folate (ng/ml)	—	6	3–25
Serum vitamin B_{12} (pg/ml)	—	70	200–900

2. Discussion

a. Initially the anemia was hypochromic-microcytic and could be attributed to iron deficiency from chronic blood loss in the gastrointestinal tract, since it fully responded to iron therapy.

b. The anemia now is macrocytic, and the patient has pancytopenia because of vitamin B_{12} deficiency.

c. The vitamin B_{12} deficiency developed because of destruction of the mucosa of the ileum by regional ileitis.

B. Polycythemia

1. Description. A 46-year-old man had a routine medical examination before employment. He had smoked cigars and cigarettes for the past 25 years and had a nonproductive cough and mild fatigue. He appeared plethoric, but otherwise the physical examination was normal. The hemogram showed hemoglobin; 19 g/dl; hematocrit, 58 percent; mean corpuscular volume, 98 fl; white blood count, $7.5 \times 10^3/mm^3$; platelets, $280 \times 10^3/mm^3$. Other laboratory data were: red blood cell mass, 44 ml/kg (increased); plasma volume, 38 ml/kg (normal); arterial oxygen pressure, 75 mm Hg; CO_2 pressure, 35 mm Hg; arterial oxygen saturation, 88 percent; carboxyhemoglobin, 10 percent (increased); P_{50}, 23 mm Hg (low). Spirometry studies were normal. He stopped smoking, and 3 months later the hemoglobin was 16 g/dl and hematocrit 48 percent.

2. Discussion

a. The polycythemia could be attributed in part to the reduced arterial oxygen saturation caused by the presence of carboxyhemoglobin.

b. In addition, the carboxyhemoglobinemia caused an increased affinity of hemoglobin for oxygen (low P_{50}), impairing oxygen release to tissues and also mediating a compensatory increase in red-cell production.

c. The diagnosis of smoker's polycythemia was confirmed, since it reversed when smoking was stopped.

Questions

More than one answer may be correct.

1. Leukopenia and thrombocytopenia would be expected to occur along with anemia if the anemia is due to:
   a. A cytoplasmic maturation defect (e.g., iron deficiency).
   b. A nuclear maturation defect (e.g., pernicious anemia).
   c. A stem-cell defect (e.g., aplastic anemia).
   d. Hemolysis (e.g., hereditary spherocytosis).
2. Measurement of the arterial oxygen saturation distinguishes:
   a. Polycythemia rubra vera from polycythemia caused by a kidney tumor.
   b. Polycythemia rubra vera from polycythemia caused by chronic lung disease.
   c. Polycythemia rubra vera from relative polycythemia.
   d. Polycythemia due to right-to-left intracardiac shunt from polycythemia caused by emphysema.

28 Neutrophil Disorders

I. **Normal physiology**

   A. **Neutrophil production, survival, and regulation.** The granulocyte-macrophage committed stem cell differentiates in response to a "granulopoietin"—more commonly referred to as colony-stimulating factor (CSF) (Fig. 28-1). This stem cell then proliferates through three to seven cell divisions over 6 to 7 days, along with progressive maturation and acquisition of specific functions of granulocytes and monocytes. The mature monocyte circulates for 1 to 2 days before entering tissues, where it remains for weeks and functions as a macrophage. The kinetics of eosinophils and basophils, representing a small fraction of the granulocyte series, are not as yet well defined. In contrast, it is well established that a large portion of mature or near-mature neutrophils, equal to 10 times the number of neutrophils generated daily by the marrow, remain held up for 6 to 7 days in a marrow neutrophil reserve pool, which can be called upon for sudden needs (Fig. 28-1). After leaving the marrow, the neutrophil remains in the circulation only some 12 hours, approximately equally distributed between a circulating pool and a pool marginated along the vascular endothelium. The neutrophil then migrates into tissues, where its survival is 1 to 2 days.

   The control mechanisms through which the normal blood neutrophil concentration is maintained are not fully understood. The blood neutrophil concentration per se is not known to mediate production or release from the marrow. The candidate humoral substance is CSF, found in bone marrow, plasma, and urine; CSF is probably produced by monocytes and macrophages in response to an undefined stimulus delivered to them by mature neutrophils. In cell cultures, this material stimulates committed stem cells to produce granulocyte colonies. A negative feedback control of neutrophil production is thought to be mediated by the bone marrow reserve pool, with release of feedback inhibition when this pool becomes depleted. A granulocyte-releasing factor in plasma appears to accelerate neutrophil flow from the marrow reserve pool into the blood in response to certain stimuli. A variety of physiologic and pharmacologic substances and diseases mediate neutrophilia through several mechanisms (Table 28-1), most of which can be viewed as physiologic in response to signaled needs for circulating neutrophils.

   B. **Neutrophil function.** Neutrophils possess three principal characteristics that define their important role in cellular defense against microorganisms: (1) *chemotaxis*—a capacity to move unidirectionally toward sites of infection, injury, or inflammation in response to certain stimuli (chemotactic factors) released by such sites, namely, bacterial products, damaged tissues, and certain complement components; (2) *phagocytosis*—the capacity to recognize and ingest foreign particles, e.g., opsonized (immunoglobin- or complement-coated) bacteria; and (3) *microbial killing*—the capacity to respond to the phagocytic event with a sequence of reactions yielding microbicidal products: degranulation, fusion of the granules with the phagosome, release of the granule contents (e.g., proteolytic enzymes and myeloperoxidase), and activation of a nicotinamide adenine dinucleotide phosphate

Figure 28-1

Regulatory circuits of neutrophil production. CSF = colony stimulating factor; GRF = granulocyte releasing factor.

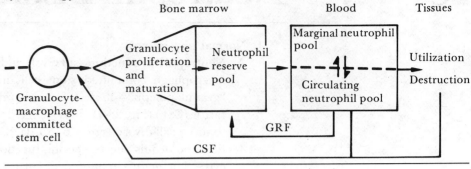

Table 28-1

Neutrophil Kinetics in Neutrophilia States

Cause of Neutrophilia	Bone Marrow		Blood		
	Dividing Pool	Storage Pool	Marginal Pool	Circulating Pool	Neutrophil Egress
Acute stress (epinephrine)	N	N	↓	↑	N
Acute infection (endotoxin), etiocholanolone	N	↓	↑	↑	N
Chronic infection, neoplasms, familial, lithium carbonate	↑	↑	↑	↑	N
Adrenocorticosteroids	N	N	↑	↑	↓

N = normal; ↑ = increased; ↓ = decreased.

Figure 28-2

Generation of oxidants (H_2O_2, OH^-, and halide) in neutrophils. G-6-PD = glucose 6-phosphate dehydrogenase; GSH = reduced glutathione; GSH-P = glutathione peroxidase; GSSG = oxidized glutathione; GSH-R = glutathione reductase; SD = superoxide dismutase; MP = myeloperoxidase; HMP = hexose monophosphate; NADPH = reduced nicotinamide adenine dinucleotide phosphate.

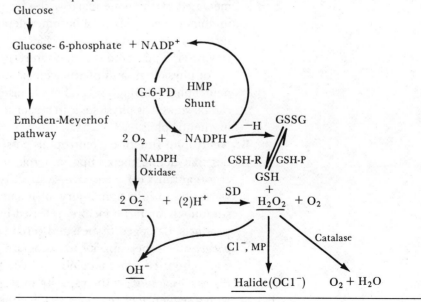

(NADPH) oxidase that generates superoxide, hydrogen peroxide, and hydroxyl radicals (Fig. 28-2).

II. Mechanisms of neutropenia

A. Decreased production of neutrophils. As in the case of erythrocytes, neutrophil production by the marrow may be impaired or may cease following stem cell damage, replacement of marrow tissue by an infiltrative process, or ineffective granulopoiesis. In contrast to erythrocytes, because the life span of circulating neutrophils is short (about 12 hr), their reduced production will quickly result in neutropenia. The relatively long period (50%) of the neutrophil's life span spent in its development makes this cell line particularly vulnerable to the commonly encountered toxic effects of drugs and ionizing radiation, which disturb the fundamental mechanisms of cell differentiation, mitosis, and growth; neutropenia develops first or more often than anemia or thrombocytopenia. Phenothiazine drugs uniquely inhibit deoxyribonucleic acid (DNA) synthesis in granulocyte precursors of susceptible persons. Many chemotherapeutic drugs inhibit various aspects of nucleic acid metabolism in all dividing cells; these effects extend to stem cells after sufficient dosage and long duration of their use. For many other drugs the mechanism by which stem-cell injury is produced is not known. Removal of most drugs usually permits prompt recovery. Rare and undefined defects of stem cells or their regulation, causing neutropenia and granulocyte hypoplasia in the bone marrow, may be inherited. One type manifests as cyclic neutropenia, occurring at intervals of 19 to 21 days. Recently, suppressor T cells inhibiting granulocyte development have been described in patients with rheumatic disorders and Felty's syndrome.

B. Increased destruction of circulating neutrophils. Neutrophil antigen-antibody reactions with consequent antibody coating of the neutrophils lead to their phagocytic destruction through the Fc fragment receptor mechanism of macrophages. Neutrophil isoantibodies are occasionally acquired during sensitization from blood transfusions or in pregnancy. Autoantibodies to neutrophils or soluble immune complexes may arise as part of autoimmune disorders (e.g., disseminated lupus erythematosus, Felty's syndrome). Drugs may act as haptens against which the host develops antibodies, causing destruction of neutrophils through agglutination, phagocytosis, or direct cytotoxicity by the antigen-antibody reaction on the neutrophil membrane. Such drug-induced neutropenia may develop quite rapidly and produce acute agranulocytosis (e.g., aminopyrine, phenylbutazone, thiouracil).

Neutropenia associated with a shortened neutrophil survival may occur as an inherited or acquired abnormality for which the mechanism is not known. Certain acute bacterial infections (e.g., typhoid, paratyphoid, tularemia) and a number of viral, rickettsial, and protozoal infections are accompanied by neutropenia, for which the mechanism is also not known. Increased utilization, as well as impaired production of neutrophils, occurs in overwhelming bacterial infections.

C. Altered distribution of neutrophils. Neutrophils, with or without erythrocytes and platelets, may be pooled in an enlarged, congested spleen (hypersplenism). In this case, neutropenia is part of a balanced leukopenia, and the ratio of neutrophils to lymphocytes and monocytes remains normal. Selective margination of neutrophils results from their increased adherence to the vascular endothelium (shift neutropenia), e.g., Felty's syndrome. Transient neutropenia develops after hemodialysis because contact of plasma with the dialyzer membrane activates complement, producing neutrophil aggregation and subsequent sequestration of these aggregates in the pulmonary microvasculature.

D. **Consequences of neutropenia.** Absolute neutropenia predisposes to infections of many kinds and recovery from infection is delayed. A decrease of neutrophils to less than 500 per cubic millimeter is termed agranulocytosis and almost invariably results in bacterial infection with a high risk of death.

III. **Mechanisms of neutrophil dysfunction**

A. **Defective chemotaxis and phagocytosis.** Inherited defects in the complement system interfere with the function of complement involved in chemotaxis and opsonization. Patients with sickle cell anemia have a defect in complement activation to opsonize pneumococci. Inherited and acquired deficiencies of immunoglobulins lead to impaired antibody coating of bacteria (opsonization). The hyperosmolar environment interferes with the chemotactic events in diabetes mellitus, particularly with ketoacidosis. The uremic environment in renal failure states inhibits chemotaxis, and adrenocorticosteroids inhibit chemotaxis and phagocytosis.

Few abnormalities that interfere with the chemotactic process have been localized to the neutrophil itself. In the "lazy leukocyte syndrome," neutrophil locomotion and neutrophil response to chemotactic stimuli are impaired along with a state of neutropenia. In allergic individuals with very high IgE levels, impaired chemotaxis is thought to be related to histamine, the chemical mediator released upon interaction of antigen with the IgE on the neutrophil membrane; H_2 histamine receptor blockade improves the chemotactic defect. A rare defect in the neutrophil contractile protein actin is accompanied by impaired phagocytosis but chemotaxis is intact.

B. **Defective intracellular killing.** The principal defects in the final microbicidal step by neutrophils are inherited abnormalities impairing generation of the oxidants (Fig. 28-2). The most prominent example is chronic granulomatous disease, which is due to deficiency or impaired activation of the membrane-bound NADPH-dependent oxidase. Severe deficiency of glucose-6-phosphate dehydrogenase or glutathione peroxidase also interferes with the oxidase, since sufficient NADPH cannot be generated. With these enzyme defects there is no defense against catalase-positive bacteria (e.g., *Staphylococcus* and *Serratia*) in that the catalase from these organisms destroys any available H_2O_2, which is essential stimulant of the HMP shunt pathway to produce NADPH necessary for the oxidase. Deficiency of myeloperoxidase makes neutrophils unable to oxidize halide (e.g., Cl^-), which is microbicidal for fungi.

IV. **Pathophysiology of leukemias.** Cytogenetic studies suggest that leukemias arise as a consequence of a genetic change in a stem cell, altering the differentiation, maturation, and proliferation characteristics of its progeny. Enzyme studies in glucose-6-phosphate dehydrogenase-deficient double heterozygotes (black females) provide further supportive evidence for the clonal (i.e., single cell) origin of a leukemic cell line. The agents modifying a stem cell's genome are probably many, primary candidates being radiation, chemicals, and viruses. Genetic factors appear to play a role in some individuals.

A. Acute granulocytic leukemia. In acute leukemia, primitive undifferentiated or differentiated leukocyte precursor cells proliferate at a normal or reduced rate but fail to mature. They accumulate because they do not respond to normal feedback regulation and are not effectively removed. Through mechanical crowding and nutritional deprivation the normal, unaffected stem cells are prevented from self-renewal, differentiation, and proliferation. This is also demonstrated in the virtual absence of granulocyte colony development in leukemic marrow-cell cultures. The consequences are progressive anemia, neutropenia, and thrombocytopenia. In time, the marrow barrier for egress of immature, leukemic (blast) cells is broken; they accumulate in the blood and in various tissues and eventually may interfere with organ functions. The accumulating leukemic cell mass raises the metabolic rate, depriving tissues of fuels. Eventual catabolism of the leukemic cells leads to increased uric acid production and uric acid nephropathy. Large amounts of lysozyme can be released into plasma, and consequent lysozymuria can produce renal tubular dysfunction with hypocalcemia, hypokalemia, and azotemia. When leukemic cell counts reach over 100×10^3 per cubic millimeter, central nervous system leukostasis, along with the thrombocytopenia, predisposes to intracranial hemorrhage. Cellular products (thromboplastic substances) in acute promyelocytic leukemia cells trigger coagulation in vivo, with consumption of clotting factors and platelets, markedly enhancing the risk for hemorrhage. Short of the less common event of vital organ dysfunction from leukemic cell infiltration, the host nearly always succumbs to hemorrhage or sepsis if the leukemic process cannot be controlled.

B. Chronic granulocytic leukemia. Here granulocyte differentiation is normal, maturation may be prolonged, and granulocyte function is normal. The underlying defect causes an excessive cell proliferation due to an expanded granulocyte-committed stem-cell pool and not infrequently also an expansion of the megakaryocyte cell line. The marker chromosome abnormality (the Philadelphia chromosome) is present in all hemopoietic cell lines, indicating a genetic change in the pluripotent or totipotent stem cell. The granulocyte regulatory mechanisms appear intact in that the leukemic cells respond to humoral regulation, and serum and urine have increased colony stimulating factor (CSF). The granulocyte mass slowly expands, crowding out erythropoiesis and thrombopoiesis, and resulting in anemia and thrombocytopenia. Granulocytes at all stages of development migrate out of the marrow and accumulate in the peripheral blood. They also proliferate in various extramedullary sites, principally in the spleen and liver, less often in other parenchymal organs, and occasionally in serous linings (peritoneum, pleura). The progressive cell proliferation raises the metabolic rate, causing weight loss, and associated hyperuricemia may precipitate clinical gout. The leukemic stem cell clone, however, appears unstable and after some 3 to 4 years acquires the inability to mature. A pathologic picture indistinguishable from acute leukemia, called the blastic transformation or blastic phase of chronic granulocytic leukemia, evolves. In the majority of cases, the blastic cell line has the morphologic and biochemical characteristics of acute granulocytic leukemia. In the minority, the blastic cell line is like acute lymphocytic leukemia, as documented by a high content of an enzyme characteristic of primitive lymphoid cells, terminal deoxynucleotidyl transferase (TdT). This latter type responds distinctly better to available chemotherapeutic agents.

V. **Clinical example of neutropenia**

A. **Description.** A 45-year-old woman was admitted with high fever (105° F) and signs and symptoms of a kidney infection. She was taking a phenothiazine (Thorazine) for psychiatric problems. Six years ago she had a gastrectomy for severe gastritis. On examination, aside from bilateral costovertebral angle tenderness, an enlarged spleen was found. Laboratory data: hematocrit, 33 percent; white blood cell count, $1.2 \times 10^3/mm^3$; white blood cell differential count—polys, 5 percent; bands, 10 percent; lymphs, 27 percent; monocytes, 58 percent; platelets, $150 \times 10^3/mm^3$; reticulocytes, 2 percent.

B. **Discussion**

1. Phenothiazine-induced agranulocytosis in a susceptible individual could predispose to the acute urinary tract infection; the bone-marrow aspirate would then show marked depression of the granulocyte cell series.

2. Severe infection and excessive utilization of granulocytes at the site of inflammation could cause the neutropenia; the bone-marrow aspirate would then show granulocytic hyperplasia.

3. Malabsorption of vitamin B_{12} consequent to the gastrectomy could cause the neutropenia as part of a megaloblastic anemia; the bone-marrow aspirate would then show megaloblastic changes.

4. The splenomegaly (at this point of unknown cause) could depress the leukocyte count through hypersplenism but is not likely to predispose to infection if it merely causes leukocyte pooling in the spleen; hypersplenism would be associated with mild hyperplasia of all marrow elements.

Questions   Select the single best answer.

1. A patient has developed agranulocytosis from a drug and there is loss of all granulocyte precursor cells in the bone marrow. After the drug is stopped the blood neutrophil count would be expected to increase at the earliest after:
   a. 6 hours.
   b. 24 hours.
   c. 7–9 days.
   d. 3 weeks.

2. Acute leukemia predisposes to infection because it is accompanied by:
   a. A lack of opsonins (immunoglobulins and complement).
   b. A lack of NADPH-dependent oxidase in neutrophils.
   c. Decreased neutrophil production.
   d. Increased neutrophil destruction.

29 Platelets

I. **Normal physiology**

A. **Platelet production (thrombopoiesis) and survival.** Platelets are produced by cytoplasmic fragmentation of megakaryocytes, the giant multinucleated cells that constitute less than 1 percent of all bone marrow cells. The megakaryoblast, the earliest recognizable precursor of the megakaryocyte cell line, arises from the megakaryocyte-committed stem cell and matures first by endomitosis (nuclear endoreduplication), in which nuclear material replicates without cell division. This results in a series of giant cells containing the equivalent of 4, 8, 16, and 32 sets of chromosomes; this number is also referred to as the nuclear number (N), e.g., 4N and 8N, or ploidy value. Thus, the megakaryocyte is a polyploid cell, as opposed to other hemopoietic cells that are diploid (2N). Megakaryocytes are recognizable only after they become polyploid; in normal marrow about two-thirds of megakaryocytes are 16N. Unlike the granulocytic and erythroid cell lines, the megakaryocyte cytoplasm matures after the nuclear replication. It grows in size and becomes acidophilic and granular, acquiring the distinctive cotton-candy appearance, and specific cytoplasmic organelles appear. Following this sequence of events, which requires 4 to 5 days, platelets are released by cytoplasmic fragmentation.

Platelets circulate as 2- to 3-micron cytoplasmic disks at a concentration of 150 to 450×10^3 per cubic millimeter. Like erythrocytes, newly formed platelets are larger (megathrombocytes) than older ones; they are also hemostatically more efficient. After 8 to 10 days, they are removed by macrophages in the liver and spleen. Of the circulating platelet mass, one-third exists as a pool in the spleen, while in slow transit through the tortuous splenic cords. The physiologic significance of this splenic pool is not known. To maintain a normal platelet count in the adult, the marrow produces 35×10^3 platelets per cubic millimeter of blood per day, but its production capacity is as high as eightfold over normal. Unlike the granulocytes, there is no ready reserve of platelets in the marrow, so that the ability of the marrow to increase platelet levels acutely is minimal.

B. **Regulation of platelet production.** Normally the platelet concentration in the blood is regulated by the hormone thrombopoietin. Thrombopoietin increases megakaryocyte differentiation from the committed stem cell, stimulates endomitosis, and thus the amount of platelet-producing cytoplasm, as well as cytoplasmic maturation and platelet release. Based on experiments in animals, secretion of thrombopoietin seems to be modulated by the blood platelet concentration. However, the lack of increased thrombopoiesis in thrombocytopenia due to excessive splenic pooling in enlarged spleens points to the platelet mass (circulating pool + splenic pool), rather than the platelet concentration as regulating thrombopoietin production. A physiologic splenic inhibitor of thrombopoiesis has also been postulated.

C. **Platelet function.** Platelets constitute the initial and foremost line of defense against accidental blood loss by their continual maintenance of vascular integrity, initial arrest of bleeding by platelet plug formation (primary hemostasis), and contribution of phospholipid to the process of fibrin formation that stabilizes the platelet plug (secondary hemostasis). Within a second or two after a break in the endothelium, platelets passing by avidly adhere to the exposed subendothelial collagen (Fig. 29-1). Adherent platelets release endogenous adenosine diphosphate (ADP), which recruits more platelets to the site by transforming them into thorny spheres that interact with one another, as well as with already adherent platelets, and in turn release more ADP. This forms a firm platelet plug. In addition, platelet factor 3 (PF$_3$), a phospholipid, is unmasked on the aggregated platelets. This factor promotes thrombin generation (see Chap. 30), leading to fibrin deposition over the platelet plug and formation of a thrombus. Thrombin also causes further platelet aggregation and promotes ADP release and prostaglandin synthesis (see the following paragraph).

In recent years, the important role of prostaglandins in platelet function has been discovered. Platelet aggregation activates a phospholipase, which releases arachidonic acid from platelet membrane phospholipids. Through a series of reactions arachidonic acid is converted to prostacyclin, thromboxane A$_2$, or inactive prostaglandins (Fig. 29-2). Prostacyclin is a potent inhibitor of aggregation and serves to balance the effects of thromboxane A$_2$. Since prostacyclin synthetase is derived from normal vessel walls, vessel injury could conceivably decrease the availability of the enzyme and impair prostacyclin formation, tilting the balance in favor of thromboxanes and hence toward platelet aggregation and clotting.

Blood flow gradually dilutes and dissipates the ADP, as well as thrombin and prostaglandins, from the site of vessel injury, halting this localized clotting. The formed clot retracts and the thrombus is consolidated by the contractile platelet-membrane protein thrombasthenin.

II. Mechanisms of thrombocytopenia

A. Decreased production of platelets. As in the case of erythrocytes and granulocytes, platelet production is impaired following stem cell damage (from drugs, chemicals, and x-rays), due to infiltrative processes in the bone marrow, or with hemopoietic cell maturation defects (see Table 29-1). Selective suppression of megakaryocyte production is seen from a few agents—namely, thiazide diuretics, alcohol, and estrogenic hormones. Upon removal of the offending agent, recovery is usual. States of thrombopoietin lack have not as yet been well described. In a few instances of congenital thrombocytopenia, the response to normal plasma infusions was believed to represent thrombopoietin deficiency.

B. Increased destruction of platelets. The two principal mechanisms for excessive platelet destruction are immunologic (antibody-mediated) removal and nonimmune consumption. Immune destruction of platelets may be autoimmune, the antibody being directed against a platelet antigen. It may occur without other disease (e.g., idiopathic autoimmune thrombocytopenic purpura) or in association with disorders predisposing to autoantibody formation (e.g., systemic lupus erythematosus lymphomas). Antibody coating damages the platelets, and they are rapidly removed by the spleen and liver macrophages. Immune destruction may also be mediated through immune complexes. Drugs are an important and common cause of immune platelet destruction by this mechanism. Drug-antibody complexes (immune complexes) nonspecifically adsorb onto the platelets, leading to complement activation on the surface of the platelets and their subsequent

Figure 29-1

Formation of the hemostatic plug. PF₃ = platelet factor 3; ADP = adenosine diphosphate.

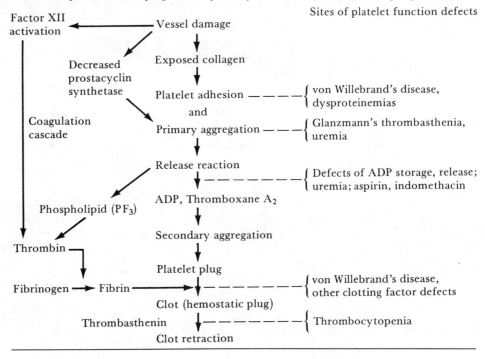

Sites of platelet function defects

Figure 29-2

Generation of prostacyclin and thromboxane. PGG₂ = prostaglandin G₂; PGH₂ = prostaglandin H₂; PGI₂ = prostaglandin I₂.

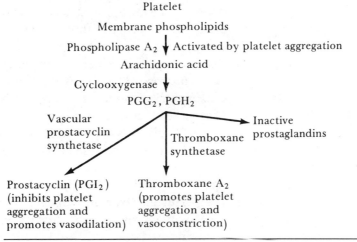

lysis. Common offenders are quinidine, quinine, and heparin; recovery upon their withdrawal is usual. Platelets may be consumed along with fibrinogen and other clotting factors in disseminated intravascular coagulation (DIC) (see Chap. 30). Selective consumption of platelets occurs in deposited fibrin strands, in association with widespread vascular injury as in vasculitis, thrombotic thrombocytopenic purpura, and the hemolytic uremic syndrome. Trauma from abnormal blood currents around vascular prostheses (e.g., prosthetic heart valves) mechanically disrupts platelets as it does erythrocytes.

C. **Altered distribution of platelets.** The normal splenic pooling of platelets may increase to 70 to 80 percent or even 90 percent when the spleen is enlarged (e.g., in portal hypertension, sarcoidosis, Gaucher's

Table 29-1   Pathophysiologic Classification of Thrombocytopenia

Mechanism	Disorder
I. Decreased production	
A. All cell lines affected	Stem cell disorders (aplastic anemia)
	Vitamin B_{12} and folate deficiency
	Hematologic malignancies (leukemia, myeloma)
	Marrow infiltration (carcinoma, lymphoma, granuloma)
B. Only megakaryocyte line affected	Ethanol
	Thiazide diuretics
	Estrogens
	Congenital thrombopoietin deficiency (rare)
II. Increased destruction or loss	
A. Immune	Drug induced (immune complex)
	Autoimmune thrombocytopenic purpura
B. Nonimmune	Disseminated intravascular coagulation
	Thrombotic thrombocytopenic purpura
	Hemolytic uremic syndrome
	Vasculitis
	Prosthetic heart valves
	Wash out
	Postperfusion
III. Abnormal distribution	Hypersplenism (portal hypertension, Gaucher's disease)
IV. In vitro platelet agglutination and satellitism	Spurious thrombocytopenia

disease). The total platelet mass is normal so that thrombopoiesis is not increased despite the thrombocytopenia. The thrombocytopenia is usually mild, and bleeding problems are uncommon.

D. Washout thrombocytopenia. When a large amount (greater than 10 units) of stored blood is used to replace massive blood loss, or with exchange transfusions, thrombocytopenia regularly occurs. Here the thrombocytopenia is caused by replacement of viable platelets with nonviable platelets in the stored blood coupled with the limited ability of the marrow to increase platelet levels acutely. A similar mechanism is operative in the thrombocytopenia seen with therapeutic plasmapheresis and leukapheresis.

E. Postperfusion thrombocytopenia. Thrombocytopenia of varying degrees is regularly seen in patients undergoing open heart surgery, requiring extracorporeal perfusion. Platelets are believed to be activated in the perfusion apparatus and to form small aggregates, which are trapped in the filters of the apparatus and in the lung. The platelet count usually returns to normal within a week.

F. Spurious thrombocytopenia. Platelets may spontaneously aggregate in vitro in the blood collection tube containing ethylenediaminetetraacetic acid (EDTA) so that the aggregates are counted as single platelets, or platelets may adhere to granulocytes in vitro (satellitism) and not be counted at all. In either case, the result will be a spurious thrombocytopenia. Although the mechanism(s) and the in vivo significance of these phenomena are not known, their recognition prevents unnecessary investigation.

III. Mechanisms and sites of platelet dysfunction

    A. Inherited defects. Most often platelet dysfunction is encountered in von Willebrand's disease, in which inherited deficiency of a platelet-binding portion of factor VIII impairs platelet adhesion to the vessel wall (see Fig. 29-1 and Chap. 30). Uncommon inherited defects of platelet function include lack of certain membrane glycoproteins (Glanzmann's thrombasthenia) and failure to store (storage pool disease) or release ADP, all impairing platelet aggregation.

B. Acquired defects. Platelet dysfunction occurs in chronic renal failure states and has been attributed to retained metabolites (e.g., guanidinosuccinic acid). Thromboxane A_2 production also appears impaired. Intensive dialysis markedly improves the platelet dysfunction. A number of drugs alter platelet function. Aspirin irreversibly acetylates cyclooxygenase, thus blocking further steps in prostaglandin synthesis, including formation of thromboxane A_2. Indomethacin and other analgesic drugs inhibit this enzyme reversibly. It is not known how very high doses of penicillins alter platelet function.

C. Hyperfunction. In vivo hyperactivity of platelets appears related to increased propensity for thrombosis. Examples of clinical settings are idiopathic recurrent venous thrombosis, myeloproliferative disorders, transient ischemic attacks, and smoking. The precise mechanisms for the hyperactive state of platelets is not known.

IV. Consequences of thrombocytopenia and platelet dysfunction. Insufficient numbers of platelets decrease the vascular integrity and primary hemostasis in capillaries, and hence cause subcutaneous and mucosal bleeding (petechiae), prolonged bleeding after trauma, a prolonged bleeding time, and impaired clot retraction. In general, hemostasis is not seriously impaired with platelet counts above 50×10^3 per cubic millimeter, especially if the platelets are young and, therefore, hemostatically more effective. If the platelet count reaches much below 50×10^3 per cubic millimeter, almost invariably excessive bleeding occurs, the major risk being intracranial hemorrhage. Platelet function defects usually produce mild spontaneous bleeding and often may only be uncovered by severe trauma, surgical procedures, or therapy with drugs that alter platelet function.

V. Mechanisms of thrombocytosis

A. Primary thrombocytosis. Hemorrhagic thrombocythemia, a myeloproliferative disorder, is an example of autonomous thrombocytosis, usually producing platelet counts of several million per cubic millimeter. A megakaryocyte stem cell clone proliferates and fails to respond to the physiologic regulatory mechanisms of thrombopoiesis. Although the resulting thrombocytosis may predispose to thrombosis, hemorrhagic manifestations are more common because the platelets produced are functionally defective. Similar thrombocytosis occurs in the more common disorders of polycythemia rubra vera and chronic granulocytic leukemia, in which pluripotent stem cell clones proliferate excessively.

B. Secondary (reactive) thrombocytosis. Thrombocytosis commonly accompanies varied conditions such as hemorrhage, inflammation, iron deficiency, and surgery. The mechanism of this platelet response is not defined. The platelet concentration remains below $1,000 \times 10^3$ per cubic millimeter, is not harmful, and subsides when the associated state is treated. Thrombocytosis also follows splenectomy, due to loss of the splenic pool and the splenic inhibition of thrombopoiesis; here it may be marked (i.e., greater than $1,000 \times 10^3/mm^3$), but it is usually transient.

VI. Clinical example of thrombocytopenia

A. Description. A 20-year-old woman noted bruises over her legs for 2 weeks; bleeding during her last menstrual period was considerably greater than usual. Six weeks ago she had a bad cold. She had multiple petechiae and several 3-cm ecchymoses over the lower extremities. The spleen was not palpable. Hemogram showed: hemoglobin, 10 g/dl; hematocrit, 32 percent; white blood count, $9 \times 10^3/mm^3$; platelets, $20 \times 10^3/mm^3$. On blood smear, platelets were markedly reduced in number and several were large. The bone-marrow aspirate revealed a striking increase in megakaryocytes, many with lack of nuclear lobulation. She was treated with prednisone, 80 mg per day, and 2 weeks later the platelet count was $250 \times 10^3/mm^3$.

B. Discussion

1. The large platelets in the blood smear along with a megakaryocytic hyperplasia indicate that the mechanism for the thrombocytopenia is increased platelet destruction.
2. The response to prednisone therapy suggests an antibody-mediated process.
3. The antecedent viral illness could have initiated the immune thrombocytopenia.
4. The anemia is probably due to iron deficiency from recent blood loss superimposed on marginal iron stores in this young, menstruating woman.

Question

Match each item in A with an appropriate one from B. You may use items in B more than once or not at all.

A	B
(1) Thrombocytopenia of B_{12} or folate deficiency	(a) Inhibits platelet aggregation
(2) Immune thrombocytopenia	(b) Normal number of megakaryocytes
(3) Petechial bleeding in a patient with normal platelet count	(c) Increased marrow megakaryocytes
(4) Prostacyclin	(d) Promotes vasoconstriction
(5) Hypersplenic thrombocytopenia	(e) Platelet dysfunction
(6) Thromboxane A_2	(f) Absent megakaryocytes

30 Disorders of Blood Coagulation

I. **Normal physiology.** The clotting factors are proteins that circulate in the plasma and are not enzymatically active until clotting is triggered. When converted from the inactive zymogen to the enzymatically active clotting factor, they are said to be activated. A typical clotting factor is shown in Figure 30-1. The small *a* denotes the active clotting factor. Notice that a peptide bond was broken to reveal the enzymatically active catalytic site. The factor Xa now goes on to take a bite out of another inactive factor, e.g., prothrombin, to convert it to the active form, thrombin.

Figure 30-2 shows the clotting cascade. The activated factor X (Xa) is at the very center of things. It can be formed in two ways: by the intrinsic pathway starting with factor XII and by the extrinsic pathway starting with factor VII. Intrinsic refers to a protein family contained in the plasma; extrinsic refers to the need for tissue factor, which is not circulating in the plasma. Figure 30-2 illustrates that a number of components are needed to activate factor X to Xa. In the intrinsic pathway factor IXa, phospholipid, factor VIII (a helper protein), and Ca^{2+} are required. The activator of prothrombin, Xa, requires the same type of components, including a helper protein, factor V. Activation of factor X by the extrinsic pathway is similar, since tissue factor contains both a phospholipid and a helper protein. Therefore, the three major steps involving vitamin K–dependent clotting factors are virtually identical (see Fig. 30-3).

The proteins involved in these reactions are all vitamin K–dependent clotting factors made by the liver (i.e., X, IX, prothrombin, and VII). Vitamin K permits the modification of these enzymes just before they leave the liver. During this modification, an extra carboxyl group is put on certain glutamic acid groups on the outside of the clotting protein (Fig. 30-4).

The modified dicarboxyglutamic acid groups allow vitamin K–dependent clotting to be activated (Fig. 30-5). If clotting had to rely on factor Xa randomly hitting prothrombin and converting it to thrombin, such an event would be very rare. In this complex, Ca^{2+} binds the double negative charge on the clotting factor to two negatively charged phosphate groups on the phospholipid. This mechanism allows Xa to bind directly next to a prothrombin and cleave it to thrombin, which then leaves the complex. The helper protein (V in this case) probably helps align the complex. The other complexes (i.e., IXa-X-VIII and VII-X-tissue factor) are similar.

Now consider the big picture. Where does the phospholipid in the complex come from? Probably from *inside* platelets that bind to exposed collagen at the site of tissue damage, release their contents, and expose the negatively charged phospholipids. The clotting process is then set in motion exactly where needed—at the site of injury.

II. **Mechanisms of common defects of coagulation factors**

  A. **Defects of specific components of the clotting complex.** If vitamin K is not available in adequate quantities (e.g., because of malnutrition, antibiotic therapy), the carboxylation step cannot take place and abnormal vitamin K–dependent clotting factors enter the circulation.

Figure 30-1   *Activation of a clotting factor.*

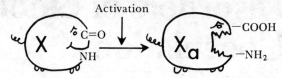

Figure 30-2   *The coagulation cascade. The vitamin K–dependent clotting factors are indicated by an asterisk.*

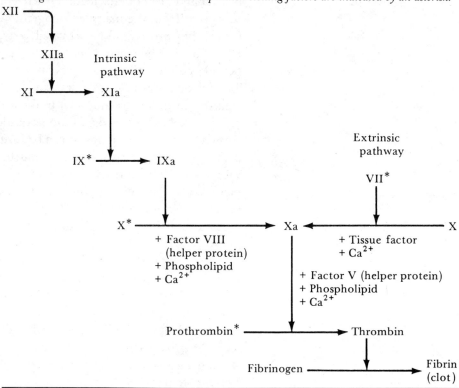

Figure 30-3   *The three analogous steps in thrombin formation.*

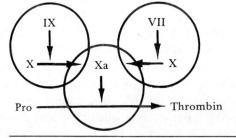

Figure 30-4   *Carboxylation of vitamin K–dependent clotting factors.*

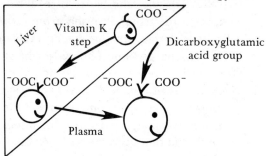

Figure 30-5

Activation of the vitamin K–dependent clotting factor prothrombin.

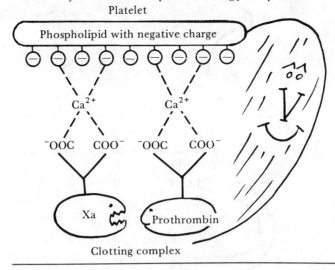

Vitamin K–dependent clotting factor in a normal individual and in a patient with vitamin K deficiency.

Figure 30-6

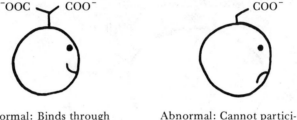

These lack the double negative charge needed to participate in the clotting complex (Fig. 30-6).

Warfarin is an oral anticoagulant drug commonly given to prevent formation of clots in veins. It blocks the action of vitamin K in the liver, and again defective clotting factors lacking the extra carboxyl group enter the circulation (Fig. 30-7).

The liver produces all the vitamin K–dependent clotting factors as well as factor V. If liver damage is so extensive (e.g., in endstage cirrhosis) that the proteins can no longer be made, clotting is similarly impaired.

The normal clotting physiology is altered each time blood is drawn and anticoagulants are added. Citrate is the most commonly used anticoagulant and acts by binding calcium; it thus removes calcium from the clotting complex (Fig. 30-8).

Some individuals are genetically deficient in one of the large helper proteins (e.g., factor VIII in classic hemophilia) or in a vitamin K–dependent factor (e.g., IX). The clotting complex cannot be formed and effective clotting cannot occur.

B. Defects in multiple components of the clotting system

  1. Disseminated intravascular coagulation. Infection can trigger the clotting system so that many components of the system are used up. Platelets are also consumed, being deposited with fibrin in the small blood vessels, and thrombocytopenia results. In this setting, the patient often begins to bleed because the normal supply of clotting factors, as well as platelets, has been reduced.

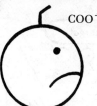

Figure 30-8   *Calcium binding to citrate.*

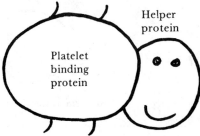

Figure 30-9   *The factor VIII complex.*

Helper protein

Platelet binding protein

2. **von Willebrand's disease.** Factor VIII has more than one function. As discussed earlier, one portion of the molecule, the helper protein (Fig. 30-9), helps the clotting complex function and is low or absent in classic hemophilia. However, there is a second portion of the molecule (platelet-binding protein) that ties platelets to damaged vessel wall surfaces and thus helps form the initial platelet plug (see Chap. 29). Patients who inherit von Willebrand's disease also have decreased levels of the platelet-binding portion of factor VIII and are unable to form platelet plugs.

C. **Consequences of coagulation factor defects.** Abnormalities of the clotting proteins, in contrast to platelet abnormalities, cause bleeding in joints and deep tissues. Following trauma, such bleeding may be delayed because the platelet plug forms normally, but the hemostatic plug (clot) is weak, if it forms at all.

III. **Clinical example of coagulation abnormality**

A. **Description.** A 59-year-old man had abdominal pain, nausea, and vomiting. Acute diverticulitis was found, and he was treated with antibiotics for 19 days. Symptoms of intestinal obstruction persisted, requiring resection of the sigmoid colon with drainage of an abscess and a diverting colostomy. Eight days postoperatively, he could have nothing by mouth and was still on antibiotics when a retroperitoneal hemorrhage developed with a drop of hematocrit from 35 percent to 25 percent. The prothrombin time (PT) was 18 sec (normal, <12 sec), the partial thromboplastin time (PTT) was 50 sec (normal, <30 sec), and the platelet count was normal. He was given 3 mg of vitamin K, and 24 hours later the PT was 11 sec and PTT was 35 sec.

B. Discussion

1. The retroperitoneal hemorrhage occurred because of clotting factor deficits, reflected in the prolonged PTT and PT (which indicate deficiencies in both the intrinsic and extrinsic pathways of coagulation, respectively).

2. The setting of no food intake for over 2 weeks, coupled with prolonged antibiotic therapy (which reduces vitamin K–forming bacteria in the intestinal tract), produced vitamin K depletion.

3. That deficiencies in vitamin K–dependent clotting factors caused this complication is confirmed by the prompt correction of the PT and PTT following vitamin K administration.

Questions

Select the single best answer.

1. An individual is discovered who lacks the enzyme necessary to carboxylate the glutamic acid groups on the vitamin K–dependent clotting factors. When this person begins to bleed, effective treatment might include:
   a. Infusion of phospholipid intravenously.
   b. Administration of large doses of vitamin K.
   c. Infusion of plasma from a normal donor.
   d. Administration of aspirin to prevent platelet aggregation, followed by intravenous calcium.

2. Warfarin works as an anticoagulant because it:
   a. Increases the rate of destruction of prothrombin, factors VIII, IX, and X in the liver and thus lowers their circulating levels.
   b. Blocks platelet participation in the formation of a hemostatic plug.
   c. Blocks the synthesis of all amino acid peptides that make up the clotting factors.
   d. Results in the formation of clotting factors, which lack dicarboxylglutamic acid groups.

VI Immunology and Rheumatology

Samuel R. Oleinick
Morris Reichlin
Russell T. Schultz
James H. Wells

31 Immediate Hypersensitivity Disease

I. Mechanisms

The major biologic value of the immune system appears to be in protective functions such as protecting against infection. The term *hypersensitivity* indicates an immunologic reaction that is harmfully overintense and often directed against an agent from which protection seems unnecessary. *Allergy,* another term for hypersensitivity, is taken from the Greek words for altered state of reactivity and refers to the change to the hypersensitive state brought about by a sensitizing exposure. The antigens involved in allergic sensitization and reactivity are referred to as allergens. Many allergens are protein in nature, although simple chemicals and drugs may sensitize haptenically. Allergic or hypersensitivity reactions may occur in response to any of the four Gell-Coombs classification mechanisms.

Immediate hypersensitivity reactions are mediated by pharmacologically active substances produced by mast cells and basophils. The classic mechanism (Gell-Coombs type I) involves the interaction of an allergen with specific IgE antibodies, which are fixed to the cell surface, thus sensitizing the cell. However, reactions that are clinically similar may be produced by other mechanisms, both immunologic and nonimmunologic, that do not involve IgE. Immunologically, subclass IgG_4 has been reported to contain antibodies that can sensitize cells in a way similar but not identical to IgE and to participate in allergic reactions in some cases. Additionally, when IgG and IgM antibodies activate the complement system (IgE does not), the produced fragments C3a and C5a are capable of releasing mediators. These fragments, called anaphylatoxins, may also be produced nonimmunologically through alternate-pathway complement activation. Some drugs act directly on the cell membranes of mast cells and basophils to release mediators; examples include opiate drugs, polymyxin, thiamine, and curare. When injected into the skin, these drugs will cause wheal and flare reactions similar to those produced by allergens in subjects with IgE hypersensitivity. In the clinical disease states to be discussed, IgE is frequently involved in mediator release. However, in some patients and with some stimuli, it is not. In such cases mediator release is thought to occur on a nonimmunologic basis, resulting in physiologic manifestations similar to those resulting from release involving IgE. The basis for the nonimmunologic release of mediators in these diseases is in some instances not well understood.

Semantically, there is lack of full agreement on whether all reactions caused by the mediators of type I hypersensitivity should be classified as immediate hypersensitivity, regardless of whether or not IgE was involved in mediator release. For the purposes of this discussion, they will be so classified.

The immediate hypersensitivity diseases include allergic rhinitis, bronchial asthma, urticaria, angioedema, and systemic anaphylaxis. Except for allergic rhinitis (by definition), IgE is of variable involvement in these diseases; it is part of the mechanism in some cases and not in others. Allergic rhinitis has a nonallergic counterpart, nonallergic eosinophilic rhinitis, in which mediators are released nonimmunologically. When IgE is involved, skin testing is useful in identifying some causative allergens.

A hereditary tendency (atopy) to develop immediate hypersensitivity diseases is often apparent but is not invariable. This tendency is most often seen in rhinitis and asthma, less frequently in urticaria and angioedema. The effect of heredity is poorly defined in anaphylaxis. It is unclear whether severe anaphylaxis, caused, for example, by penicillin or Hymenoptera stings, is more common in persons with other indications of an atopic tendency or not. However, one must realize that reactions are not confined to such individuals.

Mast cells and basophils have different cellular precursors but many functional similarities. Mast cells develop from mesenchymal precursors and are found in all subcutaneous and submucosal tissues, usually in proximity to small blood vessels, including vessels of peripheral nerves. Basophils originate in the bone marrow and circulate in the blood. Both contain histidine decarboxylase, are capable of making histamine and other mediators, and show similarities in cell membrane hormone receptor sites.

IgE antibody has a sedimentation coefficient of 8S and a molecular weight of 190,000. It is inactivated by heating at 56° C for 2 to 4 hours. IgE is synthesized primarily in those lymphoid tissues near the respiratory and gastrointestinal tracts. Its production is under control of both suppressor and helper regulator cell populations. After appearance in the circulation it remains there briefly, having a serum half-life of 2 to 3 days. Thereafter, IgE binds through the Fc portion of the molecule to specific binding sites on circulating basophils and tissue mast cells.

IgE is a homocytotropic antibody, meaning that it will fix to the tissues of man and other primates but not those of other species. The Prausnitz-Küstner (PK) procedure is performed by injecting serum that contains specific IgE antibodies into the skin of a nonsensitive recipient, allowing time for fixation of antibodies, then injecting specific allergen to demonstrate skin test reactivity. During the first few days after serum injection, 95 percent or more of the IgE content leaves the injection site by diffusion. The optimum time for fixation of the remainder is 1 to 2 days. After fixation, IgE displays a high affinity for its binding sites, with a tissue half-life of 8 to 14 days. Skin sites passively sensitized with high-titred sera may remain so for months.

The primary normal function of IgE is hypothesized to be a role in combating certain parasitic infestations, since high levels are found in patients so affected. Almost all normal persons have detectable, though low, serum IgE levels. As a group, atopic allergic patients have higher serum IgE levels than normals, although there is considerable overlap. Often, total serum IgE levels will rise temporarily after a sufficiently heavy exposure to a specific allergen, such as during a pollen season or after an IgE-mediated drug reaction.

IgE-mediated reactions are initiated by interaction of an allergen molecule with two cell-bound IgE molecules (bridging). The mediators of the reaction are produced by mast cells and basophils through a nonlytic, energy-requiring process. Some of the known and suspected mediators include histamine, slow-reacting substance of anaphylaxis (SRS-A), eosinophil-chemotactic factor of anaphylaxis (ECF-A), neutrophil chemotactic factor of anaphylaxis (NCF-A), prostaglandins, kallikrein, and platelet activating factor (PAF). As a group these mediators govern the cellular changes in the target organs affected by immediate hypersensitivity by their actions on smooth muscle, blood vessels, glandular secretion, nerves, and chemotactically responsive hematopoietic cells.

Aside from their roles in immediate hypersensitivity, these mediators normally participate in other important processes. In some instances they may be part of other inflammatory reactions. Some appear to be part of normal regulatory mechanisms for glandular, vascular, and smooth muscle function. For example, histamine is a controlling regulator of acid secretion by the stomach. It acts through cell membrane receptor sites (H2) that are functionally distinct from those involved in immediate hypersensitivity (H1) and thus are blocked by different antihistamine drugs.

As a mediator of immediate hypersensitivity, histamine has received the greatest amount of attention. It is preformed by decarboxylation of histidine and stored in the metachromatic granules of the cells. Its actions are brief and intense, and include constriction of respiratory and gastrointestinal smooth muscle, vascular dilation and increased permeability, and stimulation of secretion by mucosal glands. Histamine is probably an important mediator in virtually all immediate hypersensitivity reactions. SRS-A, a product of arachidonic acid metabolism that is distinct from the prostaglandins, has been assigned a definite role in the bronchoconstriction of asthma. ECF-A causes the influx of eosinophils, which are a hallmark of type I reactions and which to some extent may regulate these reactions. The other mediators have at this time been assigned only probable roles.

The intensity of an immediate hypersensitivity reaction is determined by several factors. The intensity of allergen exposure is important. When IgE is involved, the amount of specific antibody on the cell surface determines the degree of mediator release. Individuals vary in the histamine content of various organs and probably in other mediators as well. Also, some persons release mediators more readily than others to a given stimulus. Similarly, some individuals have target tissues that are more reactive to mediators than those of others. In some instances, autonomic reflexes, which will be discussed in the next chapter, regulate the reaction. Other regulatory systems are thought to be of additional importance, such as histaminases and eosinophil arylsulfatase, an enzyme capable of degrading SRS-A. Most of the drugs used to control such reactions do so either by affecting mediator release or by modifying the effect of mediators on target tissues, or by doing both.

II. **Clinical syndromes**

A. **Allergic rhinitis and asthma** will be discussed further in Chapter 32.

B. **Urticaria** (hives) typically appear as pruritic, reddened cutaneous elevations that blanch with pressure. Individual lesions come and go, usually lasting less than 24 hours, and disappear without residuals. Histologically, small venules and capillaries in the superficial dermis are dilated, and localized edema due to vascular permeability is present. Angioedema may occur alone or in conjunction with urticaria. It results from a similar process deeper in the dermis and subcutaneous tissues; swelling is more extensive, and erythema and itching less prominent or absent. Sometimes resolution requires as long as several days. When allergy is the cause, a food or drug is most frequently indicated and is often obvious. However, in some patients hives become a chronic problem, and in this setting allergy is seldom found. Chronic urticaria can occasionally be linked to one of a wide array of conditions; these may include infections, other inflammatory processes including collagen vascular diseases, neoplasia, emotional stress, or exposure to physical agents such as heat, cold, water, pressure, or sunlight. However, more than 80 percent of the time no causation is ever found for chronic urticaria.

C. **Anaphylaxis** is a severe, often life-threatening, systemic allergic reaction. It may variably involve the skin (hives, flushing, itching), the gastrointestinal tract (nausea, vomiting, cramps, diarrhea), the respiratory tract (wheezing, upper airway angioedema), and the cardiovascular system (hypotension). When anaphylaxis proves fatal, death is usually due to shock, asthma, or upper airway closure. Allergies to a wide variety of substances through every conceivable route of exposure have been reported as causes. Drug treatment, especially with penicillin, is the most frequent. In some cases allergic mechanisms are not involved. Such reactions are termed anaphylactoid. An example is the reaction to injected contrast medium, occasionally seen during radiographic dye studies due to nonimmunologic mediator release.

D. **Atopic dermatitis or atopic eczema** is a chronic inflammatory skin disorder that often has an association with other signs of atopy. It most typically begins during the first 2 years of life and often remits by ages 4 to 6, although it sometimes begins then. Other, less frequent times when it shows a tendency either to appear or to remit are at or about puberty or in late adolescence. Atopic dermatitis is a problem seen in only a small minority of atopically allergic persons; however, the majority who have this skin condition will at some time develop asthma or allergic rhinitis and tend to be highly allergic. In most, immediate hypersensitivity mechanisms are not thought to be directly involved in causing the dermatitis. These patients have dry, itchy skins, which itch even more after mechanical abrasion and tend eventually to thicken (lichenify) from the inflammation caused by chronic excoriation. The self-inflicted trauma that actually produces skin damage in most of these patients is termed the scratch-itch cycle.

Clinically, atopic dermatitis often affects mainly the antecubital and popliteal fossae, although the face and neck are not uncommonly involved, as well as other sites. Its usual appearance is that of a dry, scaly, chronic inflammation of the skin, which can become wet and oozing, crusted, and more inflamed when it is flared by scratching or secondary infection. Treatment of associated immediate hypersensitivity disorders usually does not benefit the dermatitis. Therapeutically, measures to reduce dryness and itching, prevent scratching, and control inflammation are valuable.

III. **Clinical example of immediate hypersensitivity disease**

A. **Description.** A patient with known valvular rheumatic heart disease was admitted for treatment of subacute bacterial endocarditis caused by an organism that antibiotic sensitivity testing indicated would require penicillin for effective treatment. History disclosed an urticarial reaction to penicillin 10 years previously. Skin testing was carried out with dilute solutions of penicillin G and penicilloyl polylysine (PPL) and was negative. Using the skin tests as the first dose, gradually increasing doses of penicillin G were given every 15 minutes until the patient was receiving 20 million units daily. On the third day he developed urticaria, which responded to antihistamines without cessation of penicillin treatment.

B. **Discussion**

1. In some patients, allergy to a drug declines spontaneously after a period of avoidance.

2. When drug allergy is suspected, the drug should be avoided if possible and an alternative treatment sought.
3. Only when the benefits of the drug outweigh the risk of a severe allergic reaction should cautious readministration be considered in a setting where therapy is immediately available.
4. Skin tests are not available for most drugs, with penicillin being an exception.
5. PPL cross-reacts immunologically with the major metabolic product of penicillin. The majority of patients with positive skin tests to penicillin G or PPL will have an IgE-mediated allergic reaction within the first 48 hours of penicillin treatment, which is the time period during which such a reaction is most likely to be fatal.
6. Skin tests with penicillin G and PPL do not identify the small percentage (less than 5 percent of patients) with penicillin allergy to other metabolites of the drug, so cautious administration is still advised. They also do not predict reactions that are not IgE-mediated (such as rashes) or that occur later than 48 hours from starting the drug (as in this case, due to an anamnestic response).

Questions

More than one answer is possible.

1. Which of the following is/are true?
   a. Anaphylactic reactions to penicillin will not occur in patients without prior hay fever, asthma, or other allergic disease.
   b. Most cases of chronic urticaria are caused by food or drug allergy.
   c. IgE is required for histamine release.
   d. Immediate hypersensitivity reactions may be nonimmunologic.
2. Death from anaphylaxis usually is *not* caused by:
   a. Shock.
   b. Angioedema of the upper airway.
   c. Asthma.
   d. Gastrointestinal bleeding.

32

Allergic Respiratory Diseases

I. **Normal structure and function of the airway.** The nose and the tracheobronchial tree may be viewed as a central duct system with the essential job during inspiration of delivering air to the alveoli, where the pulmonary blood is oxygenated and waste removed for elimination by exhalation. During inhalation, a vital function of this duct system is to serve not merely as a conduit, but also as an air conditioner. Inspired air must be properly warmed, humidified, and cleansed as it passes through these ducts to protect the more sensitive distal portions of the pulmonary apparatus.

The internal nares are separated from each other by the nasal septum. Along the lateral walls, the turbinates are formed by bony ridges, which run from front to back. Except for an area of squamous epithelium near the external nares, the nasal mucosa is a pseudostratified, ciliated, columnar epithelium. The mucosa and submucosa contain both simple and compound mucinous and serous glands. These glands normally secrete as much as 1,500 to 2,000 ml per day, to form the mucous blanket that overlies the ciliated epithelium. The mucous blanket is layered, with a thin layer of mucin lying on top of a weak electrolyte solution through which the cilia project. Over the inferior and middle turbinates the submucosa is vascular. The arteries and veins run parallel to the mucosa in the direction of the long axis of the turbinate. They are anastamotically connected by capillaries that empty into distensible venous sinusoids prior to delivery of blood to the venules. There is both sympathetic and parasympathetic innervation to blood vessels and mucous glands. Parasympathetic discharge increases glandular secretion and dilates blood vessels; sympathetic impulses do the reverse.

As air passes through the nose, particles are removed from it by impaction and trapping in the mucous blanket. During normal nasal breathing, particles larger than 20 microns are virtually all removed from the air by the nose. The beat of the mucosal cilia carries the blanket posteriorly to the nasopharynx, where it is swallowed, thus disposing of any entrapped pollutants. Heat exchange is regulated mainly by capillary blood flow, while the caliber of the turbinates is controlled by the amount of blood pooling in the venous sinusoids. When the turbinates are engorged, air turbulence is increased, thus facilitating heat exchange, humidification of the air, and removal of pollutants.

The tracheobronchial tree is also lined with a ciliated epithelium, contains both serous and mucous glandular elements, and has an overlying mucous blanket. This mucous blanket also is carried by ciliary action toward the pharynx to be discarded. Because of reabsorption of water, only about 10 ml of mucus per day normally reaches the larynx. Many small particles that have escaped removal during passage through the nose will impact in the bifurcating bronchial tree during inspiration. It is unlikely for particles larger than 5 microns in diameter to reach the alveoli.

The walls of the trachea and large bronchi are supported by horseshoe-shaped cartilaginous rings. More distally they give way to apposed cartilage plates, invested by a fibroelastic membrane also containing bundles of smooth muscle. The plates decrease progressively in size and are eventually replaced by smooth muscle, which gradually becomes abundant enough to invest the entire bronchial wall.

A comprehensive discussion of the innervation of the lung will not be attempted. However, vagal parasympathetic efferent fibers innervate smooth muscle, glands, and blood vessels. Sympathetic efferent nerves are thought to supply mainly parasympathetic ganglia. Parasympathetic discharge produces increased smooth muscle tone and increased production of watery secretions. Afferent sensory fibers to the bronchial epithelium are stimulated by irritant exposures; they trigger reflexive coughing and bronchoconstrictive vagal parasympathetic efferent discharge.

Mast cells are found in connective tissue throughout the body, including the nasal and bronchial submucosae, and in association with blood vessels in both the nose and lung. Their role in the production and release of the mediators of immediate hypersensitivity reactions was described in Chapter 31.

II. Allergic rhinitis and asthma

A. Mechanisms.
Eosinophilia is a prominent feature of both allergic rhinitis and asthma. During periods of symptomatology, increased levels of eosinophils are often noted in the peripheral blood and respiratory secretions, and the tissues of the respiratory passageways contain a cellular infiltrate that is largely composed of eosinophils. Since the mediator eosinophil-chemotactic factor of anaphylaxis (ECF-A) is responsible for the influx of eosinophils into respiratory tissues, and since the releases of individual mediators are thought usually to occur together as a group phenomenon, this eosinophilia is considered a marker for mediator release in general, regardless of whether IgE is involved.

In allergic rhinitis the mucosa is boggy and congested. Its color is typically pale due to edema, and a bluish discoloration from stasis of blood in venous sinusoids is often seen. Excessive glandular activity results in hypersecretion of watery mucus. Additionally, patients frequently complain of mucous membrane pruritus and paroxysms of sneezing.

Histamine is thought to be the important mediator of allergic rhinitis through its actions on blood vessels, glands, and afferent sensory nerves. The basis for this postulate is the beneficial therapeutic effect for many patients with allergic rhinitis of drugs that are competitive antagonists of histamine. Although other mediators are released, the extent to which they contribute to disease has not been well studied in allergic rhinitis.

In bronchial asthma both histamine and slow-acting substance of anaphylaxis (SRS-A) are assigned definite roles as mediators of disordered physiology, but evidence is mounting for the additional involvement of mediators such as prostaglandins and platelet activating factor (PAF). The parasympathetic nervous system also plays a role. When asthma is triggered by allergen inhalation, mediator release is the initial occurrence, and the mediators are thought to act directly on smooth muscle, glands, blood vessels, and other target cells. On the other hand, when asthma is triggered by various irritants (e.g., smoke, ozone, sulfur dioxide, citric acid aerosols), the initial event is reflex parasympathetic cholinergic discharge. The acetylcholine liberated from postganglionic, parasympathetic nerves is thought to have a direct bronchoconstrictive action and to increase glandular secretion.

Furthermore, since cholinergic activity enhances mediator release, and since histamine may trigger parasympathetic reflexes, mutual augmentation of these two effector systems can occur. This appears to be the case in asthma. Whether or not recruitment of parasympathetic reflexes by released mediators is a significant mechanism in allergic rhinitis has not been adequately studied.

In bronchial asthma there is increased resistance to airflow due to smooth muscle constriction in both large and small airways. Additionally, there is edema of the bronchial wall, as well as an inflammatory cellular infiltrate in which eosinophils are prominent. Hypersecretion of mucus occurs. During an attack, areas of the mucosa may be shed and the submucosa denuded. Because of impaired mucociliary clearance, ineffective coughing due to bronchospasm, and the separate but sometimes complicating factor of dehydration, mucous plugs may form and occlude both small- and medium-sized airways. These events are reflected in wheezing dyspnea, which can be chronic and unremitting, but is more likely to be episodic or to fluctuate widely in degree.

In selected circumstances—for example, to identify an allergen when skin testing is not feasible—controlled exposure of the asthmatic patient to a suspect allergen is carried out to see if it will precipitate asthma. At least three patterns of asthmatic response may be seen, either alone or in combination. Most typically, asthma occurs within minutes. Occasionally, however, a late response occurs, either 3 to 12 hours after challenge or nocturnally for several nights afterward.

During a progressive asthma attack, deterioration in pulmonary function occurs that reflects increasing airway resistance, air trapping, and reflexive hyperinflation, which tends to increase elastic forces in the lung that combat airway collapse. Thus, although vital capacity and flow rates worsen, total lung capacity tends to increase due to elevation of residual volume.

Mucous plugging and bronchospasm occlude airways, impairing ventilation of areas of the lung parenchyma. Blood flow to these areas is reduced by reflex vasoconstriction but does not stop completely. Since the blood supply to these areas cannot be oxygenated, systemic arterial hypoxemia may result; it is a common feature of asthma. If such shunting is widespread, the reflex pulmonary vasoconstriction it produces can lead to acute pulmonary hypertension. This is seen only in very severe asthma. The same is true of carbon dioxide retention. Typically, carbon dioxide elimination is not impaired even though moderate to severe hypoxemia may be present. The onset of hypercapnia is a sign that overall pulmonary ventilation has been profoundly impaired.

When asthma becomes chronic, histologic changes in bronchial tissues occur. The smooth muscle hypertrophies, the subepithelial basement membrane becomes thickened, and an increase in mucosal goblet cells and submucosal mucous glands takes place.

B. **Clinical aspects.** Clinically, allergic rhinitis affects 10 to 15 percent of the population and asthma about 3 percent. Approximately 30 percent of patients with allergic rhinitis give a history of asthma or at least episodic wheezing. Allergic rhinitis or asthma can begin at any age, but most patients have onset of symptoms before the age of 20. The most frequent causes of nasal allergy are seasonal pollens, airborne fungal spores, house dust, and animal danders. Only occasionally is food allergy a cause. The majority of asthmatic patients have similar allergies, to inhaled allergens that are causative factors. This is especially true in children and young adults. However, nonallergic causation is also common; viral infections and heavy exertion will frequently produce exacerbations. With increasing age, there is a general tendency for allergy to be less prominent and for triggers such as respiratory irritants and adverse atmospheric conditions to be more important. A minority of asthmatics can have severe flares after ingesting aspirin and certain other analgesics; allergic mechanisms have not been demonstrated, and pharmacologic idiosyncrasy is suspected. Finally, in many patients and with many flares, at times exacerbating exposures may not be apparent.

In highly industrialized societies, occupational respiratory disease is recognized as an increasing problem. Many types can occur, including allergic rhinitis and asthma. Multiple potential occupational sensitizers have been recognized. A sample of these items would include such diverse agents as molds among handlers of organic materials, drugs and biologicals in the pharmaceutical industry, vegetable gum dusts in the printing industry, flour inhaled by bakers, and simple haptenic chemicals such as toluene diisocyanate (TDI) where polyurethane is produced, and trimellitic anhydride (TMA) used in plastic manufacturing. Respiratory disease with some such agents is complex, resulting variably from immediate hypersensitivity, other immune mechanisms, primary irritant properties of the agent, or some combination. Individual susceptibility of workers and the symptom complexes they develop vary.

In differentiating allergic rhinitis and asthma from other respiratory conditions, the finding that more than 15 to 20 percent of the cells in respiratory secretions are eosinophils during symptomatic periods is helpful. This does not prove an allergic etiology but is, rather, a marker for mediator release. In a small percentage of patients with eosinophilic rhinitis, nonimmunologic mechanisms for mediator release are suspected; this commonly occurs in bronchial asthma, as mentioned previously.

With asthma, the usually fluctuating nature of symptoms is also diagnostically useful, as is the bronchial hyperresponsiveness that is a part of this disease. Asthmatics develop signs and symptoms due to bronchoconstrictive drugs and other stimuli more readily and to a greater extent than do patients with other bronchopulmonary diseases. They will also show more marked improvement in pulmonary function with bronchodilator treatment unless severe asthma is present. In severe asthma, the poor initial response to drug treatment reflects the importance of mucous plugging and bronchial edema and inflammation, in addition to the smooth muscle spasm. Severe asthma that is unresponsive to bronchodilators is termed status asthmaticus and is a medical emergency. When bronchodilators alone are insufficient, corticosteroids and other drugs may be required. With a sufficiently aggressive medical regimen, asthma that is not complicated by some other process is a potentially completely reversible form of obstructive bronchopulmonary disease.

III. **Allergic bronchopulmonary aspergillosis.** This condition can occur as a complication of asthma. It is caused by colonization of an asthmatic patient's bronchial tree by the fungus *Aspergillus* and the subsequent hypersensitivity responses that develop. This characteristically results in a marked increase in asthmatic symptoms as well as transient infiltrates on chest x-ray, marked peripheral blood eosinophilia, fever, and weight loss. These patients have much higher total levels of serum IgE antibodies than are usually seen in uncomplicated asthma. They have not only specific antibody for *Aspergillus* of the IgE class, but also precipitating antibodies that are usually IgG. Type IV cell-mediated immune mechanisms are also suspected to play a part in the inflammatory response, which often leads to bronchiectasis and pulmonary fibrosis. The treatment is long-term corticosteroid use, which is thought to eradicate the fungus by reducing production of the bronchial secretions that act as the growth medium.

IV. **Allergic alveolitis (hypersensitivity pneumonitis).** Like bronchial asthma, allergic alveolitis can be caused by hypersensitivity to various inhaled fungi and organic dusts. However, more peripheral lung tissues and different mechanisms are involved. The prototype is farmer's lung, caused by thermophilic actinomycetes in moldy hay. Many other causes have been implicated, such as pituitary snuff, pigeons and lovebirds kept as pets, and a variety of fungi from contaminated humidifiers and air-conditioning systems. Immediate hypersensitivity is usually not present, but precipitating antibodies are often demonstrable. A mixture of types III and IV hypersensitivity is suspected. Symptoms following exposure may be severe. When severe, the reaction occurs 4 to 6 hours after exposure and consists of cough, dyspnea, fever, leukocytosis, and pulmonary function changes that reflect reduction in lung air volume and increased stiffness of peripheral lung tissues. With continued or repeated exposure, pulmonary fibrosis develops. When hypersensitivity is not intense, a chronic low-level exposure can result in the insidious development of pulmonary disability without other symptoms.

V. **Clinical example of allergic rhinitis and asthma**

A. **Description.** A 14-year-old boy came to the emergency room for treatment of an acute exacerbation of asthma. He gave a history of first wheezing in infancy with respiratory infection. Since the age of 4 he has had allergic rhinitis, which is worse in the fall of the year. At the age of 5 he began having wheezing episodes that were controlled by bronchodilators given regularly in the fall and sporadically the rest of the year, except when viral respiratory infections required the addition of corticosteroids. The present episode began with fever and coughing 3 days previously. He was using both an oral bronchodilator and a nebulized bronchodilator at excessively frequent intervals. He was wheezing and very dyspneic.

Arterial blood gases on room air: $PaO_2 = 52$; $PaCO_2 = 40$; $pH = 7.40$. A chest x-ray was normal.

He did not respond to injected epinephrine and was admitted for treatment with oxygen, intravenous aminophylline, and corticosteroids. Gradual improvement began about 12 hours after admission.

B. **Discussion**

1. This patient had mixed asthma, caused partially by allergy (at least during ragweed season in the fall) and partially by nonallergic mechanisms (as with his current, probably viral respiratory infection). This is common.

2. Atopic allergy or asthma can develop at any age but most frequently has already developed by the age of 10. Although some children outgrow the diseases, many do not.

3. Overuse of inhaled bronchodilators commonly makes a flare of asthma even worse, perhaps because of irritation from the aerosol.

4. His normal $PaCO_2$ was ominous. Earlier in the attack he would have been alkalotic with a low $PaCO_2$ due to hyperventilation. When seen he was ventilating more poorly and was at high risk for rapid deterioration. Had that occurred he might have required mechanical ventilation.

Questions

More than one answer is possible.

1. Which of the following is/are seen only in severe asthma?
   a. Arterial hypoxemia.
   b. Arterial hypercapnea.
   c. Elevated right heart pressures.
   d. Lack of response to bronchodilators.
2. The pathophysiology of bronchial asthma does not necessarily include:
   a. Mediator release.
   b. Respiratory eosinophilia.
   c. Bronchial smooth muscle constriction.
   d. IgE.

33 Immunologically Mediated Disease

I. **Background.** The topic of hypersensitivity has been previously introduced in Chapter 31, on immediate hypersensitivity (type I hypersensitivity). Other mechanisms for immunologically mediated tissue alteration or tissue destruction (hypersensitivity) are categorized in the Gell-Coombs classification.

   A. **Type II hypersensitivity** involves antibodies directed against cellular or tissue antigens (e.g., red cells, platelets, basement membranes of renal glomeruli or lung alveolar capillaries) or against antigens or haptens that have become fixed to cells or tissue components. The complement system is usually but not invariably involved in producing the inflammatory process.

   B. **Type III hypersensitivity** is due to the deposition of immune complexes in blood vessels. The ensuing inflammatory response is usually preceded by activation of the complement system at the site of deposition.

   C. **Type IV hypersensitivity** is mediated by the effector cells of cell-mediated immunity. Specifically sensitized thymus-derived (T) cells are these effector cells. Destructive tissue changes occur because of cytotoxic T cells or incident to chronic inflammation mediated by lymphokines released from T cells.

   D. Several newly recognized forms of immunologically produced tissue injury do not fit into the Gell-Coombs classification and are described here. First is antibody-dependent cell-mediated cytoxicity (ADCC) where IgG antibody fixes to antigens on target cells and nonsensitized K lymphocytes bind to the antibody through a cellular Fc receptor and effect cellular lysis. Second, there are several types of antibodies to cell receptors that produce diverse pathogenic effects. Antibodies to the insulin receptor (as in acanthosis nigricans) interfere with hormone binding and lead to serious degrees of insulin resistance. Antibodies to the acetylcholine receptor are found in more than 90 percent of patients with myasthenia gravis and lead to defective neuromuscular transmission, the neurophysiologic defect in this disease. Finally, antibodies to receptors on thyroid cells drive the target cell to hyperfunction in Graves' disease (hyperthyroidism).

   In the last several years, a class of lymphocytes has been recognized that are toxic to tumor cells, virus-infected cells, and some normal cells and that do not require presensitization for their activity. They are called natural killer (NK) cells. While the pathogenic potential of all these mechanisms is clear, their actual role in mediating tissue damage will become more apparent in the future.

II. **Immune complex diseases (type III hypersensitivity).** This is perhaps the most frequent and the best-studied form of immunologically mediated disease. Type III hypersensitivity may or may not be autoimmune. The antigen in the complex may be due to either exogenous or endogenous antigens listed in Table 33-1.

   The infrequency of identifying the antigen in immune complexes is related to the fact that, without clinical leads to a possible inciting event,

Exogenous Antigens	Endogenous Antigens
Viral, bacterial, fungal, protozoan or helminthic antigens	DNA, ribosomes, RNA, various RNA proteins
Animal sera to tetanus or clostridial toxins, snake venoms, or human lymphocytes	Human IgG (the Fc is the target for rheumatoid factor)
	Thyroglobulin
Drugs such as penicillin, sulfonamides, hydantoin compounds, piperazine	Tumor antigens (e.g., CEA, melanoma, lung carcinoma antigens)
	Renal tubular proximal epithelial cell antigen (as in sickle-cell disease, Fanconi syndrome)

CEA = carcinoembryonic antigen; DNA = deoxyribonucleic acid; RNA = ribonucleic acid.

screening for all possible antigens would be prohibitive. Nonetheless, the list in Table 33-1 is surely incomplete, and one can anticipate a wider recognition of responsible antigens in the future.

A. Circulating immune complexes. Newer technology has allowed the identification and quantification of circulating immune complexes in serum or plasma and of immune complexes in effusions or in the cerebrospinal fluid.

Since antibody binding to antigen is a defensive mechanism for eliminating exogenous antigens or altered self-antigens, including senescent cells, it is not unexpected that low levels of immune complexes may be found in healthy persons. Indeed, circulating immune complexes can be identified in the absence of clinical disease, and immune complex disease histologically confirmed by tissue deposition of antibody and complement may exist in the absence of circulating immune complexes.

B. Pathogenicity of immune complexes. There are several characteristics of the antigen-antibody complexes themselves and of the host that determine the inflammatory potential of immune complexes. The ratio of antibody to antigen determines the size of the complex. Those formed at equivalence or slight antigen excess are most pathogenic: large lattice complexes are efficiently extracted from the circulation by the reticuloendothelial system; very small complexes (Ag_2Ab) do not deposit in tissues efficiently and do not activate the complement system. Certain properties of the antigen—such as (1) affinity for such particular structures as the glomerular basement membrane (e.g., DNA) and (2) stability—enhance participation in immune complex disease, while certain properties of the antibody—such as its ability to fix complement, affinity for antigen, and immunoglobulin class—determine the phlogistic potential of a particular antibody. Also playing a role in susceptibility to immune-complex–induced disease are host factors such as functional impairment of monocytes-macrophages mediated by corticosteroids or morphine, genetically determined deficiency of reticuloendothelial function (e.g., B8 DR_3 individuals), or saturation of the reticuloendothelial system by either particulate substances or prolonged exposure to circulating immune complexes.

C. Site of deposition of complexes. The site of deposition of complexes is determined by local tissue physicochemical and hydrostatic factors, anatomy of the microcirculation, affinity of the complexes for tissue

Table 33-2   *A Workable Classification of Vasculitis*

1. Polyarteritis group
   a. Classic polyarteritis nodosa
   b. Allergic granulomatosis (Churg-Strauss syndrome)
   c. Overlap syndrome of systemic necrotizing vasculitis
2. Hypersensitivity vasculitis (allergic vasculitis, leukocytoclastic vasculitis)
3. Subgroups of hypersensitivity vasculitis
   a. Serum sickness
   b. Henoch-Schönlein purpura
   c. Essential mixed cryoglobulinemia
   d. Vasculitis associated with malignancies (especially lymphomas, leukemia, and multiple myeloma)
   e. Vasculitis associated with other primary disorders (especially rheumatoid arthritis and systemic lupus erythematosus)
   f. Vasculitis associated with fulminant rheumatic fever
4. Wegener's granulomatosis
5. Lymphomatoid granulomatosis/polymorphic reticulosis
6. Giant cell arteritis
   a. Temporal (cranial) arteritis
   b. Takayasu's arteritis
7. Thromboangiitis obliterans (Buerger's disease)
8. Mucocutaneous lymph node syndrome (Kawasaki's disease)
9. Miscellaneous
   a. Behçet's syndrome
   b. Erythema nodosum

components, and perhaps local permeability factors. The site of deposition of immune complexes produces the site of clinical signs and symptoms. The preeminent sites of deposition in human disease include the glomerulus and renal tubular basement membrane, the synovium, the dermal-epidermal junction and dermal vessels of the skin, the pulmonary alveolar capillary basement membrane, the uveal tract of the eye, the choroid plexus of the brain, and the intrinsic vessels of larger vessels and of nerves.

D. Mechanisms of tissue damage. Deposition of immune complexes leads to fixation and activation of complement at tissue sites. Vascular dilatation and increased permeability occur due to the anaphylatoxin components of C3 and C5; neutrophils and monocytes attracted by complement-generated chemotactic factors result in acute (and perhaps chronic) inflammation. Activated granulocytes achieve tissue destruction through their generation or release of free oxygen radicals; prostaglandins; vasoactive peptides; proteases such as collagenase, elastase, and chymotrypsin-like enzyme; and chemotactic factors for macrophages. In some instances, the vasculitis is predominantly a lymphocyte-mediated phenomenon with mononuclear cell infiltration and progression to granulomas.

E. Classification of vasculitis. Vasculitis, a major clinical consequence of type III hypersensitivity is classified (Table 33-2) according to:
   1. Clinical presentation.
   2. Possible precipitating agents (sera, drugs, infections).
   3. Vessels involved (arteries vs. veins vs. capillaries, size and anatomic location of involved vessels, involvement of skin or lungs).
   4. Histologic appearance (leukocytoclastic vasculitis with granulocyte infiltration, fragmentation, and nuclear dust; necrotizing vasculitis; granulomatous vasculitis; or lymphocyte/plasma cell invasion as seen in lymphocytic angiitis and granulomatosis or in lymphomatoid granulomatosis).

5. Association with other primary disorders.

Vasculitis usually presents as a multisystem disorder. Typical bedside findings in vasculitis include palpable purpura, gangrene and ulceration, subcutaneous nodules, erythema nodosum, splinter hemorrhages, livedo reticularis, Raynaud's phenomenon (some instances), urticaria (some instances), and mononeuritis multiplex. These and many of the other features can be related to localized ischemia or infarction due to impairment of tissue perfusion.

III. Autoimmune diseases

A. Mechanisms of tissue injury. Autoimmunity may involve one or more of the above-described mechanisms. Type I hypersensitivity has not been recognized as an important pathway in autoimmune responses but it may be that early in the course of vasculitis, IgE-mediated responses may lead to enhanced vascular permeability and set the stage for immune complex mediated vasculitis. Type II hypersensitivity is an important cause of organ-specific autoimmune disease. In Goodpasture's syndrome, antibodies to glomerular basement membrane produce a rapidly progressive glomerulonephritis and antibodies to alveolar basement membrane are associated with pulmonary hemorrhage. Autoantibodies to red cell membrane antigens and autoantibodies to platelets are the immunopathogenetic cause of autoimmune hemolytic anemia and idiopathic thrombocytopenic purpura, respectively. Immune complex disease (type III) due to immune responses to endogenous antigens has been discussed above. Type IV hypersensitivity plays a role in Hashimoto's thyroiditis, polymyositis, and rheumatoid arthritis and may participate in the tissue damage of interstitial nephritis, myasthenia gravis, and demyelinating diseases of the nervous system.

As already mentioned, antibodies to receptors (which might be considered a form of type II hypersensitivity) play a role in the development of Graves' disease, certain forms of insulin resistance, and myasthenia gravis.

Clinical evidence for autoimmunity comes from several sources. An association with a confirmed autoimmune disease, the immunohistologic demonstration of gamma globulin and complement in tissue lesions, the histologic picture of mononuclear cells having infiltrated around blood vessels, and a clinical response to anti-inflammatory and immunosuppressive drugs all contribute indirect support for the diagnosis of autoimmunity. More direct evidence comes from the demonstration of specific autoantibodies. These data become compelling when such autoantibodies are either directly pathogenic (e.g., in type II reactions), the autoantibody level fluctuates with disease activity (e.g., anti-DNA in lupus patients), or specific antibody or the antigens are demonstrably enriched in the tissue lesions.

A number of diseases with immunologic features but where the antigen has not been identified have subsequently been shown not to be of autoimmune etiology. These include: (1) the vasculitis that accompanies some cases of hepatitis B virus infection (which may account for 20–30% of cases of polyarteritis nodosa); (2) subacute sclerosing panencephalitis (SSPE), in which a slow virus infection with measles virus seems to be operative; and (3) at least one instance of insulin-dependent diabetes mellitus in which there was Coxsackie B virus infection of the pancreatic islet cells.

B. Systemic lupus erythematosus (SLE) is a complex human disorder characterized by multisystem involvement. It is often considered the prototype autoimmune disease. Immunologically there is a breakdown of regulation of the immune system with polyclonal activation of B lymphocytes, depression of suppressor T cells during active disease, and production of antibodies against a variety of cells and soluble substances. The pathologic changes are thought to be due to immune complex deposition in the glomerulus and tubular basement membrane, the pulmonary alveolar-capillary membrane, the pleura, pericardium, myocardium, synovium, peripheral nerves, and brain. Despite the demonstration of immune deposits in some of the vessels of the above organs, there is no solid evidence in all instances to document an immune complex mechanism for tissue damage in all of these organs. The evidence for immune complex–mediated disease is strong for the renal disease and weak for all other organs.

Cytotoxic antibodies to red cells and platelets are firmly established as a pathogenic mechanism for anemia and thrombocytopenia in SLE. Antibodies to clotting factors may play a role in a hemorrhagic diathesis in some patients and antibodies to lymphocytes may play a primary role in the disordered immune regulation that is characteristic of this disease. Unregulated B cell hyperactivity to some of the antigens listed in Table 34-1 (in Chap. 34, Inflammatory Rheumatic Diseases) and deficiency of T suppressor activity are probably also important in the pathogenesis of SLE.

The roles of disordered type IV hypersensitivity, ADCC, and NK cells are as yet unevaluated and could account for some of the unexplained or poorly understood phenomena in this disease.

The clinical picture may range from mild and remittent to severe, rapidly progressive, and fatal. The preponderance of the disease in women of child-bearing age probably represents the interaction of female sex hormones on the immune system in a genetically predisposed person. Environmental or infectious agents are also suspected as playing a role as inciting causes. Flares of the disease are associated with physical and emotional stress, infections, trauma, surgery, pregnancy, exposure to sunlight, and drugs.

Therapy is directed at control of symptoms, development of a placid life style, and avoidance of precipitating factors. Corticosteroids and immunosuppressive drugs are employed in severe or difficult cases. Experimentally, plasmapheresis (to remove autoantibodies and immune complexes) and lymphopheresis to remove lymphocytes are being investigated. Anecdotally, life-threatening complications have been reversed in selected patients by these pheresis procedures.

IV. **Clinical example of immune complex disease**

A. **Description.** A 25-year-old male welder was admitted because of a 5-month history of arthralgias and arthritis, weight loss, and fever. He had used oral and intravenous recreational drugs but none for the previous 5 years.

He had been hospitalized in another city and treated with corticosteroids. At that hospital, laboratory studies and procedures revealed an elevated sedimentation rate, hematuria and proteinuria, anemia, leukocytosis and thrombocytosis, negative antinuclear antibody, positive rheumatoid factor, normal complement levels, elevated liver alkaline phosphatase, lactic dehydrogenase (LDH), and serum glutamic oxaloacetic transaminase (SGOT). Hepatitis B surface antigen was negative. Liver biopsy and bronchoscopy were negative.

Physical findings were consistent with Cushing's syndrome due to corticosteroid therapy.

Urinalysis revealed 3$^+$ proteinuria, 4$^+$ occult blood, 15–20 RBC, and 12–15 WBC/HPF. There was 1.9 g of proteinuria per 24 hours, and a creatinine clearance of 56 ml per minute. Serum studies failed to reveal immune complexes.

Arteriography revealed multiple aneurysms in the renal and hepatic arteries consistent with (probably diagnostic of) polyarteritis nodosa.

Therapy with prednisone and cyclophosphamide enabled him to return to work as a roughneck in the Texas oilfields.

B. Discussion

1. The patient had a polysystem disease with arthritis, fever, weight loss, and renal disease. Polysystem disease should direct the physician to consider infection, malignancy, collagen-vascular disease, metabolic disease, or miscellaneous diseases such as sarcoidosis and amyloidosis.

2. The diagnosis of polyarteritis is based on the clinical picture plus the finding of arteritis on biopsy (muscle biopsy, renal biopsy, etc.). The demonstration of multiple arterial aneurysms in the renal and celiac-mesenteric systems may substitute for a biopsy in selected cases.

3. Both intravenous use of amphetamines and infection with hepatitis B virus have been implicated in the etiology of polyarteritis nodosa.

4. Immune complexes may be difficult to identify in the circulation but can be found in the arteritic lesions.

5. Therapy with corticosteroids and cyclophosphamide has converted an almost uniformly fatal disease to one with a high rate of cure, including reversal of arterial aneurysms.

Questions

Select the single best answer.

1. Which microorganism has been implicated in the etiology of polyarteritis nodosa (by demonstration in circulation and in the immune deposits in involved arteries)?
   a. *Plasmodium falciparum.*
   b. *Streptococcus pneumoniae.*
   c. Hepatitis B.
   d. *Cryptococcus neoformans.*
   e. Varicella-zoster virus.

2. Which one of the following statements is *incorrect*?
   a. If immune complexes are present in the circulation, symptoms of immune complex disease will invariably exist.
   b. Immune complexes may occur in tissues and be associated with disease in patients who fail to show immune complexes in circulation.
   c. Circulating immune complexes primarily cause disease by involvement of blood vessels (vasculitis or glomerulitis).
   d. The antigen present in immune complexes may be exogenous (such as bacterial antigens) or endogenous (such as DNA).
   e. Certain autoimmune diseases are mediated by immune complexes; however, this mechanism does not explain all autoimmune disorders or all disorders with an immunologic component.

34

Inflammatory Rheumatic Diseases (Noninfectious): Mediation by Immunologic Mechanisms

I. Introduction. This chapter examines a group of rheumatic diseases in which the primary tissue lesion is inflammatory but whose etiology and pathogenesis are for the most part unknown or only incompletely understood. Included in this discussion will be rheumatoid arthritis, the seronegative spondyloarthropathies, the collagen-vascular diseases, Sjögren's syndrome, and rheumatic fever.

Invasion of joint spaces by microorganisms and deposition of crystals in joint structures are well-known mechanisms of joint inflammation. Infection of joints is referred to as infectious arthritis; gonococci, pneumococci, staphylococci, myobacteria, and fungi are some of the better-known offenders. Gout is the most common condition in which arthritis is caused by crystal deposition in joints.

Neither of these mechanisms has been demonstrated to play a role in the inflammation occurring in the diseases under consideration. Attempts to recover microorganisms from the inflammatory lesions in these diseases have been made repeatedly, using the most advanced techniques, and have given mostly negative results. Isolated reports of success have not been confirmed even when attempted again by the same investigators. Of course, it is still possible that the inflammatory reaction in these diseases is due to direct tissue invasion by microorganisms that cannot be cultivated by currently available techniques or to the dissemination of nonviable fragments of microorganisms into tissues, but these possibilities await further investigations. Histopathologic examination of the inflammatory lesions in these diseases shows them to be comprised predominantly of varying mixtures of immunologically competent cells including T and B lymphocytes, plasma cells, and macrophages. Whatever the etiology of these diseases, it is generally believed that the tissue inflammation occurring in them is mediated by immunologic mechanisms.

There are four ways in which immunologic reactions can cause tissue inflammation, injury, or dysfunction. These have been described in Chapters 31 and 33. Type II, III, and IV reactions have all been considered to play a role in the idiopathic rheumatic diseases to be considered in this section.

The often chronic and aggressive nature of the inflammatory reaction occurring in these diseases and the puzzling lack of any apparent etiologic factor have led many to consider autoimmunity as a possible cause. For these to be autoimmune diseases would require that they be the result of a destructive immunological reaction(s), which for some reason has become directed at a normal body component that is present or somehow becomes localized at the sites where inflammation occurs. Autoimmunity in the form of autoantibody formation is frequently observed in some of these diseases, especially systemic lupus erythematosus (SLE) and rheumatoid arthritis (RA).

Antibodies to nuclear antigens occur in virtually all patients with active SLE. Rheumatoid factor occurs in 80 percent of patients with RA and can be defined as an immunoglobulin of any class whose specific reactivity is directed at a portion of the Fc fragment of human IgG. These are clearly autoantibodies because their specific reactivities are with native antigens present in the host forming the antibodies. The question is whether these autoantibodies are only an epiphenomenon (a result of the disease or the generalized immunological hyperactivity that is associated with most of these diseases) or whether they, or cell-mediated immunity with corresponding specificities, are the essential feature(s) of the disease mechanism.

The problem is that most of these autoantibodies are not absolutely specific for the disease or manifestations of a disease in which they may have a role. Only some of them are specific for a given disease, and then they are not present in the disease with a 100 percent incidence. Most of them are present to some extent in a wide range of other diseases and even in presumably healthy individuals. However, it does seem likely that DNA/anti-DNA complexes mediate the renal injury in SLE, and that IgG rheumatoid factors which undergo self-aggregation into complexes may mediate some of the extraarticular manifestations of RA and also contribute to the intensity of joint inflammation. Both of these would be type III reactions.

A frequently proposed concept of autoimmunity in the rheumatic diseases, which also takes into account that many of these diseases show a varying genetic predisposition, is as follows. As a result of some environmental insult, perhaps a viral infection, the genetically predisposed individual fails to eliminate the offending agent in a normal manner. A generalized immunological hyperactivity results, possibly related to defective suppressor T lymphocyte function. Some have also postulated the presence of a polyclonal B cell activator. The loss of normal suppressor function permits autoantibody formation to occur. Whether or not disease results depends on the antigenic specificities of the autoantibodies formed, the amount and type of antibody formed, and the avidity of the antibodies for their antigen. The autoantibodies present in a given disease may then have a variable relation to the disease. Some may be only a result of the disease or the immunological hyperactivity; some may have a close relation to some etiologic factor or particular pathogenic mechanism, and then be more or less disease-specific, their detection being useful as a diagnostic test; some may be an essential part of the disease mechanism. These concepts are most applicable to SLE and RA and, although reasonable, are far from being considered as established; they leave many aspects of these diseases unexplained.

II. **Rheumatoid arthritis.** The initial lesion in rheumatoid arthritis is inflammation in the synovial membrane with a prominent perivascular component. The synovial membrane then undergoes extensive proliferation and is densely invaded by lymphocytes, plasma cells, and histiocytes. It gradually assumes the appearance of a vascular granulation tissue, referred to as pannus, which invades and destroys bone and cartilage beginning at the site of attachment of synovial membrane to bone. The destruction of joint structures is mediated by enzymes such as collagenase, cathepsins, and other proteases released by the inflammatory cells. The disease is chronic and may last for decades. It involves multiple joints in a symmetrical distribution, but not the lumbar and thoracic spine, and usually not the sacroiliac joints.

The discovery some 30 years ago that RA is associated with IgM rheumatoid factors (and more recently, IgG rheumatoid factors) represents a significant advance. Detection of IgM rheumatoid factor by simple agglutination tests is frequently done in the clinical laboratory and is a helpful diagnostic test. About 80 percent of patients clinically diagnosed as RA give positive reactions, such patients being referred to as seropositive. Seropositive RA differs from seronegative RA in being a more homogeneous disease with, on the average, more severe joint involvement and a tendency to extraarticular manifestations such as subcutaneous nodules, pulmonary fibrosis, and vasculitis. Recent tissue-typing studies reveal that seropositive RA patients have a greatly increased incidence of the DR_4 antigen specificity whereas seronegative RA patients do not. Thus, there are genetic differences between the two forms of the disease. Some patients diagnosed clinically as seronegative RA may actually have some other type of joint disease. IgM rheumatoid factors are present in a wide variety of other chronic inflammatory diseases, in some normal individuals, and in 25 percent of aged persons.

Both cellular and humoral immunologic mechanisms appear to be involved in the synovitis of RA. T lymphocytes are a prominent part of the inflammatory reaction; lymphokines have been demonstrated in the joint fluid; and thoracic duct drainage that removes mostly T lymphocytes and decreases cellular immunity has been shown to ameliorate the inflammatory reaction of RA. On the other hand, many of the plasma cells present in the rheumatoid synovium have been shown to produce rheumatoid factors. IgG rheumatoid factors, which can be considered antibodies to themselves, undergo self-aggregation. The degree to which this occurs depends on the concentration of normal IgG present, which would be expected to be low in the interstitium of the rheumatoid synovium, where the locally formed rheumatoid factors are being released. The larger complexes of this sort activate the complement system. These complexes have been demonstrated in the synovial fluid and serum of patients with RA, as have also immunoglobulin complexes with IgM rheumatoid factor. The inflammatory cells in rheumatoid synovial fluid contain ingested immunoglobulin-complement complexes; joint fluid complement levels in seropositive RA are usually much depressed. Rheumatoid factor complexes probably contribute to the intensity of joint inflammation and may mediate some of the extraarticular manifestations of RA.

III. **Seronegative spondyloarthropathies.** This designation includes ankylosing spondylitis, Reiter's syndrome, some forms of juvenile chronic arthritis, and certain other diseases. Some of these were previously referred to as rheumatoid variants; ankylosing spondylitis was previously called rheumatoid arthritis of the spine. This view was considerably changed when it was found that most of the patients with these diseases were seronegative for rheumatoid factor. This has been reinforced by the finding that these diseases are associated with the human histocompatibility antigen, HLA-B27. For example, 95 percent of Caucasians with ankylosing spondylitis are HLA-B27 positive in contrast with a 7 percent incidence of this antigen in the normal population. These conditions are now considered distinct diseases entirely separate from RA.

Ankylosing spondylitis is a chronic inflammatory disease affecting sacroiliac joints, spinal structures, and less frequently, other joints. It is clinically recognized most often in young men; in its most severe forms, it can lead to complete spinal immobility and severe postural deformity.

Reiter's syndrome is a symptom complex consisting of arthritis, urethritis, conjunctivitis, and mucocutaneous lesions. The disease often seems to be a consequence of certain infections such as chlamydial infections of the genitourinary tract, *Shigella* dysentery, and others (much as rheumatic fever is a result of streptococcal infections).

The synovitis in Reiter's syndrome is generally less cellular than in RA, but the synovitis in ankylosing spondylitis, when it affects peripheral joints, is similar to RA but with more tendency to extend to the capsule and periarticular structures. This was one of the reasons for its originally being considered rheumatoid arthritis of the spine.

The remarkable association of these diseases with the HLA-B27 antigen is the strongest disease association found for any of the histocompatibility antigens. A definitive explanation for this relation has been elusive. Some proposed explanations include: HLA-B27 itself or a closely linked gene product binds a bacterial or viral product and causes the disease; the B27 gene or a closely linked gene determines an inappropriate immune response to some agent, and this initiates the disease process; and B27-positive patients may respond excessively to inflammatory mediators such as prostaglandins.

IV. **Collagen-vascular diseases.** This designation usually includes systemic lupus erythematosus (SLE), polyarteritis nodosa (PN), dermatomyositis (DM), and progressive systemic sclerosis (PSS) also called scleroderma. SLE is a chronic disease usually affecting young women and characterized by multisystem involvement (arthritis, dermatitis, pleuritis, pericarditis, nephritis, cerebritis, etc.) and recurrent, often severe, febrile episodes. PN is also a disease affecting multiple body systems, with necrotizing vasculitis being the underlying pathologic lesion. DM is characterized by muscle inflammation and degeneration, as well as dermatitis. PSS is characterized by thickening and hardening of the skin, plus fibrosis and degeneration of synovium, digital arteries, esophagus, intestinal tract, heart, lung, and kidneys. In the latter condition, fibrosis rather than inflammation is the dominant lesion.

These diseases are usually classified together as collagen-vascular or connective-tissue diseases. It has become apparent over the years that they do have some overlapping clinical and serologic manifestations. However, the original reason for grouping them together was that early pathologic observations suggested they were characterized by a common pathologic lesion widely distributed in the connective tissues and blood vessels of the body. The common lesion was considered to be fibrinoid necrosis or degeneration of collagen fibers. The implication was that there might be some underlying abnormality in the collagen fibers or connective tissues of the body that causes these diseases. However, despite extensive efforts, this has never been demonstrated. The connective tissues and blood vessels of the body serve as sites for the inflammatory and fibrotic lesions of these diseases, but otherwise appear normal. There are some other conditions, such as the Ehlers-Danlos syndrome or osteogenesis imperfecta, that are a result of molecular abnormalities of connective tissue. These latter diseases are more appropriately referred to as connective-tissue diseases.

Antibodies to nuclear antigens are common in these diseases and are true autoantibodies; the nuclear antigens involved are multiple. The pattern of autoantibody formation in terms of the recognized nuclear antigens varies from one disease to the other. Accounting for this variation has an important bearing on attempts to explain these diseases as being

Table 34-1   *Antibodies in Systemic Lupus Erythematosus*

Antibodies against cells and particles
  Red blood cells, lymphocytes, platelets, neural membranes, mitochondria, ribo-
    somes, and lysosomes
Antibodies against soluble substances
  DNA (both native and single-stranded forms), gamma globulin, a family of RNA
    protein antigens (Sm, nuclear RNP, Ro, and La), DNA histone, RNA (both single-
    and double-stranded), cardiolipin, clotting factors, histones, and other poorly
    identified soluble antigens

autoimmune. For example, antibodies to single-stranded or denatured DNA occur in many chronic diseases and are most likely to be just a reaction to the disease. High-titered, high-avidity antibodies to native DNA are usually confined to active SLE with low complement levels and active nephritis and are believed to cause the nephritis. Antibodies specific for nucleoprotein (DNA + protein) are common in SLE, are characteristic of drug-induced SLE, and occur with some frequency in RA. Their recognition is a useful diagnostic procedure, but their role in disease activity is doubtful.

As listed in Table 34-1, a variety of autoantibodies occur in patients with SLE in addition to antibodies to DNA. Most of the listed antibodies occur most characteristically in SLE, but those with the highest specificity for the disease are antinative DNA and antiSm, although neither of these occurs in all the patients. No specific autoantibodies are known to occur in polyarteritis nodosa but in both the polymyositis syndromes and in PSS, families of antibodies occur that are characteristic of these two diseases. For example, antibodies to an antigen termed Jo_1 occurs in about 30 percent of patients with polymyositis, while antibodies to two different antigens designated PM_1 and Ku occur in patients with polymyositis-PSS overlap syndromes; and antibody to an antigen Mi occurs in patients with DM. Similarly, it has been demonstrated by the indirect fluorescent antibody technique that virtually all patients with PSS have antibodies that bind to Hep_2 cells, a long-term tissue culture line. The two antibodies with the highest frequency bind to the centromeric portion of the chromosome (approximately 60%) and to the nucleolus (approximately 25%), respectively. While these antibodies may or may not be involved in the pathogenesis of PSS, they are proving to be of diagnostic usefulness and provide clues for investigators to pursue in their quest for the etiology and mechanism of these still obscure diseases.

V. **Sjögren's syndrome.** Sjögren's syndrome is a clinical triad consisting of dry eyes (kerato-conjunctivitis sicca), dry mouth (xerostomia), and a connective-tissue disease, usually rheumatoid arthritis. The pathology of the disease is characterized by dense infiltration of affected organs by mononuclear cells composed primarily of lymphocytes, with some plasma cells and histiocytes. Two forms of the disease exist: primary, in which no connective tissue disease is present; and secondary, in which the infiltrated salivary and lacrimal glands are accompanied by either rheumatoid arthritis, PSS, SLE, or PM.

It has been recognized in recent years that many organs in addition to the lacrimal and salivary glands are infiltrated by mononuclear cells. Thus, there may be lymphadenopathy, splenomegaly, pulmonary infiltrates, and various renal lesions but principally renal tubular acidosis, interstitial nephritis, and less frequently, glomerulonephritis. There is also a remarkable incidence of vasculitis with nonthrombocytopenic purpura, vascular ulcers, peripheral neuropathy of the mononeuritis multiplex type, and even central nervous system involvement.

Aside from the obvious association with connective-tissue diseases, all of which are thought to have autoimmune features, there is an impressive array of autoantibodies in this disease. Rheumatoid factors occur in 90 to 95 percent of both primary and secondary Sjögren's syndrome. Hyperglobulinemia is the rule; antinuclear factors occur in 50 to 60 percent of these patients, and antibodies to two antigens that occur in 30 percent of SLE patients termed Ro and La occur in 60 and 30 percent, respectively, in Sjögren's syndrome. These antigens have also been termed SSA and SSB, respectively. Not surprisingly, a high proportion of patients with SLE–Sjögren's syndrome have these antibodies.

While the etiology of Sjögren's syndrome remains obscure, genetic factors play some role, since the DR_3 antigen specificity and certain B cell antigens (715, 350, and 172) are greatly increased in these patients compared with controls.

VI. Rheumatic fever. Rheumatic fever is clearly caused by group A streptococcal infections. Bacteriologic or serologic evidence of preceding streptococcal infection is invariably present in cases of rheumatic fever; prevention of streptococcal infections by prophylactic use of penicillin prevents rheumatic fever. The pathogenesis of the disease, however, remains unsettled. The streptococci possess antigens that cross-react with human heart muscle. Infection with these organisms does cause formation of antibodies reactive with human heart muscle, and this could explain the myocarditis of rheumatic fever but not the valvulitis. Deposition of immune complexes containing streptococcal antigens or tissue antigens has been suggested as a possible mechanism for the valvulitis. Rheumatic fever is a rarely made diagnosis at the present time, in sharp contrast with its wide prevalence in years up to and including World War II. Apparently, widespread use of antibiotics has altered its incidence.

VII. Clinical example of inflammatory rheumatic disease

A. Description. A 50-year-old woman noted the onset of pain and stiffness affecting her hands, wrists, and feet 6 months ago. In the previous 2 weeks her left knee and left ankle had become painful and swollen, making it difficult for her to walk. Aching and stiffness were especially severe in the morning when she first got up and were only partially relieved after being up and around for 3 hours. She took 4 to 6 aspirins a day for her symptoms, with little relief. She had been treated with a diuretic drug for mild hypertension for the last 2 years. Aspiration of the fluid from her left knee showed an inflammatory effusion with a total white blood count of 9.5×10^3 per cubic millimeter, but no urate crystals could be identified. X-rays of her hands and wrists showed only soft tissue swelling about some of the finger joints. Some of the initial laboratory results were as follows: serum uric acid, 8.5 mg/100 ml (normal range, 3.5–8.0); serum salicylate, <5 mg/100 ml; and RA agglutination test, positive at a dilution of 1:2560.

As part of her treatment, it was recommended that she increase her dose of aspirin to 12 to 16 tablets daily.

B. Discussion

1. The clinical picture was typical of rheumatoid arthritis.

2. The positive test for rheumatoid factor gave strong support for the diagnosis; it tends to be associated with more severe, sustained disease.

3. X-rays showed only periarticular soft tissue swelling, a finding which can be more accurately detected by physical examination. In rheumatoid arthritis the appearance of diagnostic x-ray changes, such as marginal erosions of bone, may not occur for many months after the first appearance of clinically detectable synovitis.

4. The presence of rheumatoid factor does not establish a diagnosis of RA, and the presence of hyperuricemia does not establish a diagnosis of gout.

Questions

Select the single best answer.

1. The direct cause of destruction of bone and cartilage in rheumatoid arthritis is most likely to be:
   a. Lymphokines.
   b. The complement system.
   c. A type III immunologic reaction.
   d. Proteolytic enzymes.
   e. An infectious agent.

2. Autoantibody formation to various cellular constituents is common in the inflammatory rheumatic disease. The presence of such autoantibodies:
   a. Establishes a role for autoimmunity in the etiology of these diseases.
   b. Excludes an infectious etiology for these diseases.
   c. Is most likely to be a result of the widespread distribution of the lesions in these diseases in the connective tissues of the body.
   d. May be a result of defective suppressor function of T lymphocytes.
   e. Excludes the possibility that these diseases may result from an ingested chemical.

Degenerative Joint Diseases and Gout

I. Degenerative joint disease (osteoarthritis) and degenerative disk disease

   A. Normal anatomy and function. The freely movable (diarthrodial) joints of the body have a characteristic anatomy, which is shown in Figure 35-1.

   The synovial membrane that lines the joint, except over the hyaline articular cartilage, is composed of a surface lining layer of modified connective-tissue cells called synoviocytes and an underlying layer of loose connective tissue. The hyaline articular cartilage does not have a blood or nerve supply and receives its nutrition by diffusion from blood vessels in adjacent structures. In order to be nourished adequately by this mechanism, hyaline articular cartilage has to be thin and, in fact, does not exceed a thickness of 6 mm in any joint.

   The opposing bone ends of a joint are usually slightly incongruous but, with load bearing, deform and become congruous. The hyaline cartilage and the underlying subchondral bone function as a shock absorber and undergo the necessary deformation with weight bearing. The hyaline articular cartilage also functions in joint lubrication. The glycosaminoglycans present in the cartilage are highly negatively charged and, when not under weight-bearing pressure, are forced by this negative charge to occupy the maximum volume permitted by the encasing collagen fibers of the cartilage. The space created by extending these molecules is occupied by water. With weight bearing, the water is forced out between the joint surfaces so that the fluid film between opposing cartilaginous surfaces of moving joints is made up of cartilaginous interstitial fluid. This highly efficient mechanism of joint lubrication under load bearing is referred to as hydrostatic. Joint lubrication under non–load-bearing circumstances is believed to be performed by a special joint-fluid glycoprotein affixed to cartilaginous surfaces that keeps them from touching. This is referred to as boundary lubrication. Substantial loss of congruity of opposing bone ends markedly interferes with these mechanisms.

   The intervertebral disks are examples of poorly movable joints; their typical anatomy is shown in Figure 35-2.

   The structure is such as to permit limited motion with good stability at each disk interspace; the nucleus pulposus functions as a shock absorber. When motion at each of the disk interspaces is combined, a substantial range of spinal motion is achieved. The joints between the superior and inferior articular facets that arise from the bony neural arches of each vertebra are typical diarthrodial joints.

   B. Pathologic changes and consequences of joint degeneration. With aging, degenerative changes occur to some extent in all individuals' joint structures and are attributed to the wear and tear that is the result of normal use. These changes, which begin in the twenties, progressively advance in some people, leading to significant pain and loss of function.

   In osteoarthritis the initially observed changes occur in cartilage at sites of maximum weight-bearing stress and consist of flaking (tangential loss of chunks of cartilage) and fibrillation (longitudinal fissuring

Figure 35-1

Diagram of normal diarthrodial joint.

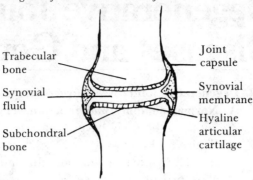

Trabecular bone

Synovial fluid

Subchondral bone

Joint capsule

Synovial membrane

Hyaline articular cartilage

Figure 35-2

Diagram of normal intervertebral disk.

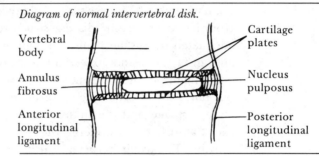

Vertebral body

Annulus fibrosus

Anterior longitudinal ligament

Cartilage plates

Nucleus pulposus

Posterior longitudinal ligament

of cartilage). Subchondral bone cysts or geodes form at points where fissures extend all the way through the cartilage into the underlying trabecular bone. These cysts are formed as a result of high intraarticular pressures being transmitted from the joint space through the opening into the marrow cavity. These bone cysts may collapse and lead to considerable deformation of bone surfaces; this is especially likely to occur in the hip. In association with loss of cartilage, reactive bone formation occurs at two sites: (1) There is increased bone formation in the subchondral bone underlying the point of maximal cartilage loss; on x-ray this appears as increased bone density or sclerosis. (2) There is also bone overgrowth at the margins of the joints, which appears to take place along lines of lateral stress from the attached ligaments. On x-ray this appears first as a sharpening of articular margins, with the margin acquiring an acute angle rather than being rounded, and then as hook-like extensions of bone from the articular margin that are in continuity with the underlying subchondral bone. These projections of bone are called osteophytes. The end result is a complete loss of the joint space, subchondral sclerosis and cyst formation, and prominent osteophytosis.

The degenerative changes that occur in the cartilaginous plates of intervertebral disks are similar to those that occur in the cartilages of diarthrodial joints. With degeneration of the disk, radial tears occur in the annulus fibrosus, and the nucleus pulposus extends into positions outside its normal confines. It is especially likely to extend up to the vertebral margins on either side of the posterior longitudinal ligament. A herniated intervertebral disk is said to occur when the disk material causes protrusion into the vertebral canal (protruded disk) or where the annulus ruptures and free disk material extrudes into the vertebral canal (extruded disk). Pressure on the spinal cord or nerve roots may occur. Herniation of the intervertebral disk often occurs, usually from trauma or strain, without preceding degeneration. Osteophytosis is a common component of degenerative disk disease and is usually of no consequence. However, posterolateral osteophytes may impinge on nerve roots in the intervertebral foramina, and posterior osteophytes extending across the posterior margin of the disks in the cervical spine (spondylosis) are sometimes identified as a cause of spinal cord compression. Extensive bony enlargement related to degenerated disks and apophyseal joints, as well as bony enlargement of the lamina, may lead to stenosis of the cervical or lumbar spinal canal and may be associated with neurologic defects.

It should be appreciated that degenerative joint and disk disease are common, and often benign, processes and that pathologic study of these conditions is usually limited to severe examples. Fortunately, x-rays give a less invasive way of studying these structures for evidence of degeneration and show varying degrees of joint space narrowing from cartilage loss, subchondral sclerosis and cyst formation, and marginal osteophytosis.

C. **Nomenclature and incidence.** There is a general tendency in the United States to refer to both degenerative joint and disk disease as osteoarthritis. The English use the term *osteoarthrosis* to escape the implication of its being an inflammatory disease. Some would say that *osteoarthritis* should be used only in relation to diarthrodial joints, which would include the spinal apophyseal joints but not the disks. But this is a convention that is frequently violated; one will often see discussions in major textbooks in which manifestations of degenerated and herniated disks are described as part of osteoarthritis of the cervical and lumbar spine. It may well be that the pathophysiology of the degenerative changes in these structures is similar; still, the intervertebral disks are different anatomically from the freely movable joints, management of these conditions is different in some respects, and the possibility of neurologic complications might be better kept in mind if the term *degenerative disk disease* is used. There is an unfortunate tendency in practice to refer to every poorly defined, painful musculoskeletal condition as osteoarthritis.

Osteoarthritis of diarthrodial joints is usually divided into primary and secondary forms. The primary form occurs without evident predisposing cause and affects only certain joints, which include the distal and proximal interphalangeal joints of the fingers, the carpalmetacarpal joint at the base of the thumb, the acromioclavicular joint, the hip, the knee, and the first metatarsophalangeal (MP) joint of the foot. In patients with numerous simultaneously affected joints, the condition has been referred to as primary generalized osteoarthritis. When changes in the hands are extensive and with more prominent inflammatory manifestations, the condition has been referred to as erosive inflammatory osteoarthritis. Secondary osteoarthritis usually affects these same joints but with definite predisposing factors—such as obesity, knock-knee or bowlegs, a congenitally incompletely formed hip joint, previous joint trauma or fracture, and a host of other conditions. The MP joints of the hands, wrists, elbows, shoulders, and ankles are less commonly affected by osteoarthritis.

II. **Gout, hyperuricemia, and crystal-induced inflammation**
A. **Definition of gout.** Gout is a form of arthritis that, in its early stages, is characterized by recurrent, paroxysmal, acute attacks of severe joint

inflammation lasting for a few days to a few weeks. The attacks are the result of deposition in joint structures of monosodium urate crystals from hyperuricemic body fluids that are supersaturated with urate. About 15 to 25 percent of hyperuricemic individuals will have acute gout at some time in their lives, the usual age of onset being the fifth and sixth decades. If the underlying hyperuricemia is not treated, 50 to 60 percent of patients who have had acute gout will tend to have progressively more frequent attacks and, finally, chronic persistent arthritis with multiple tophaceous deposits in bones and subcutaneous sites and sometimes severe incapacity. These chronic manifestations of gout are due to persisting tissue deposits of monosodium urate crystals. Uric acid renal lithiasis occurs in 10 to 20 percent of gouty patients. The occurrence of gout in man results from a lack of the enzyme uricase, so that uric acid becomes the end product of purine metabolism; this along with an inefficient renal excretory mechanism leads to mean serum urate levels that approach the calculated level of saturation. Most other mammals possess the uricase enzyme and have the more soluble allantoin as the end product of purine metabolism.

B. **Definition of hyperuricemia.** The limit of solubility of sodium urate in solutions having the sodium content of plasma, allowing for about 5 percent binding of urate to protein, is 6.8 mg/100 ml. Levels above this represent supersaturation. The mean serum urate level in men is around 5 mg/100 ml. Values are lower before puberty and in premenopausal women. Postmenopausal females have a mean level close to that of men. The mean plus 2 standard deviations would place the upper normal level of serum urate for men at about 7 mg/100 ml. The values given are for true serum urate levels measured by an enzymatic spectrophotometric method. Many clinical laboratories use automated equipment and a colorimetric method for measuring serum urate; the values obtained may be as much as 1 mg/100 ml higher than true serum urate levels. For proper interpretation, any reported value of serum urate has to be related to the mean and normal range of values obtained by the procedure being used.

C. **Relation of hyperuricemia to gout.** Gout is related to the duration and degree of hyperuricemia. In the well-known study of the adult population of Framingham, Massachusetts, it was found that only 2 percent of hyperuricemic individuals in their early thirties had gout, whereas 23 percent of those in their late fifties had gout. Only 5 percent of gouty patients are female; this can be related to the lower level of serum urate in women up to the time of the menopause. In certain conditions in which enzyme defects lead to marked overproduction of uric acid and high serum urate levels, uric acid renal lithiasis and gout are seen at an early age.

D. **Mechanism of hyperuricemia in primary gout (no evident predisposing condition).** Overproduction of uric acid is present in about 60 percent of patients with primary gout. Uric acid is removed from the body by two routes; two-thirds is excreted in the urine by the kidneys, and one-third is destroyed in the gut by the uricase activity of intestinal bacteria. A patient who shows increased levels of uric acid in a 24-hour urine specimen, preferably after being on a purine-free diet for several days, can be assumed to be an overproducer of uric acid. Some 25 percent of gouty patients can be demonstrated to be overproducers of uric acid by this simple measurement.

However, a normal value does not exclude overproduction. A patient may have normal urinary levels but still be excreting excessive amounts into the gut. Using radioisotope methods to measure urate pool size, turnover, and rate of incorporation of labeled precursors into urinary uric acid, urate overproduction can be demonstrated in over half of gouty patients. The precise mechanism for this is unknown except for a few patients with recognized congenital enzyme defects.

The remaining gouty patients, and also some of the overproducers, show underexcretion of uric acid by the kidney for a given serum urate level. They require higher serum levels to excrete the same amount of uric acid as normals. The renal handling of urate is somewhat complicated. Most of it except the small amount that is protein bound is filtered at the glomerulus. There are multiple tubular reabsorptive sites for uric acid, the principal one being in the first portion of the proximal tubule. There is a urate secretory site in a more distal portion of the proximal tubule, which apparently corresponds to the site where other weak organic acids such as salicylates are secreted. The actual amount of uric acid excreted in the urine is the sum of what is secreted and what fails to be reabsorbed; it averages about 7.5 percent of what is filtered at the glomerulus. The precise factors that cause gouty patients to be underexcretors of uric acid are unknown.

E. **Secondary gout and other mechanisms of hyperuricemia.** Gout occurs in certain hematologic diseases such as chronic leukemia, polycythemia vera, multiple myeloma, thalassemia, and pernicious anemia. Hyperuricemia is common in these diseases; it is caused by an increased turnover of nucleic acid purines as a result of marked cellular proliferation.

Administration of potent diuretics such as a thiazide or furosemide raises serum urate levels an average of 1 mg/dl and sometimes more. Apparently, volume depletion caused by these drugs enhances proximal tubular reabsorption of urates and may also indirectly suppress tubular secretion. Half of the new patients with gout who were detected in the Framingham study were patients taking diuretics for hypertension.

Chronic renal insufficiency is often associated with hyperuricemia, but gout is uncommon. However, the renal lesion from chronic lead poisoning (related to the intake of moonshine whisky with a high lead content or to use of leaded paints) is often associated with gout.

Alcoholism and salicylates affect serum urate levels, and use of alcohol is often associated with gout. Alcoholism and the associated fasting cause lactic acidemia, which suppresses tubular secretion of urate and promotes hyperuricemia. The fasting state also seems to lead to increased purine synthesis. Salicylates at low blood levels (<5 mg/100 ml) compete with urate for tubular secretion and promote hyperuricemia. At higher blood levels (>15 mg/100 ml), salicylates inhibit renal tubular reabsorption of urates and lead to hyperuricosuria and hypouricemia.

F. **Crystal-induced inflammation.** The factors that initiate urate crystallization from supersaturated fluids are largely unknown. Increased turnover and depletion of glycosaminoglycans from tissue sites have been suggested. These substances inhibit urate crystallization. At any rate, in acute gouty attacks, the initial deposition of crystals is followed by the appearance of polymorphonuclear leukocytes (PMNs), perhaps as a result of activation of the complement system by the crystals. PMNs, which have phagocytized crystals, release a potent chemotactic factor; this would appear to account for the further accumulation of PMNs. The attacks proceed in a crescendo fashion with peak intensity typically being reached within 24 hours of onset. Gouty attacks are more common in lower than upper extremities and more common in distal portions of the extremities than in proximal portions. This may be explained by the temperature gradients that exist in these areas, with lower temperatures favoring urate crystallization.

There is a second common form of crystal-induced arthritis related to the deposition of calcium pyrophosphate crystals in the synovium. This syndrome is called pseudogout and is distinguished from gout principally by the weak positive birefringence of the crystals recovered from the synovial fluid of pseudogout patients, as opposed to the strong negative birefringence exhibited by the urate crystals recovered from gouty synovial fluids. This disease was previously recognized as chondrocalcinosis; a helpful x-ray finding is a fine linear calcification in the medial meniscus of the knee joint. The mechanisms leading to the formation and deposition of calcium pyrophosphate crystals are unknown.

III. Clinical example of gouty arthritis

A. Description. A 55-year-old man reported having intermittent attacks of pain and swelling affecting multiple joints for the last 5 years. In the past year the trouble was much more persistent, and he noted the development of nodular enlargements on some of his fingers and over his elbows. He was admitted to the hospital because of an especially severe attack of arthritis affecting his ankles, knees, and left wrist. He drank alcohol moderately and had received treatment for hypertension for 10 years. Aspiration of the fluid from his left knee showed an inflammatory effusion with a total white blood count of 15,000 per cubic millimeter. Compensated polarized light microscopy of the joint fluid showed many strongly negative-birefringent, needle-shaped crystals, most of which were within leukocytes. Aspirate from the nodule on his left elbow contained densely packed aggregates of the same crystals as the joint fluid. X-rays of his feet showed multiple bone lesions around the MP joints, which had a punched-out appearance; some had overhanging cortical margins. Some of the laboratory results were as follows: urinalysis, 1^+ protein, 2–3 WBC/HPF; creatinine, 1.6 mg/100 ml; uric acid, 10.2 mg/100 ml; rheumatoid arthritis agglutination test, negative.

B. Discussion

1. The demonstration of urate crystals in joint fluid or tissue aspirates, using compensated polarized light microscopy, is the best method of establishing the diagnosis of gouty arthritis.
2. The presence of persistent osseous or subcutaneous urate deposits is the hallmark of chronic tophaceous gout (chronic gouty arthritis) and is a major indication for long-term antihyperuricemic therapy.
3. At postmortem examination untreated gouty patients may show urate deposits in renal medullary areas. However, at present it would appear that renal functional impairment in gout is most often related to age, vascular disease, nephrolithiasis, infection, and other factors.

Questions

Select the single best answer.

1. All of the following are features of osteoarthritis except:
   a. Subchondral bone sclerosis.
   b. Subchondral bone cysts.
   c. Marginal erosions.
   d. Osteophyte formation.
   e. Joint space narrowing.

2. The hyperuricemia in gouty patients may be related to any of the following except:
   a. An enzymatic defect leading to overproduction of purines.
   b. Increased turnover of nucleic acid purines.
   c. Administration of a thiazide diuretic.
   d. Chronic lead poisoning.
   e. Increased absorption of purines from a normal diet.

36 Immunodeficiency

I. **Introduction.** Resistance to infection is a well-orchestrated interaction of resistance factors—such as tissue barriers, phagocytic cells, and interferon—and components of the immune system—such as antibodies and immune lymphocytes (cell-mediated immunity). When the system works well, pathogenic organisms are denied penetration into the body from surfaces exposed to the environment. If penetration of cells occurs or if the microorganisms gain access to the internal environment, inflammation localizes the infectious inoculum, organisms are phagocytized and digested, dangerous exotoxins are neutralized, and viruses are prevented from absorbing to target cells (or having absorbed and penetrated the cell, are prevented from replicating).

To achieve a successful defense the body mobilizes white blood cells of the granulocytic and macrophage/monocyte series (eosinophils are also involved, especially in intestinal parasitic diseases) and undergoes lymphoid hyperplasia, generating antibody production and amplifying sensitized lymphocytes for the cellular immune response.

Thus, it can be seen that deficiencies of one or more components of this complicated system may lead to inordinate susceptibility to infection. The susceptibility may be to a broad range of microorganisms or to specific infectious agents. Common pathogens may be involved, or organisms of low virulence may become significant pathogens in the immunodeficient patient.

A. **Lymphocyte biology.** Lymphocyte precursors arise in hematopoietic tissue (bone marrow in the postfetal period). Differentiation and maturation of the T lymphocyte series occurs in the thymus or perhaps at a later stage under the influence of thymic factors (thymic extracts, thymic hormone, thymopoietin, etc.). A comparable organ for differentiating and maturing B lymphocytes has not been definitively identified in mammals; perhaps it is the bone marrow itself. Monocytes also arise from hematopoietic tissue.

1. **Lymphocyte subclasses.** Lymphocytes, which are morphologically indistinguishable in the light microscope, are known to have subclasses recognizable by certain surface markers and functional characteristics. B lymphocytes differentiate into plasma cells and thus represent the precursors of antibody-forming cells. T cells, or thymus-derived cells, are of at least two types, helper or amplifier cells and a cytotoxic suppressor type. There are differences in surface antigens detected by monoclonal antibodies, in proliferative response to soluble antigen (only the helper cell proliferates), and as their names imply, in functional characteristics. There are other cells, morphologically lymphocytes, which are not functional B or T cells and which mediate antibody-dependent cell-mediated cytotoxicity (ADCC) and natural killer (NK) activities; each of these cell lines is functionally discrete. These cells may derive from what was formerly designated the null cell population.

2. **Lymphocyte markers**

   a. **Cell surface markers.** A number of surface markers identify the various lymphocyte subclasses. Immunoglobulins on the lymphocyte surface identify B lymphocytes, the precursors of the antibody-forming plasma cells. HLA-D/DR transplantation (Ia) antigens are present on mature B cells, some monocytes, and activated T cells. The various T lymphocyte subclasses can be recognized by monoclonal antibodies to various surface markers designated T3$^+$ (all T cells), T4$^+$ (helper cells), and T5$^+$T8$^+$ (cytotoxic suppressor T cells). There are also monoclonal antibodies, identifying a monocyte surface antigen.

b. **Lymphocyte membrane receptors.** Most mature B cells have complement (C3b and C3d) receptors. A proportion of B cells have receptors for the Fc portion of IgG, mouse red blood cells, and Epstein-Barr virus on their surface. Most T cells have a receptor for sheep cells on their surface; distinct subpopulations have a receptor for the Fc portion of bovine IgG (Tγ) cells and a receptor for the Fc portion of bovine IgM (Tμ), respectively. Null (K) cells have a receptor for the Fc portion of IgG.

c. **In vitro functional activities of lymphocytes**

(1) Proliferation with mitogen stimulation (concanavalin A, phytohemagglutinin, pokeweed mitogen).

(2) Proliferation in mixed lymphocyte cultures.

(3) Helper function for antibody-synthesizing cells.

(4) Suppressor function for antibody-synthesizing cells.

(5) Cytotoxic function of sensitized T cells.

(6) K cell cytolytic activity in antibody-dependent cell-mediated cytotoxicity.

(7) Release of lymphokines (macrophage migration inhibitory factor; macrophage activating factor; chemotactic factors for mononuclear cells, neutrophils, and eosinophils; skin reactive factor; lymphotoxin; blastogenic factor; cloning inhibitory factor; lymph node permeability factor; interferon; and transfer factor).

(8) Natural killer cell activity against tumor cell lines.

Interaction of these various lymphocyte subclasses is a complex and highly organized system leading to antibody secretion, amplification of the immune and accessory cellular responses, inflammation, and destruction of microorganisms and tumor cells. Surveillance of self and recognition of foreignness is a function of this system, tumor cells are eliminated, and cell-mediated hypersensitivity and autoimmunity are natural or aberrant side effects.

B. **Complement.** The complement system is a complex molecular array of plasma proteins that are synthesized by liver parenchymal cells or macrophages. Some components are involved in pathways of sequential activation, and in their active form some of these molecules are enzymes. Other molecules bind to receptors on red cells, granulocytes, eosinophils, basophils, mast cells, B lymphocytes, or monocytes/macrophages. Other complement components are inhibitors. Still others are stabilizers of previously formed complement complexes.

1. The *classic pathway* involves the sequential activation of C1, C4, and C2 by antigen-antibody complexes (aggregated gamma globulin or other mechanisms may duplicate this effect).

2. The *alternative pathway* consists of the sequential interaction of C3b (a fragment of C3), activated factor D, and Bb (a fragment of factor B). This complex is stabilized by properdin (factor P). Activation of the alternative pathway can be set into motion by microbial products (bacterial cell walls, endotoxins, and yeast cell wall extracts), snake venom (cobra venom factor), aggregated immunoglobulins,

immunoglobulins that ordinarily do not activate complement through the classic pathway, an IgG immunoglobulin known as C3 nephritic factor, cellophane in dialysis coils, and radiographic contrast media. The alternative pathway may be a defense mechanism early in infection before antibodies are produced.

3. Either of these early activation pathways eventuates in the activation of C3 and the subsequent effector complement cascade (C5, C6, C7, C8, and C9).

4. Complement activation results in the generation of biologic activities by the formation of active enzymes or proteolytic fragments whose cumulative effect may be cytolysis, virus neutralization, or the mediation of inflammation. Activated C1 potentiates virus neutralization by antibody. C2b and C4a have kinin activity. C3a causes the degranulation of mast cells, smooth muscle contraction (anaphylatoxin activity), and increased vascular permeability. C3b enhances phagocytosis and immune adherence, while C5a has both anaphylatoxic and chemotactic activities. The trimolecular complex C5, C6, and C7 is a potent chemotactic agent. The activated complex C8 and C9 of the two terminal components is designated the attack complex and can lead to lysis of mammalian cells and bacteria.

   The combined effect of these processes is to mediate inflammatory and cytolytic activities at specific sites of antigen-antibody reaction.

5. Genetically acquired deficiencies of complement may lead to characteristic syndromes. C1 esterase inhibitor deficiency leads to hereditary angioneurotic edema. Homozygous C1, C2, C4, C5, and C7 deficiencies are commonly associated with connective-tissue diseases such as SLE, polymyositis, or scleroderma-like syndromes. The most common of these is C2 deficiency, in which roughly one-third of the patients develop an SLE-like syndrome. Homozygous C3 deficiency is extremely rare but is associated with recurrent bacterial infections. Deficiencies of the late complement components C6, C7, and C8 are associated with disseminated *Neisseria gonorrhoeae* and systemic *Neisseria meningitidis* infections.

II. **Classification of immunodeficiency.** Immunodeficiency states may be primary (of unknown cause) or secondary to another disease. The primary deficiency may be congenital or acquired in later life.

A. **Congenital immunodeficiencies** are usually the result of (1) failure of one or more cell lines of the immune system or the phagocytic system to develop, (2) defective function of these cells, or (3) lack of production of accessory humoral substances such as complement components. Examples of these are the absence of B lymphocytes in Bruton's agammaglobulinemia, dysfunctional granulocytes in chronic granulomatous disease, and absence of late complement components (C6, C7, or C8), leading to susceptibility to systemic dissemination of *Neisseria* infections.

   The reason for the absence of cellular elements of the immune system or dysfunction of these elements is incompletely understood. A partial listing of explanations is as follows: (1) absence or failure of stem cells, (2) defects of enzymes of the purine metabolic pathway, and (3) immune suppression of precursor cells or of the maturation of these precursor cells into functional immunocompetent cells. This absence of functional cells may thus be due to autoimmune or nonimmune causes. Also, both types of mechanisms may operate in the same patient. For example, perhaps 1 out of every 600 persons has selective deficiency of IgA in plasma and secretions. Some of these persons are unable to synthesize or secrete IgA because of defective B lymphocytes. Other such persons have T cells that suppress IgA-synthesizing B cells as well as having defective B lymphocytes.

B. **Primary acquired and secondary immunodeficiencies** may also be a result of absence of the necessary cells or their dysfunction. Autoreactive cells, which destroy precursors of differentiated lymphocytes, in addition to being generated by malignancies and by infections, may be generated by drugs, by aging, and during systemic lupus erythematosus. In other instances where autoreactive cells are found the proximate cause is not known.

In certain of the primary acquired immunodeficiencies (an example of this is the gamut of disorders collectively termed common variable immunodeficiency, formerly known as acquired agammaglobulinemia) and in certain secondary immunodeficiencies (such as anergy associated with Hodgkin's disease, polyclonal immunoglobulin deficiency seen in multiple myeloma, and anergy associated with disseminated fungal infections), suppressor cells for the immunoglobulin-synthesizing B cells or for the effector T cells of cell-mediated immunity are present. These suppressor cells may be T lymphocytes or monocytes/macrophages.

Table 36-1 summarizes some of the more prominent diseases of immunodeficiency and attempts to list etiology and mechanisms for the observed deficiency.

III. **Clinical considerations.** Immunodeficient patients come to the physician with infections; rarely, the immunodeficiency is an asymptomatic finding. A careful history often directs the physician toward a broad categorization of the defect, since certain groups of infections are associated with deficiencies of particular components of the immune response (see Table 36-2).

IV. **Clinical evaluation of the patient with immunodeficiency.** Careful history and family history should be taken, especially stressing age of onset of infections, frequency and type of infection, offending microorganism, and clues to diseases associated with immunodeficiencies. Among these associated diseases and abnormalities are: allergies; autoimmune/collagen-vascular diseases; ectodermal dysplasias of skin, hair, and nails; endocrinopathies; hematologic abnormalities; malabsorption; malignancies; skeletal abnormalities (e.g., short-limbed dwarfism); eczema; telangiectasia; and ataxia. Physical examination should especially direct attention to enumerating the sites of infection, character of associated inflammation, status of lymphoid tissues (lymph nodes, tonsils, spleen, and liver), and stigmata of cutaneous, mucosal, and skeletal abnormalities. On the basis of these results, hypotheses can be tested further by selectively performing some of the tests listed in Table 36-3.

V. **Clinical example: immunodeficiency**

A. **Description.** An 8-year-old boy was seen because of recurrent sinus infections, bronchitis, and pneumonia since infancy.

In infancy he was treated briefly with gamma globulin. He had required high-dose intravenous antibiotics for a recent pneumonia and sinusitis.

Physical examination was unremarkable except for some growth retardation and coarse rales in his lungs. No arthritis or skin rashes were noted.

Previous workup for cystic fibrosis was negative. Chest x-ray

Table 36-1   *Classification of Immunodeficiency States*

A. Primary immunodeficiency
  1. Congenital
    a. Bruton's agammaglobulinemia: defect of precursors of B cells
    b. Selective IgA deficiency*
    c. Di George syndrome: aplasia or dysplasia of the thymus with failure of maturation of T lymphocytes
    d. Chronic mucocutaneous candidiasis (T-cell defect)
    e. Severe combined immunodeficiency: defect of lymphocyte stem cells (half of these patients are defective in adenosine deaminase, which allows toxic levels of purine metabolites to poison T-cell precursors; the profound B-cell defect is unexplained as yet, as is the T-cell defect in patients with normal adenosine deaminase)
    f. Miscellaneous: ataxia telangiectasia, Wiskott-Aldrich syndrome, Chédiak-Higashi syndrome, chronic granulomatous disease, complement deficiencies, T-cell defect due to purine nucleoside phosphorylase deficiency
  2. Acquired
    a. Common variable immunodeficiency (section II*)
B. Secondary immunodeficiency
  1. Nutritional defects
    a. Protein-calorie malnutrition
    b. Vitamin deficiencies
    c. Trace metal deficiencies (especially zinc)
  2. Malignancies
    a. Multiple myeloma: suppressor monocytes/macrophages
    b. Hodgkin's disease: suppressor T cells or suppressor monocytes/macrophages
  3. Infections
    a. Disseminated fungal infections: increased suppressor T cells
    b. Tuberculosis with pleural effusions: sequestration of reactive T lymphocytes in the effusion fluids
    c. Infectious mononucleosis: increased suppressor T cells during active disease
    d. Influenza, measles, paramyxoviruses: acute self-limited depression of T-cell–mediated immunity
  4. Collagen-vascular diseases: in the prototype disease, systemic lupus erythematosus, there are autoantibodies for suppressor T lymphocytes, a decreased autologous mixed lymphocyte reaction, a decreased B-lymphocyte primary immune response, impaired clearance of antibody coated particles, and perhaps a decrease in helper T lymphocytes
  5. Burns: loss of plasma immunoglobulins
  6. Protein losing enteropathy: gastrointestinal loss of plasma immunoglobulins and circulating lymphocytes
  7. Nephrotic syndrome: loss of plasma immunoglobulins
  8. Treatment with corticosteroids or cytotoxic drugs
  9. Miscellaneous
    a. Sarcoidosis: sequestration of reactive T lymphocytes in the lung, heightened resting autologous mixed lymphocyte reaction
    b. Splenectomy: suboptimal antibody responses to particulate antigens such as the pneumococcus; absence of the major reticuloendothelial (phagocytic) organ of early life; defects of the alternate pathway of complement activation
    c. Sickle-cell disease with splenic infarction: defects of the alternate pathway of complement activation
    d. Myotonic dystrophy: hypercatabolism of IgG

*See accompanying text.

Table 36-2   *Infections Associated with Various Immunodeficiency States*

Infections associated with deficiencies of humoral immunity
    Encapsulated pyogenic bacteria
        Streptococcus
        Pneumococcus
        Meningococcus
        Haemophilus
        Pseudomonas
    Staphylococcus
    Giardia lamblia (enteritis)
    Pneumocystis carinii (pneumonia)
    Viruses having a viremic phase (hepatitis, polio, and echoviruses)
Infections associated with granulocyte defects
    Catalase-positive organisms such as *Staphylococcus aureus* and *Serratia marcescens* as
        well as other bacteria, *Candida albicans,* and *Aspergillus* are problems in chronic
        granulomatous disease
    Pyogenic bacteria are risks in neutropenia and in Chédiak-Higashi syndrome
Infections associated with a deficiency of T-cell-mediated immunity

Bacteria	Viruses
Mycobacterium	*Herpes simplex*
Salmonella	*H. zoster*
Listeria monocytogenes	Cytomegalovirus
Francisella tularensis	Rubeola (measles)
Brucella	Vaccinia
Treponema pallidum	Helminths
Pseudomonas mallei	*Schistosoma*
P. pseudomallei	*Strongyloides*
Fungi	Protozoa
Aspergillus	*Toxoplasma gondii*
Candida	*Plasmodia*
Cryptococcus neoformans	Unclassified
Phycomycetes	*Pneumocystis carinii*
Histoplasma capsulatum	
Coccidioides immitis	

showed a pneumonitis and pleural reaction. Paranasal sinus x-rays showed an air-fluid level in the right maxillary sinus (acute sinusitis). Sputum culture grew out *Haemophilus influenzae.*

White blood count varied from 7.8 to 10.8×10^3 per cubic millimeter with 50 to 62 percent polymorphonuclear leukocytes and 3 to 11 percent bands (stabs).

Serum protein electrophoresis showed almost complete absence of gamma globulin. IgG was 86 mg/100 ml (normal, 700–1,400), IgA was less than 1.1 mg/100 ml (normal, 100–350), and IgM was 11 mg/100 ml (normal, 60–220). There was no secretory IgA detected in saliva.

The patient was blood type O positive but he had no anti-A or anti-B. Agglutinins for typhoid, paratyphoid, and proteus were negative. A battery of skin tests for delayed hypersensitivity (cell-mediated immunity) was positive for functional T lymphocytes (positive PHA skin test) and for recall (anamnestic) cellular immunity (positive mumps skin test).

B. Discussion

  1. The early onset of infections, persistence of infections to present age 8, male sex, almost total absence of immunoglobulins of all classes, and intact cell-mediated immunity establish the diagnosis of Bruton's agammaglobulinemia.

A. Routine laboratory tests
  1. Complete blood count (with differential count and platelets)
  2. Serum protein electrophoresis
  3. Cultures (identify the infecting microorganism)
B. Roentgenography
  1. Chest
     a. Acute and chronic lung changes
     b. Thymus shadow
  2. Nasopharynx, for tonsillar tissue
  3. Sinuses, for inflammation
C. Test for T-cell function
  1. Screening: Delayed hypersensitivity skin testing
     a. Recall antigens (streptokinase, mumps, *Candida* especially valuable)
     b. Phytohemagglutinin (PHA)
  2. Specialized
     a. T-cell count (E-rosettes)
     b. Lymphocyte transformation (PHA, concanavalin A, specific antigens)
     c. Migration inhibition factor (MIF) production
     d. Specific immunization (DNCB, KLH)
     e. Mixed lymphocyte cultures
D. Test for B-cell function
  1. Screening
     a. Quantitative immunoglobulin levels
     b. Schick test (IgG antibodies)
     c. Diphtheria, tetanus, polio, measles, mumps antibody titers
     d. Isohemagglutinin titers (IgM antibodies)
  2. Specialized
     a. B-cell count (EAC rosettes, surface immunoglobulin-bearing cells)
     b. Immunization studies (typhoid, KLH, pneumococcal polysaccharide)
     c. Lymphocyte transformation (pokeweed mitogen)
E. Effectors of immunity
  1. Complement (total hemolytic complement, components, inhibitors, inactivators, stabilizers, etc.)
  2. Neutrophils (count, morphology, phagocytosis, bactericidal assay, NBT-test)
  3. Macrophages (morphology, phagocytosis, chemotaxis)
  4. Rebuck skin window or in vitro leukotactic or chemotactic assays
F. Tissue examination
  1. Bone marrow aspiration
  2. Lymph node biopsy
  3. Tonsils, appendix, small-bowel biopsy
  4. Rectal biopsy

DNCB = dinitrochlorobenzene; KLH = keyhole limpet hemocyanin; EAC = erythrocyte-antibody-complement; NBT = nitroblue tetrazolium.

2. Although this is a genetic X-linked disorder, fewer than half of the patients will have a positive family history. The carrier state cannot be identified.

3. Chronic respiratory infections in childhood (and especially recurrent pneumonias and unexplained bronchiectasis) should prompt an investigation for cystic fibrosis and immunoglobulin-deficiency disorders.

4. Biopsy of lymph nodes, small intestine, or rectum reveals an absence of plasma cells.

5. Treatment is lifelong replacement with gamma globulin and antibiotics as needed. Despite this, upper airway infections recur. Recurrent pulmonary infections lead to pulmonary insufficiency. Gastrointestinal infections, collagen-vascular diseases, viral hepatitis, and encephalitis may be troublesome.

1. Match the following infections (A) with the immune defect (B).

A	B
(1) Disseminated *Neisseria* infections	(a) Defective humoral immunity
(2) Fatal pneumococcal bacteremia	(b) Defective cellular immunity
(3) Recurrent pneumococcal pneumonia	(c) Splenectomy
(4) Recurrent staphylococcal pneumonia	(d) Absence of C6
(5) Chronic *Candida* infections	(e) Defective granulocyte function

2. Identify the *incorrect* statement.

   a. Antibody production to thymus-dependent antigens requires that B lymphocytes interact with helper T cells.

   b. K cells need to be primed (sensitized) to the specific target cell antigen before they can interact with the antibody for the particular cell target.

   c. T cells release lymphokines on exposure to the specific antigen to which they are sensitized.

   d. The complement system can be activated by mechanisms that do not involve antigen-antibody complexes.

   e. Suppressor cells for T and B lymphocytes have been identified in many primary and secondary immune deficiency disorders.

VII Infection

Everett R. Rhoades

37   Inflammation

There is no physiology of infections in the sense that cardiac physiology provides the basic science of cardiology. Therefore, at present it is impossible to formulate a unified pathophysiology of infectious diseases. However, there are two pathologic alterations of body function which seem consistently related to infections: inflammation and fever. Inflammation is the subject of this chapter, and fever that of Chapter 38.

I. **Introduction.** In the first century A.D., Celsus enunciated the cardinal signs of inflammation: rubor (redness), tumor (edema), calor (heat), and dolor (pain). Later, a fifth sign of inflammation called functiolaesa (loss of function) was added. For several centuries inflammation (which means "internal flame") was considered to be a pathologic process representing the end result of noxious stimuli. This concept gradually changed following the extensive observations by Metchnikoff, reported in his "Lectures on the Comparative Pathology of Inflammation" in 1892. In these studies, he described phagocytosis and its role in inflammation. The participation of cells in the inflammatory response had originally been demonstrated by Cohnheim, who showed that the cellular infiltrate arose from circulating leukocytes that crossed blood vessel walls by diapedesis. Inflammation came to be considered a defense mechanism rather than a disease process and as such was recognized by Metchnikoff as the "most important phenomenon in pathology." In addition, the concept of inflammation gradually came to embrace the idea that the basic process of inflammation was leakage of the blood vessels. These two mechanisms, vascular permeability and cellular infiltration, remain the basic components of inflammation. In the last decade the events associated with inflammation have been extensively studied, with primary attention given to various compounds that apparently serve as mediators, both augmenting and controlling the process so that it can be shut off at the appropriate time. Inflammatory responses may be categorized as acute or chronic.

II. **Vascular events**

A. **Changes in blood flow.** The initial event in inflammation, although not universally present, is transitory vasoconstriction. This seems to arise from direct injury to vessels but may in fact be neurally mediated. The period of vasoconstriction is followed by a more diffuse and pronounced vasodilatation with a sharp increase in blood flow—sometimes up to ten times the normal flow. The duration of this increased flow varies and may be followed by a return to normal flow or by a period of stasis. The stasis may yield to a return to normal flow or it may lead to necrosis. There are several potent stimulators of vasodilatation. These will be discussed below in section IV, Mediators of inflammation.

B. **Permeability.** Increased permeability of local blood vessels is one of the basic processes of inflammation and is responsible for the swelling ("tumor"). During the first several hours, the swelling is a result of transudation of plasma into the interstitial tissues. Subsequently, swelling is associated with cellular infiltration and, later still, with the production of new connective tissue, as an attempt at healing begins. Capillary endothelium acts as a filter, utilizing a variety of techniques for transport of various materials across the capillary wall while at the same time protecting the integrity of the intravascular volume. Commonly, there are spaces, or potential spaces, at the junctions of endothelial cells. Various mechanisms regulate the size of these fenestrae. In addition, in some endothelial cells there are small vesicles that ferry materials across the endothelium. Different types of endothelial lining reflect the specialized processes that occur in various tissues. For example, in capillaries with a continuous endothelium, such as those encountered in the brain and lungs, there are no obvious fenestrae. Fenestrated endothelium is found in the glomerulus of the kidney and in various endocrine organs. The third type of endothelium, because of larger openings between cells, is termed discontinuous and is found in bone marrow.

The maintenance of the circulatory volume depends upon an equilibrium between the hydrostatic pressure inside the vessels and the osmotic pressure of tissue proteins (both of which tend to cause fluid to move out of vessels) and counteracting forces that tend to hold fluid within the vessels. The latter include the osmotic pressure of plasma proteins and the hydrostatic pressure of tissue surrounding the vessels. The net balance of forces favors a slight movement of fluid across vessels into the surrounding tissues, where it is ultimately recirculated through lymph channels. The vascular leak either occurs in response to direct injury or is stimulated by chemical mediators. The action of these mediators results in an increase in the size of the fenestrae and an outpouring of plasma into the perivascular tissue. The increase in size of fenestrae appears to be caused by contraction of the endothelial cells. It is obvious that this exudation of plasma must be controlled or else the circulation of blood might stop. A major factor which limits exudation is the aggregation of platelets which plug the fenestrae. Another limiting factor is the increase in extravascular pressure that results from the accumulation of edema fluid.

C. **Pavementing of leukocytes.** Concomitant with the vasodilatation and stasis of flow, circulating leukocytes begin to accumulate along the periphery of vessels and stick to the venular endothelium. At first, they stick for only a moment, then detach and continue to circulate. Soon, however, the sticking becomes more prolonged, and the venules become covered with a layer of leukocytes—the pavementing of Cohnheim. This adherence appears to be a function of the endothelium rather than of the leukocytes themselves. The leukocytes involved are neutrophils, eosinophils, and monocytes. Lymphocytes are strikingly absent.

III. **Cellular infiltration.** The predominant histologic change in inflammation is an intense collection of leukocytes, especially neutrophils. Indeed, the whole process of inflammation appears to be directed at the accumulation of large numbers of these cells, with the preparatory process being the pavementing of leukocytes in the venules. Few leukocytes cross *capillary* endothelium; rather, they migrate through *venular* endothelium by amoeboid movement (diapedesis). The transit through the venular wall takes from 2 to 9 minutes and occurs between endothelial cells. The transit through the basement membrane is not completely understood and may be mediated to some extent by various enzymes that temporarily open the basement membrane to passage.

One might suppose that the increased vascular permeability also facilitates emigration of leukocytes. However, these phenomena seem to be separate and independent, as can be shown by time studies. Similarly, the phenomenon of emigration is distinct and separable from leukocyte chemotaxis, but the latter clearly plays a role in emigration of leukocytes. After diapedesis, neutrophils move about in either a random or a directed manner in the tissues.

IV. Mediators of inflammation

A. Intravascular. A number of compounds have been found that profoundly influence inflammation. Many of these are formed inside the vessels from circulating precursors. Some of these are attractants for leukocytes, such as kallikrein and fibrinopeptides. Fibrinogen and endoperoxides cause activation and aggregation of platelets, which may serve to control edema and prevent blood leakage. Activated platelets release 5-hydroxytryptamine, a potent permeability mediator. Associated with platelet aggregation, prostaglandin E2 not only increases permeability but potentiates a variety of other mediators.

Bradykinin is one of the most potent mediators of inflammation, playing a major role in venule dilatation. The bradykinin system is activated by proteolytic enzymes acting on circulating kininogens present in serum globulins. In addition, bradykinin increases permeability and may also increase stickiness of the venular endothelium for leukocytes. Finally, bradykinins are potent pain stimulators.

Hageman factor (coagulation factor XII) is similarly activated from circulating precursors and is responsible for a number of augmenting effects. For example, it probably activates the bradykinin system, initiates the reactions converting prothrombin to thrombin, and activates plasmin. Thus, it plays a role in stimulating both clotting and fibrinolytic processes.

Finally, the complement system (C3, C5, and combined C5, C6, and C7) stimulates vascular permeability and chemotaxis. It also seems to stimulate release of neutrophils from the bone marrow.

There are undoubtedly other intravascular mediators of the inflammatory process. It is not surprising that many, if not all, of these are interrelated, sometimes in seemingly paradoxical ways. The net result is to produce a cascade effect but also, equally importantly, to provide for proper homeostasis.

B. Tissue mediators. Histamine is perhaps the major mediator of inflammation. It is found in basophils, mast cells, and platelets. Histamine release is stimulated by physical injury, toxins, and lysosomal proteins. Histamine is a particularly active vasodilator and permeability stimulator. Mast cells of some animals also release 5-hydroxytryptamine (serotonin), which has action similar to histamine. Prostaglandins are released from a variety of cells, including phagocytosing neutrophils. Prostaglandins E1 and E2 increase vascular permeability, exert chemotactic effects, and induce pain. A variety of important mediators, called lymphokines, are derived from lymphocytes. These exert their greatest effect on neutrophils, seemingly to regulate their accumulation, by substances that cause migration and by other substances that stop migration. Many of the factors modulating the inflammatory response act inside as well as outside the vasculature. A separation of these myriad factors and events into the two components is done mostly to help simplify somewhat the discussion of their effects. Some of the most important mediators are shown in Table 37-1.

V. Chronic inflammation

A. Definition. *Chronic inflammation* is most readily defined chronologically. In general, the term refers to inflammation that lasts more than several weeks. Chronic inflammation may arise from acute inflamma-

Table 37-1

Mediator	Origin	Major Action
INTRAVASCULAR ORIGIN		
Bradykinin	Activated from plasma precursors	Dilatation of venules Increases permeability Pain
Hageman factor	Activated from plasma precursors	Coagulation Activates kallikrein
Complement (C3, C5, C5, C6, C7)	Activated from plasma precursors	Increases permeability Chemotaxis Attacks bacteria
Fibrin	Activated from plasma precursors	Acts as matrix for phagocytosis
TISSUE ORIGIN		
Histamine	Mast cells (and platelets)	Dilatation of venules Increases permeability Chemotaxis (eosinophils) Inhibits motility of leukocytes Inhibits release of lysosomal enzymes
Serotonin	Mast cells	Dilatation of venules Increases permeability
Platelet-activating factor	Mast cells	Hemostasis
Prostaglandins	Variety of cells Leukocytes	Dose-regulated modulating functions Potentiate histamine and bradykinin
Migration inhibition factor	Lymphocytes	Accumulation of macrophages or monocytes
Chemotactic factors	Lymphocytes	Accumulation of neutrophils, eosinophils, and basophils

tion or may appear without an observable acute phase. It is easy to understand that acute inflammation may become chronic when contact with the noxious agent is prolonged.

The hallmark of chronic inflammation is the predominance of mononuclear cells in the infiltration. The other major histologic feature of chronic inflammation is the presence of connective tissue, manifested in its early phase by granulation tissue (not granulomata). In addition to monocytes, there are often lymphocytes, plasmacytes, and eosinophils. Usually, redness, heat, and swelling are less pronounced in chronic inflammation than in acute.

B. **Granulomatous inflammation.** Although in fact a form of chronic inflammation, granulomatous inflammation is sufficiently distinctive and has such important etiologic implications that it is often considered separately. The term *granulomatous* originally referred to small nodules, visible to the naked eye, present in infected tissues. It has gradually come to designate a microscopic appearance characterized by epithelialization of monocytes, the formation of localized collections of these epithelialized monocytes called tubercles, and the presence of multinucleated giant cells.

Certain microorganisms typically elicit granulomatous inflammation. These include mycobacteria, fungi, and certain parasites. Many foreign bodies—such as oils, talc, and sutures—also commonly stimulate granulomatous inflammation.

In chronic inflammation, the monocytes arise from circulating cells but also to some degree from cell division in the local tissues. Much of chronic inflammation is closely associated with the immune system, especially that dependent upon the thymus, which seems to act as the major mediating influence.

VI. Disturbances of inflammation

A. Vascular. The major disorders affecting the intravascular events have to do with disturbances of circulating volume and of hemostasis. It is obvious that extensive loss of plasma decreases circulatory volume. In addition, the vasodilatation causes pooling of blood in the affected capillary bed. When this is extensive, it may result in considerable relative loss of circulating volume. The stasis also results in hypoxia of cells in the area.

Activation of the Hageman factor not otherwise controlled may produce widespread intravascular clotting, especially when combined with platelet aggregation. These effects may result in exhaustion of clotting factors with resultant, seemingly paradoxical bleeding. Disturbances may arise from overproduction of clotting factors or from failure of the normal fibrinolytic system. The syndrome thus produced is termed disseminated intravascular coagulation. It represents a serious disturbance of grave prognostic significance.

B. Exaggerated inflammation. Persistent inflammation may result from failure of the inflammatory process to dispose of foreign material. Certain organisms, such as the tubercle bacillus, are also difficult to dispose of and lead to chronic inflammation. Sometimes antigen-antibody complexes deposit in tissues such as the glomerulus and stimulate persistent, damaging inflammation. Another example of disordered inflammatory response is seen in rheumatoid arthritis, in which cartilage is damaged by the inflammation. This may lead to deformity or other crippling effects.

Many noxious substances, while stimulating inflammation, cause an excess release of proteolytic enzymes from leukocytes, which in turn damage normal tissues. This may be seen in the lung, for example, after the inhalation of silica particles. It is thought that similar mechanisms may be responsible for the pathogenesis of emphysema. Inflammation may thus exceed its intended protective effect and actually become part of a pathologic process of considerable cost to the host.

Exaggerated inflammatory responses may occur when large numbers of bacteria within the vascular space itself stimulate intravascular inflammation, with increased toxicity and uncontrolled activation of clotting mechanisms. These intravascular events may also be triggered by circulating antigen-antibody complexes.

C. Leukocyte function

1. Neutropenia. Obviously, a deficient number of leukocytes results in an inadequate inflammatory response. Neutropenia may arise from a number of circumstances. For example, malignancies such as leukemia may displace normal leukocytes from the bone marrow. Many drugs, such as chloramphenicol and phenylbutazone, interfere with the production of leukocytes. Certain infections, especially those caused by viruses, are associated with neutropenia.

2. **Decreased migration of leukocytes.** Certain intrinsic deficiencies within leukocytes result in decreased migration. A rare condition, the Chédiak-Higashi syndrome, is associated with decreased locomotion and abnormal granules that fail to function normally. Job's syndrome, characterized by repeated infections, is also associated with decreased cell migration. Leukocytes of diabetic patients may migrate poorly, as do those of severe alcoholics.

VII. **Clinical example of abnormal functioning of inflammatory process**

A. **Description.** A 75-year-old man was found by a nurse to be unconscious in bed about 4 hours after undergoing repeated attempts of bladder catheterization to relieve urinary obstruction. He had a hot, dry skin, pulse 130 per minute, and blood pressure of 60/0. White blood cell count was 3,000 per cubic millimeter with normal differential. A diagnosis of septic shock was made, and he was placed on intravenous colloidal fluids and dopamine in an effort to maintain his circulation. Appropriate antibiotics were given. He did not respond to this regimen, and after 12 hours petechiae and ecchymoses developed over the extremities, spreading to the trunk. Blood began to ooze from his bladder and intravenous catheters.

His platelet count fell to 35,000 per cubic millimeter; the partial thromboplastin time (PTT) became prolonged, as did the prothrombin time (PT). Fibrin split products became elevated. Chest x-ray revealed increasingly diffuse radiodensities and assisted ventilation was required. Pulmonary wedge pressure was normal. His condition continued to deteriorate, and he died 48 hours later.

Autopsy revealed extensive necrosis of organs with proteinaceous fluid in the interstitium and alveoli of the lungs. Microembolization was noted in pulmonary vessels.

B. **Discussion**

1. The load of gram-negative bacteria and their products (including endotoxin) stimulated a massive release of vasoactive peptides, including bradykinins. These caused increased vascular permeability (as shown in his lungs), with resultant decreased blood volume and decreased cardiac output. The decreased perfusion of tissues increased local hypoxia and led to necrosis.

2. The endotoxin also stimulated at least two other events: (1) activation of Hageman factor, which probably contributed to the diffuse intravascular coagulopathy; and (2) activation of the complement cascade system, which under normal circumstances enhances inflammation, undoubtedly leading to intravascular coagulation through activation of plasma thromboplastin antecedent.

3. The low white blood count (WBC) can be explained on the basis of local sticking of WBC along venules and sequestration in tissues.

4. The normal pulmonary capillary wedge pressure indicates that the pulmonary edema was not of cardiac origin.

5. This case represents an exaggerated response of the normal inflammatory processes, which resulted in poor organ perfusion, blockage of oxygen transport from alveoli to capillaries, bleeding, and finally death.

Select the single best answer.

1. In the microvasculature, pavementing and emigration of neutrophilic leukocytes during inflammation occur basically along:
   a. Arterioles.
   b. Capillaries.
   c. Venules.
   d. Closed capillary channels.
   e. None of the above.

2. The principal perivascular phenomenon associated with acute inflammation is:
   a. Migration of eosinophils.
   b. Activation of Hageman factor.
   c. Increased size of fenestrae in capillaries.
   d. Accumulation of neutrophils.
   e. None of the above.

38 Hyperthermia and Fever

I. **Introduction.** The thermometer was the first instrument of precision in medical practice (Fahrenheit produced his mercury thermometer in 1714). Modern clinical thermometry began with the studies by Wunderlich, who recorded the temperature of all patients entering his clinic with a foot-long thermometer held in the axilla for 20 minutes. He published his findings in a monograph, "On the Temperature in Disease," in 1868. Since that time, knowledge of fever and elevated body temperature has played a central role in the study of human disease. An understanding of clinical medicine requires an understanding of how body temperature is regulated, situations in which it is disturbed, and the special situation called fever. Because there is often confusion about hyperthermia and fever, certain important definitions are listed in Table 38-1.

II. **Normal body temperature.** The definition of *normal body temperature* can be given only in terms of probabilities and ranges, much to the discomfiture of those who hold firmly to the idea that the "normal" body temperature is 37° C and not anything else. Actually, the distribution of mean temperature in a group of young, healthy adults follows the normal bell-shaped distribution and at rest varies from 36.5° to 37.5° C. The median temperature for this group is really 36.7°, not 37° C. The outside tolerable limits of body temperature are about 36° to 40.5° C. The temperature of different parts of the body varies, and body temperature also varies with time. A number of factors influence the normal body temperature, as shown in Table 38-2.

The highest body temperature is reached in striated muscle during repetitive contraction and may reach 42° C. The core body temperature averages about 37.5° C, and in resting conditions the highest temperature occurs in the liver. Nearly the same levels are present in aortic blood, the esophagus, and the tympanic membrane; oral temperatures are ordinarily about 0.4° C lower; skin temperature is about 1.0° C lower. The basal heat production of human adults averages about 1,650 calories per day. It results from a number of metabolic processes, such as digestion and the maintenance of transcellular ionic gradients. When these mechanisms produce insufficient body heat, other means are enlisted to supply it. The major mechanism for this is muscular activity, often manifested by shivering.

A. **Temperature homeostasis.** The maintenance of a more or less constant body temperature depends upon a balance between heat production and heat loss. Since virtually all heat loss occurs through surface phenomena between the body and the environment, it is easy to understand the importance of the integument in the conservation or dissipation of heat from the body core. By far the most important mechanism for this is regulation of blood flow through the skin: increased blood flow to dissipate heat and decreased blood flow to conserve body heat. Skin blood flow is regulated by neural mechanisms in which afferent nerves detecting either warmth or cold conduct impulses to the hypothalamus and efferents from the hypothalamus direct either skin vasoconstriction or vasodilatation.

Which technique the body utilizes for temperature homeostasis depends upon the ambient temperature. In ambient temperatures between 22.5° and 30.5° C, the normal person at rest regulates body

Table 38-1   *Definitions*

Hyperthermia	Elevated body temperature arising from a variety of causes. May be normal but often abnormal.
Fever	A special kind of hyperthermia produced by endogenous pyrogen.
Set point	A concept relating to the integrative function located in the hypothalamus that controls the balance between heat loss and heat gain, and directs the maintenance of constant body temperature. In fever, the set point remains intact but is turned up. In most hyperpyrexia, it remains unchanged. In heat stroke, it is deranged.
Heat illness	Disturbances of body function induced by failure of the body to adapt to a heat load. There are three types: heat cramps, heat exhaustion, and heat stroke.

Table 38-2   *Factors Influencing Normal Body Temperature*

Time of day or night
Age
Ingestion of food
Emotional state
Pregnancy
Menstrual cycle
Exercise
State of hydration
Thyroid status

Table 38-3   *Factors Governing Body Temperature Regulation*

Heat Gain	Heat Loss
Basal metabolic rate	Radiation
Cell membrane and ionic pump	Convection
Vasoconstriction in skin	Decreased ambient temperature
Striated muscle contraction	Vasodilatation in skin
Muscle tone increase	Hyperpnea
Exercise	Sweating
Shivering	
Increased ambient temperature	

AMP = adenosine monophosphate.

temperature by means of heat *loss*. This is accomplished by radiation (about 60%), convection (about 15%), and evaporation (about 15%). Other insensible losses, such as breathing, contribute in a minor way.

Above an ambient temperature of 30.5° C, more elaborate mechanisms come into play. The evaporative mechanism becomes paramount, accounting for up to 98 percent of heat loss, while the convective and radiant losses contribute proportionately less.

Thus, the major mechanism for producing body heat in cold conditions is muscular activity, and the greatest mechanism for dissipating heat in hot conditions is sweating. All the other mechanisms contribute considerably less than these (Table 38-3).

In addition to the *physiologic* mechanisms discussed above, a number of *behavioral* techniques are used by man to regulate body temperature. In fact, clothing is so important that an unclothed individual may die of exposure to cold at surprisingly mild temperatures. In addition, warm-blooded animals mimic poikilothermic animals by moving to locations where a more suitable ambient temperature may be found. The integration of behavior modifications used for temperature regulation is poorly understood.

B. **Integrative mechanisms.** We have seen that fairly complicated processes are at work to maintain the body core temperature within a rather narrow range. Integration of these processes depends upon a thermostat-like mechanism, which for want of a better term is currently called the set point. This set point is located in the anterior portion of the hypothalamus. Unmyelinated nerve receptors for warmth and cold located in various parts of the body, but especially in the skin and central nervous system, are linked to the hypothalamus as afferent conductors. In the hypothalamus, the various afferent impulses are integrated in such a way that efferent impulses then direct the appropriate change in physiologic or behavioral modifications. The steps in this process are largely unknown, but a number of mediators appear to be capable of changing the set point.

Direct stimulation of the hypothalamus of experimental animals by heat or by electrical current results in tachypnea, vasodilatation, and sweating. Norepinephrine injected into the hypothalamus causes a drop in body temperature; serotonin causes an elevation. Increases of these compounds have been detected in the hypothalamus of experimental animals after exposure to changes in ambient temperature. Prostaglandins of the E series cause alpha-adrenergic receptors to release cyclic adenosine monophosphate (AMP), which in turn alters the Ca^{2+}/Na^+ ratio. This alteration results in firing of efferent neurones in the anterior hypothalamus. The present consensus is that the prostaglandins play a major role in mediating events within the hypothalamus that are concerned with temperature regulation.

III. **Hyperthermia.** It is important to distinguish between hyperthermia, which represents simply an increase in body temperature, and fever, which is a special hyperthermal situation. Hyperthermia may result from changes within the body or by changes in the environment. Endogenous factors include exercise, dehydration, certain metabolic derangements, damage to the central nervous system, and response to medications such as certain anesthetics. Exogenous factors include increases in ambient temperatures such as occur in sauna baths or boiler rooms. With extreme hyperthermia (heat stroke) the integrative processes and effector organs fail, so that the individual may in fact become poikilothermic. Death may readily ensue if the patient's temperature is not reduced promptly.

IV. **Fever**

A. **Mechanisms.** In contrast with ordinary hyperthermia, *fever* results from a change in the set point or the thermoregulatory center in the hypothalamus, regardless of the ambient temperature. In the case of fever, there seems to be a top level beyond which it is uncommon for the temperature to rise. With hyperthermia, body temperature may rise considerably higher than is ordinarily seen with fever, and temperatures may reach lethal levels.

The mechanisms for gaining or dissipating heat remain the same with fever as with hyperthermia. In fever the thermoregulatory center is turned up to a higher point, so that a new balance is achieved between heat gain and loss. This alteration results from the action of endogenous pyrogen.

Endogenous pyrogen is formed by a variety of body cells, but especially the granulocytic leukocytes. It is released from leukocytes following ingestion of endotoxin, viruses, bacteria, or other foreign materials. There seems to be little evidence to support the idea that infectious agents and most other foreign material act directly on the thermoregulatory center. They seem to act only by stimulating the release of endogenous pyrogen from the above-mentioned cells. (Hence they are termed exogenous pyrogens.) When human leukocytes are exposed in vitro to various noxious agents, a heat-labile pyrogen is recovered from the supernate. Endogenous pyrogen does not seem to be stored preformed in leukocytes, but is rapidly manufactured by the leukocytes.

Other cells capable of producing endogenous pyrogen include eosinophils, monocytes, Kupffer cells, tissue macrophages, and certain tumor cells. However, not all phagocytic cells produce endogenous pyrogen, at least in vitro. Lymphocytes do not appear to be a source of endogenous pyrogen, but activated lymphocytes produce lymphokines, which stimulate endogenous pyrogen production by granulocytes.

Endogenous pyrogen derived from neutrophils is a polypeptide of 15,000 daltons. That derived from macrophages seems to be made up of two types of molecules, one of 15,000 daltons and one of approximately 40,000 daltons. Endogenous pyrogen is destroyed by heating for 30 minutes at 60° C and is inactivated by proteolytic enzymes. The larger molecule seems to be associated with a more prolonged temperature elevation. The site of action of endogenous pyrogen appears to be in the anterior hypothalamus. Injection of endogenous pyrogen into this area increases the firing rate of thermosensitive neurones, resulting in heat conservation. Whether the other mediators are stimulated directly by endogenous pyrogen as the only mechanism is not yet clear. It is likely that they have a secondary augmenting role in elevating body temperature. Antipyretics such as aspirin inhibit prostaglandin synthesis. Indeed, this may be the mechanism by which certain antipyretic agents act. Certain adrenal steroids, such as etiocholanalone, are pyrogenic and rarely cause persistent fever.

B. **Role of fever in disease.** There is a great deal of discussion about whether fever is beneficial or harmful to humans. A number of observations utilizing poikilothermic animals indicate that the occurrence of elevated body temperature is beneficial and results in improved survival in experimental infections. This effect, of course, may not be applicable to humans. There are a few pathogens that are directly injured by elevated temperatures. For example, both *Neisseria gonorrhoeae* and *Treponema pallidum* are killed by temperatures of 38° to 40° C. In fact, "fever" was widely employed for therapy of these conditions in the preantibiotic era (and occasionally resulted in heat stroke). During fever, the liver produces acute phase reactants, such as C-reactive protein and ceruloplasmin, which bind to carbohydrates in bacterial cell walls and are utilized in complement fixation. Hence, they may assist in phagocytosis. Serum iron and zinc decrease during fever, but except for the fact that bacteria require iron for multiplication, a beneficial effect has not been described.

There is a prevalent attitude, not founded on experimental observation, that patients with fever should be treated with antipyretics. In view of the fact that fever may be of some benefit, perhaps one should be less enthusiastic about lowering milder levels of fever. However, the discomfort that often accompanies fever may be relieved by mild analgesics, which are often also antipyretic.

Occasionally, fevers may persist for long periods of time. Often the cause cannot be determined. Most prolonged fevers are associated with infections, autoimmune diseases, or certain malignancies. When the cause cannot be found, the condition is termed fever of undetermined origin (FUO). This is an important clinical syndrome that requires special evaluation.

V. Disturbed function. Disturbances of function related to abnormalities of the heat-regulating system are called heat illnesses. There are one major and two minor heat illnesses. One minor type, termed heat cramps, results presumably from electrolyte disturbances during physical exercise in a hot environment. The mental status is clear, and body temperature is not ordinarily elevated. Heat exhaustion is also associated with dehydration and electrolyte imbalance. The patient may have dizziness, weakness, syncope, nausea, vomiting, or cramps and may exhibit confusion. Body temperature may be slightly elevated, but the patient will usually exhibit moist, pale skin. These conditions are rarely fatal and do not merit further consideration here.

The major dangerous heat illness is termed heat stroke. In this condition there is serious derangement of temperature regulation. It arises from a failure to adapt to an increase in environmental temperature or from failure to dissipate an endogenous heat load. The failure may occur over the course of several hours or days, depending upon a number of circumstances. Conditions that dispose to heat stroke include: obesity, poor physical condition, fasting, alcoholism, chronic skin conditions interfering with increased sweating, and congestive heart failure. External factors favoring the development of heat stroke include a prolonged heat wave, high humidity, improper clothing, and sauna baths. Several drugs interfere with sweating. These include all compounds with anticholinergic activity, such as benztropine, trihexyphenidyl, atropine, phenothiazines, and antihistamines. An acute febrile illness may predispose to heat illness if other factors are present, but fever, per se, rarely leads to heat stroke. General anesthesia occasionally results in severe hyperthermia, which can lead to heat stroke.

An important process in heat adaptation is an increase in aldosterone secretion, which decreases the amount of sodium lost in sweat and urine; nonetheless, significant depletion of extracellular fluid may occur. Also, proportionately more potassium is lost, and significant potassium depletion may result. Some consider loss of potassium to be the central defect in severe heat illness. Typically, cutaneous vasoconstriction occurs in an attempt to maintain perfusion of vital organs. This vasoconstriction adds to the elevated body core temperature. As the body core temperature rises to dangerous levels (about 41° C), other body functions begin to falter. For example, patients with heat illness are in a hypermetabolic state; hence, cardiac rate and output are increased. Rhabdomyolysis may occur and contribute to renal damage. In addition, hemoconcentration, elevated serum sodium, decreased serum potassium, and metabolic acidosis are likely. Pulmonary edema may occur, especially if intravenous fluids are given very rapidly. At about 42° C definite damage to cells may be seen. This includes denaturation of proteins, damage to mitochondria, and damage to membranes.

Delayed organ failure may occur in those who survive the initial hours of heat stroke. Renal failure, hepatic failure, or congestive failure may ensue. Disseminated intravascular coagulation is a rare complication. Heat stroke should be regarded as a complex metabolic derangement associated with extreme elevation of temperature.

VI. Clinical example of heat stroke

A. **Description.** The patient, a 21-year-old recruit from Ohio, arrived at an Air Force base in San Antonio, Texas, on August 23. He was taken to the emergency room at 6:30 A.M. on August 26 after fainting in the breakfast line. In the emergency room he was noted to be confused and was referred to the mental health clinic, where he spent most of the morning. At about noon a physician noted the patient to be shaking and to be hyperextending his neck. Because of this, he was returned to the emergency room, where his rectal temperature was found to be 108° F (42.2° C). At this time the patient was incoherent. He was immediately placed in an ice bath, with a femoral venipuncture to deliver intravenous fluids. After 9 minutes in the bath, rectal temperature had fallen to 101° F, so he was removed from the bath. After removal, his temperature continued to fall, reaching a level of 96.5° F (35.8° C).

He was then admitted to the intensive care unit, where his blood pressure varied from 60 to 90/0. Pulse was 120. He became comatose and developed cyanosis of arms and legs. The blood urea nitrogen, 40 mg/100 ml on admission, rose to 128 mg/100 ml in a few days, along with serum creatinine of 10.6 mg/100 ml. Hematocrit on admission was 52, and hemoglobin was 17 g/100 ml. Serum sodium was 158 mEq/L; potassium, 3.8 mEq/L; chloride, 119 mEq/L; and CO_2, 10 mEq/L. The serum potassium rose to 6.3 mEq/L. During the first few days in the hospital, the patient never excreted more than 100 ml of urine per day. He required careful dietary, fluid, and electrolyte management and frequent hemodialysis treatments but recovered without sequelae.

B. **Discussion**

1. Heat stroke occurred when this man traveled from a location of moderate temperature to a hot, humid environment and began vigorous physical training.

2. The symptoms of heat stroke are variable. The patient had a period of a few hours in which the only obvious abnormality was mental change. Only when his behavior became almost completely involuntary was his temperature taken and found to be dangerously high. It is easy to see how such a person could die without a diagnosis of heat stroke being made.

3. During and immediately after his cooling, he exhibited a certain degree of poikilothermia in which his temperature dropped to abnormally low levels. (He was wrapped in blankets for warmth!)

4. The elevations of serum sodium, chloride, hematocrit, and hemoglobin were manifestations of hemoconcentration, occurring as a result of depletion of sodium and water.

5. Acute renal failure occurred from the combined effects of renal hypoperfusion and myoglobinuria resulting from rhabdomyolysis. Only a previously healthy person receiving the best medical attention would be expected to survive such a catastrophic illness.

Questions

Select the single best answer.

1. In fever, the set point circuitry:
   a. Is unresponsive to stimuli.
   b. Is activated directly by endotoxin.
   c. Is damaged and therefore unresponsive to stimuli.
   d. Remains intact but behaves in such a way that body temperature is raised.
   e. Causes a decreased secretion of sodium in sweat.
2. Which one of the following is true?
   a. Only fever associated with exogenous pyrogens may be called hyperthermia.
   b. All hyperthermia is fever.
   c. Fever is a special kind of hyperthermia that arises from release of endogenous pyrogens.
   d. Hyperthermia is a special aspect of fever in which endogenous pyrogen acts upon bacteria to produce exogenous pyrogen.
   e. None of the above is true.

VIII Nephrology

Anthony W. Czerwinski
Arnold J. Felsenfeld
Christian E. Kaufman, Jr.
Henry F. Krous
Francisco Llach
James A. Pederson
Laura I. Rankin

39 Disorders of Sodium and Water Metabolism

I. **Volume and composition of the body fluid compartments.** As shown in Figure 39-1, total body water averages about 60 percent of body weight. Of this total, approximately two-thirds is confined to the intracellular space and one-third constitutes the extracellular space. The extracellular space consists of the interstitial compartment and the plasma. Although total body water may vary, according to the fat content of the body, from as low as 50 percent to as high as 70 percent of body weight, the percentages shown in Figure 39-1 are adequate approximations for clinical purposes. The composition of the extracellular fluid includes sodium as the major cation and chloride and bicarbonate as the major anions. Consequently, the concentration of sodium correlates closely with the osmolality of the extracellular fluid. The compositions of the plasma and of the interstitial fluid are virtually identical with the exception of the higher protein content of the plasma. In the intracellular space, potassium and magnesium are the major cations, phosphate and proteins the major anions. In this compartment, the osmolality will parallel the concentration of the potassium and magnesium. Since almost all cell membranes are freely permeable to water, the osmolality is identical (about 285 mOsm/kg) in the extracellular and the intracellular compartments.

II. **Fluid compartment volume and osmolar changes that occur with the loss or gain of sodium or water from the body.** An understanding of disorders of sodium and water metabolism depends on a clear concept of how the volume and osmolality of body fluid compartments change in response to loss or gain of sodium and water from the body (Fig. 39-2).

The addition of solute-free water to the extracellular space (Fig. 39-2A) lowers the osmolality and increases the volume of this compartment. Water then moves along an osmotic gradient into cells until the osmolality is equal in both compartments. Thus, a new equilibrium is established whereby osmolality is decreased and volume is increased in both compartments. The magnitude of these changes is proportional to the increase in total body water. Similarly, loss of solute-free water results in opposite changes (decreased volume, increased osmolality) in both compartments.

The addition of a hypertonic sodium solution to the extracellular compartment (Fig. 39-2B) increases the osmolality of the extracellular fluid. Since sodium is confined to the extracellular space, water moves along the osmotic gradient out of the cells. Thus, extracellular volume increases while intracellular volume decreases; both changes are proportional to the increase in osmolality of the body fluids. When an isotonic sodium solution is added to the extracellular space (Fig. 39-2C), no osmotic gradient is generated between the extracellular and the intracellular fluid. Therefore, the increase in extracellular fluid volume is equal to the administered volume of isotonic saline. Likewise, loss of isosmotic fluid from the extracellular space does not change volume or composition of the intracellular fluid compartment.

Loss of sodium without the net loss of water results in the changes depicted in Figure 39-2D. Since sodium cannot be lost from the body without a concomitant loss of water, the changes in Figure 39-2D generally result from the replacement of sodium-rich fluid losses with solute-

Figure 39-1

Approximate volume of body fluid compartments.

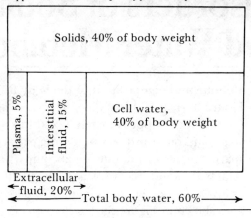

Figure 39-2   *Changes in volume and osmolal concentration of intracellular (I) and extracellular (E) fluids. A = addition of water to the body; B = addition of hypertonic salt solution; C = addition of isotonic salt solution; and D = loss of sodium chloride. Compartments enclosed by solid lines represent initial normal state; those enclosed by dashed lines represent the final experimental state. Height of compartment represents osmolal concentration; width represents volume. (From D. C. Darrow and H. Yannet, Changes in volume and osmolal concentration of intra- and extracellular fluid. J. Clin. Invest. 14:266, 1935. Reproduced by permission of the publisher, Rockefeller University Press.)*

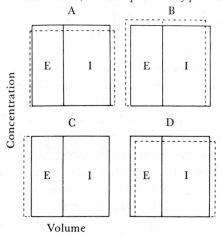

free water. Figure 39-2D can be envisioned as the result of loss of isotonic saline (reverse of Fig. 39-2C) and the subsequent addition of an equal quantity of solute-free water (Fig. 39-2A). At equilibrium the osmolality is decreased throughout body fluids, and the intracellular volume is increased to the same extent that extracellular volume is decreased. In effect, water moves from extracellular to intracellular compartments because of a net loss of extracellular solute.

III. **Normal regulation of sodium balance.** The principal factor determining the extracellular fluid volume is the amount of sodium present in the body. Normally the extracellular fluid volume is closely regulated by the kidneys, and any tendency toward expansion of the extracellular space results in excretion of the excess sodium. In the same way, loss of sodium and contraction of the extracellular space promptly cause excretion of sodium-free urine. Since sodium is confined to the extracellular space, loss or gain of sodium will be reflected by contraction or expansion of the extracellular compartment. This occurs because the change in sodium balance induces a secondary passive movement of water across cell mem-

Figure 39-3

Influence of sodium content on the volume of the body fluid compartments.

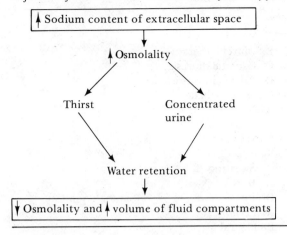

Table 39-1

Mechanisms Controlling Renal Sodium Excretion

I. Glomerular filtration rate
II. Aldosterone
III. Third factor
    A. Composition of blood
    B. Renal hemodynamics
       1. Perfusion pressure
       2. Venous pressure
       3. Renal vascular resistance
       4. Intrarenal distribution of blood flow and glomerular filtration rate
    C. Autonomic nervous system
    D. Natriuretic hormone(s)

branes (Fig. 39-2B, D) and because of changes in total body water. As illustrated in Figure 39-3, an increased amount of sodium in the extracellular space will result in positive water balance (increased total body water). This is because the increased osmolality that occurs stimulates both thirst and the secretion of antidiuretic hormone (ADH), resulting in greater water intake and less water loss. Hence, the sodium content determines the volume of the extracellular compartment, which in turn is the major factor influencing renal sodium excretion. The mechanisms by which changes in extracellular fluid volume control renal sodium excretion are listed in Table 39-1. Alterations of these mechanisms are undoubtedly important in the pathogenesis of the abnormal sodium retention that occurs in a variety of disease states.

IV. **Disorders of extracellular fluid volume**

    A. **Sodium depletion (contraction of extracellular volume).** The terms *sodium depletion* and *contraction of extracellular fluid volume* are virtually synonymous. They refer to a deficit of sodium and not to a decrease in the concentration of sodium (hyponatremia) in the extracellular fluid. A sodium deficit may or may not be associated with hyponatremia (see section VI below, Disorders of water metabolism).

        1. **Pathogenesis.** Sodium depletion results from abnormal loss of sodium-containing fluids. The potential mechanisms are listed in Table 39-2. The normal renal response to even mild sodium depletion is avid reabsorption of virtually all the filtered sodium (mechanisms listed in Table 39-1). Since normal fecal and sweat

Table 39-2   *Causes of Sodium Loss*

I. Urinary
  A. Renal disease
  B. Diuretic therapy
  C. Osmotic diuresis
  D. Adrenal insufficiency
II. Gastrointestinal
  A. Vomiting
  B. Diarrhea
  C. Drainage
III. Skin
  A. Sweating
  B. Burns
IV. Drainage
  A. Peritoneal
  B. Pleural

Table 39-3   *Effects of Sodium Depletion (Decreased Extracellular Volume)*

I. ↓ Plasma volume
  A. Renal
    "Prerenal azotemia"
    ↓ Urine Na^+, volume
    ↑ Urine osmolality
    ↓ Diluting capacity (hyponatremia)
  B. Cardiovascular
    ↓ BP, ↑ pulse
    ↓ Pulse pressure
    Orthostatic hypotension
  C. CNS—↓ cerebral function
  D. Liver, muscle—lactic acidosis
II. ↓ Interstitial volume
  Poor skin turgor
III. Hemoconcentration
  ↑ Hgb, Hct
  ↑ Plasma proteins

BP = blood pressure; CNS = central nervous system; Hb = hemoglobin; Hct = hemocrit; ↓ = decreased; ↑ = increased.

losses of sodium are minimal, inadequate sodium intake alone cannot result in significant sodium depletion.

2. **Effects of sodium depletion.** Contraction of the extracellular space results in proportional changes in the plasma and interstitial volume. The subsequent decrement in blood volume by reduction of cardiac output impairs tissue perfusion. The clinical and laboratory manifestations of sodium depletion (contraction of extracellular fluid volume) can therefore be attributed to the effects of hemoconcentration and, most importantly, a reduced plasma and interstitial volume (Table 39-3). A common result is prerenal azotemia (an elevation of blood urea nitrogen [BUN] that is not secondary to renal disease). Prerenal azotemia may result from any event (including sodium depletion) that reduces renal blood flow. Renal hypoperfusion may impair the glomerular filtration rate and thereby elevate the serum creatinine concentration as well as the BUN. Typically, however, a disproportionate increase in BUN occurs as a result of the greatly enhanced tubular reabsorption of

Figure 39-4

The effects of sodium depletion on the renal capacity to excrete a dilute urine. ADH = antidiuretic hormone.

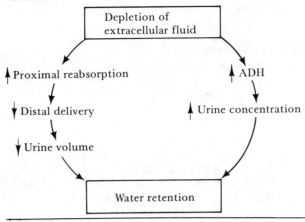

sodium, water, and urea that occurs whenever renal perfusion is impaired. Since ADH is also released under these circumstances, the renal response to depletion of extracellular fluid volume (or any state of hypoperfusion) is the excretion of a scanty, concentrated urine virtually free of sodium (Fig. 39-4).

As described above, sodium depletion results in enhanced renal sodium reabsorption and a reduced renal capacity to excrete a dilute urine, as outlined in Figure 39-4. Continued water intake in the wake of impaired excretion may result in dilution of body fluids and the development of hyponatremia (Fig. 39-2D). However, since sodium depletion generally results from loss of hypotonic sodium-rich fluids, hyponatremia is not a necessary feature of sodium depletion; if water losses exceed sodium losses, the concentration of plasma sodium will tend to rise. Therefore, salt depletion is commonly accompanied by a normal or high serum-sodium concentration, and the serum-sodium concentration is of little value in deciding whether a patient is sodium depleted (see section VI below, Water metabolism).

B. Sodium excess (expansion of extracellular space). Any tendency for expansion of the extracellular space normally results in excretion of the excess sodium through the renal control mechanisms listed in Table 39-1. Failure of these mechanisms, which may result from conditions listed in Table 39-4, causes an overt increase in extracellular fluid volume. This is recognized by the presence of edema, the clinical hallmark of an expanded extracellular space.

Edema represents an increase in the interstitial fluid volume. Since the interstitial space composes three-fourths of the total extracellular space, the latter is also increased when edema is clinically evident. Edema results from an imbalance of the capillary Starling forces shown in Figure 39-5. In renal or cardiac failure, edema results primarily from an increase in hydrostatic pressure. It may also result from a reduced plasma oncotic pressure, from nephrotic syndrome, or as in cirrhosis, from the combined effects of increased hydrostatic and decreased oncotic pressure. Occasionally, edema results from a damaged capillary endothelium, which leaks plasma proteins into the interstitial space (some examples of lung edema). Impairment of lymphatic drainage can also cause edema.

Table 39-4

Causes of an Expanded Extracellular Space

I. Impaired sodium excretion
   A. Heart failure
   B. Hepatic cirrhosis
   C. Renal failure
   D. Nephrotic syndrome
II. Excessive sodium intake
   A. Iatrogenic (intravenous saline)
   B. Accidental salt poisoning

Figure 39-5

Capillary Starling forces that influence fluid distribution between plasma and interstitial compartments. (From R. W. Schrier, Renal and Electrolyte Disorders (2nd ed.). Boston: Little, Brown, 1980, p. 81. Reproduced with permission of R. W. Schrier and the publisher.)

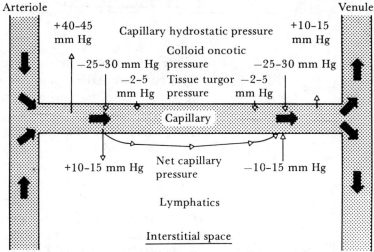

V. Normal regulation of water balance. Water moves freely across cell membranes, quickly abolishing any potential osmotic gradients between the intracellular and the extracellular compartments. In health, the tonicity of body fluids is closely regulated to maintain a concentration of total solute of 280 to 290 mOsm per kilogram by adjustments in water intake (thirst) and water excretion (urinary). Whereas sodium balance regulates the volume of the extracellular compartment, water balance is adjusted according to the osmolality of body fluids. The renal capacity to adjust body fluid tonicity is quite remarkable, in that normal kidneys can produce as little as 400 cc of concentrated urine or excrete as much as 20 liters of solute-free water each day as needed to regulate water balance.

   A. Renal concentrating mechanisms. Hypothalamic neurons secrete ADH in response to elevation of body fluid osmolality or depletion of blood volume. As a result of the action of ADH, the permeability to water of the distal convoluted tubule and the collecting duct is markedly enhanced. This system provides the mechanism for water to diffuse into the hypertonic medullary interstitium as fluid traverses the distal convoluted tubule and collecting duct. Hence, the presence of sufficient ADH permits normal kidneys to conserve water by excreting the daily solute load in as little as 400 ml of highly concentrated (up to 1,200 mOsm/kg) urine.

   B. Renal diluting mechanisms. By contrast, in the absence of ADH, a normal consequence of hypotonic body fluids, the distal tubule and collecting duct are rendered impermeable to water (Fig. 39-6). There-

Figure 39-6

Renal diluting mechanisms. The sites of sodium chloride and water reabsorption in the absence of antidiuretic hormone (ADH) are indicated in this composite nephron. With a glomerular filtration of 144 L/day, approximately 45 L of filtrate would remain at the end of the proximal tubule and 28 L would remain at the tip of Henle's loop. In the absence of ADH, little water is reabsorbed beyond this point, and up to 20 L of solute-free water can be excreted in the urine.

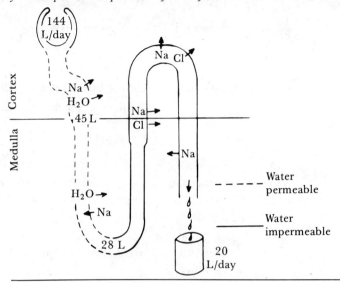

fore, water reaching the tip of Henle's loop does not back-diffuse into the medullary interstitium and is virtually all excreted in the urine. Hence, water excretion can be adjusted to match intake by changes in ADH secretion. If necessary, up to 20 liters of solute-free water can be excreted each day to maintain water balance.

VI. Disorders of water metabolism. Since water balance is normally adjusted to maintain a constant osmolality of body fluids, disorders of water metabolism are defined with reference to the osmolality. Therefore, two potential disorders exist: too much water in relation to solute (hypoosmolality) and too little water in relation to solute (hyperosmolality).

    A. Hyperosmolality (hypernatremia). Since sodium is the predominant cation in the extracellular fluid, any significant increase in sodium concentration indicates hyperosmolality of the body fluids. Osmolality may also be increased secondary to a high concentration of other solutes (i.e., glucose, mannitol) that are confined to the extracellular space. Under these circumstances the serum-sodium concentration is not necessarily increased and the hyperosmolar state must be confirmed by measurement of plasma osmolality. Although hypernatremia is occasionally associated with an increased sodium content of the extracellular space, most commonly the sodium content is normal or low and there is an even greater water deficit. Because intracellular solute content remains relatively constant, hyperosmolality causes cells to shrink (Fig. 39-2B). Therefore, the hyperosmolar state is almost always associated with both a relative and an absolute water deficit throughout the body fluid compartments.

    By assuming that any increase in sodium concentration (or osmolality) is proportional to changes in total body water (TBW), we can estimate the magnitude of the water deficit from the formula:

$$H_2O \text{ deficit} = BW(0.6)\left(1 - \frac{140}{Na_{obs}}\right).$$

The derivation of this formula, where

Normal serum sodium concentration = 140 mEq/L
Na_{obs} = serum sodium concentration observed
BW = body weight
TBW = 0.6 (BW)

$$\text{Present TBW} = \text{Normal TBW} \left(\frac{140}{Na_{obs}} \right)$$

is as follows:

$$
\begin{aligned}
\text{H}_2\text{O deficit} &= \text{Normal TBW} - \text{Present TBW} \\
&= \text{BW} (0.6) - \text{BW} (0.6) \left(\frac{140}{Na_{obs}} \right) \\
&= \text{BW} (0.6) \left(1 - \frac{140}{Na_{obs}} \right)
\end{aligned}
$$

If the patient's usual weight is accurately known, a comparison with current body weight will allow another means of estimating the water deficit.

EXAMPLE: Calculate the water deficit of a man whose usual weight is unknown. Current body weight = 70 kg, and serum Na = 170 mEq/L. Thus:

$$
\begin{aligned}
\text{H}_2\text{O deficit} &= 0.6 \, (70) \left(1 - \frac{140}{Na_{obs}} \right) \\
&= 42 - 34.6 \\
&= 7.4 \text{ L}
\end{aligned}
$$

It is apparent that since water is lost from the intracellular and extracellular spaces the magnitude of the deficits may be substantial.

1. **Pathogenesis of hypernatremia.** The mechanisms by which hypernatremia may occur are listed in Table 39-5. A water deficit may potentially develop from inadequate water intake or excessive water loss. Since a normal, alert adult will adjust water intake to match losses, hypernatremia (hyperosmolality) usually implies an impairment of water intake. In most patients with hypernatremia, both inadequate water intake and excessive loss are present. Hypernatremia can also result from the addition of a hypertonic sodium solution to the extracellular fluid. However, the hyperosmolar state will not be sustained unless water intake is also impaired.

2. **Effects of hypernatremia.** Since water is lost proportionally from all compartments and the blood volume normally constitutes one-twelfth of total body water, a pure water deficit will have little tendency to produce hypovolemia. For example, in a 70-kg man with a pure water deficit causing serum Na of 170 mEq/L, the blood volume would be reduced by 600 cc. Calculation:

$$
\begin{aligned}
\text{Total H}_2\text{O deficit} &= 7.4 \text{ L (see above)} \\
\text{Blood volume} &= \frac{1}{12} \, (7.4) \\
&= 600 \text{ cc}
\end{aligned}
$$

A reduction of the blood volume by 600 cc often will not be detected on clinical evaluation. Hence, with a pure water deficit the features of a reduced blood volume listed in Table 39-3 are not prominent and, if present, suggest coexisting sodium depletion.

Table 39-5   *Mechanisms of Hyperosmolality (Hypernatremia)*

   I. Inadequate water intake
     A. Impaired consciousness
     B. Impaired thirst (rare)
     C. Weakness, physical restraints
  II. Excessive (solute-free) water loss
     A. Renal losses (concentrating defect)
     B. Extrarenal—i.e., sweat, gastrointestinal, respiratory
 III. Addition of hypertonic sodium solution to the extracellular fluid
     A. Hypertonic NaCl, or $NaHCO_3$
     B. Massive sodium ingestion

Figure 39-7

The brain in hypertonic states. In the top section the dashed line separates the brain (exaggerated in its relative size) from the rest of the ICF. Early in hypertonic states, the brain shares proportionally the water loss incurred by the rest of ICF. Later (middle section), appearance of idiogenic osmoles (solid square) causes the brain to expand toward its normal volume. Correction of hypertonicity by rapid replacement of water deficit (bottom section) results in brain swelling due to the extra solute. (From P. U. Feig, The hypertonic state. N. Engl. J. Med. 297:1445, 1977. Reprinted by permission of the New England Journal of Medicine and P. U. Feig.)

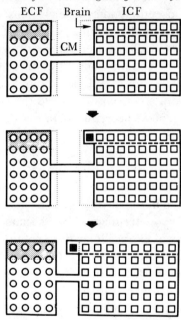

The major effects of water depletion are due to the effects of hypertonicity on brain function. Acute hypernatremia, whether due to addition of hypertonic saline or loss of water, results in cell shrinkage throughout the body (Fig. 39-2B). In the brain, a change in cell size and tonicity is particularly disruptive. Not surprisingly, acute hypernatremia is often associated with encephalopathy. In chronic states of hypernatremia the brain can protect cell volume by generating new intracellular solute called idiogenic osmoles (Fig. 39-7). In experimental hypernatremia, this mechanism allows return of brain volume to normal in about 7 days. The development of idiogenic osmoles, although protective of cell volume during hypernatremia, may result in cell swelling when osmolality is rapidly returned toward normal (Fig. 39-7). This may explain the neurologic deterioration that sometimes occurs during rapid correction of hypernatremia. These considerations suggest that in se-

Table 39-6   *Causes of Impaired Water Excretion*

Sodium depletion (contracted extracellular space)

Drugs

Endocrine disorders (deficiency of aldosterone, cortisol, or thyroxine)

Congestive heart failure

Hepatic cirrhosis

Renal failure

Emotional and physical stress

Positive pressure ventilation

Syndrome of inappropriate ADH secretion

ADH = antidiuretic hormone.

vere, chronic hypernatremia, water replacement should be gradual, with correction in 48 to 72 hours.

B. Hypoosmolality (hyponatremia). Since sodium is the major cation in the extracellular fluid, hypoosmolality is invariably accompanied by hyponatremia. Although the osmolality of body fluids is usually reflected by the serum-sodium concentration, one should be aware of so-called pseudohypoosmolality. This results when glucose, or any substance of small molecular weight, is present in a high concentration in the extracellular space; water is drawn from the intracellular space, lowering the sodium concentration of the extracellular fluid. In this circumstance there will be a significant discrepancy between the serum-sodium concentration and the serum osmolality.

1. Pathogenesis of hypoosmolality (hyponatremia). Hypoosmolality indicates excess water relative to the solute content of the fluid compartments. Since the intracellular solute content remains relatively constant, hyponatremia causes generalized cell swelling. However, the volume of the extracellular space is subject to marked variation in the disease states associated with hyponatremia. Therefore, hyponatremia may be associated with an increased, decreased, or normal extracellular fluid volume and sodium content.

As described earlier, hypoosmolality should inhibit ADH and induce renal excretion of the excess water (Fig. 39-6). Therefore, the occurrence of hyponatremia implies impairment of the normal mechanisms for eliminating water. In fact, hyponatremia must result whenever the intake of solute-free water exceeds the renal capacity to eliminate it. The disease states associated with impairment of water excretion are listed in Table 39-6.

A useful clinical approach is to classify causes of hyponatremia according to the clinical state of extracellular volume. All of the causes of sodium depletion and volume expansion discussed in section IV (Disorders of extracellular fluid volume) may be associated with hyponatremia. Hyponatremia may also be associated with an approximately normal extracellular fluid volume (Table 39-7). In this circumstance the total body sodium content is also approximately normal. Therapy follows logically: sodium depletion requires repletion. Otherwise, restriction of water intake and treatment of the underlying cause are the basic elements of management.

2. Effects of hypoosmolality (hyponatremia). The effects of hyponatremia are due to the resultant increase in brain water. There is

Hypothyroidism
Drugs
Positive pressure ventilation
Pain, emotional stress
Syndrome of inappropriate ADH secretion

ADH = antidiuretic hormone.

Table 39-8   *Effects of Hyponatremia*

Nausea and vomiting
Confusion
Lethargy
Stupor
Coma
Seizures

evidence that acute hyponatremia, developing in hours, produces more severe brain swelling than does chronic hyponatremia. Presumably, this is due to an adaptive loss of solute from brain cells chronically exposed to a low osmolality.

The major clinical features of hyponatremia are listed in Table 39-8. Most, if not all, can be attributed to the increased brain water. Permanent brain damage may result.

VII. Clinical example of disorders of sodium and water metabolism

    A. Hypernatremia

        1. Description. An 84-year-old woman was brought to the hospital from a nursing home because she was lethargic and refused to drink fluids. On admission, her blood pressure was 100/60, the pulse was 110 per minute, and skin turgor was poor. Laboratory work revealed a BUN of 100 mg/dl, sodium of 170 mEq/L, potassium of 4.0 mEq/L, Cl of 105 mEq/L, and CO_2 of 24 mEq/L. Serum creatinine was 2.5 mg/dl. Urinalysis showed a specific gravity of 1.030; no protein, glucose, or acetone was present. Urine sodium was 5 mEq/L and urine osmolality 726 mOsm/kg. She weighed 60 kg.

        2. Discussion. The following conclusions can be justified from these data:

        a. There was severe hyperosmolality of body fluids.

        b. Inadequate water intake, not excessive water loss, was the primary reason for the negative water balance this patient experienced.

        c. The water deficit was approximately 6.4 liters. Calculations:

$$\text{Water deficit} = 0.6 \,(\text{BW}) \left(1 - \frac{140}{\text{Na}_{obs}}\right)$$
$$= 36 - 36\left(\frac{140}{170}\right)$$
$$= 36 - 29.6$$
$$= 6.4 \text{ L}$$

Of this deficit, approximately one-third, or 2 liters, was lost from the extracellular space and two-thirds (4 L) from cell water.

   d. Since there was no evidence of expansion of extracellular fluid volume and no evidence of sodium loss, the sodium content of the extracellular space was probably close to normal. Furthermore, since about 2 liters of water was lost from the extracellular fluid (see above), significant sodium depletion was unlikely since a further contraction of extracellular fluid volume would have induced circulatory collapse (shock).

B. **Sodium depletion and hyponatremia**

1. **Description.** A 42-year-old woman with chronic renal disease was seen on return to the nephrology clinic. She complained of nausea and vomiting for the previous week. She appeared chronically and acutely ill. Blood pressure was 118/90 supine, 90/60 standing; weight was 64 kg. The neck veins were flat; there was no edema. The remainder of the physical exam was unremarkable. Review of the record revealed that 3 weeks previously she had been feeling good. Blood pressure then was 138/86 supine, 134/88 standing. She weighed 63 kg on that visit.

   Blood chemistries were:

	3 weeks ago	This visit
Na^+ (mEq/L)	139	122
K^+ (mEq/L)	5.5	3.9
HCO_3^- (mEq/L)	20	15
Cl^- (mEq/L)	105	94
BUN (mg/dl)	29	56
Glucose (mg/dl)	104	111
Hemoglobin (g/dl)	10.4	11.1

2. **Discussion**

   a. The history of vomiting coupled with the reduction in blood pressure, orthostatic hypotension, and worsening azotemia indicated depletion of extracellular fluid volume.

   b. The presence of hypoosmolality indicated that continued water intake coupled with impairment of water excretion from depletion of extracellular fluid volume resulted in dilution of body fluids (Fig. 39-4).

   c. The increase in weight indicated that the decrease in extracellular volume must have been associated with a greater increase in intracellular fluid volume, so that there was a net increase in total body water. Figure 39-2D schematizes this situation.

Questions

Select the single best answer.

1. Sodium depletion is virtually always associated with:
   a. Hyponatremia.
   b. Contraction of the intracellular space.
   c. Contraction of the extracellular space.

d. Expansion of the extracellular space.
e. None of the above.

2. What would be the effect of intravenous infusion of 1 liter of isotonic saline in an anuric patient?
   a. Expansion of the interstitial space by about 1 liter.
   b. Expansion of the intracellular space by about 670 cc.
   c. Expansion of the blood volume by about 670 cc.
   d. Essentially no effect on the size of the intracellular space.
   e. None of the above.

40 Potassium Homeostasis

I. **Background: normal physiology**

   A. **Potassium content and distribution.** Potassium is the most abundant cation in the human body. In young adult males the total body potassium is approximately 50 mEq per kilogram of body weight. However, the amount of potassium relative to body weight decreases with age because of decreasing muscle mass and increasing amounts of adipose tissue. In normal persons, more than 98 percent of the body potassium is located intracellularly. If we assume an extracellular fluid volume of 14 liters and an extracellular potassium concentration of 3.5 to 5 mEq per liter, the quantity of potassium in the extracellular space in a 70-kg man would be 49 to 70 mEq. The remainder of the potassium (about 3,500 mEq), is intracellular in location.

   B. **Role of potassium in the body.** The intracellular-to-extracellular potassium concentration ratio is of major importance in the maintenance of the resting cell membrane potential. Changes in this potential alter the capacity of the individual cell to polarize or depolarize. The majority of symptoms that occur in association with acute changes in serum potassium concentration are related to changes in the cell membrane potential. A second major function of potassium is the maintenance of the intracellular osmolality. Potassium and its attendant anions are the major contributors to intracellular osmolality. Because the intracellular and extracellular compartments are in osmotic equilibrium, an increase in intracellular potassium concentration will result in the flow of water into the cell and an increase in cell volume; the converse occurs with a decrease in intracellular potassium. In addition to these functions, potassium is an important cofactor in the regulation of certain enzymes.

   C. **Potassium balance.** Potassium homeostasis involves an external balance related to total potassium intake and excretion and an internal balance related to the intracellular-extracellular distribution.

      1. **External balance.** The average American adult ingests 100 mEq of potassium daily, the bulk of which is excreted by the kidney (90 percent), while a small amount, approximately 10 percent, is excreted in the stool. In patients with chronic renal failure, this relation changes because of a decrease in the ability of the kidney to excrete potassium; in these patients the bowel may become an important route of potassium excretion.

        a. **Renal potassium handling.** The kidneys maintain the external potassium balance through the process of glomerular filtration, tubular reabsorption, and tubular secretion. The proximal tubule reabsorbs 50 to 60 percent of the filtered potassium, another 30 to 40 percent is then reabsorbed in the ascending limb, and the remainder is reabsorbed in the distal tubule and collecting duct. Tubular secretion occurs in the distal convoluted tubule down an electrochemical gradient from the cell into the nephron lumen. Normally, potassium excretion is determined by the rate of tubular potassium secretion, and little of the filtered potassium appears in the urine.

        b. **Factors governing renal potassium secretion.** There are three major factors controlling renal potassium secretion. The first is the intracellular potassium content. An increase in the intracellular potassium concentration (by whatever means) is associated with an increase in potassium secretion. Conversely, a decrease in intracellular potassium content is associated with a decrease in renal tubular potassium secretion. One of the mechanisms of aldosterone's action is through its influence on the intracellular potassium concentration; this occurs because aldosterone causes an increased influx of potassium into the cell from the basolateral portions of the cell membrane. A second factor regulating potassium secretion is the urinary flow rate; in general, the greater the urinary flow rate, the greater the amount of potassium secreted. A final factor is the negative charge within the tubular lumen fluid. For example, the greater the distal tubular reabsorption of sodium and the more anions that remain in the urine, greater the amount of potassium secreted. Thus, a second mechanism by which the aldosterone can influence distal tubular potassium excretion is through its ability to increase sodium reabsorption in the distal tubule and thus to increase the intraluminal negativity.

2. **Internal balance.** An understanding of those factors controlling intracellular and extracellular potassium distribution is incomplete. The factors involved include alterations in acid-base homeostasis, changes in body fluid osmolality, and the modulating effects of certain hormones.

   a. In general, an increase in the extracellular fluid hydrogen ion concentration and a decrease in bicarbonate concentration will increase the plasma potassium concentration. Conversely, a decrease in hydrogen ion concentration or an increase in bicarbonate concentration will decrease the plasma potassium concentration. The magnitude of the change in potassium concentration depends on the type of acid or alkali and whether the primary disorder is of metabolic or respiratory origin. While these changes are often seen with acute acid-base disturbances, chronic acid-base disturbances are more complex and involve changes in external balance as well as potassium redistribution.

   b. The hormones primarily involved with potassium distribution include insulin and the catecholamines. Thus, an increase in serum potassium enhances the release of insulin, and an increase in insulin concentration increases the influx of potassium into the cell. Conversely, potassium depletion and hypokalemia decrease insulin release, and this will result in less potassium being transferred into cells. The effect of the catecholamines depends on whether they are predominantly alpha- or beta-adrenergic agonists. Alpha-adrenergic agonists cause an increase in serum potassium by increasing the release of potassium from the liver. Beta-adrenergic agonists cause a decrease in serum potassium by stimulating potassium influx into liver and muscle cells.

II. **Hypokalemia.** Hypokalemia is operationally defined as a serum potassium less than 3.5 mEq per liter. Hypokalemia can occur with a reduction in intracellular potassium (potassium depletion) or with a normal intracellular potassium, i.e., potassium redistribution. The signs and symptoms of hypokalemia are in general related to the magnitude of the deficit and rapidity with which hypokalemia develops. Table 40-1 presents an esti-

Table 40-1

Serum Potassium Concentration (mEq/L)	Adult Deficit (mEq)
3.0	100
2.5	300
2.0	500
1.5	700
1.0	1,000

Approximate Size of Potassium Deficit

Table 40-2   *Causes of Hypokalemia*

Potassium redistribution
  Acute respiratory or metabolic alkalosis
  Familial hypokalemic periodic paralysis
  Hyperalimentation
Potassium depletion
  Impaired potassium intake
  Increased gastrointestinal losses
    Protracted vomiting
    Diarrhea
    Laxative abuse
    Villous adenoma
  Increased urinary loss
    Primary or secondary hyperaldosteronism
    Excessive glucocorticoids
    Licorice abuse
    Diuretic therapy
    Renal tubular acidosis
    Magnesium depletion
    Congenital or acquired renal tubular defect
    Bartter's syndrome
Potassium depletion without hypokalemia
  Metabolic acidosis
  Uremia

mate of total body potassium deficits as related to the degree of hypokalemia.

  A. **Mechanisms of hypokalemia.** Table 40-2 lists some of the causes of hypokalemia. The first major category is related to potassium redistribution from the extracellular to the intracellular space. Thus, with respiratory or metabolic alkalosis, hypokalemia is a common finding. Acute alkalosis may not be associated with any change in total body potassium; however, with chronic metabolic alkalosis, severe potassium depletion can develop because of increased renal excretion. Familial hypokalemic periodic paralysis is a rare disease manifested by episodes of paralysis and hypokalemia without any change in total potassium content. Hyperalimentation, especially with high-glucose solutions, causes transcellular potassium shifts because of an increase in insulin secretion. While this occurs in all patients, it is much more likely to be associated with hypokalemia in a person who is concurrently potassium depleted. Potassium depletion can also be associated with a decrease in potassium intake, e.g., alcoholism or anorexia nervosa. Much more commonly, potassium depletion and hypokalemia occur because of the excessive loss of potassium either through the gastrointestinal tract or through the kidneys. Potassium depletion may occur without hypokalemia. Thus, in diabetic ketoacidosis, an increase in urinary potassium excretion results in cellular potassium depletion with a normal or elevated serum potassium. This becomes potentially very important during treatment of ketoacidosis, when insulin causes the movement of potassium back into the cells and a rapid decrease in serum potassium. Likewise, in chronic uremia, potassium depletion can be associated with either a normal or an elevated serum potassium.

B. Consequences of hypokalemia. There are multiple consequences of hypokalemia, but the principal ones involve the neuromuscular system, the cardiovascular system, and the kidney.

1. **The neuromuscular effects** are related to an increase in the intracellular-to-extracellular potassium ratio, and associated with this there is an increase in the resting membrane potential and a decrease in neuromuscular excitability. In skeletal muscle this is associated with weakness and occasionally with complete paralysis. In the gastrointestinal tract an adynamic ileus may result. With severe potassium depletion muscles can undergo degenerative changes with alterations in the mitochondria, transverse tubules, and sarcoplasmic reticulum. These changes can be associated with rhabdomyolysis and the replacement of muscle with fibrous tissue.

2. **The cardiovascular effects** are also related to the change in resting membrane potential. The electrocardiogram reflects these changes with a decrease in the T-wave amplitude, an increase in the U-wave amplitude, and an increased incidence of arrhythmias, which include atrial tachycardia, ventricular premature contractions, ventricular tachycardia, and ventricular fibrillation. Severe potassium depletion and hypokalemia can result in myocardial cell necrosis and fibrosis and in peripheral vasoconstriction with ischemia.

3. **Renal effects.** If the kidneys are not the source of the hypokalemia, they will respond by decreasing urinary potassium. In general, if the potassium intake is stopped and the kidneys are normal, the expected change in the potassium excretion is as follows: in approximately 4 to 7 days the urinary potassium excretion will decrease to less than 20 mEq/24 hr and in 10 to 15 days the urinary potassium usually decreases to less than 5 mEq/24 hr. In all patients with hypokalemia a urinary potassium concentration should be obtained. If the urinary potassium concentration is low (<10 mEq/L), it can be concluded that the cause of the hypokalemia does not directly involve the kidney, i.e., the loss of potassium is extrarenal, and that the hypokalemia is of more than 2 weeks' duration.

   The earliest adverse effect on the *kidney* is an inability to maintain a hypertonic renal medulla and, consequently, a decrease in the ability to concentrate the urine. With severe hypokalemia, other renal functions are variably impaired—i.e., a decrease in glomerular filtration rate, an increase in renal ammonium excretion, and at times, an increase in the urinary phosphate excretion. Microscopic urinalysis can be normal or can show pyuria, hematuria, or cylindruria. Kidney size is normal and most of these functional changes are reversible. However, with severe and chronic potassium depletion, some patients can develop a chronic interstitial renal disease and renal failure. In addition, there is some evidence that with potassium depletion the kidneys are more susceptible to infection and acute tubular necrosis.

4. Other consequences of potassium depletion include: a decrease in insulin release leading to impaired glucose tolerance, impairment in growth, polydipsia, and (occasionally) edema.

III. **Hyperkalemia**

A. **Mechanisms of hyperkalemia.** Hyperkalemia is defined as a serum potassium greater than 5.5 mEq per liter. The causes for hyperkalemia are listed in Table 40-3. There are two major categories, pseudohyperkalemia and true hyperkalemia. With pseudohyperkalemia the laboratory value is elevated; however, the actual concentration of potassium in vivo is normal. The most common cause of falsely elevated serum potassium measurements is the in vitro breakdown of red blood cells, white blood cells, or platelets. In addition, serum potassium measurements can be elevated if the tourniquet is tightly applied, especially if the blood is drawn from a vigorously exercising extremity. The mechanisms of true hyperkalemia include redistribution of potassium from the cells into the serum, a sudden increase in potassium intake and a decrease in urinary potassium excretion. The increase in serum potassium following a rapid increase in extracellular fluid osmolality is unusual, but this can occur in diabetic patients who have been given a large bolus of hypertonic glucose intravenously. In this situation the sudden increase in the extracellular osmolality causes a rapid flow of water from inside the cell; with this bulk flow there is also a passive transfer of potassium from cells. Regarding the causes of decreased urinary potassium excretion, the following should be noted: Hyperkalemia is a common accompaniment of acute renal failure. However, in chronic renal failure, hyperkalemia does not occur until less than 20 percent of normal kidney function remains, unless there is a concomitant increase in potassium input or some disorder in potassium regulation, e.g., hypoaldosteronism.

B. **Consequences of hyperkalemia.** The primary consequences of hyperkalemia relate to the neuromuscular and cardiovascular effects, although there are renal and metabolic consequences as well.

1. **Neuromuscular consequences of hyperkalemia.** With the decrease in intracellular-to-extracellular potassium concentration ratio, there is a decrease in the resting cell membrane potential. This is manifested as weakness, which can proceed to generalized flaccid paralysis including the muscles of respiration. In addition to weakness, patients may experience paresthesias and a sense of anxiety.

2. **Cardiovascular consequences of hyperkalemia.** In the heart the membrane effect is associated with an increased velocity of repolarization and a decreased velocity of depolarization, producing characteristic ECG changes. These changes include: peaking of the T waves, prolongation and eventual disappearance of the P waves, widening of the QRS complex, heart block, asystole, and ventricular fibrillation. The presence of ECG changes due to hyperkalemia is considered a medical emergency.

3. **Renal and metabolic consequences of hyperkalemia.** Other effects of hyperkalemia include a stimulation of aldosterone, insulin, and epinephrine secretion, all of which tend to drive potassium into cells. Normal kidneys also respond to any increase in serum potassium so that a rise in serum potassium is minimized. In addition, the kidney has the ability to adapt to chronic high potassium loads

Table 40-3   *Causes of Hyperkalemia*

I. Pseudohyperkalemia
  A. Prolonged or tight tourniquet
  B. Vigorous hand gripping
  C. In vitro hemolysis
  D. Extreme leukocytosis or thrombocytosis
II. True hyperkalemia
  A. Potassium redistribution
    1. Acute respiratory or metabolic acidosis
    2. Hyperkalemic familial periodic paralysis
    3. Drugs, succinylcholine, digitalis intoxication
    4. Rapid increase in osmolality of extracellular fluid
    5. Insulin deficiency
  B. Increased input
    1. Exogenous
      a. High potassium diet
      b. Potassium supplements
      c. Salt substitutes
    2. Endogenous
      a. Hemolysis
      b. Rhabdomyolysis
  C. Decreased urine losses
    1. Renal failure
    2. Potassium-sparing diuretics
    3. Decrease in mineralocorticoids
      a. Addison's disease
      b. Hypoaldosteronism
    4. Decrease in renal tubular potassium secretion
      a. Familial
      b. Sickle-cell disease
      c. Systemic lupus erythematosus

so that when challenged, a given potassium load is excreted much more rapidly in the patient who is on a high-potassium intake as compared to the patient on a lower-potassium intake. This *adaptation* involves aldosterone and changes in the intracellular potassium concentration and is of major importance in potassium homeostasis in the patient with kidney failure.

IV. Clinical examples of hypo- and hyperkalemia

  A. Hypokalemia

    1. Description. A 21-year-old female who had been repeatedly hospitalized because of hypokalemia was admitted because of weakness and difficulty in walking. She denied vomiting, diarrhea, or diuretic use. On examination the patient was thin, weighed 38 kg, had a blood pressure of 90/60 mm Hg, a pulse of 104 per minute, and demonstrated an orthostatic fall in blood pressure. The only significant finding on physical examination was significant weakness of both upper and lower extremities.

    2. Laboratory results

Sodium	139 mEq/L
Potassium	2.0 mEq/L
Chloride	85 mEq/L
HCO_3^-	40 mEq/L
Arterial pH	7.54
pCO_2	50 mm Hg

pO$_2$	86 mm Hg
BUN	25 mg/100 ml
Serum creatinine	0.6 mg/100 ml
Urine specific gravity	1.010
Urine potassium	80 mEq/L
Urine sodium	100 mEq/L

ECG showed sinus tachycardia with occasional ventricular premature contractions and an apparent increase in the Q–T interval. •

3. Discussion

a. Factors which may have played a role in this patient's hypokalemia include the systemic alkalemia, which favors the movement of potassium into the cell and the high rate of urinary potassium excretion.

b. In addition, although the patient denied a poor oral intake, her appearance and weight of 38 kg suggest inadequate intake.

c. The increase in the urinary potassium suggests that the primary route of loss is the kidney. The other possibility is that this is an acute disorder and that the kidney has not yet responded to the decrease in serum potassium. This seems unlikely in view of the severe degree of the hypokalemia.

d. The lack of hypertension makes primary hyperaldosteronism unlikely. However, the urinary findings would be compatible with either diuretic abuse or a primary renal tubular disorder. The decreased blood pressure and increased pulse rate suggest that the patient has a decrease in extracellular fluid volume and this is supported by the increased ratio of blood urea nitrogen to serum creatinine (prerenal azotemia). Surreptitious diuretic use is the most likely explanation for this constellation of findings.

B. Hyperkalemia

1. **Description.** A 73-year-old male had a many-year history of proteinuria and hypertension. Four months before hospitalization, the patient developed edema, and he was started on a potent diuretic, sodium restriction, and potassium supplements. The patient now is in a stuporous state, with a pulse of 52 per minute and shallow respirations.

2. Laboratory at admission

Sodium	139 mEq/L
Potassium	8.6 mEq/L
Chloride	100 mEq/L
HCO$_3^-$	16 mEq/L
Arterial pH	7.23
pCO$_2$	41 mm Hg
pO$_2$	56 mm Hg
BUN	150 mg/100 ml
Serum creatinine	7.5 mg/100 ml

ECG showed P–R interval, 0.30; QRS, 0.20; Q–T interval, 0.52; peaked T waves.

3. Discussion

a. Factors which may be playing a role in the patient's high serum potassium include: the use of potassium supplements, the decreased renal function, the increased arterial H^+ concentration, and the decreased HCO_3^- concentration.

b. The cardiac effects of the hyperkalemia are profound, and in this patient a fatal arrhythmia is possible.

c. Immediate therapy should include administration of intravenous calcium to counteract the cardiac toxicity. Potassium should be redistributed into cells by correcting the acidosis with bicarbonate and giving insulin and glucose. Dialysis therapy may also be needed to control the hyperkalemia.

Questions

Select the single best answer.

1. Renal potassium secretion is enhanced by all except which *one* of the following?
   a. An increase in intracellular potassium content.
   b. An increased urine flow rate.
   c. Increased concentrations of aldosterone.
   d. A decrease in distal tubular sodium reabsorption.
   e. An increase in potassium intake.
2. Potassium depletion may cause all except which *one* of the following?
   a. Cardiac arrhythmias.
   b. Impairment of urinary diluting ability.
   c. Neuromuscular paralysis.
   d. Impaired glucose tolerance.
   e. Polyuria.

41 Hydrogen Ion Homeostasis: Metabolic Acidosis and Alkalosis

I. **Background: normal physiology.** The normal metabolism of carbohydrates, lipids, and certain amino acids yields carbon dioxide (CO_2) and water, which combine to form carbonic acid. This compound is commonly called a volatile acid; as long as respiratory function is normal, the CO_2 is excreted by way of the lungs. Normal humans excrete approximately 200 to 300 mM of carbon dioxide per kilogram per day; a 70-kg man would excrete 14,000 to 21,000 mM of volatile acid each day. Other potential sources of hydrogen ion include the oxidation of organic sulfates to sulfur-containing acids and the oxidation of organic phosphates to phosphoric acid. In disease states, the incomplete oxidation of fat can result in increased amounts of beta-hydroxybutyric acid or acetoacetic acid (diabetic ketoacidosis), and the incomplete oxidation of carbohydrate can produce lactic acid. If the patient is to remain in hydrogen ion balance, these nonvolatile or fixed acids must be excreted by the kidney.

Normal humans excrete approximately 1 mEq of nonvolatile acid per kilogram per day. In certain disease states, more than 700 mEq of nonvolatile acids are produced; when this overwhelms the capacity of the kidney to excrete the acid load, the hydrogen ion concentration of blood increases.

At a blood pH of 7.4, the hydrogen ion concentration is 40 nanoequivalents per liter (nEq/L) (4×10^{-9} Eq/L). The relation of pH to H^+ concentration is presented in Table 41-1.

Cellular metabolism continuously adds hydrogen ion to the body fluids; hydrogen ion accumulation is prevented by the excretion of volatile and nonvolatile acids (Fig. 41-1).

Temporary fluctuations in hydrogen ion concentration are minimized by a series of buffers that can either accept or donate a hydrogen ion. Some of these buffer systems are intracellular (e.g., hemoglobin in the red blood cells) and others are predominantly extracellular (e.g., bicarbonate–carbonic acid buffer system); however, all buffer systems are in equilibrium with one another.

$$[H^+] \sim \frac{H_2CO_3}{HCO_3^-} \sim \frac{H_2PO_4^-}{HPO_4^-} \sim \frac{H\,Hb}{Hb^-} \sim \frac{H\,protein}{Protein^-} \sim \frac{H\,apatite}{Apatite^-} \sim etc.$$

The importance of the bicarbonate–carbonic acid buffer system is that it is the principal extracellular buffer. It is also a major source of hydrogen or bicarbonate ions. Thus, during the process of hydrogen ion secretion by the kidney and stomach, the source of the hydrogen ion is carbonic acid; consequently, bicarbonate ions are released into the extracellular fluid. Similarly, pancreatic production and secretion of bicarbonate into the intestinal lumen is coupled with hydrogen ion secretion into the blood. An additional reason that the bicarbonate–carbonic acid system is important is that the body has physiologic mechanisms to control the concentrations of hydrogen ion and bicarbonate; that is, the kidney regulates the bicarbonate concentration and the lung regulates the con-

Table 41-1	Relationship of pH to H^+ Concentration	
	pH	nEq(H^+)/L
	4.5	31,600
	7.0	100
	7.1	79
	7.2	63
	7.3	50
	7.4	40
	7.5	32
	7.6	25

Figure 41-1   *Control of hydrogen ion concentration ($[H^+]$).*

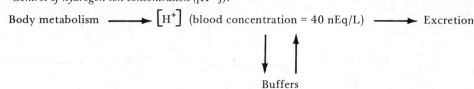

Body metabolism $\longrightarrow$ $[H^+]$ (blood concentration = 40 nEq/L) $\longrightarrow$ Excretion

Buffers

centration of carbonic acid through the control of the partial pressure of CO_2 in the arterial blood ($PaCO_2$).

II. Disorders of hydrogen ion homeostasis

A. Definitions. The following definitions are useful for understanding any discussion of hydrogen ion homeostasis:

Acidemia. An increase above normal in the blood hydrogen ion concentration.

Alkalemia. A decrease below normal in blood hydrogen ion concentration.

Isohydremia. A condition in which the hydrogen ion concentration of blood is normal, 40 nEq per liter, and the pH is 7.4.

Acidosis. A pathophysiologic process that if unopposed can result in acidemia.

Alkalosis. A pathophysiologic process that if unopposed can result in alkalemia.

B. Types of acid-base disturbances. There are four simple types of acid-base disturbance. The respiratory acid-base disturbances involve an alteration in alveolar ventilation that results in a primary change in the $PaCO_2$ and therefore in the blood carbonic acid concentration. In *respiratory acidosis* there is a primary increase in the $PaCO_2$, and in *respiratory alkalosis* there is a primary decrease in $PaCO_2$. In the metabolic acid-base disturbances, the initiating factor causes a primary change in the blood bicarbonate concentration; thus, in *metabolic acidosis* there is a primary decrease in the bicarbonate concentration, and in *metabolic alkalosis* there is a primary increase in blood bicarbonate concentration.

Figure 41-2 presents an operationally useful method for dissecting the pathophysiology of acid-base disturbances. Initially there is a disturbance in hydrogen ion concentration. This change immediately involves the various buffer systems in a way that minimizes the change in hydrogen ion concentration.

In the metabolic disorders, the increase or decrease in blood bi-

Figure 41-2

Phases of an acid-base disturbance.

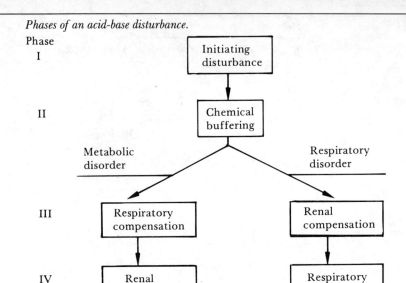

carbonate concentration is associated with a predictable change in alveolar ventilation (respiratory compensation) that further minimizes alterations in blood hydrogen ion concentration. Finally, in the correction of metabolic disorders the blood bicarbonate concentration is returned to normal, because the kidneys excrete the nonvolatile acids and regenerate the bicarbonate that was lost (metabolic acidosis) or excrete the excess bicarbonate (metabolic alkalosis). In the respiratory acid-base disorders, renal compensation occurs in response to a primary increase or decrease in $PaCO_2$, but the acid-base abnormality is corrected only when alveolar ventilation returns to normal. Thus, any description of a simple acid-base disturbance should consider not only the initiating disturbance (the factors causing a primary change in $PaCO_2$ or bicarbonate) but also the compensatory responses.

In many instances, two or more simple acid-base disturbances can occur simultaneously. When this situation arises, the term *mixed acid-base disturbance*, or *complex acid-base disturbance*, is used. For example, respiratory acidosis and metabolic alkalosis commonly occur in patients who have both chronic CO_2 retention resulting from pulmonary disease and congestive heart failure requiring diuretics. In these patients, the diuretic can cause metabolic alkalosis, and, depending on which of the disorders of acid-base metabolism predominate, the patient could have acidemia, alkalemia, or isohydremia.

III. Metabolic acidosis

A. **Etiology.** Metabolic acidosis represents a primary decrease in plasma bicarbonate concentration that, if unopposed, can result in acidemia. The decrease in bicarbonate can occur because of a direct loss of bicarbonate from the body, because of an increase in bicarbonate utilization, or because of a decrease in bicarbonate generation by the kidneys.

Some of the causes of metabolic acidosis are listed in Table 41-2. In most instances of diarrhea, the stool has a relatively high concentration of bicarbonate; this represents the initiating disturbance that causes a decrease in blood bicarbonate level. Increased bicarbonate utilization occurs with lactic acidosis. In this condition, there is increased production and decreased removal of lactic acid; during

Table 41-2   *Causes of Metabolic Acidosis*

Primary bicarbonate loss
   Gastrointestinal losses by diarrhea, fistula, or ureterosigmoid anastomosis
   Renal losses, congenital or acquired proximal renal tubular acidosis
Increased bicarbonate utilization
   Ketoacidosis (diabetic or starvation)
   Lactic acidosis
      Tissue hypoxia
      Impaired oxygen utilization
      Associated with hepatic cirrhosis
      Idiopathic
   Exogenous acid input
      Ammonium chloride
      Hydrochloric acid or sulphur containing amino acids
      Salicylate intoxication
      Ethylene glycol intoxication
      Methanol intoxication
Decreased renal bicarbonate generation
   Renal failure
   Distal renal tubular acidosis

chemical buffering, bicarbonate is utilized to minimize the change in serum hydrogen ion concentration. The third major cause of metabolic acidosis is associated with impaired renal function and with the impaired excretion of nonvolatile acid.

Regardless of the initiating disturbance, the decrease in bicarbonate concentration results in an increase in hydrogen ion concentration. This relationship is depicted by the following formula:

$$[H^+]\ (nEq/L) = \frac{24\ PaCO_2\ (mm\ Hg)}{HCO_3^-\ (mM/L)}$$

The increase in hydrogen ion interacts with other buffer systems within the body, and therefore the change in pH is minimized.

The next line of defense involves the lung. There is a predictable increase in alveolar ventilation and a corresponding decrease in $PaCO_2$. This relationship is represented by the following formula:

$$PaCO_2 = 1.5\ (HCO_3^-) + 8$$

Respiratory compensation begins within minutes but does not reach a steady state until 12 to 24 hours after the initiation of acidemia. It lowers the hydrogen concentration, but does not return it to normal.

The final step in any metabolic acid-base disturbance involves the kidney, since the lungs cannot add bicarbonate to the extracellular fluid and cannot excrete nonvolatile acids. The kidney regulates the serum bicarbonate concentration by:

1. **Reclaiming all the filtered bicarbonate.** Reclamation occurs in both proximal and distal tubules, but 80 to 90 percent of the bicarbonate is reclaimed in the proximal tubule. The magnitude of this process is exemplified as follows: If we assume that the normal bicarbonate concentration is 25 mM per liter and that the glomerular filtration rate is 120 ml per minute, then 4,320 mM of bicarbonate is filtered and reclaimed by the kidney each day. The calculation illustrating this is: 0.025 mM/ml $\times$ 120 ml/min $\times$ 1,440 min/day = 4,320 mM/

24 hr. Urine with a pH of less than 6.4 has a negligible concentration of bicarbonate.

   2. **Generating bicarbonate.** In addition to reclaiming the bicarbonate that is filtered, the kidney also generates bicarbonate. This process, occurring in the distal tubule, is dependent on the ability of this tubule to develop a steep hydrogen ion gradient between the tubular lumen and the blood. Each hydrogen ion excreted results in the generation of one bicarbonate ion, which is then returned to the blood. The hydrogen ion secreted into the urine is excreted in one of three forms:

   a. Free hydrogen ion. Urine having a pH of 4.5 contains 0.03 mEq of free hydrogen ion per liter; thus, the amount of hydrogen ion excreted in this way is minuscule. The importance of the free hydrogen ion is that it titrates urinary buffers and traps ammonium (NH_4^+) within the tubular lumen.

   b. The second form in which hydrogen ion is excreted is as buffered hydrogen ion, or so-called titratable acid (TA). The major urinary buffer system involves $HPO_4^=$ and $H_2PO_4^-$. Approximately one-third to one-half of the hydrogen ion excreted each day is in this form.

   c. The third way hydrogen ion is excreted is as ammonium. The tubule cell produces ammonia (NH_3) by the deamidation of certain amino acids, the most important of which is glutamine. The NH_3 produced diffuses from the cell into the lumen of the tubule and, in an acid urine, combines with H^+ to form NH_4^+. Normally, one-half to two-thirds of the hydrogen ion is excreted as ammonium.

   As mentioned previously, normal adults excrete approximately 1 mEq of hydrogen ion per kilogram per day; under the stress of acidemia, the amount of hydrogen ion excreted in the urine can increase to 6 to 10 mEq per kilogram per day. Much of this adaptation occurs because of an increased production of ammonium. Renal adaptation, as compared to respiratory compensation, is slower and may require 5 days to achieve the maximum response.

B. **Consequences.** The consequences of acidemia are often interrelated with the effects of the disease causing the acidosis. At a blood hydrogen ion concentration of 50 nEq per liter (pH 7.3) the patient can be asymptomatic, but if the acidemia occurs rapidly may show apathy, mental confusion, or altered neuromuscular activity. At a hydrogen ion concentration of 100 nEq per liter (pH 7.0) the acidemia is potentially life threatening. Myocardial contractility and peripheral resistance decrease, and there is also a decrease in responsiveness to sympathomimetic amines, which may cause hypotension and even shock. With chronic metabolic acidosis, acidemia is usually better tolerated and symptoms may be less apparent. However, bone buffers are titrated in chronic metabolic acidosis; this may play a role in the development of renal osteodystrophy.

IV. **Metabolic alkalosis.** This condition represents a primary increase in bicarbonate concentration that, if unopposed, will result in alkalemia. Any discussion of the pathophysiology of metabolic alkalosis must consider those factors that initiate and those that maintain the metabolic alkalosis. The kidney is pivotal in the maintenance of the disorder.

Table 41-3   *Causes of Metabolic Alkalosis*

Primary gain of bicarbonate
  Excess bicarbonate intake
  Metabolism of bicarbonate precursors, i.e., lactate, acetate, citrate
  Post-hypercapnia alkalosis
Net loss of H$^+$ (associated with the endogenous generation of
    bicarbonate)
  Renal H$^+$ loss
    Excess mineralocorticoid activity
      Hyperaldosteronism
      Increased deoxycorticosterone
      Licorice gluttony
    Thiazide and loop diuretics
    Hypercalcemia
    Hypoparathyroidism
  Gastrointestinal H$^+$ loss
    Vomiting or nasogastric suction
    Chloride diarrhea
    Villous adenoma

A. Etiology. An increase in bicarbonate concentration can occur because of the direct addition of bicarbonate or because of the net loss of hydrogen ion from the body with the secondary generation of bicarbonate. The major source of hydrogen ion for the body is the dissociation of carbonic acid to hydrogen ion and bicarbonate. Hence, loss of hydrogen ion will result in a net accumulation of bicarbonate. Some of the more common causes of metabolic alkalosis are listed in Table 41-3.

In some patients there is a direct gain of bicarbonate through the chronic ingestion of sodium bicarbonate or calcium carbonate. An indirect addition of bicarbonate can occur from the metabolism of citrate, lactate, or acetate, all of which serve as bicarbonate precursors. This may result from exogenous administration of these anions or during the correction of certain disease states, e.g., ketoacidosis or lactic acidosis, when the accumulated endogenous acids and their salts are metabolized to bicarbonate and hydrogen ion. The hydrogen ion is excreted, and there is a net addition of bicarbonate to the extracellular fluid.

Bicarbonate can also be added to the extracellular fluid by the kidney. Thus, patients with impaired ventilation of more than a few days' duration have an increase in extracellular fluid bicarbonate. With mechanical ventilation, the PaCO$_2$ can rapidly fall to normal. However, the bicarbonate may not be excreted as rapidly, and thus, with the correction of hypercapnia, metabolic alkalosis can ensue.

Metabolic alkalosis can also occur because of an increase in hydrogen ion loss by the kidneys or the gastrointestinal tract. It should be noted that villous adenoma can be associated with either metabolic acidosis or metabolic alkalosis. This would depend on whether the tumor secretes a bicarbonate-rich solution or whether the fluid is high in chloride and low in bicarbonate. In most instances of diarrhea, whatever the cause, the stool is rich in bicarbonate; however, in certain patients with villous adenoma and in patients with familial chloride diarrhea, the stool is high in chloride, and this may result in metabolic alkalosis.

Table 41-4 *Factors Maintaining Metabolic Alkalosis*

Decrease in effective arterial blood volume (EABV)

Increased tubular H^+ secretion
  Potassium depletion
  Increase in $PaCO_2$
  Increased serum calcium, phosphate

Increase in the intraluminal negative potential
  Increased cation reabsorption, e.g., increased Na^+ reabsorption in
    hyperaldosteronism
  Decreased anion reabsorption, e.g., increased chloride loss associated with loop
    diuretics

B. Compensatory mechanisms. The increase in serum bicarbonate initiates chemical buffering to minimize the fall in free hydrogen ion concentration. Also, the decrease in hydrogen ion concentration results in a predictable decrease in alveolar ventilation and increase in $PaCO_2$. The relationship between bicarbonate and $PaCO_2$ is shown in the following:

$$PaCO_2 = 0.9\,(HCO_3^-) + 14.5$$

Respiratory compensation begins in minutes and requires 12 to 24 hours for complete compensation. In contrast with metabolic acidosis, the degree of compensation is limited by the requirement for oxygen; thus, in most patients the $PaCO_2$ does not rise above 55 mm Hg.

C. Maintenance of metabolic alkalosis. Correction of metabolic alkalosis would require that the kidney excrete the excess bicarbonate. The addition of bicarbonate to the extracellular fluid should result in an increase in the plasma bicarbonate concentration and a corresponding increase in the glomerular filtration of bicarbonate. If tubular bicarbonate reabsorption were unchanged, the increased bicarbonate would rapidly be excreted. However, if there is a decrease in bicarbonate filtration (e.g., renal failure), or an increase in tubular bicarbonate reclamation or generation, then any increase in serum bicarbonate will be maintained until those factors that favor bicarbonate retention are corrected. Factors that favor bicarbonate reclamation and generation are listed in Table 41-4. They are responsible for the maintenance of chronic metabolic alkalosis.

D. The consequences of alkalemia. With mild alkalemia, the patient may be asymptomatic; however, with severe alkalemia, the symptoms and signs may include an increase in neuromuscular irritability, with tetany and hyperactive deep-tendon reflexes. Serious cardiac arrhythmias and impairment in alveolar ventilation with resulting hypoxemia may also occur. Some of these features may be due to the leftward shift of the oxyhemoglobin dissociation curve, with impairment of oxygen delivery to the tissues.

V. Clinical examples

  A. Metabolic acidosis due to diarrhea

  1. Description. A 36-year-old male was hospitalized with a 3-day history of fever and watery diarrhea (Fig. 41-3). On examination, he was acutely ill with a blood pressure of 90/60 mm Hg, a pulse of 112 per minute, a respiratory rate of 24 per minute, and a temperature of 37.5° C. The abdomen was distended and hyperresonant on

Figure 41-3

Pathogenesis of metabolic acidosis associated with diarrhea.

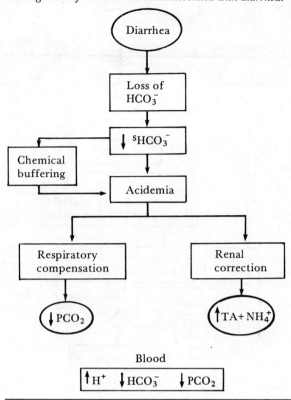

percussion, without localized tenderness, and on auscultation rushes of bowel sounds were heard.

The following laboratory results were obtained:

Venous blood	Arterial blood	Urine
Na^+ 135 mEq/L	pH 7.21	Specific gravity 1.028
K^+ 2.0 mEq/L	H^+ 62 nEq/L	pH 4.5
Cl^- 110 mEq/L	$PaCO_2$ 26 mm Hg	Na^+ 2.0 mEq/L
HCO_3^- 12 mEq/L		

2. **Discussion.** The patient's problems included extracellular volume depletion, metabolic acidosis, and hypokalemia. Analysis of the metabolic acidosis follows.

  a. Initiating disturbance. Diarrhea usually results in the loss of hypotonic fluids, which may contain large amounts of bicarbonate (e.g., 40–80 mM/L) and potassium. The loss of bicarbonate would initiate changes in the blood pH, which would then be minimized by chemical buffering.

  b. A rise in the blood hydrogen ion concentration would stimulate respiratory ventilation, which would further limit the rise in the hydrogen ion concentration. This patient had an appropriate respiratory response for the decrease in blood bicarbonate.

$$PaCO_2 = 1.5(HCO_3^-) + 8$$
$$26 = 1.5 \times 12 + 8$$

  c. The kidney response is slower; the maximum renal response may not occur until 5 days after the onset of the acid-base distur-

Figure 41-4

Pathogenesis of metabolic alkalosis associated with vomiting.

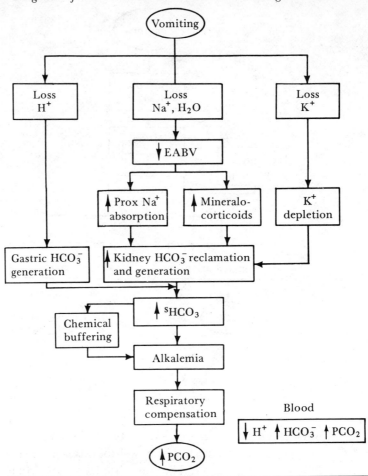

bance. The predominant renal response would be the formation of an acid urine that contains little bicarbonate and has an increased amount of titratable acid and markedly increased amounts of ammonium. The increased renal hydrogen ion production would generate bicarbonate, which would be added to the extracellular fluid. If bicarbonate generation equaled bicarbonate loss, there would be no change in blood hydrogen ion concentration. If bicarbonate loss in diarrhea exceeded the renal generation of bicarbonate, a progressively more severe acidemia would ensue.

B. Metabolic alkalosis due to vomiting

1. **Description.** A 32-year-old male was seen because of vomiting of 1 week's duration (Fig. 41-4). On initial examination, he was apathetic and demonstrated a supine blood pressure of 90/60 mm Hg and a pulse of 116 per minute.

   The following laboratory results were obtained:

Venous blood	Arterial blood	Urine
Na^+ 143 mEq/L	pH 7.55	Specific gravity 1.028
K^+ 2.7 mEq/L	H^+ 28 nEq/L	pH 5.0
Cl^- 93 mEq/L	$PaCO_2$ 46 mm Hg	Na^+ 5 mEq/L
HCO_3^- 36 mEq/L		K^+ 46 mEq/L

2. Discussion

a. The patient was alkalemic, with an increased serum bicarbonate concentration, and therefore had metabolic alkalosis. Respiratory compensation is appropriate for the serum bicarbonate.

$$PaCO_2 = 0.9 \, (HCO_3) + 14.5$$
$$46.9 = 0.9 \, (36) + 14.5$$

Thus, the data are compatible with a vomiting-induced metabolic alkalosis. There was also evidence of a decrease in extracellular fluid volume, including hypotension, tachycardia, a urine specific gravity of 1.028, and urine sodium of 5 mEq/L.

b. Vomiting is associated with the loss of water, hydrogen ion, chloride, and small amounts of sodium and potassium. The source of the hydrogen ion is the parietal cell, which dissociates carbonic acid to hydrogen ion and bicarbonate. The hydrogen ion is secreted into the stomach and lost with the vomitus. The bicarbonate ion is added to the blood, leading to an increase in serum HCO_3 ($^SHCO_3^-$) concentration and alkalemia. Initially, there is an increase in the renal filtration of bicarbonate, so that early during the development of the metabolic alkalosis, there is an increased urinary excretion of bicarbonate and also its attendant cation, sodium.

c. The decrease in blood hydrogen ion concentration initiates chemical buffering within the body and also induces hypoventilation so that there is an increase in $PaCO_2$. These adjustments, although not so predictable as those that occur in metabolic acidosis, tend to limit the decrease in the hydrogen ion concentration.

d. The kidneys maintain the metabolic alkalosis because of decreased effective arterial blood volume and potassium depletion, which favor increased reclamation and generation of bicarbonate. The cause of the decreased effective arterial blood volume is the loss of water and sodium in the vomitus, as well as a loss of sodium during the period of initial bicarbonate diuresis. The cause of the potassium depletion includes the small loss of potassium in the vomitus and a much larger cumulative loss of potassium in the urine that is enhanced by the secondary hyperaldosteronism. Thus, the kidney is pivotal in the maintenance of the metabolic alkalosis. Renal correction of the metabolic alkalosis cannot occur until those factors that maintain the increased bicarbonate generation and reclamation are corrected. When these factors are no longer operative, the excess bicarbonate would be excreted. During the period when all the filtered bicarbonate is being reabsorbed, the urine will be acid (paradoxical aciduria) despite systemic alkalemia.

Questions

1. The following statements are related to the role of the kidney in H^+ homeostasis. Which *one* of the following is false?
   a. The amount of free H^+ in urine is less than 1.0 mEq/L.
   b. The bulk of H^+ secretion is involved in bicarbonate reclamation.
   c. The kidney is capable of correcting acidemia rapidly (within hours).

d. The kidney is the major organ for the excretion of nonvolatile acids.

e. At a pH of 6.0, the amount of HCO_3 in urine is negligible.

2. A 24-year-old man is brought to the hospital in a confused state with a rapid respiratory rate. Examination demonstrates blindness and hyperemic optic disks. The initial laboratory studies:

Venous blood	Arterial blood
Na^+ 136 mEq/L	pH 6.98
K^+ 5.5 mEq/L	$PaCO_2$ 30 mm Hg
Cl^- 100 mEq/L	
HCO_3^- 4 mEq/L	

BUN is 25 mg/100 ml; Cr, 1.2 mg/100 ml. Which of the following statements is false?

a. The patient has metabolic acidosis.

b. The respiratory response is appropriate.

c. There is an increased utilization of HCO_3^-.

d. An acid urine pH is anticipated.

e. This represents a life-threatening problem.

Calcium, Phosphate, and Vitamin D

I. **Background: normal physiology.** Approximately 99 percent of total body calcium (Ca) and 85 percent of body phosphate (P) are located in bone. They compose 1.9 percent and 1.4 percent of total body weight, respectively.

A. **Calcium homeostasis.** Normal total serum Ca is 10 mg/dl (8.5–10.5 mg/dl). Of the total Ca concentration, about 50 percent exists in the ionized form; 40 percent is bound to serum protein, chiefly albumin; and 5 to 10 percent is complexed with citrate and other organic ions. The ionized and the citrate-bound fractions, but not the protein-bound fraction, are filterable at the glomerulus. The most closely regulated moiety is the ionized fraction (Ca^{2+}), which expresses the biochemical activity of Ca. It is this fraction upon which many vital bodily functions are dependent. By contrast, the albumin-bound fraction may demonstrate considerable variation, depending upon the concentration of serum albumin. Diseases characterized by depressed levels of serum albumin frequently have decreased total serum-calcium concentration, while the ionized level of calcium remains normal.

Calcium is a strongly positive ion that binds tightly to anions. Being divalent, it possesses the ability to cross-link two separate negative charges. As a consequence of these chemical properties, calcium serves to maintain the stability of cell membranes. By linking negative phosphate groups in phospholipid membranes, Ca stabilizes lipid membranes and reduces their permeability. Calcium also competes with sodium for entry sites in nerve cells; thus, it plays a role in the gating of sodium fluxes across the cell membrane during the conduction of the nerve impulse. Hence, neuromuscular function is dependent on the fine regulation of ionized Ca^{2+} concentration. An elevated, ionized Ca^{2+} concentration in the serum reduces neuromuscular irritability; a low concentration has the opposite effect.

The concentration of Ca^{2+} ions in the extracellular fluid depends on the delicate balance maintained by the absorption of Ca from the gut, bone deposition and resorption, and excretion through the kidney and the gut. The usual American diet contains approximately 1 g of elemental Ca daily. The principal source of the calcium is dairy products; exclusion of dairy products reduces the daily intake to 200 mg. Approximately 30 percent of ingested calcium is absorbed by the intestine, and the remainder excreted in the feces. The primary site of calcium absorption is the proximal small intestine. Modulation of calcium homeostasis occurs principally through vitamin D metabolites and parathyroid hormone. The intestinal absorption of Ca is dependent on the presence of vitamin D, principally 1,25-dihydroxycholecalciferol ($1,25[OH]_2D_3$). There are two mechanisms responsible for intestinal Ca absorption: (1) active transport and (2) a passive or diffusion-related process. In the presence of an adequate concentration of $1,25(OH)_2D_3$, calcium is transported from the mucosa to the serosa against a concentration gradient. The overall data indicate that the intestinal cells must contain a pump mechanism capable of moving Ca against an electrochemical gradient. There is also evidence indicating that passive permeability or simple diffusion also plays a quantitatively important role in the absorption of Ca; this process is regulated by vitamin D metabolites. The exact mechanism of the role of vitamin D in augmenting intestinal calcium absorption has yet to be completely unraveled. Both calcium-binding protein and calcium adenosine triphosphatase (ATPase) may have a role.

Intestinal absorption of calcium is usually adjusted to the amount of Ca intake. The lower the calcium intake, the greater the fractional calcium absorption by the intestine. The ability of the intestine to modulate the fractional calcium absorption is presumably secondary to changes in renal synthesis of $1,25(OH)_2D_3$. The changes in $1,25(OH)_2D_3$ synthesis result, in turn, from changes in parathyroid hormone secretion.

In the kidney only the non–protein-bound calcium is filtered. If the serum calcium falls below 7.5 mg/dl with normal serum proteins, urinary calcium excretion falls to zero as a result of enhanced reabsorption of filtered Ca stimulated by parathyroid hormone. Any reduction in glomerular filtration rate will diminish renal Ca clearance. Of the approximately 10 g of Ca filtered through the glomeruli daily, about 98 percent is reabsorbed. Most of the Ca is reabsorbed in the proximal tubule, 20 to 25 percent is absorbed in the loop of Henle, and about 10 percent further distally. The concentration of Ca in the luminal fluid in the proximal tubule remains unchanged from the ultrafiltrate of plasma, indicating that, like sodium, Ca is absorbed with water in the same proportion that exists in the glomerular filtrate. Active reabsorption of calcium does occur in the loop of Henle and in the distal nephron.

Administration of most diuretics results in an increased excretion of both sodium and Ca. The thiazide diuretics are exceptions. Thiazides will produce a sodium diuresis while increasing calcium reabsorption from the glomerular filtrate. The increased Ca reabsorption occurs in the proximal nephron, as a consequence of contraction of the extracellular fluid volume. Another major modulator of urinary calcium excretion is parathyroid hormone, which enhances tubular reabsorption of Ca in the distal nephron.

B. **Phosphate homeostasis.** In contrast with Ca, phosphate is widely distributed in nonosseous tissues both in inorganic form and as a component of various functional macromolecules, including phospholipids, phosphoproteins, nucleic acids, and intermediates of carbohydrate metabolism. Soft tissue P composes only about 15 percent of the total body content. The remainder is deposited as inorganic P in the mineral state of bone, primarily as calcium hydroxyapatite, but also less tightly bound as amorphous calcium phosphate. Only a small fraction of cellular phosphate is present in the form of inorganic P; however, this fraction is important since it is the source of adenosine phosphate (adenosine monophosphate [AMP], adenosine diphosphate [ADP], and adenosine triphosphate [ATP]) formation.

Phosphorus plays an important role in many biologic functions. It is critical for the structural integrity of cells; it regulates enzymatic activity; it is involved in fuel storage, as well as transformation of energy; and it plays an important role in the delivery of oxygen to tissues according to the level of 2,3-diphosphoglycerate (2,3-DPG) and ATP in the red blood cells. In adults, the concentration of serum P varies between 2.5 and 4.5 mg/dl. The serum P tends to decrease after the ingestion of a carbohydrate meal and in the presence of respiratory alkalosis. Conversely, volume depletion, acidosis, and exercise may elevate the serum P levels. In children, the serum P concentration varies between 4 and 7 mg/dl. In plasma, only a small fraction (12%) is protein-bound; the remainder exists as a free ion in association with various cations. Serum P concentration may exhibit a daily variation of as much as 50 percent, which suggests that the evolution of the hormonal regulation of phosphate has not been driven by the need to regulate this mineral within narrow limits.

The average dietary intake of phosphate, derived largely from dairy products, cereals, and meats, is 800 to 900 mg per day; approximately 50 to 65 percent of the ingested P is absorbed in the gut. Available evidence suggests that absorption occurs primarily in the jejunum and may be augmented by the presence of $1,25(OH)_2D_3$. Because of dietary abundance and efficient absorptive adaptation to dietary restriction, P deficiency is rarely attributable to inadequate intake.

Inorganic P is freely filtered at the glomerulus, and a variable amount is reabsorbed in the proximal tubule. This is an active process, and the transport mechanism appears to be subject to saturation. Of great importance is the fact that parathyroid hormone (PTH) inhibits the proximal reabsorption of P. The phosphaturic action of PTH occurs within minutes after administration and results in an increased urinary excretion of P as the serum P falls. Whether there is a distal nephron site for P reabsorption that is affected by PTH remains uncertain.

A normal adult excretes about 500 to 800 mg of phosphate daily, depending on the dietary intake. With the normal serum P of 3.5 mg/dl, and a glomerular filtration rate of 180 liters per 24 hours, 6,000 mg per day are filtered. Thus, by reabsorbing 90 percent of the filtered P, 600 mg can be excreted, which is roughly the daily intake. If the glomerular filtration rate should fall to only 17 liters per 24 hours, then the daily intake of 600 mg of P could be excreted without elevating the serum P concentration only by completely suppressing tubular reabsorption. Any further fall in glomerular filtration rate would prevent the excretion of the 600-mg intake unless an increase in serum concentration occurs. As serum P rises, serum Ca falls, with resultant stimulation of PTH secretion. However, the low glomerular filtration rate prevents the physiologic action of the hormone to increase phosphate clearance. In such secondary hyperparathyroidism of renal failure, the hormone continues to have some effect on bone metabolism, although its renal effects are severely blunted or abolished.

C. **Hormonal regulation of calcium and phosphate**

1. **Parathyroid hormone (PTH)** is the principal regulator of Ca homeostasis. A decrease in the blood levels of Ca perfusing the parathyroid gland is the main factor in the stimulation of PTH secretion. The increased PTH secretion in response to hypocalcemia tends to restore the serum Ca concentration to normal. This is achieved by an increased bone resorption, increased tubular reabsorption of Ca from the glomerular filtrate, and increased $1,25(OH)_2D_3$ synthesis, which then increases intestinal Ca absorption. These direct effects of PTH on both the kidneys and skeletal system are mediated by cyclic AMP.

2. **Vitamin D.** Vitamin D is the other principal hormonal factor in the maintenance of normal Ca homeostasis. This sterol, cholecalciferol, is produced naturally in the skin when 7-dehydrocholesterol is exposed to sunlight (wavelength 290–320 nm). Vitamin D is also ingested in the diet, mainly in dairy products and fortified foods. The first principal metabolic conversion occurs in the liver, where 25-hydroxylation produces 25-hydroxy vitamin D_3 (25-OHD$_3$). A significant amount of 25-OHD$_3$ undergoes enterohepatic circulation and is reabsorbed in the distal small intestine. When in the circulation, 25-OHD$_3$ is bound to an alpha globulin (MW 58,000). A second major metabolic conversion of vitamin D occurs in the renal cortex, where $1,25(OH)_2D_3$ is formed; $1,25(OH)_2D_3$ is the vitamin D metabolite that induces the most rapid and greatest increase in intestinal calcium absorption and, in conjunction with PTH, augments bone calcium resorption. The two major regulators of $1,25(OH)_2D_3$ synthesis are PTH and hypophosphatemia (low level of serum phosphorus). Hypocalcemia is not directly responsible for increased $1,25(OH)_2D_3$ synthesis, but achieves this result because of increased PTH secretion. (In parathyroidectomized animals, hypocalcemia does not increase $1,25(OH)_2D_3$.) However, hypophosphatemia has been shown to stimulate $1,25(OH)_2D_3$ production independent of PTH. In addition to 25-OHD$_3$ and $1,25(OH)_2D_3$, there are other measurable vitamin D metabolites, such as $24,25(OH)_2D_3$ and $1,24,25(OH)_3D_3$. Some evidence exists that $24,25(OH)_2D_3$ may play a role in regulating PTH production; however, it must be stressed that this evidence is quite preliminary and incomplete. At present, $1,24,25(OH)_3D_3$ is believed to be a degradation product of $1,25(OH)_2D_3$.

II. **Hypercalcemia**
   A. **Pathogenesis of hypercalcemia.** The most common cause of hypercalcemia is primary hyperparathyroidism. Malignancy with metastasis to bone is the second most frequent cause of hypercalcemia. Certain malignancies produce hypercalcemia through the release of some humoral substances such as osteoclast-activating factor (multiple myeloma and lymphoma) and possibly prostaglandins. Vitamin D excess is another cause of hypercalcemia. With vitamin D overdose, the hypercalcemia is due to a marked increase in the intestinal absorption of Ca. Approximately 10 percent of patients with sarcoidosis will have hypercalcemia. The cause is believed to be secondary to increased levels of $1,25(OH)_2D_3$; consequently, these patients have a high Ca absorption in the gut. Immobilization may produce hypercalcemia in those patients with a high rate of bone turnover, such as patients with Paget's disease or thyrotoxicosis or the growing child. The precise mechanism for the development of hypercalcemia in these situations is unclear. Finally, increased ingestion of Ca may sometimes induce hypercalcemia, e.g., in patients who are treated for peptic ulcer disease with an excessive amount of milk and alkali, such as Ca carbonate.
   B. **Consequences of hypercalcemia**
      1. **Soft tissue calcification.** Hypercalcemia, especially in the presence of elevated serum P, may induce metastatic calcification of the soft tissues. Calcification occurs earliest in the more alkaline areas of the body. There are alkaline sites on the contraluminal side of the acid-secreting epithelia: gastric mucosa, renal tubules, and the lung alveoli. In these tissues, metastatic calcifications may develop quickly. Periarticular soft tissue calcifications are also common sites. The

cornea of the eye is another place where metastatic calcification occurs. Usually the Ca crystals deposited in the cornea are visible only by slit-lamp examination, but if extensive, the deposits may be visible as a band keratopathy along the lateral margin of the cornea. This type of calcification is also commonly seen in patients with chronic renal failure and secondary hyperparathyroidism.

2. **Renal effects.** Acute hypercalcemia may induce acute renal failure, most likely due to increased renal vascular constriction. Chronic hypercalcemia frequently causes polyuria and a vasopressin-resistant impairment in urine concentration. Other complications relate to the deposition of calcium within the renal parenchyma. The associated inflammation and fibrosis can result in chronic interstitial nephritis and renal failure.

3. **Gastrointestinal effects.** Anorexia, nausea, and vomiting are frequent; an increased incidence of peptic ulcers and pancreatitis has also been reported in these patients.

4. **Cardiovascular effects.** With moderate to severe hypercalcemia, there is shortening of the Q–T interval in the electrocardiogram, increased susceptibility to digitalis-induced arrhythmias, and occasionally varying degrees of heart block. Hypertension is often found in patients with hypercalcemia. This may be partly due to the nephropathy but also can occur in the presence of normal renal function. A mechanism may be increased peripheral resistance caused by the hypercalcemia and increased cardiac output caused by the positive ionotropic effect of Ca.

5. **Neurologic effects.** High serum Ca has an inhibitory effect on neuromuscular activity and frequently is manifested in patients by apathy, lack of energy and spontaneity, anxiety, or depression. In severe hypercalcemia, there are varying degrees of mental confusion and disorientation progressing to delirium, loss of contact with reality, hallucinations, depression of consciousness, and coma.

III. **Hypocalcemia**

A. **Pathogenesis of hypocalcemia.** The recent advances in the metabolism and action of PTH and the various vitamin D metabolites have changed the approach to the hypocalcemic patient. The various causes of hypocalcemia are currently classified in the following manner.

1. **PTH deficiency.** The hypocalcemia is secondary to lack of PTH, resulting in a decrease in bone resorption and impaired renal tubular reabsorption of Ca. Besides the hereditary form of hypoparathyroidism, there are other causes of PTH deficiency, such as thyroid surgery with accidental removal of the parathyroid glands. The hypoparathyroid patient has a low serum Ca and a high P. The levels of plasma $1,25(OH)_2D_3$ are low because of both the low PTH and the high P.

2. **Resistance to the actions of PTH.** There are two entities in which resistance to PTH occurs. The most common is renal failure, in which the level of parathyroid hormone is high but there is resistance at the bone level to the calcemic action of PTH. The second entity is called pseudohypoparathyroidism, where there is resistance to the skeletal and renal actions of PTH. The basic defect in pseudohypoparathyroidism is the failure of PTH to generate a cyclic AMP response.

3. **Vitamin D deficiency.** This major group of hypocalcemic disorders includes so-called nutritional rickets. The vitamin D stores can become depleted with decreased intake of vitamin D, lack of exposure

to sunlight, malabsorption syndromes, and some agents that bind vitamin D, e.g., cholestyramine. The plasma level of $25(OH)D_3$ is low in these patients.

4. **Abnormal metabolism of $25(OH)D_3$.** Diffuse parenchymal liver disease and abnormalities of the biliary tract may affect calcium and vitamin D homeostasis. Low levels of $25(OH)D_3$ have been found in patients with diffuse liver disease as well as biliary tract abnormalities. Impaired production of $25(OH)D_3$ by the liver is the most likely explanation, although abnormal intestinal absorption of vitamin D may be another factor. The prolonged administration of anticonvulsant drugs may result in hypocalcemia and osteomalacia because they induce hepatic microsomal enzyme activity, resulting in products that are biologically inactive.

5. **Defective production of $1,25(OH)_2D_3$.** Hypocalcemia is a common finding in patients with chronic renal failure. The kidney is the only site of production of $1,25(OH)_2D_3$; thus, patients with advanced kidney disease usually have low levels of $1,25(OH)_2D_3$, accounting for a decrease in intestinal Ca absorption and also skeletal resistance to the calcemic action of PTH. The Fanconi syndrome, characterized by proximal renal tubular dysfunction with impaired reabsorption of various solutes, may also result in decreased synthesis of $1,25(OH)_2D_3$.

6. **Miscellaneous.** Chelation by various agents such as ethylenediaminetetraacetic acid (EDTA) and citrates may induce hypocalcemia. Acute pancreatitis can induce hypocalcemia; the mechanism is not known. Finally, acute hyperphosphatemia may lead to significant hypocalcemia, especially in those patients with renal function deterioration. Also, chemotherapy for the treatment of acute leukemia and lymphoma has been noted to induce severe hyperphosphatemia and hypocalcemia.

B. **Consequences of hypocalcemia.** The clinical signs of hypocalcemia are more dramatic than those of hypercalcemia. Spontaneous muscle cramps may be an early manifestation of mild hypocalcemia. Tetany and generalized tonic-clonic seizures will develop with more severe reduction in the concentration of serum Ca. Evidence of hypocalcemia may be elicited by simple bedside tests. Tapping with the finger over the supramandibular portion of the parotid gland causes spasm of the muscle innervated by the seventh nerve; this is Chvostek's sign. Another, perhaps more specific, test is that of Trousseau. In this test, a blood pressure cuff is inflated around the upper arm of the patient and maintained until a carpopedal spasm develops (flexion contraction of wrists and metacarpal phalangeal joints with fingers held straight and grouped with tips together). If no carpopedal spasm develops within 3 minutes, the test is regarded as negative. Spontaneous tetany may be a life-threatening problem if the pharyngeal or respiratory muscles are affected.

IV. **Hypophosphatemia**

A. **Pathogenesis of hypophosphatemia.** Hypophosphatemia can result from decreased intake, a transcellular phosphate shift, or increased loss. Since phosphate is widely distributed in food, decreased intake is a rare cause of hypophosphatemia. With starvation, malabsorption syndrome, or vigorous use of phosphate-binding antacids, phosphate depletion is possible. Transcellular shift of phosphate is common and related to the formation of phosphate intermediates of glycolytic metabolism, e.g., glucose 6-phosphate, 1,3-diphosphoglycerate, and high-energy phosphate compounds. This can help to explain the hypophosphatemia of intravenous hyperalimentation, alcoholism, and respiratory alkalosis as well as that occurring during the treatment of diabetes ketoacidosis. Causes of increased phosphate loss include acquired and congenital renal tubular defects (e.g., Fanconi syndrome, hypomagnesemia, x-linked hyphophosphatemic rickets) and functional changes that increase renal phosphate loss (e.g., hyperparathyroidism, volume expansion, and diuretic use).

B. **Consequences of hypophosphatemia.** Severe hypophosphatemia (serum concentration <1.0 mg/dl) produces dysfunction in blood cells, the central nervous system, and skeletal and cardiac muscle. The erythrocyte may show a decreased concentration of ATP and 2,3-DPG. With profound deficiencies these changes may result in hemolysis. Since 2,3-DPG affects the erythrocyte oxygen-transport capacity, low concentrations of 2,3-DPG are associated with impaired tissue oxygen release. Thus, hypophosphatemia causes dysfunction through tissue anoxia and decreased high-energy phosphate compounds. In vitro, hypophosphatemia impairs leukocytic, chemotactic, phagocytic, and bacteriocidal activity. Central nervous symptoms include paresthesias, lethargy, convulsions, and coma. The effect in skeletal muscle typically appears after starvation followed by refeeding without phosphorous supplements. In this situation weakness, rhabdomyolysis, myoglobinuria, and (rarely) acute respiratory failure have occurred. Hypophosphatemia can adversely affect myocardial performance, decreasing the stroke volume and even causing heart failure. With phosphate repletion the cardiomyopathy is reversible.

V. **Clinical example of hypercalcemia**

A. **Description.** A 35-year-old woman was discovered to have a blood pressure of 150/105 and was placed on a thiazide diuretic. She had passed a kidney stone 6 months previously. After 18 months of using the diuretic, her serum calcium was 11.8 mg/dl and serum phosphorus was 2.1 mg/dl. The patient was requested to discontinue her thiazide diuretic and return in 4 weeks with a 24-hour urine.

Lab results

Serum		Urine	
Na	138 mEq/L	Ca^{2+}	350 mg/24 hr
K^+	3.6 mEq/L	P	800 mg/24 hr
Cl^-	114 mEq/L	TRP	70%
HCO_3^-	21 mEq/L		
Ca^{2+}	11.9 mg/100 ml		
P	2.0 mg/100 ml		

B. **Discussion**

1. The most likely diagnosis in this patient is primary hyperparathyroidism. Features supporting this diagnosis are: (a) hypercalcemia, (b) hypophosphatemia, (c) hypercalciuria, (d) hyperphosphaturia, and (e) elevated serum chloride and depressed serum bicarbonate.
2. The thiazide diuretic was discontinued because thiazides have been reported to cause hypercalcemia. However, with thiazides, the serum calcium level is rarely above 11 mg/100 ml, and the effect of thiazide diuretics is to decrease urinary calcium excretion.

3. The history of kidney stones is quite common in primary hyperparathyroidism. Parathyroid hormone increases $1,25(OH)_2D_3$ levels, resulting in increased intestinal calcium absorption, and also mobilizes calcium from bone. Even though the effect of PTH on the kidney is to increase calcium reabsorption, hypercalciuria results because of the high filtered load of calcium. The hypercalciuria is believed to be the major cause of kidney stones.

4. Hypercalcemia increases the peripheral vascular resistance; thus, hypertension is common with primary hyperparathyroidism.

5. Hypophosphatemia is produced because increased PTH levels result in a marked phosphaturia. The tubular reabsorption of phosphorus (TRP) is calculated by the following formula:

$$1 - \frac{\text{Phosphate clearance}}{\text{Creatinine clearance}}$$

A TRP of less than 85 percent frequently reflects increased PTH levels, especially when renal function is normal.

Questions

Select the single best answer.

1. The following statements regarding calcium are true except:
   a. Approximately 50 percent of the total serum calcium exists in the ionized form.
   b. The extracellular concentration of calcium depends upon a balance between Ca absorption from the gut, the deposition in bone, and excretion through the kidney and gut.
   c. $1,25(OH)_2D_3$ augments calcium absorption from the gut.
   d. In parathyroidectomized animals, hypocalcemia will increase $1,25(OH)_2 D_3$ production.
   e. Acute hypercalcemia may induce renal failure.
2. The following statements regarding phosphorus and vitamin D are true except:
   a. Hypophosphatemia is a stimulus for increased $1,25(OH)_2D_3$ production.
   b. Parathyroid hormone increases phosphorus excretion by the kidney.
   c. More than 50 percent of the plasma phosphorus is protein bound.
   d. Vitamin D is produced in the skin upon exposure to sunlight.
   e. The production of $1,25(OH)_2D_3$ occurs in the renal cortex.

43 Glomerulonephritis and the Acute Nephritic Syndrome

I. **Introduction.** Over the last few years, advances in immunology, the development of experimental animal models, and the clinical use of renal biopsy in the early stages of renal disease have increased understanding of the pathogenesis of the various types of glomerulonephritis.

II. **Immunopathogenesis of glomerulonephritis.** In the majority of types of glomerulonephritis, glomerular injury is the result of glomerular capillary deposition of circulating antigen-antibody complexes. Various antigens, both endogenous and exogenous, have been demonstrated in human immune-complex glomerulonephritis. Other less frequent causes of glomerular injury include anti-glomerular basement membrane nephritis and so-called in situ antigen-antibody complex nephritis.

A. **Immune complex disease.** Experimental animal models have greatly contributed to a better understanding of this disease. One model involves the exogenous administration of bovine serum albumin to a rabbit, with resulting acute serum sickness. The sequence of immunologic events is outlined in Figure 43-1. After the experimental rabbit receives a single injection of a large amount of a purified radio-labeled bovine serum albumin, three phases can be identified: (1) an early and rapid decrease of radio-labeled albumin (antigen) due to equilibration between the intravascular and extravascular protein pools; (2) a second, slower decline of the radio-labeled antigen due to a nonimmune metabolism of the albumin; and (3) a later, rapid decrease of the radio-labeled albumin due to the formation of antigen-antibody complexes. At the time these complexes appear in the circulation, the serum complement levels decrease and inflammatory lesions are demonstrable in the kidney, heart, arteries, and joints. In the kidney this is manifested by an acute diffuse glomerulonephritis (Fig. 43-2).

The various components of immune complexes can be demonstrated by immunofluorescent microscopy. This technique utilizes tissue sections treated with fluorescein-labeled antibodies. Thus, various antibodies and complement can be demonstrated in the glomerulus in the form of granules localized in the mesangium and along the glomerular basement membrane. A granular or lumpy-bumpy pattern of immunoglobulin and complement depositions is characteristic of immune-complex disease (Fig. 43-3). By electron microscopy these deposits can be shown as electron-dense, finely granular precipitates, usually located on the subendothelial side of the basement membrane, in the mesangium, and along the subepithelial side of the basement membrane. The lesions observed in the acute-serum-sickness model of immune-complex disease are similar to if not identical with those observed in acute glomerulonephritis in humans (Fig. 43-4).

A variety of renal lesions can be induced by changing the method of bovine serum albumin administration from a single dose to daily low doses of antigen given over several weeks. Thus, continued formation of immune complexes may result in a variety of glomerular lesions, including focal lesions, mesangial lesions, and diffuse proliferative glomerulonephritis. However, in the chronic model, the

Figure 43-1

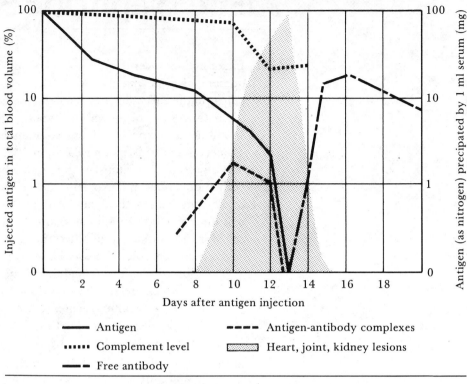

Immunologic sequence after injection of albumin antigen in the rabbit. (From C. G. Cochrane and F. S. Dixon, Cell and tissue change through antigen-antibody complexes. In P. A. Miescher and H. F. Muller-Eberhard [Eds.], Textbook of Immunopathology. *New York: Grune & Stratton, 1968, vol. 1, p. 94. Reproduced by permission of the publisher and C. G. Cochrane.)*

Figure 43-2

Acute postinfectious immune-complex glomerulonephritis. The capillary loops are narrowed conseequent to neutrophilic infiltration and swelling of endothelial and mesangial cells. (Hematoxylin and eosin, original magnification 250×.)

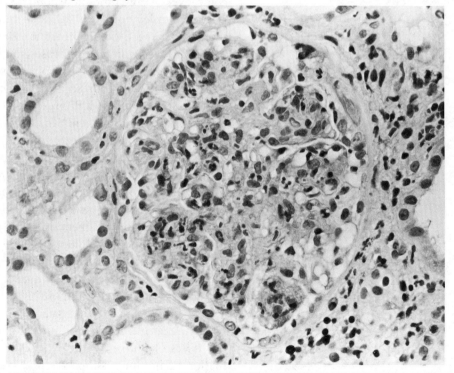

Figure 43-3

Acute postinfectious immune-complex glomerulonephritis. The glomerular capillaries show lumpy-bumpy immuno-fluorescence against IgG.

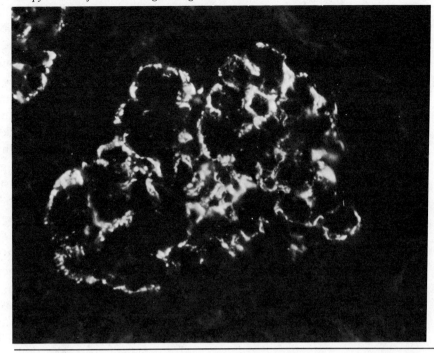

Figure 43-4

Acute postinfectious immune-complex glomerulonephritis. Numerous electron-dense deposits are situated upon a normal glomerular capillary basal membrane. Tertiary podocytes have surfaced these deposits. A neutrophil is present within the capillary lumen. (Uranyl acetate and lead citrate, original magnification 5,200×.)

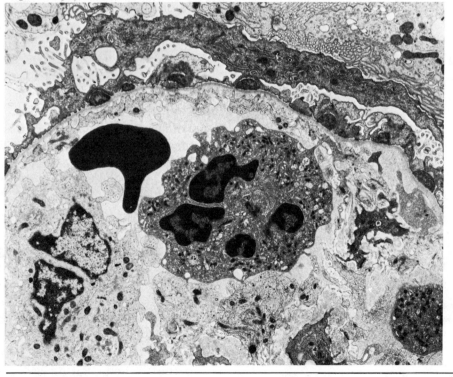

glomerular disease occurs only when there is a state of antigen-antibody equivalence or mild antigen excess. If the experimental animal responds to the chronic antigen administration with marked antibody production, a state of antibody excess will result, and the large antigen-antibody complexes are readily removed by the reticuloendothelial system without inducing glomerular injury. Similarly, if a large amount of antigen is administered and there is a poor antibody response, the result will be the formation of small complexes that do not result in glomerular injury. From these observations it becomes clear that other factors, in addition to the type of antigen-antibody complexes, may determine the nature of glomerular injury. These factors include the degree of glomerular permeability, renal blood flow, and the hydrostatic pressure in various renal compartments. Finally, genetic factors may also be important in the susceptibility to various types of glomerulonephritis.

1. **Viral-induced immune-complex disease.** Certain experimental animals develop circulating antigen-antibody viral complexes and glomerular lesions. In man, glomerulonephritis can result from hepatitis B virus infection, vaccinia, and measles.

2. **Immune-complex disease associated with parasitic disease** has been found in both experimental animals and in humans. Thus, acute and chronic parasitic infections such as schistosomiasis, malaria, and toxoplasmosis are associated with immune-complex glomerulonephritis. In these cases the specific parasitic antigen has been shown to be present within the immune complexes.

3. **Immune-complex disease in inbred New Zealand mice** causes a spontaneous syndrome that resembles systemic lupus erythematosus. It has been shown that this nephritis is induced by glomerular deposition of immune complexes, and the antibodies have been shown to be directed against nuclear antigens.

B. **Anti-glomerular basement membrane (anti-GBM) disease.** The glomerular injury in anti-GBM disease is the result of antibodies reacting against a component of the glomerulus, the basement membrane. In one animal model, rat glomerular basement membrane is injected into a rabbit, generating antibodies to the glomerular basement membrane. Rabbit serum containing these antibodies is then injected back into the rat; the antibodies react with the rat glomerular basement membrane and severe glomerulonephritis develops. A similar glomerular injury can be induced by the injection of heterologous glomerular basement membrane with Freund's adjuvant. Both experimental models are characterized by severe glomerulonephritis with epithelial cell proliferation, the formation of crescents usually associated with necrosis of the glomerular tuft, and glomerular infiltration with polymorphonuclear leukocytes (Fig. 43-5). The glomerular lesions usually develop within days of a single injection. Immunofluorescent microscopy demonstrates linear deposition of immunoglobulin G and complement along the glomerular basement membrane (Fig. 43-6). No dense deposits are found at electron microscopy. It is important to note that the glomerular deposition of immunoglobulin G in a linear pattern is not specific for anti-GBM disease; this pattern occurs in other renal diseases, particularly diabetic nephropathy. However, in diabetic nephropathy, circulating anti-GBM antibodies are absent and the immunoglobulins eluted from the glomerulus do not bind to the basement membrane when incubated with normal renal tissue. This suggests

Figure 43-5

Anti-GBM glomerulonephritis with crescent formation. An epithelial crescent has compressed the glomerular tufts, which show multifocal disruption of their capillary basement membrane. Bowman's membrane is reduplicated, attenuated, and fragmented. (Jones-methenamine-silver, original magnification 250×.)

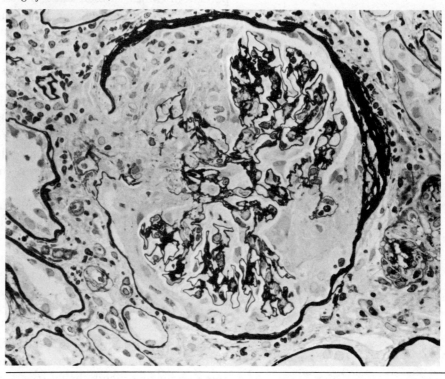

Figure 43-6

Anti-GBM glomerulonephritis. The capillary basement membrane stains linearly against IgG.

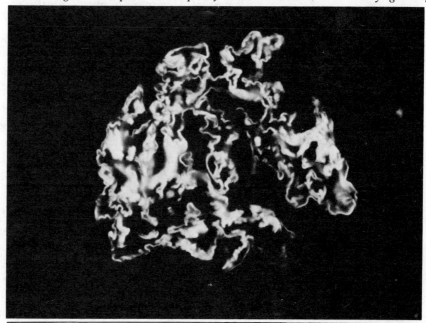

that the deposition of immunoglobulin G in diabetes may represent nonspecific protein trapping by the glomerulus. Anti-GBM nephritis is less common than immune-complex nephritis and accounts for 5 percent of clinical cases of acute glomerulonephritis. Some cases begin as a rapidly progressive glomerulonephritis; the presence of anti-GBM antibodies in the circulation is diagnostic in these cases. Other patients have Goodpasture's syndrome, i.e., the association of anti-GBM nephritis and pulmonary hemorrhage. In these patients, both glomerular and pulmonary injury occur because alveolar and glomerular basement membranes have similar antigenic characteristics.

C. **In situ immune-complex disease.** The repeated administration of small doses of heterologous antigen to experimental animals usually results in basement membrane thickening and in a granular pattern of immune deposits along the basement membrane. Until recently, it was believed that the granular pattern was always caused by deposition of circulating immune complexes, and membranous nephropathy was considered a model of chronic circulating immune-complex glomerulonephritis. However, recent evidence suggests that this granular pattern may be caused by the in situ deposition of antigen, which later is complexed to an antibody within the glomerulus. In support of this hypothesis is the observation that the majority of patients with membranous nephropathy fail to show circulating immune complexes. In addition, in experimental animals the injection of immune complexes does not result in a granular pattern of localization along the basement membrane, but instead in the deposition of the complexes in the mesangium or subendothelial space. Experimental data demonstrating that circulating antibody may combine with antigen previously deposited in the glomerulus are provided by an experimental animal model, Heymann nephritis. In this model, rats previously immunized with a proximal tubule brush-border antigen develop granular immune deposits along the basement membrane within 10 minutes of antibody injection. Presumably the antibody reacts in situ with an antigenic component in the glomerulus. Thus, it would seem that in situ immune-complex glomerulonephritis is a pathogenic mechanism that may be operative in membranous nephropathy in man. Membranous nephropathy is the most common cause of nephrotic syndrome in the adult population. However, the nature of the antigen is usually unknown. The histologic picture of membranous nephropathy is characteristic and includes: as seen by light microscopy, a membranous thickening due to diffuse spike formation of GBM material with deposits located between the spikes (Fig. 43-7); as shown by immunofluorescence, a granular deposition of immunoglobulin G and complement along the glomerular basement membrane (Fig. 43-8); and as shown by electron microscopy, subendothelial and intramembranous electron-dense deposits (Fig. 43-9). There is no cellular proliferation.

D. **Other immunologic mechanisms.** The role of cell-mediated glomerular damage in the experimental animal and in man is not clear. Lymphocytes from patients with glomerulonephritis have been shown to have increased blastogenic reactivity when incubated with glomerular basement membrane antigens, suggesting that lymphocytes already sensitized may contribute to the renal damage.

III. **Mediators of glomerular injury.** The deposition of antigen-antibody per se may be sufficient to cause glomerular injury. However, there are certain mediators activated by the antigen-antibody complexes that are of

Figure 43-7

Membranous nephropathy. The glomerular basement membrane shows diffuse spike formation; epimembranous deposits are situated between the spikes. The mesangial regions are relatively normal. (Jones-methenamine-silver, original magnification 400×.)

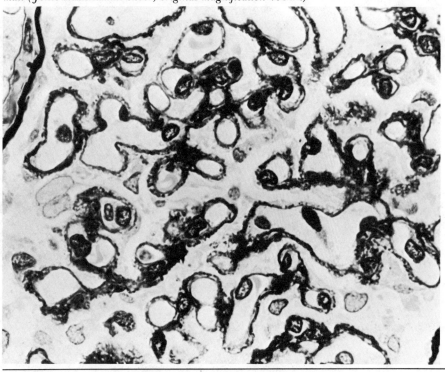

Figure 43-8

Membranous nephropathy. Granular deposits of IgG are diffusely present along the capillary basement membrane.

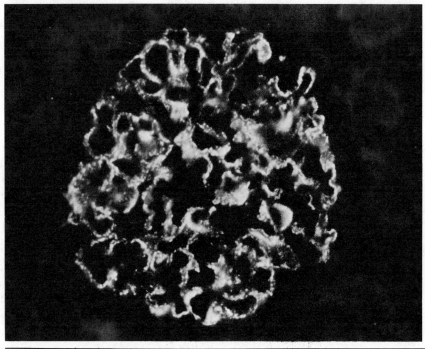

Figure 43-9

Membranous nephropathy. Extensions of capillary basal lamina project outward between the numerous epimembranous electron-dense deposits. Some deposits have been surfaced by neomembrane and are intramembranous. (Uranyl acetate and lead citrate, original magnification 5,940×.)

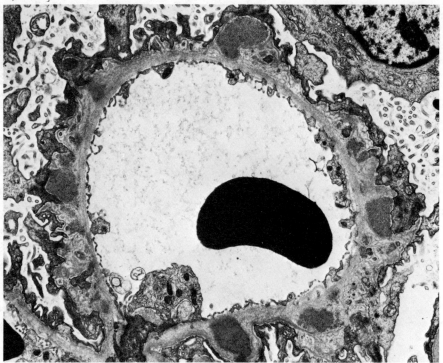

importance in the causation of glomerular damage. These include complement, polymorphonuclear leukocytes, platelets, vasoactive amines, and fibrin.

A. Activation of the complement cascade. The complement cascade may be activated by either the classic or the alternate pathways, as shown in Figure 43-10. The classic activation of the complement system involves the binding of the first component of complement, C1, to the immune complex; this reacts with C4 and then C2 to form an enzyme, C3 convertase, which then cleaves C3 into two fragments, C3a and C3b. C3b then activates the remaining components of the complement cascade, C5 through C9. The alternative pathway of complement activation is initiated by factors B and D and magnesium; this results in the cleavage of C3 without the intervention of C1, C4, and C2 (Fig. 43-10). The C3b formed from the cleavage of C3 then combines with activated factor B to form an enzyme, C3bBb. This enzyme in turn splits C3 into C3a and C3b. This self-perpetuating cycle is known as the amplification loop.

The complement system contributes to glomerular injury in two ways. First, it increases vascular permeability (anaphylatoxin activity), which facilitates immune-complex deposition. Second, these proteins attract polymorphonuclear leukocytes into the glomerulus, where they can directly damage the glomerular capillary wall.

B. Platelets and vasoactive amines also play an important role in the glomerular damage. The mechanisms that lead to glomerular basement membrane damage will also result in the aggregation of platelets and increased platelet consumption. Platelet consumption releases vasoactive amines (e.g., serotonin and histamine) and activates the clot-

Figure 43-10

Complement activation cascade. Sequence of activation of complement components both in the classic and alternate pathways. (From B. D. Rose, Pathophysiology of Renal Disease. New York: McGraw-Hill, 1981, p. 111. Copyright © 1981; used with the permission of McGraw-Hill Book Company.)

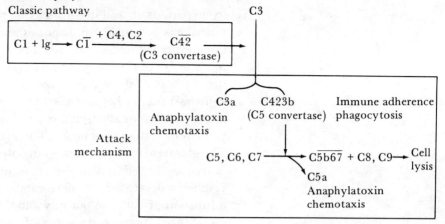

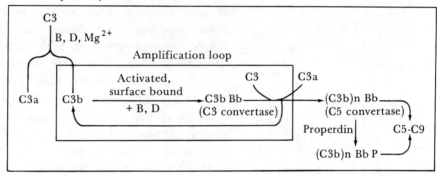

ting system; this, in turn, may contribute to glomerular injury. Antiplatelet agents have been reported to have beneficial effects in certain types of glomerulonephritis, e.g., focal sclerosis and membranoproliferative glomerulonephritis, but observations need to be confirmed.

C. **The coagulation system** may also be an important mediator of glomerular injury. Thus, fibrin and fibrin-degradation products are usually present in the glomerulus of patients with glomerulonephritis, and fibrinogen may leak into Bowman's space, where it stimulates epithelial cell proliferation and crescent formation. The formation of crescents may impair glomerular filtration by compression of the glomerular tuft. In addition, the accumulation of fibrin may impair renal blood flow and glomerular filtration. The importance of fibrin as a mediator of glomerular injury has been demonstrated by treating animals with anticoagulants or defibrinating agents that prevent the development of proliferative glomerulonephritis. Heparin and warfarin have also been reported to be beneficial in some patients with rapidly progessive glomerulonephritis; however, controlled studies on the use of these agents have not been done.

D. **Role of monocytes in glomerular injury.** Recently, the presence of monocyte infiltration in the glomerulus has been demonstrated in some forms of glomerulonephritis. Depletion of monocytes by irradiation prevents the proteinuria and glomerular damage in experimental nephritis. This observation suggests that monocytes may play a role in the production of glomerular injury.

IV. Clinical characteristic of the acute nephritic syndrome. Patients with acute glomerulonephritis often develop edema, hypertension, gross hematuria, and diminished urine output. This symptom complex is known as the nephritic syndrome. In addition, symptoms resulting from severe hypertension and uremia may be present.

A. **Urinalysis** is valuable in diagnosis and usually demonstrates cellular casts, especially red blood cell casts, a rather characteristic finding in the acute nephritic syndrome. However, in a minority of patients the urinalysis may show only proteinuria or hematuria. The abnormal urinalysis occurs because disruption in the capillary wall results in filtration of normally unfiltered red and white blood cells and large protein molecules (primarily albumin).

B. **The glomerular filtration rate** estimated from the creatinine clearance is frequently reduced in the acute nephritic syndrome. This is the result of a decrease in the permeability coefficient of the capillary wall, a function of both the porosity and the surface area of the basement membrane. In the early stages of experimental glomerulonephritis, the decrease in permeability coefficient is usually the result of a decrease in effective surface area. Later, with increased cell proliferation, fibrin deposition, and fibrosis, there is a reduction in the capillary lumen size; this diminishes both the capillary blood flow and the hydrostatic pressure, thus decreasing the glomerular filtration rate. A decrease in plasma oncotic pressure secondary to hypoalbuminemia may also lead to a reduction in the plasma volume and a secondary decrease in the glomerular filtration rate. The decrease in plasma oncotic pressure will shift fluid out of the vascular space into the interstitial space, leading to a decrease in plasma volume plus a reduction in cardiac output, renal blood flow, and glomerular filtration rate.

C. **The edema** that is common in patients with the acute nephritic syndrome is the result of renal sodium and water retention. Patients with acute glomerulonephritis have a decreased glomerular filtration rate and normal renal tubular function. This glomerular tubular imbalance causes such patients to show the symptoms of prerenal failure, with increased tubular sodium and water reabsorption, as well as edema formation. Finally, the presence of hypoalbuminemia may be associated with edema even in the presence of an adequate glomerular filtration rate. The hypoalbuminemia causes the translocation of fluid into the interstitial space, a decrease in plasma volume and in renal blood flow, and increased tubular sodium and water reabsorption.

D. **Hypertension** is another common manifestation of the acute nephritic syndrome. Volume expansion and the presence of vasoconstrictive substances (e.g., renin) may both participate in the genesis of the hypertension. In most patients with acute glomerulonephritis, the hypertension is due to fluid retention and the removal of the excess of fluid usually returns blood pressure to normal. A minority of patients have severe glomerular ischemia, which may be associated with increased renin secretion and hypertension. This may be the case in patients with vascular diseases, e.g., the hemolytic uremic syndrome and malignant nephrosclerosis. In these diseases, fibrin deposition induces arteriolar occlusion. Renin-related hypertension usually does not respond to fluid removal and may require the use of agents that lower renin secretion (propranolol) or agents that block angiotensin II generation (converting enzyme inhibitor).

V. Clinical example of acute nephritic syndrome

A. Description. A 32-year-old Caucasian man was hospitalized because of proteinuria, edema, and a blood pressure of 200/110. Two weeks previously the patient had a sore throat and a mild fever. Urine sediment on admission revealed multiple red blood cell casts. Renal biopsy was performed, and light microscopy demonstrated diffuse endothelial and mesangial cell proliferation without crescent formation. There were multiple polymorphonuclear leukocytes within glomerular capillaries. Immunofluorescence showed a lumpy-bumpy pattern of immunoglobulin G and complement deposition. Electron microscopy demonstrated the presence of electron-dense deposits in the subendothelial and subepithelial space.

B. Discussion. The presence of proteinuria, edema, and hypertension is suggestive of the acute nephritic syndrome. This is further confirmed by an abnormal urinalysis revealing multiple red blood cell casts. The history of a sore throat is indicative of pharyngitis, most likely streptococcal, which led to the development of an acute glomerulonephritis. This is confirmed by the renal biopsy findings of glomerular cell proliferation with multiple polymorphonuclear leukocytes. The lumpy-bumpy pattern at immunofluorescence and the presence of electron-dense deposits are characteristic of an acute immune-complex glomerulonephritis.

Questions

More than one answer may be correct.

1. Mediators of glomerular injury include:
   a. Platelets.
   b. Monocytes and polymorphonuclear leukocytes.
   c. Serotonin and histamine.
   d. Fibrin.
   e. All of the above.
2. Which of the following conditions is *not* typically associated with the acute nephritic syndrome?
   a. Red blood cell casts in the urine sediment.
   b. Hypertension.
   c. Polyuria due to a defect in renal concentrating ability.
   d. Glomerular injury from immune complexes.
   e. Edema.

The Nephrotic Syndrome

I. **Introduction.** The most famous physician who studied the nephrotic syndrome and its close relatives was Dr. Richard Bright, a young physician at Guy's Hospital in London in the early 1800s. In his *Reports of Medical Cases* (1827), he stated: "I have never yet examined the body of a patient dying with dropsy [massive edema] attended with coagulable urine [now known to mean proteinuria], in whom some obvious derangement was not discovered in the kidneys . . . In all cases in which I have observed the albuminous urine, it has appeared to me that the kidney has itself acted a more important part, and has been more deranged both functionally and organically than has generally been imagined."

An anonymous poem illustrates the genesis of the term *Bright's disease:*

Doctor Richard Bright of Guy's
Had several patients large in size.
Their legs were swollen as could be;
Their eyes so puffed they could not see.
To this edema Bright objected,
And so he had them venesected.
He took a teaspoon by the handle,
Held it above a tallow candle,
And boiled some urine o'er the flame
(As you or I might do the same).
To his surprise, we find it stated,
The urine was coagulated.
Alas, his dropsied patients died.
Our thoughtful doctor looked inside;
He found their kidneys large and white,
The capsules were adherent quite.
So that is why the name of Bright is
Associated with nephritis.

II. **Definition of nephrotic syndrome.** A clinical situation in which the patient has heavy proteinuria (in children, >2 g/m^2/day; in adults, >3 g/day), *and* hypoalbuminemia (normal, 3.5–5.5 g/dl; nephrotic, <3 g/dl), *and* edema. They may also have elevated triglycerides and cholesterol (hyperlipidemia). The proteinuria is almost always associated with changes in the glomeruli.

III. **Normal physiology.** The level of any serum protein is defined by the balance between synthesis and loss or degradation of that protein. The primary protein in nephrotic syndrome is albumin, which is synthesized in the liver. In the kidney the glomerular basement membrane allows a small amount of albumin and proteins of lower molecular weight to pass into the ultrafiltrate. The tubule has a limited capacity to break these proteins down into peptides and amino acids, which then are reabsorbed into the blood. The balance between filtered protein and reabsorbed protein metabolites determines the urinary protein excretion, normally less than 150 mg per 24 hours. The protein concentration in the blood determines the plasma oncotic pressure. If the protein concentration, and thus oncotic pressure, decreases, Starling's forces change, with resultant translocation of water and sodium from the plasma to the interstitial spaces.

IV. **Pathophysiology of nephrotic syndrome.** The basic defect in diseases causing the nephrotic syndrome is altered glomerular permeability, so that more protein passes through the glomerular basement membrane. This protein may be primarily albumin and lower-molecular-weight proteins (an exaggerated loss of the usual urinary proteins known as selective proteinuria); or larger proteins may also be lost, such as beta-lipoprotein, transferrin, and alpha-2 macroglobulin (nonselective proteinuria). Some of the protein is metabolized and reabsorbed, giving the liver the necessary components to resynthesize the proteins; however, some is excreted in the urine. As the amount of filtered protein increases, several things occur: (1) proteinuria increases; (2) the tubules reabsorb more peptides and amino acids—at least up to a point; and (3) the liver increases its production of albumin and the other proteins. The next change occurs when the liver cannot further increase its protein production. Under that condition, as protein loss continues, the serum concentration of albumin decreases; Starling's forces then shift, with increasing interstitial fluid volume. Initially, this may be evidenced only as an otherwise unexplained increase in weight. Later, one sees dependent edema, in the legs at the end of the day or in the periorbital area and fingers at the end of the night, or the edema may localize in the scrotum, labia, or abdominal wall, as either unilateral or bilateral. When severe, it may be in body cavities (pleural or pericardial effusion, ascites, within joints). It can also accumulate in body organs, resulting in pale, swollen kidneys and in edematous mucosa in the gastrointestinal tract. As fluid shifts out of the intravascular compartment, the kidneys are perfused less. This results in a slight decrease in renal filtration and a compensatory increase in tubular reabsorption of salt and water. This attempt to increase blood volume partially backfires, since additional salt and water are then lost into the interstitial space, worsening the edema.

Accompanying the increased production of albumin by the liver is a nonspecific increase in its production of other substances, notably lipoproteins, cholesterol, and clotting factors. Early in the nephrotic syndrome, an elevation in high-density, low-density, and very-low-density lipoproteins occurs (HDL, LDL, and VLDL, respectively). Later, HDL and LDL decrease to normal while VLDL continues to increase. The clotting factors that increase are fibrinogen and factors V, VII, VIII, and X. Platelet number and adhesiveness are also increased.

A. **Clinical results of pathophysiologic changes**
  1. **Proteinuria.** Patient may note foamy urine.
  2. **Hypoalbuminemia and edema.**
  3. **Other plasma protein concentrations** decrease if lost into urine.
  4. **Plasma renin activity and aldosterone concentration** increase (due to decreased blood volume).
  5. **Cholesterol and triglycerides (lipoproteins)** increase, resulting in milky serum.
  6. **Casts** in urine. Protein concentrates form solid impressions of tubules, which appear in the urine.
  7. **Cells** in urine. White cells and red cells escape from the blood into the urine; they may also be incorporated into cellular casts.
  8. **Fat** in urine appears in cells, casts, or as droplets or crystals.
  9. **Susceptibility to infection** increases, partly because gamma globulins (antibodies) are lost in urine.

10. **Malnutrition** occurs due to protein loss in urine, malabsorption from gastrointestinal tract due to edematous absorption surface, and general malaise with poor appetite.

11. **Hypercoagulable tendency** exists with increase in clotting factors, platelet number, and platelet function. Nonspecific factors of edema and decreased activity, as well as decreased blood volume, add to this tendency; the result is increased incidence of leg vein thrombosis, pulmonary embolism, and renal vein thrombosis.

12. **An increased incidence of atherosclerosis** occurs, possibly due to changing lipoproteins.

B. **Primary renal diseases associated with the nephrotic syndrome.** The nephrotic syndrome is associated with a primary (idiopathic) renal disease in about 80 percent of adult cases and about 95 percent of childhood nephrosis.

1. **Lipoid nephrosis (minimal change disease).** Proteinuria is selective, glomerular filtration rate is approximately normal, and hypertension or hematuria is usually absent. The kidney is histologically normal except for fused foot processes (a nonspecific sign related to proteinuria). Lipoid nephrosis accounts for 50 to 75 percent of pediatric cases and 15 percent of adult cases. It responds to corticosteroid therapy.

2. **Focal sclerosis.** Nonselective proteinuria, hematuria, and hypertension occur more often than in lipoid nephrosis. Focal sclerosis typically affects teenagers and young adults. It begins in the juxtamedullary nephrons and gradually advances to destroy all renal function. It may recur in the transplanted kidney.

3. **Membranous nephropathy.** Nonselective proteinuria and microscopic hematuria are typical. Hypertension and decreasing renal function occur late. The histologic appearance includes a thick glomerular basement membrane without cellular proliferation. It is not uncommon in middle-aged and older patients and can be associated with cancer of the colon, stomach, or lung.

4. **Membranoproliferative glomerulonephritis.** Nonselective proteinuria and hematuria are usually present, with hypertension and decreasing renal function, usually occurring over 1 to 5 years. Histologically, glomerular cell proliferation and thickened basement membrane are found.

C. **Secondary causes of nephrotic syndrome (5% pediatric cases, 20% adult cases)**

1. **Collagen-vascular disease,** especially systemic lupus erythematosus.

2. **Metabolic/inherited disease,** i.e., diabetes mellitus, amyloidosis, hereditary nephritis.

3. **Malignant disease,** i.e., Hodgkin's disease, leukemia, lymphoma, multiple myeloma, solid tumors (stomach, colon, liver, breast). The histologic changes may include minimal change, membranous nephropathy, and myeloma kidney.

4. **Drugs and other causes** include mercurial diuretics, gold, penicillamine, heroin, bismuth, probenecid; bee sting, pollen, poison ivy or oak, snake venom; allergen and serum therapy.

5. **Infections**
   a. Bacterial—streptococcal, staphylococcal, syphilis, tuberculosis.
   b. Protozoan—malaria, toxoplasmosis.
   c. Helminthic—filariasis, schistosomiasis, trypanosomiasis.

      d. Viral—hepatitis B, cytomegalovirus, Epstein-Barr virus (mononucleosis), Herpesvirus.

    6. Miscellaneous causes include malignant hypertension, transplant rejection, toxemia of pregnancy.

V. Clinical examples

A. Child with nephrotic syndrome

1. Description. A 4-year-old boy was brought to the hospital because of puffy eyes. There was no history of recent infections, medication use, or familial renal disease. The child had gained 4 pounds in the preceding week. The blood pressure was 100/60. Edema of face, scrotum, penis, and legs was noted. Chest examination revealed dullness to percussion and decreased breath sounds in both bases. The abdomen was distended and demonstrated shifting dullness and a fluid wave. Lab studies: urine with 3^+ protein, hyaline casts, occasional fat bodies, 0–2 RBC, and 0–1 WBC/HPF. Blood studies: total protein, 4.0 g/dl; albumin, 1.9 g/dl; cholesterol, 300 mg/dl; BUN, 28 mg/dl, creatinine, 0.8 mg/dl; hemoglobin, 14.5 g/dl; hematocrit, 55 percent.

2. Discussion.

  a. This child had nephrotic syndrome, as indicated by marked proteinuria; low serum albumin; edema, including ascites and pleural effusion; and high cholesterol.

  b. His renal function was not normal. BUN and creatinine were increased (normal for a 4-year-old would be <10 mg/dl and 0.5 mg/dl, respectively). One reason for azotemia is intravascular volume depletion (the high hemoglobin and hematocrit suggested hemoconcentration due to loss of plasma volume). The most likely diagnosis was lipoid nephrosis.

  c. A renal biopsy was not needed to prove the diagnosis because the child fit the typical picture of minimal-change disease. If the blood pressure had been increased or if there had been more than 10 to 20 RBC/HPF, a biopsy would have been indicated.

  d. The child was placed on a regimen of bed rest and a low-salt diet to lessen edema. Prednisone, a corticosteroid (2 mg/kg/day), was given; in 10 days, the patient lost 6 pounds and no longer had edema, ascites, or pleural effusion. Urinalysis showed no protein. The BUN was 8 and the creatinine 0.5 mg/dl. A quick response to steroids is typical of minimal-change disease.

B. Nephrotic-range proteinuria

1. Description. A 64-year-old man came to a physician's office because he had been told at a recent health fair that his blood pressure was too high and that his urine contained protein. He admitted to a 15-pound weight loss over the preceding 3 months, but denied dieting. He denied edema, shortness of breath, foamy urine, or serious past medical problems. Physical exam was entirely normal except for a blood pressure of 160/105. Lab studies revealed: urine, 3^+ protein; 2 to 4 RBC/HPF. A 24-hour urine specimen contained 5.0 g of protein, the plasma creatinine was 1.8 mg/dl, and creatinine clearance was 42 ml/min. Additional blood studies included: albumin, 3.2 g/dl; BUN, 25 mg/dl; hemoglobin, 11 g/dl; Hct, 34%; cholesterol, 253 mg/dl.

2. Discussion

  a. This man did not have nephrotic syndrome. He had enough protein in his urine to qualify but did not have edema or hypoalbuminemia. Some would call this nephrotic-range proteinuria. However, the same diseases that cause the full-blown nephrotic syndrome should be considered.

b. His renal function was not normal, although some decrease in creatinine clearance may be associated with aging.

c. Troubling features in this initial workup included weight loss, mild anemia, proteinuria, hypertension, and impaired renal function.

d. Sigmoidoscopy and roentgenograms of the upper gastrointestinal tract and colon were done to search for any underlying malignancy, but the studies showed no abnormalities. Chest x-ray was also negative. Next, a renal biopsy was performed; the changes were typical of membranous disease. Remembering that it may take months for a tumor to be clinically evident, the physician followed the patient closely, looking for clues to the cause of his renal disease and meanwhile controlling blood pressure.

Questions

More than one answer may be correct.

1. Which of the following statements is/are true?
   a. Proteinuria of greater than 4 g per day can result from infection.
   b. In adults, the nephrotic syndrome is easily treated even if the cause is unknown.
   c. Most cases of nephrotic syndrome in adults are associated with a systemic disease.
   d. Membranoproliferative glomerulonephritis has a worse prognosis than membranous glomerulopathy.
   e. If a patient has a serum albumin of 4 g/dl and excretes 4 g protein per 24 hours, he may not have edema.
2. Which of the following statements is false?
   a. Selective proteinuria is more characteristic of lipoid nephrosis than of focal sclerosis.
   b. Gamma globulin loss may increase susceptibility to infection in nephrotic patients.
   c. Nephrotic patients have an increased tendency to form blood clots.
   d. The prognosis of minimal change disease is much better than that of focal sclerosis.
   e. None of the above.

45 Acute Renal Failure

I. **Introduction.** Sudden increases in serum concentrations of nitrogenous metabolic wastes, such as urea and creatinine (acute azotemia), in subjects with previously normal function characterize diverse disorders that abruptly and often reversibly impair renal function (Table 45-1). Altered cardiocirculatory physiology (prerenal azotemia) and obstruction of urine excretion (postrenal azotemia) due to ureteral, bladder, or urethral pathology indirectly impair renal function. Both function and renal integrity may also be directly impaired (renal parenchymal azotemia) by ischemic, toxic, inflammatory, or immune insults. Accompanying symptoms and urine volumes are variable, but urine composition (Table 45-2) is often distinctive for each group of azotemic disorders. The clinical course varies with the type and severity of the initiating event, prior state of renal function, state of hydration, or type of therapy employed. The spectrum may range from transient dysfunction, with few symptoms and signs, to irreversible renal failure, leading to death or requiring life support by an artificial kidney.

II. **Normal renal physiology.** A renal blood flow (RBF) exceeding 1.0 liter of blood per minute (25% of cardiac output) is required for a normal renal function. This RBF sustains a glomerular filtration rate (GFR) in excess of 100 ml per minute and delivers sufficient renal oxygen for the various tubular functions (metabolic, synthetic, and transport) that determine final urine composition. Autoregulation allows marked variances in renal perfusion pressures to develop before either RBF or GFR are substantially altered.

III. **Mechanisms of azotemia**

A. **Prerenal azotemia.** Failure of autoregulatory processes to sustain GFR as the effective circulating blood volume (ECBV) decreases appears to explain the observed features of prerenal azotemia. The neural and humoral vasoconstrictive activities that impair autoregulation affect the GFR, leaving tubular function intact, and produce low volumes (oliguria, <400 ml/day) of concentrated urine. Occasionally, a nonoliguric (>400 ml/day), prerenal azotemia is encountered in the presence of coexisting, impaired antidiuretic hormone response (central nervous system trauma, lithium, demethylchlortetracycline) or an impaired renal-medullary concentrating gradient (loop diuretics or solute diuresis).

Treatment depends on restoration of an ECBV by expanding intravascular volume and improving cardiac output. However, persistent renal hypoperfusion may predispose to overt renal damage and sustained renal failure.

B. **Postrenal azotemia.** Acute obstruction of the urinary tract appears to initiate a transient increase in intratubular pressures, which is followed by vasoconstriction. Inflammation and pressure necrosis may subsequently develop with sustained obstruction. The extent to which each factor contributes to the observed reduction in GFR and tubular function will depend on the duration and severity of the obstructive process. Significant azotemia develops only when the obstructive process is bilateral or involves previously damaged kidneys or a unilateral kidney. Complete absence of urine (anuria, <100 ml/day) characterizes complete obstruction. The anuria may be intermittent with interven-

Table 45-1	Causes of Acute Azotemia

Type of Azotemia	Mechanism	Clinical Associations
Prerenal	Impaired renal perfusion	Shock, dehydration, congestive heart failure
Renal parenchymal		
Vascular	Ischemia	Emboli, thrombi, vasculitis, hemolytic-uremic syndrome, malignant hypertension
Glomerular	Immune deposits	Acute glomerulonephritis
Interstitial	Inflammatory or toxic process involving interstitium	Pyelonephritis, allergic (penicillin, sulfonamides, diuretics)
Tubular	Obstruction	Crystals (urate) or protein (myeloma)
	Toxins	Hemoglobin, myoglobin, aminoglycosides, radio-contrast agents
	Severe ischemia	Same as prerenal
Postrenal	Obstruction	Stones, clots, prostatic obstruction, extrinsic ureteral compression

Table 45-2	Urine Composition in Acute Azotemia

Type of Azotemia	Urine Sediment	Urine Sodium (mEq/L)	$FE_{Na}(\%)$*
Prerenal	Normal or increased granular casts	<20	<1.0
Renal parenchymal			
Vascular	Red blood cells and RBC casts	Variable	—
Glomerular	RBC, RBC casts, lipid droplets	Variable	<1.0 early >2.0 later
Tubular and interstitial	WBC, eosinophils, RBC, cellular casts (all but RBC casts), renal tubular epithelial cells, granular and pigmented casts	>40	>3.0
Postrenal	Variable—can be normal or can have crystals, RBC, WBC	Variable	<1.0 early >3.0 later

*FE_{Na} = Fractional excretion of sodium:

$$FE_{Na} = \frac{\text{Clearance Na}}{\text{Clearance of creatinine}} = \frac{C_{Na}}{C_{cr}}$$

$$FE_{Na} = \frac{U_{Na}\, V}{P_{Na}} \cdot \frac{P_{cr}}{U_{cr}\, V} \qquad FE_{Na} = \frac{U_{Na}}{P_{Na}} \cdot \frac{P_{cr}}{U_{cr}}$$

P_{Na} = plasma Na$^+$ concentration (mEq/L); P_{cr} = plasma creatinine concentration (mg/dl); RBC = red blood cells; U_{Na} = urine Na$^+$ concentration (mEq/L); U_{cr} = urine creatinine concentration (mg/dl); V = urine flow rate (cc/min); WBC = white blood cells.

ing nonoliguric volumes. The urine volume may be relatively normal or even polyuric in the presence of partial obstruction. Treatment requires relief of the obstructive lesion.

C. **Renal parenchymal azotemia.** A major reduction in the GFR may be due to any severe injury to the renal parenchyma. Acute glomerulonephritis, vasculitis, or interstitial nephritis will be associated with typical histologic changes. However, ischemia or toxic insults may result in so-called acute renal failure (ARF), which is accompanied by histologic changes that vary from essentially normal to acute tubular necrosis (ATN). Clinical features are highly variable. Urine volumes range from persistent anuria with renal cortical necrosis through oliguric volumes to nonoliguria or polyuria. The oliguric type of ARF is most often noted with ischemic insults, whereas nonoliguric ARF is most frequently seen after toxic renal injuries.

The pathophysiologic mechanisms that initiate and sustain acute renal failure are not completely known, but a number of factors have been investigated in both humans and experimental animals.

1. **Tubular theories** of ARF assume that a normal GFR is sustained, at least initially. Suggested tubular mechanisms include:

   a. **Back leak** of the filtered solutes through tubular cells damaged by ischemia or toxicity could give the appearance of a depressed GFR and promote the interstitial edema with tubular collapse frequently noted in ARF. The lack of concentration of filtered solutes by the renal tubule and incomplete distal recovery of proximally injected nonresorbable solutes are findings that support the back-leakage hypothesis. Finally, some models of ARF do demonstrate a normal single-nephron GFR in the face of a depressed total GFR, but in other circumstances GFR is demonstrably depressed before tubular damage occurs (inconsistent with the back-leakage hypothesis).

   b. **Obstruction** of renal tubules by casts (cellular or pigmented), together with dilatation of the tubules proximal to the casts, is also a frequently observed abnormality in ARF. It is possible that obstruction could generate sufficient back pressure to prevent glomerular filtration. Experimental evidence, however, shows that the intraluminal pressures are actually low in some models and that the pressure required to dislodge the casts is usually less than that generated by normal filtration. The casts then seem to be a consequence of ARF rather than a cause.

2. **Vascular theories** propose that the functional and histologic abnormalities of ARF follow a primary reduction in GFR. Proposed vascular mechanisms are:

   a. **Afferent (preglomerular) vasoconstriction** is proposed as a dominant factor responsible for the severe reduction in GFR seen in many cases of ARF. Vasoconstriction may develop in response to any insult that enhances adrenergic discharge or releases catecholamines and renin. Reactive vascular endothelial edema may also be a contributing factor. Supporting observations include demonstrable renocortical ischemia; at least transient increases in concentrations of catecholamines, renin, and angiotensin in ARF; and the protective effect of intravascular volume expansion or alpha-adrenergic blockade.

   b. **Efferent (postglomerular) vasodilatation** has been investigated as an alternative possibility explaining a reduced GFR as a conse-

Figure 45-1

Typical course and treatment of acute reversible renal failure, divided according to dominant clinical features and treatment requirements. The magnitude of clinical problems and the intensity with which support treatment is required throughout the various phases of acute renal failure are indicated by the notations within diamonds.

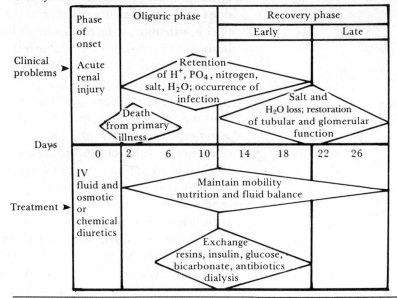

quence of accelerated postglomerular runoff and decreased glomerular filtration pressure. Renocortical ischemia and measurably decreased efferent blood flow argue against this concept.

c. **Impaired glomerular capillary permeability** has also been evaluated as a possible mechanism for reduced GFR in ARF. Limited functional and microscopic evidence supporting this concept is currently available.

3. **Factors that modify the course of acute renal failure.** The interaction of certain modifying factors—e.g., the extracellular fluid volume, vascular resistance, and prostaglandin activity—often determines whether a given insult will provoke renal failure. Once renal failure has occurred, it may be sustained by a combination of factors, including reduced renal blood flow, continued vasoconstriction, the tubular back leak of filtrate, tubular obstruction, and altered glomerular permeability. The clinical course of acute renal failure is dictated largely by the inciting events and subsequent complications (Fig. 45-1).

IV. **Clinical example of acute renal failure**

A. **Description.** A 25-year-old laborer sustained multiple fractures of both legs when scaffolding collapsed at work. He denied prior health problems. His blood pressure was 90/60 mm Hg, his pulse 130 per minute, and popliteal artery bleeding was noted. The blood pressure stabilized with 2 liters of Ringer's lactate solution and a unit of blood. After repair of the arterial laceration and stabilization of his fractures, he was transferred to a hospital ward, where he passed 300 ml of dark brown urine that gave a positive benzidine test for blood but contained no red cells on microscopic examination. A serum sample was colorless. Admitting laboratory data showed a BUN of 20 mg/100 ml, potassium of 4.9 mEq/L, and a hemoglobin of 13 g/100 ml. Severe oliguria developed during the next 24 hours. Serum chemistries included a BUN of 55 mg/100 ml, a creatinine of 8 mg/100 ml, a potassium of 6.9 mEq/L, and a creatinine phosphokinase (CPK) of 12,000 units. An electrocardiogram showed tall, peaked T waves and depressed P waves, consistent with hyperkalemia. Hemodialysis was repeated several times during the next 3 weeks to control his serum potassium concentration and azotemia. Urine volumes slowly increased, reaching 3.5 liters daily during his fourth hospital week, at which time chemical abnormalities began returning toward normal values.

B. **Discussion.** The patient's good health and normal serum chemistries before severe injury indicate that the renal failure is acute; the history also suggests that renal failure was precipitated by the combined events of hypotension and myoglobinuria associated with the injury. The colorless serum, dark benzidine-positive urine, and greatly increased concentration of muscle enzymes (CPK) support the diagnosis of myoglobinuria, which was probably an important factor in the development of the renal injury.

The subsequent course demonstrates one of the serious complications of ARF, e.g., hyperkalemia, which can result in death due to cardiac toxicity. Other common complications include infection, congestive heart failure due to fluid retention, gastrointestinal bleeding, anorexia, nausea, and vomiting. The case also demonstrates recovery of renal function after a period of oliguria; this is typical, providing the patient survives the insult that caused the renal failure.

Questions

Select the single best answer.

1. The rate of sodium excretion from a patient with oliguric parenchymal acute renal failure is commonly:
   a. 0.1 percent of filtered sodium.
   b. 0.5 percent of filtered sodium.
   c. 1.0 percent of filtered sodium.
   d. More than 2.0 percent of filtered sodium.
   e. None of the above.
2. If a patient is intermittently anuric, i.e., variable urine volumes with intervals of zero urine, the most likely diagnosis is:
   a. Acute tubular necrosis.
   b. Prerenal failure.
   c. Ureteral obstruction.
   d. Renal infarction.
   e. Bladder outlet obstruction.

46 The Uremic State

I. **Background.** In addition to excreting nonvolatile metabolic wastes (urea, creatinine, etc.), the kidney regulates the volume of body fluids and preserves the concentration of various solutes (e.g., potassium, inorganic phosphorus, and magnesium), within narrow limits. It also maintains acid-base balance, excreting excess acid or alkali and replenishing the alkali used to buffer acid metabolic products. The kidney degrades a number of peptide hormones and synthesizes several hormones. These include: renin, which influences blood flow and mineral metabolism; 1,25-dihydroxycholecalciferol, important for skeletal mineral metabolism; and erythropoietin, which influences red blood cell production by the bone marrow. As disease processes destroy the kidney, these diverse renal functions are impaired, resulting in adverse effects in virtually every organ system (see Table 46-1). Thus, abnormalities of the neurologic, gastrointestinal, cardiovascular, hematologic, skeletal, endocrine, and integumentary systems become prominent features of chronic renal failure. However, symptoms are frequently unrecognized until 85 to 90 percent of normal renal function is lost, and certain chemical abnormalities may not appear until virtually all renal function is lost. Except for minor details, the consequences are similar for all patients experiencing progressive loss of renal mass and are independent of the type of chronic renal disease (e.g., cystic, hypertensive, infectious, obstructive, glomerulonephritis, diabetic). Indeed, while examination of renal tissue early in the disease process may show specific histologic changes, later tissue samples tend to show similar disorganization (diffuse fibrosis and atrophy with focal hypertrophy and scars) irrespective of the initial insult.

II. **Effects of chronic renal disease on renal function**

A. **General clinical observations.** The fact that symptoms and overt chemical abnormalities are so long delayed in the presence of progressive renal destruction demonstrates the remarkable capacity of the kidney to adapt. This functional deterioration and adaptation can be classified into several distinctive stages that reflect the degree of nephron loss. *Diminished renal reserve* implies function mildly reduced but sufficient to maintain a normal internal milieu. *Renal insufficiency* appears when impaired capacity first becomes evident, being manifested by mild azotemia, impaired urinary concentrating ability, or mild anemia. The stress of infection, dehydration, heart failure, trauma, and so on can greatly increase the prominence of these abnormalities. *Renal failure* is recognized when chemical abnormalities are accompanied by overt functional alterations. Renal failure is usually evident when the creatinine clearance has declined to 10 to 15 percent of the normal value (100–120 ml/min). Finally, the *uremic syndrome* is evidenced by a constellation of signs and symptoms reflecting toxinlike effects on the nervous, cardiovascular, and gastrointestinal systems that are not attributable to concurrent electrolyte, hypertensive, or hematologic abnormalities. Although glomerular filtration rate is generally less than 5 percent of normal at the onset of these symptoms, the point at which symptoms occur varies from patient to patient.

B. **Adaptation in renal failure**

1. Two theories, based on clinical observations and experimental study, help explain the adaptations by which a diseased kidney may continue to function in an orderly manner.

Table 46-1   *Systemic Effects of Chronic Renal Failure*

Neurologic
  Abnormal electroencephalogram
  Fatigue
  Insomnia or somnolence
  Headaches
  Lethargy
  Seizures
  Coma
  Depression
  Anxiety
  Psychosis
  Asterixis
  Akathisia
  Paresthesia
  Paralysis
  Muscle irritability
  Muscle weakness
Hematologic
  Anemia
  Hemolysis
  Bleeding
  Thrombasthenia
  Anergy

Gastrointestinal
  Anorexia
  Nausea
  Vomiting
  Halitosis
  Diarrhea
  Bleeding
  Ulcerations
  Parotitis
Cardiovascular
  Hypertension
  Heart failure
  Atherosclerosis
  Pericarditis
  Myocarditis
  Pulmonary edema
Integument
  Pallor
  Pigmentation
  Pruritus
  Ecchymosis
  Calcification

Endocrine-Metabolic
  Hyperparathyroidism
  Amenorrhea
  Infertility
  Impotence
  Hyperglycemia
  Hyperlipemia
Skeleton
  Osteodystrophy
Urinary
  Nocturia
  Polyuria

a. **The theory of glomerular-tubular balance** assumes that tubular reabsorption decreases as the solute load per residual nephron is increased. This applies primarily to renal sodium handling.

b. **The intact nephron hypothesis,** advanced by Bricker, states that the net function in chronic renal disease resembles that which would be expected if fewer nephrons continued to function in an appropriate manner. Consistent with this theory, several types of adaptations occur.

   (1) No tubular adaptation is noted for solutes primarily excreted by glomerular filtration, e.g., urea, creatinine.

   (2) Partial tubular adaptation, by enhanced tubular secretion or decreased reabsorption, maintains the serum concentration near normal until the glomerular filtration rate is less than 25 percent of normal (e.g., hydrogen ion, uric acid, calcium, and phosphate).

   (3) Complete tubular adaptation maintains normal balances until nearly all the nephrons are destroyed, e.g., sodium, potassium, water, magnesium.

2. **The trade-off hypothesis** implies that such adaptations or adjustments by the diseased kidney are accomplished through increased concentrations of regulatory factors, at a cost which adversely affects other organs in the body. Secondary hyperparathyroidism of chronic renal failure is the best example supporting this hypothesis. This effector of phosphate balance (parathyroid hormone [PTH]) reduces renal reabsorption of phosphate. The trade-off for this balance is the parathyroid effect on the skeleton (osteodystrophy) and perhaps the anemia, neurologic abnormalities, cardiac dysfunction, and calcium deposition noted in patients with chronic renal failure.

III. **Pathogenesis of the uremic syndrome.** Many of the signs and symptoms that mark the uremic syndrome are of obscure origin. Suggested mechanisms for these clinical features include retention of toxic metabolic wastes, depletion or impaired synthesis of essential metabolites, and enhanced synthesis or impaired degradation of bioactive substances participating in the trade-off scheme of adaptation.

   A. **Toxicity** is demonstrated experimentally with high concentrations of small-molecular-weight (<500 daltons) metabolic wastes.

    1. Phenols, guanidines, and indoles have produced weight loss, anemia, hyperlipemia, neural toxicity, nausea, reduced oxygen consumption, enzyme inhibition, coagulation defects, leukocyte impairment, glucose intolerance, and impaired immunoglobulin synthesis.

    2. Phosphates and sulfates can impair folic acid metabolism and are associated with anemia, hyperparathyroidism, and bone destruction.

    3. Aliphatic amines increase hepatic acetylation of several drugs, a common feature of uremia, and may be associated with asterixis.

Other potentially toxic substances include the middle-molecular-weight substances (500–5,000 daltons) that are identified only in the plasma of uremic subjects. Clinically, these compounds correlate with the neurologic, gastrointestinal, and cardiovascular signs and symptoms that characterize the uremic syndrome.

   B. **Nutrient depletion or impaired synthesis** of bioactive compounds is associated with several problems also noted in uremia.

    1. Caloric malnutrition is accompanied by apathy, lethargy, cold intolerance, and growth failure.

    2. Protein starvation is followed by hypoproteinemia, hypoaminoacidemia, anemia, muscle wasting, and neuropathy.

    3. Folic acid and pyridoxine deficiencies promote anemia, impaired neurologic function, and altered immune responses.

    4. Depressed synthesis of somatomedin, vitamin D, and erythropoietin is accompanied by growth failure, osteomalacia, and anemia, all features of uremia.

   C. **Enhanced synthesis or impaired degradation of bioactive compounds** that might become toxic and contribute to uremic symptoms includes:

    1. **Vitamin A** excess produces irritability, itching, and hyperostosis; it may be complicated by fractures.

    2. **Cortisol** accelerates tissue catabolism, impairs glucose tolerance, and may promote hypertension.

    3. **Gastrin** levels, increased in uremia, promote gastrointestinal bleeding.

    4. **Insulin,** also increased in uremia, stimulates hepatic triglyceride synthesis, promoting hyperlipemia.

    5. **Parathyroid hormone** promotes osteodystrophy and soft tissue calcification and may be toxic to cardiac and nervous tissue.

    6. **Natriuretic hormone substances** may diffusely impair sodium-transport enzymes, with numerous adverse effects on cellular metabolism and integrity.

IV. **Effects of dialysis in uremia.** A major source of support for the concept that retention of water-soluble toxic wastes is involved in the etiology of uremic symptoms is the effect of dialysis on many of these symptoms. Dialysis removes many metabolic waste products and corrects alterations in the concentrations of ionic substances normally present in the body fluids. Symptoms which are corrected or improved on dialysis include:

encephalopathy, volume-dependent hypertension, pulmonary edema, pericarditis, platelet and leukocyte dysfunction, anorexia, nausea, vomiting, gastrointestinal bleeding, uremic halitosis, hyperkalemia, hyponatremia, carbohydrate intolerance, and malnutrition. Other symptoms do not improve or actually progress in many patients supported by chronic dialysis care. Some of these progressive uremic problems include renal osteodystrophy, growth impairment, weakness, anemia, peripheral neuropathy, atherosclerosis, hyperlipidemia, hyperparathyroidism, and vitamin D deficiency.

V. Clinical example of chronic renal failure

A. Description. A 23-year-old female computer programmer was found to have asymptomatic hypertension and azotemia (BUN, 35 mg/100 ml; creatinine, 2.8 mg/100 ml) on an employment examination. She had no known history of prior renal disease but had noticed nocturia during the previous 4 years. An intravenous pyelogram was normal. Her blood pressure was initially controlled with diuretic agents. Although feeling mildly fatigued, she remained working and socially active until after some dental surgery, when she experienced progressive nausea and occasional vomiting. Evaluation showed: BUN, 192 mg/100 ml; creatinine, 12 mg/100 ml; inorganic phosphate, 10.5 mg/100 ml; calcium, 9.0 mg/100 ml; uric acid, 10.6 mg/100 ml; and hemoglobin, 6.5 g/100 ml. Her examination was remarkable for a blood pressure of 170/100 mm Hg, pallor, a pericardial friction rub, excoriations over the arms and legs, and hypoactive reflexes at the ankles. She appeared to be having difficulty concentrating on various topics discussed in her history. Urinalysis disclosed 3^+ protein, 20 RBC, and occasional WBCs/HPF as well as broad granular and waxy casts containing occasional cells. Additional studies included echographic measurement of the kidneys (8.5 cm) and an echocardiogram showing a small posterior pericardial effusion. A kidney biopsy was not done because of the small size of the remnant kidney tissue.

B. Discussion

1. This case illustrates the subtle nature of the onset of chronic renal failure and the fact that progression of symptoms can be fairly rapid. Certain types of disease may proceed much less rapidly, for example, polycystic disease may progress for 20 to 40 years.

2. An early clue to the presence of renal disease was a history of nocturia. This occurred because of a decrease in urine-concentrating ability. Later, diluting ability may become impaired as well.

3. The fact that the patient remained active with few symptoms until nitrogenous waste concentrations had increased tenfold points out the capacity of all body systems to adapt to the progressive burdens imposed by chronic renal failure.

4. Often, overt symptomatic renal failure (uremia) follows a period of stress such as the dental surgical procedure, where infection, use of toxic antibiotics, or anorexia promotes rapid increases in waste product levels because of protein catabolism.

5. The laboratory data in this case are typical of chronic renal failure, regardless of the cause or rate of development.

Questions

Select the single best answer.

1. Select the true statement regarding the retention of phosphate, magnesium, and uric acid that occurs in chronic renal failure:

a. Serum levels rise in proportion to the reduction in glomerular filtration rate.
b. Retention of these ions is modified by tubular functional adaptation.
c. These ions are directly responsible for uremic symptoms.
d. Retention occurs only in the preterminal phase.
e. Retention is of no pathophysiologic significance.

2. The clinical features of the uremic syndrome may be related to which of the following:
   a. Accumulation of toxic metabolic waste products.
   b. Malnutrition.
   c. Alterations in biosynthesis.
   d. Increased hormone levels.
   e. All of the above.

47 Metabolic Bone Disease

I. **Introduction.** The most obvious function of the endoskeleton is to provide structural support and protection for internal organs. Such a durable frame allows locomotion across the surface of the land, preventing the natural action of gravity from collapsing the protoplasmic mass. A less evident, but vital, role for the mammalian endoskeleton is its function as a mineral reservoir. Approximately 99 percent of total body calcium and 85 percent of phosphorus are located in bone. In addition, large quantities of other substances—such as magnesium, sodium, and carbonate—are contained in bone.

The endoskeleton is often incorrectly conceptualized as a static edifice. However, the endoskeleton is constantly being remodeled and repaired. While structure remains an important function of the endoskeleton, this must be accomplished even as minerals are deposited and removed. Growth must be accomplished without an alteration of form, and repair of microfractures is in all likelihood a continuous process.

II. **Normal bone physiology**

   A. **Bone matrix.** Collagen is the principal organic component of bone. Other organic constituents include glycoprotein, protein polysaccharides, and lipids. Bone collagen, as well as the collagen of skin and tendons, consists of two identical alpha-1 chains and an alpha-2 chain. These three chains are arranged together as a triple helix. In alpha chains every third amino acid is glycine, and approximately one-fourth are either proline or hydroxyproline. Aside from collagen, elastin, and the C1q component of complement, hydroxyproline is not found in other proteins. Once the collagen is extruded from the cell, it becomes the principal component of the unmineralized bone matrix known as osteoid. When viewed with polarized light, normal collagen (osteoid) possesses a lamellar arrangement (see Fig. 47-1). However, accelerated deposition results in a disorganized pattern, and when viewed with polarized light, a haphazard or woven arrangement can be appreciated (see Fig. 47-2).

   B. **Bone mineral.** At the interface of osteoid and mineralized bone, the process of mineralization occurs. The precise details of the factors promoting and inhibiting mineralization still require considerable elaboration. Nonetheless, it does appear that the initial phase results in deposition of amorphous calcium phosphate, which upon completion of the mineralization process emerges as hydroxyapatite, $Ca_{10}(PO_4)_6(OH)_2$. The apatite crystals are small and furnish a large surface for exchange of various elements with an affinity for bone. In addition to the actual components of the apatite crystals, bone possesses large quantities of sodium, carbonate, potassium, and magnesium. Exposure to toxic substances such as strontium, lead, plutonium, uranium, radium, and aluminum will also result in increased bone content of these elements.

   C. **Bone cells**

      1. **Osteoblasts.** The osteoblasts are the cells responsible for the synthesis of bone matrix that is deposited as osteoid. The osteoblasts probably originate from the flat cells lining the bone surfaces. When active, the osteoblasts are cuboidal or columnar, mononuclear cells that are present in a monolayer along the surface of

Figure 47-1   *Normal bone is arranged in a lamellar pattern when viewed with polarized light (×200).*

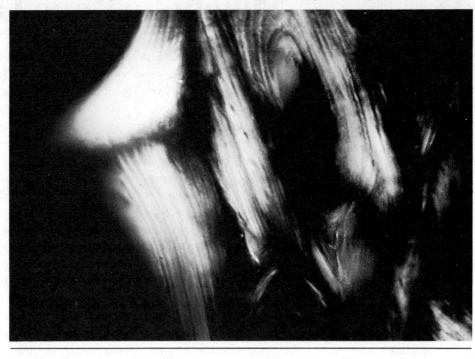

Figure 47-2   *Accelerated deposition of bone results in a disorganized pattern. When viewed with polarized light, a haphazard or woven arrangement is observed (×200).*

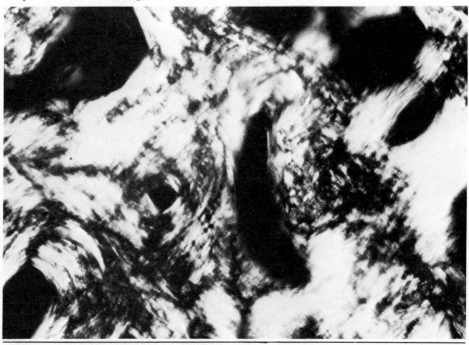

Figure 47-3

The osteoblast is a mononuclear cell that synthesizes and secretes collagen. Cuboidal osteoblasts (A) are present along the surface of an osteoid seam (B) (× 1200).

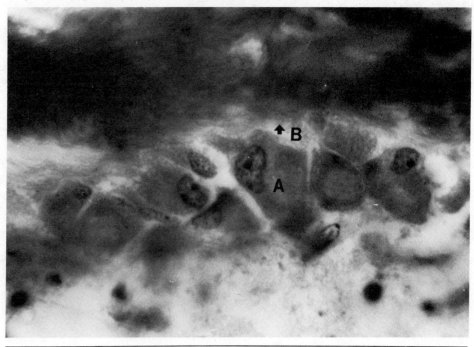

osteoid (see Fig. 47-3). In certain pathologic alterations of bone resulting in accelerated deposition, the monolayer may be replaced by osteoblasts several layers deep.

2. **Osteocytes.** The osteocytes are the cells within the mineralized bone (see Fig. 47-4). They are derived from osteoblasts which have penetrated from the bone surface into the mineralized bone. One of their outstanding features is an extensive canal system crossing an enormous surface of bone and forming a syncytium. While the osteoblast is responsible for bone deposition and the osteoclast for bone resorption, the exact role of the osteocyte in these processes remains controversial. In response to a hormonal stimulus, such as parathyroid hormone, the lacuna (nucleus) of the osteocyte will increase in size. Thus, little doubt exists that these cells are active and responsive to stimuli, but their function in bone deposition and resorption requires further study.

3. **Osteoclasts.** The osteoclasts are single- to multi-nucleated giant cells capable of resorbing bone (see Fig. 47-5). Their precursor is probably cells of the macrophage line. Osteoclasts are migratory cells rich in enzymes such as acid phosphatase and collagenases. Parathyroid hormone both activates the osteoclast and results in the migration of the osteoclast to the mineralized bone surface. The dissolution of bone by osteoclasts can be visualized, but the mechanism of mineral transport is unknown.

III. **Metabolic bone diseases.** In these disorders, the actions of vitamin D metabolites, parathyroid hormone, thyroid hormone, and probably calcium and phosphorus are very important in the pathogenesis of the bone disease. However, since the hormones and minerals involved in bone homeostasis are interrelated, a deficiency or excess in one may frequently result in major alterations in another. Thus, in osteomalacia secondary to malabsorption, bone histology generally reveals both evidence of de-

Figure 47-4   *The osteocyte is present within mineralized bone. A characteristic feature includes an extensive system of canals (canaliculi) (×500).*

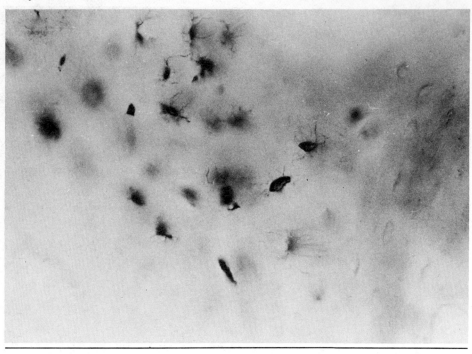

Figure 47-5   *The osteoclast is a multinucleated cell capable of bone resorption. Many large osteoclasts are observed within a resorption cavity (×500).*

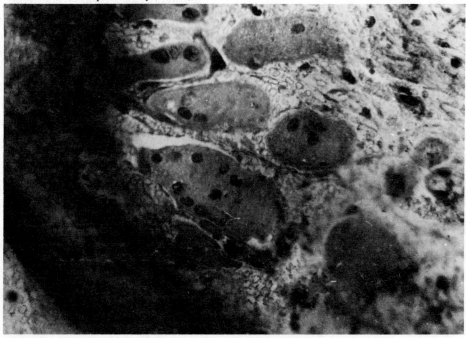

creased mineralization secondary to low levels of 25-hydroxycholecalciferol $(25(OH)D_3)$ and bone-marrow fibrosis secondary to a compensatory parathyroid hormone response. In addition to the interactions of the hormonal and mineral influences, the clinical expression of the skeletal disorder may depend upon age. While malabsorption acquired in the adult will frequently result in osteomalacia, the same deficiency in the child will generally result in rickets. In a similar manner, metabolic bone disease in children with chronic renal failure may be different from that observed in adults. Therefore, it is important to realize that the same deficiency may result in a clinically different disorder, depending upon the age of the afflicted individual; also, the histologic expression of a bone disease may be identical even though the etiologic factors are different.

A. **Rickets.** Rickets is a disease of children in which the primary problem is a failure to mineralize bone. The etiology is a deficiency of vitamin D. Once a common disease because of inadequate exposure to sunlight and intake of vitamin D, dietary rickets is rarely seen in technologically advanced countries because of fortification of some food products with vitamin D. However, rickets, secondary to vitamin D deficiency, may be observed in children with malabsorption syndromes. In these disorders, there exists an inability to absorb vitamin D and the enterohepatic circulation of $25(OH)D_3$ results in additional losses. Another cause of rickets is anticonvulsant therapy, which probably results in accelerated metabolism of the $25(OH)D_3$ produced by the liver, leading to deficiency of this vitamin D metabolite.

The vitamin D deficiency in rickets results in a failure to mineralize the deposited osteoid. Histologically, broad irregular osteoid seams that are not mineralizing are characteristically found. In addition, the mineralization defect also involves the growth plate (junction of epiphysis and metaphysis), resulting in structural instability and bowing of the long bones. Treatment is predicated upon correction of the underlying problem and providing adequate vitamin D supplementation.

1. **Vitamin D–resistant rickets (X-linked hypophosphatemic rickets).** Vitamin D–resistant rickets is a familial disorder and is transmitted by an X-linked dominant gene. The clinical presentation of patients includes short stature and bony deformities similar to other forms of rickets; the only exception is that muscular weakness is not a characteristic finding. The biochemical hallmark is severe hypophosphatemia. Histologically, a profound mineralization defect is found. However, blood levels of 1,25-dihydroxycholecalciferol $(1,25(OH)_2D_3)$ are usually normal. Recent therapeutic trials employing high-dose $1,25(OH)_2D_3$ or $1,25(OH)_2D_3$ plus phosphates have resulted in marked improvement.

2. **Vitamin D–dependent rickets.** This autosomal recessive disease is also refractory to physiologic doses of vitamin D. However, the levels of $1,25(OH)_2D_3$ are low, and the pathogenesis is probably secondary to the lack of 1-alpha-hydroxylase, the enzyme which converts $25(OH)D_3$ to $1,25(OH)_2D_3$. Physiologic doses of $1,25(OH)_2D_3$ produce healing.

B. **Osteomalacia.** Osteomalacia is characterized by a failure to mineralize bone. The prime difference from rickets is that the growth process has been completed. The cause of osteomalacia is the lack of or an abnormal processing of vitamin D. Etiologies include (1) deficient intake of vitamin D or lack of sunlight exposure (uncommon in technologically advanced societies except in the elderly); (2) malabsorption syndrome; (3) increased metabolism of $25(OH)D_3$ secondary to anticonvulsants or loss of $25(OH)D_3$ secondary to nephrotic syndrome; and (4) defective production of $1,25(OH)_2D_3$ secondary to a presumed inhibitor (tumor induced). The most common cause of overt clinical disease is malabsorption syndrome. In addition to low levels of $25(OH)D_3$, secondary hyperparathyroidism is commonly observed.

The primary criterion for the diagnosis of osteomalacia is the histologic demonstration of defective mineralization. This is best ascertained by the use of a tetracycline label. Because of certain physicochemical properties, tetracycline is localized at the interface of osteoid and mineralized bone only with active mineralization. Hence, in osteomalacia, the deposition of tetracycline is diminished. When secondary hyperparathyroidism is an accompanying feature, other histologic characteristics include bone-marrow fibrosis and increased osteoclastic activity.

C. **Renal osteodystrophy.** The metabolic bone disease associated with renal failure is complex and multifactorial. The interaction among serum calcium and phosphorus, parathyroid hormone, vitamin D metabolites, collagen maturation, and uremic toxins is incompletely understood. Before renal-failure patients become dialysis dependent, major histologic bone changes are seen. A prime stimulus for secondary hyperparathyroidism is believed to be phosphate retention. The traditional concept holds that phosphate retention results in hypocalcemia; the hypocalcemia stimulates parathyroid hormone production, which normalizes both serum calcium and phosphorus (increased excretion) but results in a higher baseline parathyroid hormone concentration. Another major contributing factor in the etiology of skeletal disease concerns the metabolism of vitamin D. The kidney is responsible for the production of both $1,25(OH)_2D_3$ and 24,25-dihydroxycholecalciferol. Decreased levels of these metabolites affect calcium absorption from the gut (especially $1,25(OH)_2D_3$) and may affect bone formation and resorption. Other factors, such as skeletal resistance to the calcemic action of parathyroid hormone and altered collagen synthesis, are also major components in the evolution of renal osteodystrophy.

In patients with end-stage renal disease requiring regular dialysis, a spectrum of disease is observed. Osteitis fibrosa—characterized by increased bone resorption, extensive osteoclastic and osteoblastic activity, and bone-marrow fibrosis—is a common finding. This group of patients will generally have high levels of parathyroid hormone as measured by radioimmunoassay. The other major disorder is osteomalacia. The histologic features include extensive and broad osteoid seams devoid of cellular activity, minimal osteoclastic activity, and in general, the absence of bone-marrow fibrosis. Tetracycline, given as a label of mineralization, will reveal almost the complete cessation of bone formation. The osteomalacic patients are characterized by levels of parathyroid hormone that range from undetectable to only minimally elevated.

Osteitis fibrosa is generally believed to result from the high levels of parathyroid hormone. As already outlined, multiple factors may produce a state of secondary hyperparathyroidism. However, with osteomalacia the etiology is less well understood. Since all dialysis patients probably have absent or decreased circulating levels of

$1,25(OH)_2D_3$, this deficiency does not explain why only some patients have osteomalacia. Also most osteomalacic patients have normal levels of $25(OH)D_3$. Recently, aluminum has been suggested as a cause of osteomalacia. The presumed source of the aluminum is the dialysis water supply and the phosphate-binding antacids which are usually recommended in these patients.

D. **Primary hyperparathyroidism.** In primary hyperparathyroidism, the parathyroid hormone levels are increased, which often results in hypercalcemia and hypophosphatemia. The latter as a consequence of the phosphaturic effect of parathyroid hormone. There are two distinct groups of patients with primary hyperparathyroidism—one with extensive bone disease and the other with renal calculi. The group with calculi have increased intestinal calcium absorption and marked elevations of $1,25(OH)_2D_3$, whereas the patients with bone disease have neither increased intestinal calcium absorption nor elevated levels of $1,25(OH)_2D_3$. The reasons for the existence of two separate groups with similar levels of increased parathyroid hormone is unclear.

With respect to bone histology, increased bone resorption, bone marrow fibrosis, and increased osteoblastic activity are frequently present, but generally the involvement is localized to small areas and may be recognized only when quantitative analysis is undertaken.

E. **Osteoporosis.** The term *osteoporosis* must be differentiated from *osteopenia,* a general term meaning a loss of bone mass. *Osteoporosis* is accurately defined as a loss of bone mass with a normal ratio of unmineralized matrix (osteoid) to mineralized bone. Conversely, other disease processes, such as osteomalacia or osteitis fibrosa, may result in osteopenia, but such osteopenia should not be considered osteoporosis.

Although there are several causes of it in the child or young adult, osteoporosis is primarily a disease of aging, particularly in females. In both males and females, an increase in skeletal mass normally occurs through approximately the third decade. After age 30 to 40 years there appears to be a decrease in skeletal mass of approximately 8 percent per decade in women and 3 percent per decade in men. After the menopause, the loss in bone mass in females is accelerated. In addition, the maximal bone mass achieved in young adults is greater in males than females. Considering these factors, the higher incidence of osteoporosis in women is not surprising. Two basic questions which should be addressed concern (1) finding a mechanism to prevent loss that appears to be part of the normal aging process and (2) discovering a means to increase bone mass in the individual with severe osteoporosis.

F. **Hyperthyroidism.** Thyroid hormone is not often considered a hormone with specific skeletal actions. However, hypercalcemia occurs in hyperthyroidism, and bone turnover has been found to be increased with hyperthyroidism. Both bone resorption and formation are increased, and osteopenia is common. In addition, it has been shown that thyroid hormone in bone culture can directly increase bone resorption. From this evidence, it would appear that thyroid hormone has a direct effect on bone and calcium metabolism.

IV. **Clinical example of metabolic bone disease**

A. **Description.** A 40-year-old woman experienced 9 months of diarrhea, lost 25 pounds, and developed diffuse musculoskeletal pain during the 3 months immediately before her clinic appointment. Prior to the onset of diarrhea, the woman had been in excellent health. When seen by her physician, she had difficulty arising from a chair and experienced musculoskeletal pain only with movement. The patient was admitted to the hospital for evaluation. The admission chest x-ray revealed several rib fractures. Laboratory tests documented the presence of intestinal malabsorption. To evaluate the reason for musculoskeletal pain and the nontraumatic rib fractures, an anterior iliac crest bone biopsy was obtained. Additional tests included plasma parathyroid hormone (PTH) and 25(OH)D$_3$ and 24-hour urine for creatinine and phosphorus.

Lab results

Serum calcium	7.2 mg/dl
Serum phosphorus	1.9 mg/dl
Serum albumin	2.9 g/dl
Plasma PTH	1.1 ng/ml (normal, <0.5)
25(OH)D$_3$	4 ng/ml (normal, 15–80)
Tubular reabsorption of phosphorus	55%

Bone biopsy report showed a marked increase in amount of trabecular surface osteoid, and a moderate increase in osteoid seam width. There was also an increase in both osteoblastic and osteoclastic activity. Areas of bone-marrow fibrosis were present where cellular activity was increased. Mineralization, as assessed by tetracycline labeling, was decreased.

B. Discussion

1. Malabsorption was documented during the hospital admission, and the clinical history suggests its presence for at least 9 months. The presence of diffuse musculoskeletal pain with malabsorption leads the physician to consider the possibility of osteomalacia.

2. The characteristic pain of osteomalacia includes a muscular component in addition to skeletal pain. Typically, the patient complains of pain mostly with movement and not at rest. In addition, an unexplained profound muscular weakness is often an accompanying finding.

3. Spontaneous, nontraumatic fractures of the ribs or pelvis are frequently seen with osteomalacia. In some osteomalacic patients, osteopenia will be an additional finding, but not always. The fractures probably occur because effective bone remodeling ceases in osteomalacia, and repair of naturally occurring microfractures cannot be accomplished.

4. Several laboratory results deserve comment. The serum calcium was decreased because of (a) decreased calcium absorption in the gut and (b) the diminished ability to liberate calcium from bone. In addition, 40 percent of serum calcium is bound to albumin, and decreased serum albumin will result in a lower total serum calcium. The hypophosphatemia may also be secondary to decreased absorption and ineffective bone resorption, but in addition, secondary hyperparathyroidism results in excessive phosphaturia. Tubular reabsorption of phosphorus is an index of renal phosphate handling. A value less than 85 percent, in the presence of hypophosphatemia, is distinctly abnormal. The secondary hyper-

parathyroidism is most likely to have occurred in response to the hypocalcemia.

5. The 25(OH)D$_3$ level is markedly reduced and is a major cause of the osteomalacia. The principal sources of vitamin D are dietary and sunlight activation of 7-dehydrocholesterol present in the skin. Since vitamin D is a fat-soluble vitamin, fat malabsorption will preclude effective intestinal transport. However, the principal source of vitamin D occurs as a result of cutaneous photoactivation, followed by transport to the liver. Thus, after conversion to 25(OH)D$_3$, an enterohepatic circulation of this metabolite ensues. Hence, with malabsorption, loss of 25(OH)D$_3$ synthesized in the skin may also occur.

Questions

Select the single best answer.

1. Which of the following is *not* a factor involved in the evolution of renal osteodystrophy?
   a. Phosphate retention.
   b. High PTH levels.
   c. Altered collagen synthesis.
   d. Increased levels of 24,25-dihydroxycholecalciferol.
   e. Skeletal resistance to the calcemic action of PTH.
2. Which of the following statements about osteoporosis is false?
   a. Osteoporosis is a loss of bone mass with a normal ratio of unmineralized matrix to mineralized bone.
   b. *Osteopenia* is another name for osteoporosis, and the terms can be used interchangeably.
   c. Osteoporosis is more frequently observed in females than males.
   d. After the third decade there is a decrease in skeletal mass of 8 percent per decade in females.
   e. Menopause results in an accelerated loss of skeletal mass.

Renal Cell Carcinoma: Mechanisms of Clinical Manifestations

I. **Background.** Renal cell carcinomas are also called hypernephromas because of the similarity of the tumors to adrenocortical tissue. They constitute approximately 90 percent of the malignant renal neoplasms and account for roughly 2 percent of cancer deaths in the United States. The death rate appears to be increasing. Roughly twice as many men as women develop the tumor. Possible predisposing factors include cigarette smoking and obesity. Tumors may involve either kidney and typically involve a single pole. They arise from proximal renal tubular epithelium. A favorable prognosis is implied by cystic degeneration and calcification (spontaneous degeneration). Extension into the renal vein does not notably affect prognosis, but extension through the capsule and distant metastases is relatively ominous. Metastatic spread is most common to lungs, bone, and liver. This malignancy has long stirred the interest of physicians because of the multiple clinical manifestations that it may produce. The following discussion will focus on current understanding of the mechanisms of these clinical features.

II. **Clinical manifestations due to the physical effects of the tumor**
  A. **Hematuria.** Tumor invasion of the collecting system results in microscopic or, less commonly, gross bleeding.
  B. **Pain.** Pain occurs with stretching of the collecting system or capsule, or from obstruction of the urine flow due to blood clots or, rarely, tumor fragments. Pain may also occur if the tumor bleeds into itself and the surrounding tissue.
  C. **Abdominal or lumbar mass.** With enlargement of the tumor, a mass may be palpated in the abdomen.
  D. **Varicocele.** Because the left spermatic vein joins the left renal vein, invasion of the renal vein by tumor may result in the development of a left varicocele.
  E. **Edema.** Extension of tumor or thrombus into the inferior vena cava may occlude the cava, resulting in massive leg edema. The hepatic vein may also become occluded.
  F. **Bruit.** Renal arteriovenous fistulas may occur with this highly vascular tumor, and this can cause a bruit over the tumor. In addition, the fistula may result in high-output congestive heart failure or hypertension.

III. **Clinical manifestations due to production of hormone-like substances**
  A. **Polycythemia** occurs in a small number of patients. It is due to secretion of erythropoietin by the tumor. Eosinophilia, leukocytosis, and thrombocytosis have also been reported.
  B. **Hypertension** due to renin production by the tumor is rarely seen.
  C. **Hypercalcemia** may occur for several reasons.
    1. The most common cause is metastatic destruction of bone, with calcium liberation.
    2. The tumor may produce prostaglandins, which can cause resorption of bone and, thus, hypercalcemia.

3. A cause which is now largely disproved is that parathyroid hormone (PTH) or a PTH-like substance may be produced by the tumor, resulting in hypercalcemia.

D. Cushing's syndrome due to production of adrenocorticotropic hormone (ACTH) may occur. This is manifested primarily by hypokalemic metabolic alkalosis.

E. Other unusual manifestations referable to hormone production by the tumor include:

1. **Galactorrhea** due to prolactin production.
2. **Hypotension** due to prostaglandin production.
3. **Feminization or masculinization** due to gonadotropin production.

IV. Clinical manifestations due to immunologic mechanisms. Glomerulonephritis due to immune complexes has been reported. Tumor-specific antibody and antigen have been demonstrated in some cases. The glomerulopathy may be manifested with proteinuria, hematuria, red cell casts, and low serum complement levels.

V. Clinical manifestations with unknown pathogenesis

A. Peripheral neuropathy or myopathy

B. Thrombophlebitis

C. Reversible liver function abnormalities and hepatomegaly occur in 15 percent of patients, in the *absence* of liver metastases. These include hypoalbuminemia, elevated alkaline phosphatase and indirect bilirubin, hypercholesterolemia, prolongation of the prothrombin time, and hyperglobulinemia (especially alpha-2 and gamma fractions). The pathologic findings in the liver are those of a chronic nonspecific hepatitis, with proliferation of Kupffer cells, hepatocellular degeneration, and periportal inflammation.

D. Fever. Fever may occur, unassociated with hemorrhage, infection, or tumor necrosis. This symptom occurs in about 25 percent of patients. Endogenous pyrogen has been demonstrated in tissue slices from some of these patients.

E. Elevated erythrocyte sedimentation rate. Elevated erythrocyte sedimentation rate occurs in 50 percent of patients and returns to normal after tumor removal. Later elevation implies metastases. The mechanisms have not been established, but may be due to coating of the red cells by glycoprotein resulting in aggregation and faster precipitation of the red cells.

F. Anemia. Anemia is common in renal cell carcinoma. It may be iron-deficient anemia due to hematuria but usually is normocytic, with increased iron in blood and bone marrow. Again, the mechanism for the latter is uncertain, but may be bone-marrow suppression due to a toxin produced by the tumor.

VI. Clinical example of renal cell carcinoma

A. Description. A 68-year-old man entered the hospital because of lethargy and pain in the lumbar spine despite pain medicine. Past history and review of systems were noncontributory. Physical examination was unremarkable except for slight tenderness in the right midabdomen, which was also obese. Neurologic exam was unremarkable except for obtundation.

Laboratory results

Hb	16.1 g/100 ml	WBC	$13.5 \times 10^3/mm^3$
Hct	48.2%		

Urinalysis
Protein   2+
RBC/HPF   40–50
Serum Chemistries

Na	136 mEq/L	Ca	19.7 mg/100 ml
K	3.2 mEq/L	P	3.3 mg/100 ml
Cl	93 mEq/L	Total protein	8.5 mg/100 ml
HCO_3	35 mEq/L	Albumin	3.7 mg/100 ml
BUN	53 mg/100 ml	Uric acid	10.0 mg/100 ml
Creatinine	2.7 mg/100 ml		

Chest x-ray was normal, except for erosion of one rib; skull x-rays showed several radiolucent areas in the calvarium.

B. Discussion

1. This patient demonstrated several signs and symptoms that would lead to the diagnosis of malignancy: eroded rib, skull lesions, decreased mental status, and bone pain.

2. Hypercalcemia in this setting with a high globulin and normal to low albumin could suggest multiple myeloma. However, serum protein electrophoresis was normal except for an increase in alpha-2 globulin. Hypercalcemia could be due to primary hyperparathyroidism, but the bone lesions on x-ray were not those of hyperparathyroidism. Cancer can also be associated with severe hypercalcemia. Lung cancer is a possible candidate, but this patient's chest x-ray was clear. Another tumor that can cause hypercalcemia is renal cell carcinoma.

3. The presence of red cells in the urine dictated an intravenous pyelogram, which showed a large right kidney with decreased function. The collecting system was not seen well, but appeared to be distorted in the right lower pole. The presence of a tumor was confirmed by arteriogram. Bone scan showed multiple areas of uptake, consistent with metastatic cancer.

4. The hypercalcemia could be due to a hormonal effect of the tumor or direct bony destruction from metastasis. The bone-scan results suggested the latter mechanism but did not exclude the former.

5. The presence of widespread metastasis indicated a poor prognosis.

Questions

Select the single best answer.

1. The most common cause of hypercalcemia in a patient with hypernephroma is:
   a. Immobilization.
   b. Prostaglandin production.
   c. Bone invasion.
   d. Parathyroid hormone production.
   e. Thyroid hormone production.

2. Which of the following serum electrolytes would be likely in a patient with renal cell carcinoma?
   a. K^+ 4.0, Cl^- 100, HCO_3^- 25
   b. K^+ 5.7, Cl^- 114, HCO_3^- 15
   c. K^+ 2.8, Cl^- 90, HCO_3^- 35
   d. *a* and *b*
   e. *a* and *c*

IX Neurology and Pain

C. G. Gunn
John W. Nelson

49 Pain

I. Significance of pain. Pain is the conscious interpretation of sensory signals from nociceptors that warn of potentially injurious bodily changes from either the internal or external environment.

  A. Acute pain is an early warning system prompting the organism to avoid or alter the noxious stimuli—in other words, to fight or flee. It is a primary survival mechanism and is best treated by relieving the underlying cause. In people with congenital absence of pain, who have no sense of acute pain, the small continually recurring inflammations and injuries of daily living are unnoticed and result in severe infections and permanent injuries, destructive and crippling arthritis, blindness, and potentially early death.

  B. Chronic pain is defined as a persistent or frequently present sensation of hurting that has not been relieved for months or longer. It has lost its biologic function; no longer a symptom, it tends to become the disease itself. It eventually brings severe physical, emotional, social, and financial decompensating stresses on the patient, his or her family, and society as a whole. It is regarded as intractable pain when it can no longer be prevented except for very short periods.

II. Acute pain mechanisms

  A. Nociceptors are the specialized terminal networks of the free-nerve endings of pain fibers. These receptors are associated with vascular beds and sympathetic plexes in every part of the body except brain tissue. They are activated by mechanical, thermal, and chemical stimuli.

    1. The nociceptors in smooth and striated muscles are activated by persistent ischemia or excessive contractile or stretched tone.

    2. All nociceptors are prompted to fire by release of endogenous substances at injury sites (K^+, H^+, bradykinin, histamine, prostaglandins, and serotonin). Prostaglandins can either directly excite nociceptors or sensitize them to the other agents listed, especially serotonin. These mediators can act synergistically, in concert, or alone.

    3. Heat not only activates nociceptor discharge but also potentiates chemically and mechanically mediated nociceptor discharge.

    4. Sympathetic efferent fibers facilitate nociceptor stimulation indirectly by producing vasospasm in the microcirculation and directly by noradrenalin release, which potentiates nociceptor free-nerve endings.

    5. Therapeutic efforts at peripheral sites include mild stretching exercises to relax spastic muscles, cold packs to decrease early pain and inflammation, and anti-inflammatory compounds, which block prostaglandin synthesis at nociceptor sites.

  B. Afferent pain fibers. These are of two kinds; the lightly myelinated A-delta fibers carry sharp, stabbing, easily localizable pain. These are common in the external somatic nerves. The small, slower-conducting, unmyelinated C fibers carry information eventually perceived as dull, burning, and diffusely localizable pain. These afferent pain fibers enter the dorsal roots of the spinal cord and synapse in the dorsal horn. Many of these fibers release substance P as a nociceptive neurotransmitter. Under pathologic conditions of trauma or nerve compression, afferent nerves may themselves be stimulated, producing pain that is perceived as originating at the distal peripheral origin of those nerves.

C. Spinal cord circuitry. The synapses and neuronal interaction in the dorsal horn permit the first opportunity for modification of transmission by both facilitating and inhibiting mechanisms. These include local interactions as well as descending influences that are related to attentiveness, alertness, orientation, past memories, and judgement.

1. At dorsal column synapses, C and A-delta neurons from peripheral nerves are excitatory to the next pain pathway neuron as they discharge acetylcholine and substance P.

2. At the same synapse, descending neurons from the brain stem and locally excited internuncial neurons block pain impulses. These inhibitory neurons possess enkephalinergic, noradrenergic, and serotoninergic transmitter systems that are inhibitory to pain information transfer. These mechanisms permit behavioral and biofeedback influences to modify acute and chronic pain at the spinal cord level. It is interesting to note that serotonin is a pain facilitator at the peripheral nociceptor but is an inhibitor at central pain synapses in the brain stem and spinal cord. Similarly, noradrenalin systems are central inhibitors to pain and also depress blood pressure. Peripheral noradrenergic sympathetics, however, are pain potentiators and raise blood pressure by arterial vasoconstriction. When large somatosensory afferent fibers are fired into the dorsal column neuronal pools—as a result of either a transcutaneous nerve stimulator, acupuncture, or counterirritation by the patient's own devices—the small fiber pain input is blocked by activation of inhibitory neuronal systems, many of which are enkephalinergic. This is a physiologic gate mechanism, an important natural mechanism of pain modification.

3. **Brain stem pain pathways** are twofold.

   a. A large fiber system with few interruptions progresses to the thalamic nuclei and then to cortex through the lemniscal system. This classic sensory pathway subserves sharp pain and the ability to localize and recognize pain and thereby avoid injury.

   b. The small-fiber, slow-traveling, multisynaptic pathways run through the reticular formation into the brain stem, hypothalamus, and the limbic nuclei and forebrain cortex. This system influences the expression of acute pain in terms of tolerance, behavior, and sympathetic autonomic responses shown in Table 49-1. It is most important in chronic pain, mediating the associated autonomic vegetative responses, the emotional behavior, and lowered pain thresholds which often occur. It is referred to as an affectational and motivational nociceptor system.

   c. The mesencephalic periaqueductal gray formation (PAG) has many autonomic and sensory functional relationships with the reticular formation and its ascending and descending connections. This area has high enkephalin levels. The cells in periaqueductal gray, dorsal horn of spinal cord, and medial raphe nuclei also have specific receptor sites for enkephalins. Exogenous narcotic agents as well as narcotic antagonists, such as naloxone, also bind to these neuronal receptor sites. Opiates and opioids block pain. Naloxone therefore blocks inhibition and increases pain. The effect of morphine and natural endogenous enkephalins and endorphins in blocking pain and altering the autonomic responses undoubtedly involves these pathways.

Affective State	Acute Pain	Subacute Pain	Chronic Pain
Anxiety ⇌	Increased heart rate Increased blood pressure Increased cardiac output Increased pupillary dilation Palmar sweating Hyperventilation Escape behavior		
Anxiety-depression ⇌		*Continued* intermittent sympathetic manifestations mixed with early onset of behavioral (vegetative) changes	
Depression ⇌			Sleep disturbances Appetite changes Constipation Psychomotor retardation Decreased pain tolerance Irritability Withdrawal Abnormal illness behavior

Table 49-1. *Affective Psychophysiologic Signs Associated with Pain Disorders*

    d. These inhibitory pathways in the periaqueductal gray, reticular formation, raphe nuclei, and dorsal horn of spinal cord are interrelated with forebrain, hypothalamus, and brain stem autonomic and cognitive mechanisms. They are involved in the conscious, subconscious, and conditional inhibitory influences on pain transmission to the cortex.

  4. Forebrain mechanisms mediate the perception of pain. The meaning of the sensation influences its perceptual quality. For example, acute onset of pain in the left arm and shoulder evokes entirely different responses in a person with a history of myocardial infarction than the same kind of pain in this person's right arm or in the left arm of a person without a prior history of heart disease. Anxiety markedly increases acute pain and changes the patient's description of and response to painful stimuli (see Table 49-1).

    There is much evidence that the meaning of the pain, the environmental situation, emotional and personality factors, and interpersonal relationships with family, friends, and health care providers all influence the unwanted progression of acute pain resulting from a disease or injury to chronic pain, which then tends to become the disease itself (Table 49-1).

III. Referred pain is seen in both acute and chronic pain states. It may occur when both visceral and somatic pain fibers share a common central nervous system integrative neuronal pool; hence, visceral pain may be perceived by the patient at a corresponding somatic location. Common examples include:

  A. Anginal and myocardial ischemic pain being referred to neck, jaw, and left medial upper arm.

  B. Diaphragmatic irritation producing ipsilateral shoulder pain.

  C. Gallbladder irritation producing subscapular back pain.

IV. Chronic pain represents one of the major inadequacies of medicine. It has been nearly impossible to measure and investigate scientifically, frustrating to evaluate clinically, and difficult to treat.

Table 49-2   Causes of Chronic Intractable Pain

Medical disorders
  Invasive cancer and compressive mechanisms
  Organ ischemias (intractable angina)
  Inflammatory disorders (vasculitis, arthritis)
Neurologic disorders
  Neuropathies of inflammation, entrapment and damage (reflex sympathetic dystrophies, phantom limb pain, myositis syndromes, arachnoiditis, compression and diabetic neuropathies, trigeminal and glossopharyngeal neuralgias)
Musculoskeletal disorders
  Muscle contraction myalgias, including headache and fibrositis
Psychologic disorders
  Depression
  Hysteria
  Compensation neuroses
  Munchausen syndrome
  Psychoses with somatic delusions

A. **Importance of psychologic mechanisms.** The largest problems are based on ignorance and an unwillingness on the part of the physician and patient alike to deal with social, economic, psychologic, and psychophysiologic mechanisms that have become major factors determining the severity and debility of the syndrome as well as the negative response to most therapeutic ventures.

In every patient, no matter how chronic or intractable the pain may seem, treatment directed toward the etiology should be done *if feasible.* In most instances, however, chronic intractable pain does not exist without psychosocial and psychophysiologic factors acting to facilitate pain. This is true in disorders with obvious pain mechanisms, such as cancer, as well as in those with no discernible physiologic mechanisms (Table 49-2).

By the same token, positive psychophysiologic mechanisms, if activated, can markedly diminish the pain and alter the chronic illness syndrome.

B. **Peripheral mechanisms**
  1. **Adrenergic mechanisms** facilitate peripheral pain in conditions such as chronic tension and vascular headaches, where vasoconstriction and increased muscle tone add to pain intractability. Here, biofeedback, relaxation therapy, and adrenergic blockade can be useful therapeutic measures.
  2. **Chronic nerve injuries,** including amputation, may produce neuromas, where regenerating nerves form a tangled skein of sensory, motor, and sympathetic neurons. Inappropriate stimulation exists in neuromas by pathologic synapses called ephapses. Pathophysiologic cross-talk may also occur in demyelinated nerves; this is called causalgia. These injured nerves are easily excited by compression stimulation and sympathetic catechols. Phantom limb sensations and pain may have a similar etiology.

C. **Spinal cord mechanisms** in chronic pain are similar to the acute situation except that the descending inhibitory mechanisms are deficient and less active. Acupuncture and transcutaneous nerve stimulation operate at this level of interaction.

D. **Brain stem integrative mechanisms** in chronic pain utilize mostly the slow-firing, diffuse pathways traveling to the affective-motivational systems of the limbic cortex and nuclei, the amygdala, and hippocampus. Chronic pain alters recent memory and affective and cognitive functions, and it produces vegetative disturbances through limbic and hypothalamic pathways. In turn, these changes lower the perceptual threshold of pain itself. By these feedback loops pain may become self-perpetuating.

E. **Thalamic and other central neural pain mechanisms.** Neither acute inflammation nor other injury of the central nervous system tissue is usually capable of producing a pain sensation. However, on rare occasions ischemic injury, such as a stroke, may produce stimulation of sensory projection systems such as dorsal horn areas or brain stem reticular and thalamic areas, with resulting burning dysesthesias localized to the periphery. These sensations are secondary to inappropriate seizure-like discharges. They are difficult to treat and respond better to anticonvulsants than to narcotics.

F. **Depression** is the affective cohort of pain perception. It produces social withdrawal, irritability, psychomotor retardation, and decrease in all pain thresholds. These factors destroy effective and rewarding life, whereas the initial disorder would or could not be so destructive (Table 49-1). Antidepressant drugs may be helpful at this level of neuropsychophysiologic intervention, as well as exercise and behavioral modifications, all utilizing patient self-help techniques and activities.

G. **Behavioral determinants** in chronic pain include increased medicinal use and dependence on others, including family and physicians. The reduced activity due to pain leads to reduced income and its chronicity leads to requests for compensation, disability, and early retirement. Losing status and becoming an economic liability may now turn a depressed patient into an irritable, self-pitying, and manipulative tyrant. Here socioeconomic factors become important in the chronic illness behavior, and the pathology of illness may now be almost unrelated to the primary disease itself.

V. **The placebo effect.** For years, the relief of pain by the inert chemical was regarded as proof that the pain was not real or purely psychologic. This is quite incorrect, since placebos are effective in postoperative pain states and cancer pain and they actually alter the vasodilation attending migraine headaches. Recent investigations have shown an increase of cerebrospinal fluid levels of enkephalins when placebos were successful in relieving pain.

Hypnosis may operate at a similar or higher level of pain modification, but so far no enkephalin increases have been demonstrated. Hypnosis does block acute and chronic pain, and the accompanying autonomic reactions but its use is impractical except in special instances.

VI. **Clinical example of chronic pain**

A. **Description.** A 52-year-old married woman had a 10-year history of muscle contraction headaches, which were occipital and frontally located. Continual and daily for 4 years, the pain had become increasingly severe in the past 2 years so that she had quit work as a secretary and stayed at home. She had seen numerous physicians and took an impressive list of medications, including tranquilizers and narcotics. Trips to emergency rooms for narcotic injections had been more frequent in the past year. She was increasingly withdrawn, and her interaction with family and friends was almost totally pain-oriented. She had experienced a 15-pound weight loss in the past year. Evaluation in the hospital during a severe headache disclosed slurred speech and mild incoordination. Although she denied using alcohol or diazepam, she had elevated blood levels of both. After investigation revealed no evidence of neurologic or medical disorders, the psychologic factors of depression and her anxieties and fears were carefully explored. The severe muscle tension and myalgias were first approached by local anesthetic blocks with complete relief of pain; then a regimen was established including twice-daily physical therapy, local heat treatment, hourly special head and neck exercises, and walking (for exercise). A tricyclic antidepressant and aspirin were given for pain, and psychotherapy sessions were scheduled twice daily. All efforts were designed to make the patient an active self-therapist. She was discharged free of headaches for the first time in 4 years. At home she experienced mild headaches controlled by her own exercise and aspirin. She returned to work and did not resume taking alcohol or tranquilizers.

B. Discussion. The patient had only a high school education. Her husband had become wealthy in the petroleum industry. Their social and business status created many feelings of inadequacy, unresolved anxiety, and depression due to her perceived inferiority from a lack of education and social graces. The locus of head and neck pain was related to her sleeping on her abdomen with neck turned to the side and to chronic neck flexing while watching television in a supine position. Her chronic high level of tense motor anxiety added muscle tension in the whole body but especially the head and neck muscles. Psychologic retardation only enhanced her chronic illness behavior, since she avoided reality with tranquilizers and alcohol. The aspirin was helpful in controlling the myalgias of continual muscle contraction by prostaglandin blockade in muscle nociceptor fields. Stretching exercises relaxed these muscles. The greatest benefit was probably produced by her psychologic reorganization based on reassurance, antidepressants, muscle-relaxation exercises, and a willingness to work toward her own recovery. These were all possible because the patient had excellent support from her family, who helped her to realize she was not inadequate and pushed her to continue her self-help program.

Questions

More than one answer may be correct.

1. Select the correct statement(s) regarding acute pain.
   a. It is different from chronic pain, since it involves no psychologic factors.
   b. Painful muscle injury involves stimulation of nociceptors by released cellular constituents such as K^+ and histamine.
   c. Tissue levels of bradykinins and prostaglandins are often elevated, which adds to nociceptor stimulation.
   d. Sympathetic stimulation of the smooth muscles and blood vessels in the area of injury decreases the pain input to the spinal cord.

2. In chronic pain:
   a. Strong pain medications are needed because the pain threshold is lower.
   b. Placebos, if successful, prove that the pain is purely psychologic.
   c. Enkephalins are inhibitory to pain transmission toward the cortex; they are elevated after acupuncture, transcutaneous nerve stimulation, and even with the belief that a placebo will be effective.
   d. Depression is a major factor in most, if not all, chronic intractable pain states.

I. Review of normal cerebral physiology

  A. Cellular anatomy and physiology. Neurons vary tremendously in size and shape, but the basic structure is the same for all. The *cell body* or soma contains the nucleus, Golgi apparatus, and Nissl substance (ribonucleic acid [RNA]). *Dendrites* arise from the soma, branch repeatedly, and receive inputs from other nerve cells through numerous synaptic connections. *Axons* send impulses from the soma to other nerve cells by finally dividing and forming synapses on the soma, dendrites, or axons of other cells. *Synapses* are specialized interfaces between two nerve cells whose membranes are separated by a narrow cleft (typically 200 Å wide).

    1. Neuronal electrical activity. The resting membrane potential is a consequence of differences of ion concentrations (primarily sodium and potassium) inside and outside the cell. However, nerve cell membranes of the central nervous system are continually influenced by activity arising from other neurons and are never completely at rest. The action potential is a transient disturbance of the resting potential, which is propagated along the fiber, transmitting information from one end to the other.

      In myelinated fibers, current flow is restricted to the nodes of Ranvier, thereby speeding conduction. In unmyelinated fibers, conduction is slow, rarely exceeding 1 to 2 m per second.

      At the synapse, a presynaptic transmitter substance evokes postsynaptic permeability change. Specialization of the postsynaptic junction determines whether the induced permeability change will be excitatory or inhibitory.

    2. Origin or electrical activity detected by the electroencephalograph. Using a battery of highly sensitive amplifiers attached to the scalp (electroencephalograph), a record of electrical activity originating from the underlying cortex (electroencephalogram [EEG]) can be made. This surface activity is believed to represent summated synaptic potentials generated by the pyramidal cells of the cerebral cortex located only 1 to 4 mm from the surface.

  B. Regional neurophysiology. Functional subdivisions of the brain have been identified. While not absolute, the importance of these areas is indicated by numerous neurophysiologic studies and clinical conditions.

    1. Motor areas. The primary motor area is located mainly in the precentral gyrus of the cortex and is responsible for most upper-motor-neuron motor activity.

    2. Sensory receiving areas. The somatosensory area is located mainly in the postcentral gyrus of the cortex and processes or interprets information from somatosensory receptors. The auditory areas, where auditory information is interpreted and over which potentials evoked by auditory stimuli can be detected on the scalp, are located mainly in the temporal lobes. The visual areas, where the contralateral visual field is represented and over which potentials evoked by visual stimuli can be detected on the scalp, are mainly in the occipital lobes.

3. **The association areas** are located mainly in the frontal lobe anterior to the motor area, in a large area of the parietal lobe behind the postcentral gyrus, and in the temporal lobe. These areas integrate a continuous flow of information from various sensory receptors and presumably interpret new data in the light of previous experience.

II. **Pathophysiology of epilepsy**

   A. **General principles.** Epilepsy may be defined as a sudden alteration of central nervous system function resulting from abnormal excessive discharge of cortical neurons (anywhere in the forebrain and perhaps in the brain stem). The symptoms of any particular attack depend on the function of the area of the brain that is being interrupted by the excessive neuronal discharge.

      1. **Etiology.** Spontaneous paroxysmal discharges may occur from diseased neurons (glial scars, tumors, degenerations, infections, ischemia, etc.) or normal neurons may be stimulated electrically (electroshock therapy) or chemically (toxic or metabolic disorders) and result in seizures.

      2. **Seizure types.** Epileptic seizures are classified according to symptoms referable to a presumed functional area of the brain and to whether they begin locally, are generalized at onset, or begin locally and become secondarily generalized. Seizures beginning locally (referred to as partial seizures) may manifest only simple motor (Jacksonian) or sensory phenomena without impairment of consciousness, or as more complex motor, sensory or psychic phenomena, usually with some impairment of consciousness. Generalized seizures are bilaterally symmetrical and without focal onset. Absence attacks (formerly called petit mal) and generalized diffuse tonic-clonic seizures (grand mal) are examples of generalized seizures.

   B. **Evaluation and management of seizure patients**

      1. **Search for a treatable etiology.** A careful and continuing search for a treatable cause should be carried out in all patients with seizures. This includes searching for intracranial causes—such as tumor, abscess, hematoma, and degenerative diseases—and metabolic causes—such as hyponatremia, hypocalcemia, hypoglycemia, and drug withdrawal.

      2. **Use of the electroencephalogram.** Epileptiform spike and sharp waves have a high correlation with the presence of clinical seizures. Other interictal EEG patterns do not. Recording the EEG during a clinical seizure and simultaneously video recording the seizure are sometimes necessary for accurate diagnosis.

      3. **Role of antiepileptic drugs.** Treatment should be started with one drug only. The choice of drug should match the seizure type. Serum antiepileptic drug level determinations should be used to monitor drug treatment.

III. **Clinical examples**

   A. **Complex partial seizures as the presenting symptom in a patient with a brain tumor**

      1. **Description.** A 32-year-old man began to have episodes in which he would suddenly begin to look about in a bewildered manner while fumbling aimlessly at his clothes, smacking his lips, and drooling saliva. The episodes lasted only a few seconds, and the patient was unaware of their occurrence afterward. Neurologic examination

was normal, and EEG revealed a spike focus over the left anterior temporal region. A computerized tomography (CT) scan revealed a mass lesion in the left anterior temporal region. The patient was placed on the antiepileptic drug phenytoin (Dilantin) at a dosage sufficient to achieve therapeutic drug levels. Surgical exploration was undertaken, revealing a meningioma over the left temporal area of the cortex.

2. **Discussion**

   a. The patient's symptomatology was consistent with complex partial seizure activity primarily manifested by psychomotor phenomena, suggesting a focal process in one of the temporal lobes of the cortex.

   b. A search was made for an etiology utilizing careful neurologic examination, EEG, and CT scan. A mass lesion was found.

   c. Antiepileptic drug therapy was begun using phenytoin (Dilantin) sufficient to achieve therapeutic blood levels.

   d. Surgical exploration was carried out to determine whether the mass lesion was treatable. It was discovered that this was the case.

B. **Absence seizures in an 8-year-old girl**

1. **Description.** An 8-year-old girl was noted to be having staring spells in school, which were interfering with her studies. These episodes lasted from 10 to 20 seconds and were sometimes accompanied by blinking of the eyes. Neurologic examination was normal. A typical episode was reproduced by having the patient hyperventilate. The patient was noted to stop hyperventilation and stare blankly for approximately 10 seconds with some blinking of the eyes. She was unable to repeat numbers said to her at that time. Computerized tomography of the head was normal. An EEG revealed three-per-second, generalized spike-wave activity of a type typical of absence seizures (petit mal). The patient was placed on ethosuximide, an antiepileptic drug often helpful in absence seizures and the episodes stopped.

2. **Discussion**

   a. The description of staring episodes in an 8-year-old girl who is otherwise normal is strongly suggestive of seizure activity of the so-called absence type.

   b. No demonstrable intracranial or extracranial disease was discovered.

   c. An electroencephalogram revealed features classic for absence seizures (petit mal).

   d. Treatment with one of the drugs usually effective in the control of absence seizures was undertaken and was successful. Another drug considered by many to be the drug of choice in this condition is valproic acid.

Questions   Select the single best answer.

1. The origin of electrical activity detected by the electroencephalogram is most likely to be:
   a. Potentials arising from axonal activity in the cerebral cortex.
   b. Potential arising from the cerebellum.

c. Summated synaptic potentials generated by the pyramidal cells of the cerebral cortex.

d. Potentials arising from electrical activity in the periaqueductal gray matter.

2. Partial seizures with complex symptomatology:

a. Formerly were called Jacksonian seizures.

b. Are rarely if ever associated with impairment of consciousness.

c. Are not related to focal cerebral dysfunction.

d. Generally are accompanied by impairment of consciousness.

51 Cerebrovascular Disease

I. Normal physiology

A. Anatomy. Four arteries carry the blood flow to the head, two vertebral arteries and two common carotid arteries. Each common carotid artery divides into an internal and an external branch. The external carotid artery supplies extracranial structures, but can also supply the brain through anastomoses with the internal carotid artery, for example, the ophthalmic artery. The internal carotid artery through its branches supplies the anterior two-thirds of the brain.

The vertebral arteries join to form the basilar artery. This vertebral-basilar system supplies the brain stem and the posterior portion of the cortex.

Superficial and deep cerebral veins drain from the brain into venous sinuses. The major venous sinuses with clinical significance are the superior sagittal sinus, the lateral sinus, and the cavernous sinus. The jugular veins drain the venous system of the brain.

B. Physiology. Autoregulation maintains a constant cerebral blood flow, which fails only when the mean arterial pressure falls below 60 mm Hg. Elevated carbon dioxide tension (PCO_2) produces vasodilatation of cerebral vessels, while oxygen has minimal effect on cerebral perfusion. Glucose has no known effect on cerebral blood flow, even when low enough to produce coma. Body temperatures in the range of 35° to 40° C do not affect blood flow. Increased blood viscosity, as in patients with polycythemia, may produce decreased blood flow. The effect of the sympathetic control of cerebral blood flow is controversial.

The metabolism of the brain is such that oxygen is consumed at a rate of approximately 3.3 ml/100 g per minute. Glucose, the major substrate, is consumed at about 5 mg/100 g per minute.

II. Pathophysiology

A. Infarction (necrosis of tissue secondary to impairment of blood supply) may occur from focal vascular occlusion or from conditions in which the cerebral blood flow is generally reduced.

1. **Occlusive arterial disease** may occur as total occlusion of one of the major arteries, such as the internal carotid artery, or as narrowing of an artery sufficient to impair blood flow. The usual cause is atherosclerosis, although any vasculopathy affecting large and medium-sized arteries may produce a similar result. Often, there is a superimposed arterial thrombosis at the site of the underlying lesion.

   Arterial occlusion may also result from emboli, which may be of cardiac origin (myocardial infarction with mural thrombi, atrial fibrillation, paradoxical emboli complicating congenital heart disease, etc.) or of arterial origin as the result of rupture of an atheromatous plaque with release of cholesterol emboli. Any of these conditions may produce focal infarction, with corresponding lasting deficit in neurologic function or transient ischemia with associated transient focal neurologic signs or symptoms. The latter are often called transient ischemic attacks (TIAs). Transient cerebral ischemia is frequently the result of cholesterol or platelet emboli from an atheromatous plaque in a carotid artery. In these instances, cholesterol particles are sometimes visible upon ophthalmoscopic examination of the fundus of the eye.

2. **Vasospasm** associated with subarachnoid hemorrhage or migraine may result in cerebral infarction.

3. **Venous thrombosis** may also cause cerebral infarction. Thrombosis of the cavernous sinus is often related to infection. Sagittal sinus thrombosis may occur with debilitating states or postpartum states. Lateral sinus thrombosis may occur in association with infection of the ear or mastoid.

4. **Generalized cerebral hypoperfusion.** Diffuse necrosis of the cortex may result from conditions in which overall cerebral blood flow is reduced (hypotension) or conditions in which severe hypoxia or hypoglycemia occurs. Widespread small-vessel occlusion may also produce diffuse multiple areas of cortical infarction.

B. **Hemorrhage.** Symptoms of an intracranial hemorrhage may result from bleeding into the subarachnoid space, from hemorrhage into the substance of the brain with the formation of a mass of blood (hematoma), or from reduced blood flow in the distribution of the involved artery.

1. **Major causes.** The usual causes of spontaneous arterial hemorrhage are rupture of an aneurysm of a large artery in the circle of Willis or rupture of a small intracerebral penetrating artery or arteriole. Hemorrhage associated with an arteriovenous malformation also occurs. Less frequently encountered conditions associated with intracranial hemorrhage are hematologic disturbances (leukemia, aplastic anemia, hemophilia, thrombocytopenic states, anticoagulant drug therapy, and disseminated intravascular coagulopathies). Also, mycotic aneurysms resulting from septic emboli associated with bacterial endocarditis, or a primary or metastatic brain tumor, may bleed into the brain substance.

2. **Mechanisms producing neurologic signs and symptoms**
   a. **Acute increased intracranial pressure** associated with bleeding may result in headache and unconsciousness.
   b. **Reduction of blood supply** to a given area of the brain will produce focal signs, depending on the function of the involved area.
   c. **Clinical changes** characteristic of an expanding intracranial hematoma associated with hemorrhage or characteristic of cerebral edema associated with a large area of infarction. In this situation, consciousness becomes progressively impaired, the pulse progressively slows, and the systolic blood pressure may rise. There may be pupillary dilatation on the side of the mass effect. Death from brain herniation will result unless the condition is corrected.

III. **Clinical examples of cerebrovascular disease**

A. **Subarachnoid hemorrhage secondary to ruptured aneurysm of the circle of Willis**

1. **Description.** A 26-year-old woman sought medical attention immediately following the abrupt onset of an excruciating headache, followed shortly by double vision. A neurologic examination revealed nuchal rigidity, ptosis of the left eye, an enlarged left pupil that did not react to light, and paralysis of the extraocular muscles innervated by cranial nerve III. A computerized tomographic scan was normal. A lumbar puncture revealed a bloody spinal fluid under increased pressure with a xanothochromic supernatant after centrifugation. Cerebral angiography revealed a saccular aneurysm

of the posterior communicating–posterior cerebral arterial junction. The aneurysm was successfully treated surgically and the patient returned home without neurologic deficit.

2. **Discussion**

   a. The abrupt onset of severe headache suggested a subarachnoid hemorrhage. The headache probably resulted from the meningeal irritation and increased intracranial pressure.

   b. The third-nerve palsy suggested an aneurysm of the posterior communicating–posterior cerebral artery junction, since a mass in this location could compress the third nerve.

   c. Because the patient was conscious without other significant deficit, surgery on the aneurysm could be carried out promptly in order to prevent further bleeding from the aneurysm.

B. **Transient cerebral ischemia due to an atheromatous plaque of the internal carotid artery**

   1. **Description.** A 55-year-old man began to have episodes consisting of weakness of the right-upper and right-lower extremities and inability to speak (aphasia) lasting usually 15 to 20 minutes. Sometimes these were accompanied by a loss of vision in the left eye, which came on as though a shade were being drawn down over the eye. At the time the patient was seen, examination was negative except for a bruit at the bifurcation of the left common carotid artery. Computerized tomographic scan was normal. Angiography revealed an ulcerated plaque of the internal carotid artery just past the bifurcation of the common carotid artery. The patient remained asymptomatic following an operation to remove the plaque.

   2. **Discussion**

      a. The history of transient focal neurologic deficit in a patient of this age strongly suggested the possibility of cerebrovascular occlusive disease.

      b. The coincidental occurrence of right hemiparesis and aphasia suggested focal involvement in the distribution of the left internal carotid artery.

      c. The occurrence of transient blindness confined to the left eye suggested transient ischemia in the distribution of the left ophthalmic artery, which is a branch of the left internal carotid artery.

      d. The underlying cause was platelet or cholesterol emboli originating in an ulcerated atherosclerotic plaque.

Questions

Select the single best answer.

1. The internal carotid artery through its branches supplies:
   a. The entire cerebral cortex, including the occipital lobes.
   b. Only the anterior portions of the cerebellum.
   c. The anterior two-thirds of the brain.
   d. The brain stem and the posterior portions of the cortex.

2. A patient complains of sudden severe headaches and rapidly loses consciousness. Examination reveals a progressive slowing of the pulse, a rising systolic blood pressure, and a dilated, nonreacting left pupil. Of the following types of cerebrovascular disease, which appears to be the most likely?
   a. Cavernous sinus thrombosis.
   b. Diffuse cortical infarction from hypoglycemia.
   c. A cerebral hemorrhage with an associated intracerebral hematoma.
   d. Transient cerebral ischemia due to an atheromatous plaque of the internal carotid artery.

The Upper Motor Neuron System and the Motor Unit

I. **Normal physiology**

A. **Upper motor neuron.** Cell bodies of the upper motor neuron system are located in the motor cortex just anterior to the rolandic fissure, where areas of the contralateral body, extremities, and face are topically represented.

Axons of those cells that are destined to innervate lower motor neuron cell bodies in the spinal cord pass downward through the internal capsule and anterior brain stem, cross to the opposite side at the medullocervical junction, and pass down the cord in the lateral corticospinal tract.

Axons of those cells destined to innervate lower motor neuron nuclei pass down through the internal capsule and anterior brain stem, where they decussate at the level of the cranial nerve motor nuclei that they are destined to innervate.

B. **The motor unit.** The motor unit consists of the motor neuron cell body, its axons, and the muscle fibers that it innervates (see Fig. 52-1).

1. **Axon.** Axons of the motor unit are myelinated. The speed of conduction is enhanced in myelinated nerves because of saltatory conduction. The nerve impulses jump from node to node, thus increasing the conduction velocity.

2. **Synapse.** The axonal tip and the muscle fiber that it innervates are separated by synaptic cleft called the motor end plate (neuromuscular junction or synapse) (see Fig. 52-2). Arriving axonal impulses cause the release of acetylcholine into the cleft. The acetylcholine finds acetylcholine receptors on the muscle side of the cleft. Attachment of sufficient acetylcholine to acetylcholine receptors produces depolarization and subsequent contraction of the muscle fiber. Acetylcholinesterase constantly acts to police the area of acetylcholine, preventing excessive build-up of acetylcholine.

3. **Muscle fiber.** Each muscle fiber is composed of hundreds to thousands of smaller units called myofibrils. Myofibrils contain proteins, actin, and myosin. These are the sliding myofilaments that constitute the contractile mechanism activated during muscle contraction.

II. **Pathophysiology of disorders affecting the upper motor neuron system and motor unit**

A. **Disorders of the upper motor neuron.** Destruction of any portion of the upper motor neuron before its destination will produce negative symptoms (deficits of purposeful movement distal to the site of destruction) or positive symptoms (exaggerated brain stem or spinal cord reflex behaviors released from neural control of higher central nervous system levels) distal to the site of the lesion. Examples are hyperreflexia, spasticity, and the extensor plantar response (Babinski sign).

B. **Disorders of the motor unit.** Destruction or impairment of any portion of the motor unit will result in absent muscle contraction, with subsequent muscle atrophy if regeneration does not occur. Disease of the muscle fiber will result in lack of function and the atrophy of the

Figure 52-1

Diagram of myelinated motor nerve showing saltatory conduction.

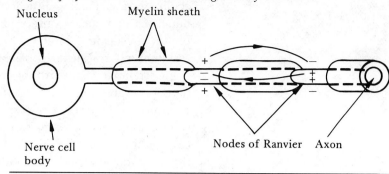

Figure 52-2

Diagram of neuromuscular junction.

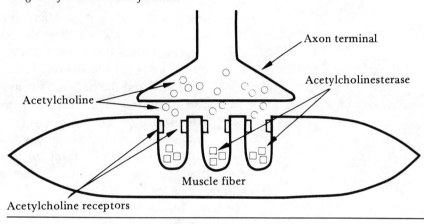

muscle. The muscle stretch reflex will be reduced or absent, depending on the severity of involvement (i.e., the number of motor units involved).

1. **Impairment of axonal function.** Axonal function may be affected by peripheral neuropathies or by local compression of peripheral nerves. Segmental demyelination may occur (segmental demyelinating neuropathy) so that conduction of the nerve impulse is slowed. This may progress to a total lack of function, as in the case of the acute polyneuritis associated with the Guillain-Barré syndrome. Spot demyelination (entrapment syndrome) with focal conduction slowing may result from local nerve compression. Primary axonal death (dying back neuropathy), beginning distally, may occur. It usually results from toxic agents or metabolic disturbances.

2. **Disorders of neuromuscular transmission.** Failure of neuromuscular transmission may result from any change that reduces the probability of interaction of acetylcholine (ACh) and receptors.

   a. Impaired release of ACh may be the cause of failure of neuromuscular transmission. This mechanism is responsible for the muscle weakness in the pseudomyasthenic syndrome and in *Clostridium botulinum* poisoning.

   b. Competitive displacement of ACh from ACh receptors can cause failure of neuromuscular transmission. The number of available receptors may be reduced by drugs such as *d*-tubocurarine or by receptor antibody, as in myasthenia gravis. Depolarizing blocking agents, such as decamethonium bromide and succinylcholine, mimic ACh but are not destroyed by acetyl-cholinesterase. Finally, anticholinesterases—such as physostigmine, neostigmine, a variety of nerve gas, and organic phosphate insecticides—inhibit or inactivate acetylcholinesterase, resulting in a so-called depolarizing block.

Certain clinical neurophysiologic tests are helpful in identifying the presence and type of impairment of neuromuscular transmission. The evoked response of muscle after repetitive stimulation of its nerve may show progressive decrement in the case of myasthenia gravis or facilitation in the pseudomyasthenic syndrome and in botulism. Single-fiber electromyography is a recently developed procedure that allows the mean of consecutive differences in the intervals between single-fiber discharges (jitter) to be determined. Jitter is increased in myasthenia gravis.

3. **Impairment of muscle fiber function.** Disturbances of muscle membrane conduction or of the contractile mechanism occur. Examples of disorders of muscle membrane mechanisms are the myotonic states (myotonia congenita, myotonic dystrophy, and paramyotonia) and the periodic paralyses (hyperkalemic, hypokalemic, and normokalemic). Disturbances of the contractile mechanism are present in the hereditary myopathies (pseudohypertrophic, limb-girdle, or fascioscapulohumeral muscular dystrophies, and myotonia dystrophica) and in the acquired myopathies (inflammatory, collagen-vascular, endocrine, toxic, and metabolic).

III. **Clinical examples**

A. **Acute inflammatory motor polyradiculoneuropathy (Guillain-Barré syndrome).** A 45-year-old bus driver began to notice muscle weakness when climbing steps and when using his ticket punch. About 2 days earlier, he had noted a transitory sensation of numbness of his feet, and 10 days earlier, he had suffered a nonspecific febrile illness apparently viral in nature. Examination revealed bilaterally symmetric mild weakness of the upper and lower extremities and absent muscle stretch reflexes throughout. There were no clear-cut objective sensory changes. Cranial nerve function was not impaired. A spinal fluid examination revealed a protein of 120 mg/100 ml and no white cells. The patient was placed in the intensive care unit for observation because of fear that he might develop paralysis of respiratory muscles. Fortunately, this did not occur, and after a few days, he was released. After receiving physical therapy, he slowly recovered.

1. **Discussion**

a. The onset of symmetric muscle weakness and arreflexia following a nondescript febrile illness suggested the Guillain-Barré syndrome. An elevated spinal fluid protein without an associated increase of white cells in the spinal fluid (albuminocytologic disassociation) often accompanies this syndrome.

b. Patients with Guillain-Barré syndrome are in danger of respiratory involvement and may need respiratory support.

c. Most patients with Guillain-Barré syndrome recover completely. The pathophysiology of the disorder is probably autoimmune involvement of the myelin sheath with relative sparing of the axon. Since axonal regeneration is not necessary for recovery, function returns when myelin is restored.

B. Diabetic peripheral neuropathy

1. **Description.** A 45-year-old man with insulin-dependent diabetes mellitus complained of burning pain in the feet and calves and some numbness and tingling in the toes. He also noticed some slapping of the feet when walking. Examination revealed reduction of all sensory modalities on the distal portions of both feet, and he had difficulty walking on his toes and heels. There was some atrophy of the intrinsic muscles of the feet bilaterally. The ankle stretch reflexes were absent, and the patellar reflexes were barely obtainable. Nerve conduction studies revealed a marked slowing of motor nerve conduction velocity in the peroneal nerves bilaterally and slowing of sensory nerve conduction velocity in the sural nerves bilaterally.

2. **Discussion**
   a. Peripheral neuropathy is a common complication of diabetes mellitus.
   b. Symptoms of distal sensory alteration and burning pain in a diabetic patient are apt to be the result of peripheral neuropathy.
   c. Weakness of distal muscles of the lower extremities of this patient suggested involvement of the motor neurons.
   d. Nerve conduction studies showed marked slowing of conduction in both motor and sensory nerves of the lower extremities, confirming the diagnosis of involvement of the peripheral nerve.
   e. The marked slowing suggests that at least some components of the peripheral neuropathy were demyelinating in nature.

Questions

Select the single best answer.

1. Saltatory conduction:
   a. Results in *increased* nerve conduction velocity in *unmyelinated* nerves.
   b. Results in *decreased* nerve conduction velocity in *unmyelinated* nerves.
   c. Results in *increased* nerve conduction velocity in *myelinated* nerves.
   d. Results in *decreased* nerve conduction velocity in *myelinated* nerves.
2. The principle cause of failure of neuromuscular transmission in myasthenia gravis is:
   a. Competitive displacement of acetylcholine from its receptors by antiacetylcholine receptor antibody.
   b. Reduced destruction of acetylcholinesterase.
   c. A deficiency of acetylcholinesterase.
   d. Impaired release of acetylcholine from the axon terminal.

X

Nutrition

Don P. Murray
Robert Whang

53 Clinical Malnutrition

I. **Introduction.** Malnutrition continues to be one of the world's major health problems. In addition, hospital surveys have determined that as many as 50 percent of general medical and surgical service patients are malnourished. This is due to a combination of factors that include the anorexia accompanying chronic disease, periods of no oral intake while hospitalized, and the catabolic effects of stress. These patients have a poorer prognosis than adequately nourished patients, unless the nutritional deficits can be repaired. It is therefore important to understand the biochemistry and pathophysiology of protein-calorie malnutrition.

Nutritional requirements include: (1) carbohydrates, which serve primarily as an energy substrate; (2) fats, which can be utilized as an energy source and are required for membrane structure and integrity as well as the structure of certain molecules; (3) proteins, which are required for structure and function of numerous molecules, including enzymes and carrier systems, and in addition may serve as an energy source; (4) vitamins, which are required as components of certain molecules and as coenzymes for various enzymatic processes; and (5) minerals and trace elements, which are required for structure of certain tissues and metabolic processes.

Protein-calorie malnutrition is defined as inadequate intake of either protein or calories to meet normal energy, tissue growth, or tissue maintenance requirements. This term encompasses a spectrum of disease entities, ranging from kwashiorkor (the deficiency of protein intake with maintenance of normal caloric intake) to marasmus (deficiency of both caloric and protein intake). As might be expected, when caloric or protein intake is inadequate, other nutrient deficiencies frequently coexist.

The pathophysiologic consequences of kwashiorkor differ from those of marasmus. In addition, the consequences of these specific nutritional deficiencies may vary depending upon the age group involved. The consequences of kwashiorkor or marasmus upon growth are far more striking in the infant than in the adolescent or adult. In each, however, the basic event is depletion of cellular energy and molecular stores, leading to impairment of cellular function.

II. **Types of nutritional disorders**

A. **Marasmus.** A diet deficient in calories necessitates use of body energy stores. Glycogen stores can be depleted over a relatively short period of time. Fat provides more calories per gram than carbohydrate, and fat stores are more slowly depleted. When glycogen and fat stores are inadequate to meet the energy requirements of the organism, catabolism of tissue protein (primarily skeletal muscle) occurs and amino acids are used for energy production. Amino acids released in this process also replenish the serum amino acid pool and can be used in the synthesis of serum and visceral proteins. It is therefore possible to maintain normal or near-normal serum protein levels during the catabolic process. In children, the most obvious manifestation of marasmus is impaired growth of all tissues.

B. **Kwashiorkor.** A diet deficient in protein, but with normal or excessive caloric content, can to a certain extent spare tissue protein from being broken down for energy production. However, in the absence of protein intake, tissue catabolism is the inevitable source of amino acids for synthesis of somatic and visceral protein. Albumin production is readily affected, and the resulting decreased plasma oncotic pressure is a contributing factor to the peripheral edema or ascites that commonly occurs.

C. **General features of combined protein-calorie malnutrition.** Since most individuals with malnutrition have features of both kwashiorkor and marasmus, the pathophysiologic manifestation of this combined protein-calorie malnutrition will be described in some detail. As in most areas of medical science, clinical and laboratory investigations of human and animal malnutrition do not always agree and in many instances are in direct conflict. Although in some cases derived from animal studies, information presented here is likely to be applicable to human malnutrition.

III. **Systemic effects of combined protein-calorie malnutrition**

A. **Immune system.** Perhaps the most striking effect of protein-calorie malnutrition is on the body's defense mechanisms (the integument and the immune system). Malnutrition and infection frequently coexist. It is sometimes difficult to differentiate the effects of malnutrition from the effects of infection upon the immune system, but the following points can be made.

There is in vitro evidence of abnormal T lymphocyte function, in that there is impaired peripheral lymphocyte blast transformation in response to mitogen and diminished rosette formation in the presence of sheep red blood cells. Total peripheral lymphocyte counts are decreased, usually to less than 1.5×10^3 per cubic millimeter. There is poor recall to prior sensitization to antigen, as demonstrated by skin test reactivity. The clinical consequences may be a higher incidence and more severe course of tuberculosis, as well as viral and fungal infections in malnourished individuals.

Serum antibody response appears to be normal or exaggerated, with the most common immunoglobulin elevation being in the IgA class. These immunoglobulin elevations are most likely to be a nonspecific reaction to infection that is frequently present. Secretory IgA, however, appears to be diminished. It has been postulated that this IgA deficiency may account for the increased frequency of small-bowel bacterial overgrowth and diarrheal syndromes in malnourished children. Although polymorphonuclear phagocytosis appears normal in malnutrition, there is impaired chemotaxis and defective bactericidal activity. The precise metabolic defect responsible for the malfunction of polymorphonuclear killing is unknown.

B. **Integument.** A large proportion of the epidermis, dermis, and dermal appendages are protein products. In protein-calorie malnutrition, pigment production and keratinization are impaired. Hair and nail growth is impeded. In severe malnutrition exfoliation and fissuring occurs; this, in combination with impaired immunocompetence, results in frequent cutaneous infection.

C. **Gastrointestinal.** Small bowel biopsies of individuals with protein-calorie malnutrition frequently reveal villous atrophy. Disaccharidase levels may be decreased, and there is evidence of impaired carbohydrate and fat absorption. The pancreas retains the ability to secrete normal amounts of water and bicarbonate in response to stimulation, but enzyme output is diminished. It is as yet unclear to what extent maldigestion and malabsorption contribute to the diarrhea seen in children with protein-calorie malnutrition, since other factors, including bacterial overgrowth and parasitic infestation, also come into play.

D. Endocrine. There is a decrease in basal metabolic rate, although free thyroxine levels are probably unchanged. Levels of growth hormone are variable, but growth hormone response to hypoglycemia is blunted. Plasma insulin levels are low, and insulin response to glucose load is depressed. Serum cortisol is increased, but this may be the result of impaired degradation rather than increased production.

E. Neurologic. Animal studies using the rat model and infant human autopsies have shown decreased brain weight, neuron numbers, and myelin synthesis in instances of malnutrition. Little is known, however, about the functional significance of these findings in humans.

F. Hematologic. Anemia is a common finding in malnutrition. There is evidence that protein depletion alone may impair erythrogenesis, but more often the cause is multifactorial (iron, folate, and B_{12} deficiencies). The effects of malnutrition on leukocyte function have been discussed in section III, A, above.

IV. Nutritional assessment

A. History and physical examination. The nutritional status of patients is estimated from the medical interview, physical examination, and selected anthropometric and laboratory measurements. Adequate dietary history should include an estimate of usual daily calorie consumption and a description of recent eating habits. Vomiting and anorexia should also be noted.

A thin habitus and the appearance of recent weight loss are obvious clues to malnutrition. However, not all malnourished patients are thin; obesity often hides evidence of muscle wasting and may promote complacency regarding the possibility of visceral protein deficiency. From the history and physical examination, conditions that are often associated with malnutrition can be identified. These include:

1. Gastrointestinal diseases characterized by malnutrition, maldigestion, or inadequate intake, including alcoholism, head and neck cancer, pancreatic insufficiency, Crohn's disease, short-bowel syndrome, postgastrectomy states, celiac disease, or any condition requiring prolonged periods of intravenous dextrose and electrolyte solutions.

2. Conditions characterized by abnormal protein losses, such as fistula, abscesses, effusions, draining wounds, and protein-losing enteropathy.

3. Increased metabolic needs, as seen in infection, hyperthyroidism, trauma, burns, pregnancy, and fever. These may also predispose the patient to malnutrition.

B. Anthropometric measurements. Three measurements are commonly employed: (1) Triceps skin-fold (TSF) thickness, which assesses the fat compartment; (2) mid-arm circumference (MAC); and (3) mid-arm muscle circumference (MAMC), which assesses the somatic protein stores.

   1. **Triceps skin-fold thickness** is obtained by using calipers to measure the thickness of the fat layer of the upper arm.

   2. **The mid-arm circumference**, determined by using a tape measure, is used to assess somatic muscle protein in the same nondominant upper arm.

   3. **The mid-arm muscle circumference**, which is also a measurement of somatic muscle protein stores, is then calculated using the following formula: $MAMC = MAC - \pi$ (TSF in cm).

C. Laboratory assessment. The laboratory is helpful in evaluating the somatic and visceral protein stores.

1. Somatic protein stores can be assessed by calculating the creatinine-height index (CHI) from the following formula:

$$\text{CHI} = \frac{\text{24-hr urine creatinine}}{\text{Ideal 24-hr urine creatinine}} \times 100$$

The usefulness of the creatinine-height index is based on the close relation between daily creatinine production (hence excretion) and muscle mass.

2. Visceral protein stores are assessed by determining serum albumin concentration, total lymphocyte count (TLC), serum transferrin level, total iron-binding capacity, and reaction to a battery of skin antigens, including purified protein derivative (PPD), mumps, streptokinase-streptodornase (SK-SD), and *Candida albicans*.

V. **Nutritional support.** The provision of adequate nutrition in the ill, hospitalized patient is pivotal in determining outcome. For example, there is a good correlation between depletion of visceral protein stores and increased surgical morbidity and mortality. An abnormal serum albumin is associated with a fourfold increase in complications and a sixfold increase in deaths. An abnormal total lymphocyte count is associated with a fourfold increase in deaths. When both serum albumin and TLC are abnormal, there is nearly a fourfold increase in complications and a tenfold increase in deaths. It is reasonable to assume that correction of these abnormalities will improve the outcome.

Nutritional support of the ill patient requires estimation of caloric requirements and nitrogen balance, both of which can be easily calculated.

A. **Formula for assessing nutritional requirements**

1. **The Harris-Benedict formula** provides a means of estimating the basal energy expenditure (BEE), taking into consideration the patient's sex, weight (W), height (H), and age (A).

BEE for men = $66 + 13.7W + 5H - 6.8A$
BEE for women = $655 + 9.6W + 1.7H - 4.7A$

W = weight in kilograms (use ideal body weight if patient is thin)
H = height in centimeters
A = age in years

There are correction factors that need to be taken into consideration over and above the basal state:

Correction factor

Activity factor	
Confined to bed	BEE × 1.20
Out of bed	BEE × 1.30
Injury factor	
Minor operation	BEE × 1.20
Trauma	BEE × 1.35
Sepsis	BEE × 1.60
Severe burns	BEE × 2.10

Thus, the total of calories needed is the product of: BEE × activity status × injury factor.

2. **Nitrogen balance** is calculated from the following considerations:
   a. Protein content of the diet.
   b. Urine urea nitrogen (UUN).

    c. Knowledge that 16 percent of protein is nitrogen.

    d. A correction factor of 3 g for nonurinary nitrogen loss. Thus, nitrogen balance = (grams dietary protein × 0.16) − (UUN + 3).

  3. Rules of thumb for providing nutritional support. In addition to characterizing depletion, determining caloric requirements, and assessing nitrogen balance, the following rules of thumb are useful in planning a prescription for nutritional support:

    a. About 1 to 2 g of protein per kilogram body weight is needed in adults.

    b. The optimum ratio of nonprotein calories to grams of nitrogen (N) is 140 : 1 or greater.

    c. With normal intake of food, calories are partitioned as follows: 40 percent carbohydrates, 40 percent fat, 20 percent protein.

    d. Potassium, phosphorus, and magnesium, the major inorganic intracellular ions, must be provided in relatively large quantities during repletion of protein and calorie deficits.

VI. Clinical example of sepsis

  A. Description. The patient was a 45-year-old male admitted with a ruptured appendix and peritonitis. He had been operated on 10 days previously at another hospital. Postoperatively, the patient continued to be febrile despite antibiotics. He had received only standard intravenous fluids, primarily 5 percent dextrose and 0.45 percent saline with KCl. His normal weight was 155 pounds. Physical examination revealed a febrile (temperature, 102° F), cachectic, acutely ill patient with a tender, distended abdomen and no bowel sounds. Further evaluation indicated the presence of a subdiaphragmatic abscess.

  B. Nutritional assessment

    1. Weight, 125 lb

    2. Height, 5 ft 10 in.

    3. Triceps skin fold, 10 mm

    4. Mid-arm circumference, 19 cm

    5. Mid-arm muscle circumference

$$\text{MAMC} = 19 - (\pi \times 1.0 \text{ cm})$$
$$\text{MAMC} = 19 - 3.1$$
$$\text{MAMC} = 15.9 \text{ cm } (<70\% \text{ of standard})$$

    6. Serum albumin, 2.4 g/dl

    7. Total lymphocyte count, 900/mm^3

    8. Skin antigen responses, <5 mm

    9. Creatinine-height index, 63%

    This septic, catabolic patient had received no protein for 10 days, but a hypocaloric intake of intravenous fluids. He had lost 30 pounds. There was evidence of both visceral protein depletion (decreased albumin, TLC, anergy) as well as fat and somatic muscle protein depletion. Nutritional support was needed to allow the patient to withstand surgery and overcome the severe infection.

$$\begin{aligned}
\text{BEE} &= 66 + 13.7\text{W} + 5\text{H} + 6.8\text{A} \\
&= 66 + 13.7(60 \text{ kg}) + 5(178 \text{ cm}) - 6.8(45) \\
&= 1{,}595
\end{aligned}$$

Activity status, 1.2 (in bed). Injury factor, 1.6 (sepsis). Calories needed = 1,595 × 1.2 × 1.6 = 3,062 Kcal/day.

C. Discussion. Because of the inadvisability of using the gastrointestinal tract (peritonitis, subphrenic abscess) for nutritional purposes, central vein hyperalimentation was utilized. The patient was given 2.5 liters of hyperalimentation fluid per day, providing approximately 3,400 calories and 125 g of protein. Potassium, phosphorus, and magnesium, as well as vitamins and trace metals, were also provided in adequate amounts. These nutrients provided the minimum needs; hence, the hyperalimentation infusion might be gradually advanced to permit more rapid repletion of energy and protein stores.

Questions

More than one answer may be correct.

1. Which of the following items may be useful in the nutritional assessment of a malnourished patient?
   a. History.
   b. Serum albumin concentration.
   c. Physical examination.
   d. Intradermal skin tests, including PPD, mumps, *Candida albicans*.
   e. Triceps skin fold.
   f. Total lymphocyte count.
   g. Mid-arm muscle circumference.
   h. History of recent weight loss.
   i. Creatinine-height index.
   j. All of the above.
2. Calculate nitrogen balance for a patient whose protein intake is 100 g and whose urinary urea nitrogen is 10 g per 24 hours.
   a. +90 g
   b. +9 g
   c. +3 g
   d. −3 mg
   e. None of the above

XI Oncology

E. Randy Eichner
Robert B. Epstein
J. Lee Murray
Robert B. Slease

54 Carcinogenesis, Cell Kinetics, and Tumor Immunology

I. **Carcinogenesis.** The term *cancer* has evoked numerous definitions in the attempt to explain a complex problem. The simplest definition is that of disordered cellular homeostasis with loss of the normal growth-controlling mechanisms. The transformation of normal to malignant tissue is not necessarily an all-or-none phenomenon and may be dependent on a number of factors in the host. For instance, a cell may have some of the characteristics of malignancy but lack the potential for invasiveness and metastatic spread (carcinoma in situ).

   A. **Structural and metabolic differences between normal and malignant cells.** Cancer cells differ from normal cells in several ways. One theory of carcinogenesis is that through initial viral- or carcinogen-induced alterations in nuclear deoxyribonucleic acid (DNA), the cancer cell undergoes cytoplasmic and membrane alterations that account for its malignant properties. Normal cells have an orderly array of membrane glycoproteins embedded in a lipid bilayer. The glycolipids act as antigens or receptors that, upon stimulation, can transmit signals from the outside to the inside of the cell. Structural proteins similar to those responsible for muscle contraction are present, which allow directed movement of membrane glycoproteins in response to external stimuli. The density and the distribution of membrane glycoproteins are important in maintaining normal communication between adjacent cells.

   In contrast, tumor cells lack a normal cytoskeleton and, therefore, have a more irregular distribution of protein constituents. Random movements of abnormal glycoproteins not only may facilitate hormone-binding sites, leading to derangements in cellular metabolism, but also may be responsible for the loss of cohesiveness between adjacent cells. In clinical terms, this may account for the infiltrative nature of cancer cells and also their increased metastatic potential.

   Tumor cells have an increase in anaerobic glycolysis with high adenosine triphosphate (ATP) turnover and are less dependent on mitochondrial oxidation than normal cells. For these reasons, mitochondria and endoplasmic reticulum are often decreased or abnormal. In addition, cancer cells contain high levels of proteolytic enzymes and other proteins that may cause abnormalities in amino acid, ion, and glucose transport. These abnormal proteases, along with other chemical mediators, such as angiogenesis factor, may allow the cells both to invade host tissues and to develop their own blood supply. It should be stressed that abnormal DNA synthesis, membrane perturbations, and cytoplasmic alterations are all irrevocably linked in accounting for the tumor cell's abnormal metabolism and growth.

   Characteristics of both benign and malignant tumor cells are shown in Table 54-1.

   B. **Etiologic mechanisms.** Both viruses and chemical carcinogens have been implicated in causing cancer. Whatever the trigger leading to abnormal DNA synthesis, the end result is a somatic mutation of ge-

Characteristics	Benign	Malignant
Growth	Expansile (capsule)	Infiltrative (not encapsulated)
Vascularity	Slight	Increased (angiogenesis factor?)
Metastases	None	Present (loss of cohesiveness)
Ulceration	Unusual	Common
Cytologic	Normal nuclear to cytoplasmic ratio	Increased nuclear to cytoplasmic ratio
	Few mitoses	↑ Mitoses (abnormal)
Ultrastructure	Normal	↓ Mitochondria
		↓ Endoplasmic reticulum
		Scattered RNA particles
		Simplified cell membrane

↑ = increased; ↓ = decreased.

netic material, resulting in the phenotypic characteristics of malignant cells.

1. **Tumor viruses.** In animals both DNA- and, more commonly, ribonucleic acid (RNA)–containing viruses cause tumors. However, few viruses have been directly implicated in the cause of human cancer.

   a. **Oncorna viruses** (RNA-containing) are responsible for numerous animal tumors. The virus particle has been found in several species of mammalian embryos. It is speculated that viral enzymes serve as a mechanism of gene exchange during embryogenesis, forming new sequences of DNA nucleotides, and that an oncogene may be formed in the process. Although theoretical, this may explain why many viral antigens cross-react with fetal tissues, and why tumors in different species share common viral-induced antigens.

   RNA viruses affect DNA synthesis through an interesting mechanism. The RNA virus enters the cell cytoplasm, where it produces an enzyme, RNA-dependent DNA polymerase. Using its own RNA as a template, the polymerase copies complementary base pairs to make single-stranded DNA, which then replicates to form the whole molecule. The virus is thus able to insert complementary base pairs into host DNA (the reverse of what occurs during normal synthesis; hence, the term *reverse transcriptase*). Through this mechanism, a virus induces the cell to synthesize its own unique proteins and tumor antigens. This enzyme has been isolated in some human leukemias.

   Interferon, a natural substance produced by the cell during viral invasion, acts as a messenger to inhibit viral penetration in surrounding tissues. Its possible role as an anti-cancer agent is undergoing extensive investigation.

   b. **Epstein-Barr virus** is the only known DNA virus directly associated with human neoplasia. Infection with Epstein-Barr virus also causes the benign condition of infectious mononucleosis. The factors controlling the development of either benign or

Table 54-2

Class	Example(s)	Tumor
Direct-acting	Alkylating agents (H_2N) Sodium arsenite (Fowler's solution)	Skin cancers Gastrointestinal cancers
Activated metabolites	Aromatic hydrocarbons Dyes Coal tar products	Lung cancer Bladder cancer Skin, gastrointestinal tract cancers
Metals	Chromium, nickel (often in combination with activated metabolites) Asbestos	Lung Mesothelioma
Mold products	Aflatoxin, bracken fern, cycad nut	Gastrointestinal cancers

malignant disease associated with this common virus are thought to relate to immunologic responses of the host.

2. **Chemical carcinogenesis.** The list of chemicals with demonstrated carcinogenic potential in man is small (Table 54-2). Most chemical carcinogens damage DNA either directly or following metabolic activation in the liver. Most compounds are only weakly carcinogenic and require synergism with other substances to exert their effect. Modifying factors such as age, diet, sex, and immunologic competence of the host are important. Chemical carcinogens may be classified as follows:

a. **Direct-acting chemicals.** Industrial chemicals, along with cytotoxic drugs (e.g., nitrogen mustard), are in this group. These compounds, highly toxic and metabolized rapidly, act by directly alkylating DNA.

b. **Chemicals carcinogenic after metabolic activation.** Certain chemicals are only carcinogenic following metabolic modification in vivo. Most carcinogens are in this class, which includes soot, coal tar, petroleum products, and cigarette smoke. They are characterized by a polynuclear aromatic hydrocarbon structure. Metabolic activation is often dependent on endogenous factors (promoters) related to diet, sex, species, and the presence of other compounds.

c. **Metals and inorganic substances.** Several metals, chiefly nickel and cadmium, along with asbestos fibers, are toxic in large quantities over time. The hazards of asbestos exposure in the insulation and shipping industries have come under intense scrutiny.

d. **Food products.** Aflatoxin is a product of various plant molds that may contaminate vegetables; it has been associated with liver tumors, primarily in Africans and Asians. Other offenders include cycasin (cycad nut), bracken fern, and American food additives such as safrol (sassafras oil), tryptophan derivatives, and cyclamate. Many of these contain nitrites, which are converted to nitrosamines by intestinal flora; they have recently been implicated in several types of gastrointestinal cancer.

II. **Cell kinetics**

A. **The cell cycle.** All renewing cells that synthesize DNA go through a series of distinct growth phases (Fig. 54-1).

Figure 54-1

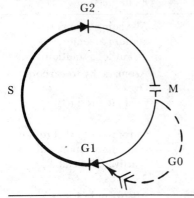

The normal cell cycle. S = DNA synthesis; G₂ = premitotic resting phase; M = mitosis; G₀ = cells not in cycle; G₁ = postmitotic resting phase.

1. **Mitosis (M).** During this stage, chromatin aligns itself along spindle fibers, following which two genetically identical daughter cells are formed.

2. **G_1.** Following mitosis, DNA synthesis ceases. RNA and protein synthesis continues, and the cell enters a rest (G_1) period. The length of G_1 may vary among cancer cells within the same tumor mass.

3. **G_0.** In both normal and tumor cells, an additional resting stage (G_0) has been described in which the cell loses its proliferative capacity and may or may not reenter the cell cycle.

4. **S Phase.** Late in G_1 an unknown signal initiates a burst of RNA synthesis; at that point the cell is committed to division. DNA replication then occurs in the S phase. The length of the S phase varies among different tumors.

5. **G_2.** After the S phase, DNA synthesis stops prior to entry into mitosis, although RNA and protein synthesis continue unabated.

   Different anti-tumor agents act at different phases of the cell cycle. Part of the success of combination drug therapy is based on the strategic timing of drugs in order to promote maximum tumor kill. For example, the administration of vincristine, a mitotic inhibitor, causes a backup of cells from G_1 through S phase, allowing for greater cell kill by agents effective in these stages.

B. **Growth kinetics**

   1. **Growth characteristics of normal and malignant tissues.** With few exceptions, all living tissues have the ability to multiply. In man, intricate homeostatic mechanisms exist to prevent cellular overgrowth. Under normal circumstances cell birth equals cell death. Cancer cells lack growth-restraining signals, such as adjacent cell contact, and proliferate toward a critical mass (10^{12} cells or 1 kg of tumor) before killing the host. Starting from the earliest clinical recognition of tumor (10^9 cells or 1 g), cancer cells grow in exponential fashion. As tumor mass increases, the time it takes for a tumor to double in size also increases (Gompertzian growth, shown by dotted line in Fig. 54-2). Two mechanisms are evoked to explain the increasing doubling time.

      a. **Increase** in cell cycle time (time from mitosis to the next phase).

      b. **Decrease** in the growth fraction, or cells participating in active division within the tumor.

   2. **Drugs' effect on cell growth.** The majority of drugs used in cancer therapy are active during cell division (Fig. 54-3); hence the per-

Figure 54-2

Growth kinetics of both normal and malignant cells. (Modified from S. K. Carter, M. T. Bakowski, and K. Hellmann, Chemotherapy of Cancer. *New York: Wiley, 1977, p. 9. By permission of S. K. Carter and the publisher.)*

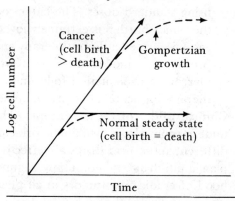

Figure 54-3

Compartmented divisions representing cell types in an individual tumor mass; cells in cycle are susceptible to most anticancer drugs. (Modified from S. K. Carter, M. T. Bakowski, and K. Hellmann, Chemotherapy of Cancer. *New York: Wiley, 1977, p. 12. By permission of S. K. Carter and the publisher.)*

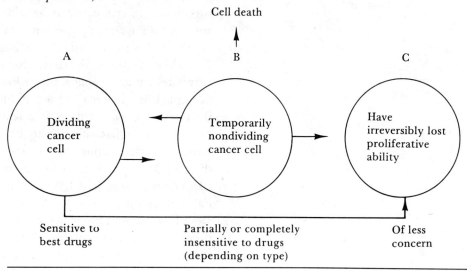

centage of cell kill is proportional to the mitotic index. Rapidly growing tumors (those with a short doubling time and high mitotic index) are often curable with chemotherapy, whereas slow-growing tumors have a greater likelihood of responding when the tumor burden is low. Therefore, the sensitivity of a tumor to therapy is based on three basic parameters: the number of cells in cycle; tumor doubling time; and tumor size.

C. Log-kill hypothesis. In studying animal leukemia, H. E. Skipper noted several principles that form the basis of successful cancer therapy:

1. **Drug efficacy.** A relation exists between drug dose and its ability to kill tumor cells. Drugs with a high therapeutic index kill a maximum fraction of cancer cells without injuring host tissues. Drugs with a low therapeutic index, plus considerable host toxicity, are unacceptable as cancer agents.

2. **Hypothesis of log-kill kinetics.** A given dose of drug kills a constant *fraction* of tumor cells, not a constant *number;* this follows first-

order kinetics. To eradicate a tumor population completely, one must either increase drug concentration within the limits of host tolerance or begin treatment when cell number is small enough, using standard doses. The latter concept, treating a patient when the tumor burden is extremely low (10^3 cells—submicroscopic disease), is termed adjuvant therapy and has been highly successful in preventing tumor recurrences in women with breast cancer. Bone marrow transplantation following sublethal radiation and chemotherapy for acute leukemia embodies the former concept.

D. **Clinical utility of these concepts.** There are several advantages to understanding basic cytokinetic principles. First, knowledge of where different anti-cancer drugs are effective in the cell cycle allows one to plan multi-drug chemotherapy regimens that have a greater likelihood of eradicating tumors in all phases of growth. Second, a basic understanding of the concept of doubling time allows the oncologist to determine which tumors would be most likely to respond to drug therapy and possibly to predict how well the patient will do following treatment.

1. **Response measurement.** In the clinical setting a reduction in measurable tumor size is an approximation of cell kill. These measurements are crude, for in actuality a complete clinical disappearance of tumor encompasses only a three-log kill (i.e., from 10^{12} to 10^9 cells). Beyond this point subclinical disease exists, and one must use other measures as criteria for cell death. In man a high kill correlates with a *prolonged disease-free interval*, as well as *survival*. For example, the greater the fraction of cells killed, the longer it takes the tumor (providing there is at least one tumor cell remaining) to undergo enough doublings to be clinically visible. Patients who have a complete remission (i.e., complete disappearance of clinical disease) are more likely to have a prolonged survival (and possibly a cure) than persons who have a lesser reduction in tumor mass (partial remission).

2. **Doubling time.** The majority of human tumors have doubling times of from 30 to 70 days. Cancers that are most responsive to therapy—such as testicular cancer, non-Hodgkin's lymphoma, and Ewing's sarcoma of the bone—have a mean doubling time shorter than 30 days. Hodgkin's disease and osteosarcomas have doubling times of 1 month, whereas common solid tumors—such as breast cancer, colon cancer, and most lung cancers—have doubling times greater than 70 days. Tumors with short doubling times (testicular tumors) are more responsive to therapy and theoretically can be cured with intense, aggressive treatment (Fig. 54-4A, bottom). On the other hand, in slow-growing cancers, such as colon cancer, fractional cell kill is small (<20%), producing a shallow response followed by early recurrence (Fig. 54-4B, top). Hence, cure is theoretically impossible and palliative therapy is indicated. In tumors with slow doubling times, for which the likelihood of fractional cell kill is less than 50 percent (breast cancer), cures are theoretically possible with treatment of minimal disease (Fig. 54-4B).

E. **Clinical examples of the concept of doubling time and response to therapy**

1. **Clinical example of Burkitt's lymphoma**

    a. **Description.** A 20-year-old white woman was admitted to the hospital, complaining of fever, chills, and easy bruising. On

Figure 54-4

Relationship between doubling time and response to therapy. A. The bottom line shows a rapidly growing tumor; fractional cell kill is large with repeated courses of therapy (dotted line). The top line shows poor response to therapy, with increasing tumor mass. B. The bottom line shows a partially sensitive tumor with intermediate doubling time. The top line indicates a tumor with a long doubling time—relatively insensitive to therapy. (From S. E. Shackney, G. W. McCormack, and J. Cuchural, Jr., Growth rate patterns of solid tumors and their relation to responsiveness to therapy: An analytical review. Ann Intern Med, 89:117, 1978. By permission of S. E. Shackney and the publisher.)

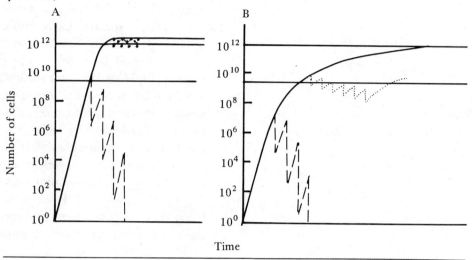

physical exam she had a large abdominal mass and a white blood count of 200,000. Most of the white cells were large, vacuolated-appearing lymphocytes, diagnostic for Burkitt's lymphoma. She underwent intensive therapy with Adriamycin, vincristine, and cyclophosphamide and had a complete disappearance of disease. Despite intensive consolidation therapy following this remission, she had a recurrence of her tumor 6 months later and died of central nervous system metastases.

b. Discussion. Burkitt's lymphoma has the most rapid doubling time known (approximately 6 days). Although quite responsive to chemotherapy, due to its rapid growth it tends to recur within a year and is usually fatal. Therapy strategy includes intensive chemotherapy to effect greatest fractional cell kill, followed by extensive consolidation therapy to prevent regrowth. Unfortunately, the development of resistance to chemotherapeutic agents eventually leads to relapse and death.

2. Clinical example of colon cancer

a. Description. A 70-year-old painter had noted blood in his stools for several months. Barium enema revealed a large apple-core lesion in the sigmoid colon; he was taken to surgery, where a large adenocarcinoma was removed. He did well until 12 months later, when he complained of nausea, weight loss, and decreased appetite. Liver scan revealed a large tumor mass in the left lobe, and he was begun on therapy with 5-Fluorouracil. Despite treatment he continued to have progression of his tumor and died 6 months later in hepatic coma.

b. Discussion. Colon cancer has doubling time in excess of 70 days, and the greatest sensitivity to any single drug is only 15 to 20 percent. Cure is unlikely, and treatment with tolerable doses of medication is acceptable practice.

III. Tumor immunology

A. Historical aspects

1. **Clinical evidence of immunologic response to tumors.** Clinicians had often recognized host immunologic responses in the prevention of tumor growth. Patients with draining abscesses in tumors tended to live longer; women with breast cancer who had benign inflammatory infiltrates surrounding tumor masses or adjacent lymph nodes had better prognoses.

2. **Early animal studies.** Early studies in animals demonstrated that tumors in one strain of mouse were rejected if implanted in another strain that had been previously immunized with a low dose of tumor cells. However, later studies using inbred strains (i.e., genetically similar) revealed that transplanted tumors were not rejected, raising serious doubts concerning the existence of tumor-specific antigens. Earlier studies were actually a reflection of genetic differences among outbred animals rather than a demonstration of tumor immunogenicity. Nevertheless, these observations gave birth to the field of transplantation immunology.

   In the 1950s, E. J. Foley induced sarcomas in inbred animals, using the carcinogen methylcholanthrane. Mice of the same strain did not develop tumors when inoculated with the chemical if they had been previously sensitized. Moreover, immune serum and lymphocytes from these animals, when injected into another inoculated animal, prevented tumor takes. Repeat experiments have confirmed these findings and represent in vivo evidence for the existence of tumor-specific antigens.

B. Tumor antigens.
Several types of antigens exist in both viral and carcinogen-induced tumors. Antigens are capable of stimulating B-lymphocyte responses (antibody synthesis) or T-lymphocyte responses (cellular immunity). The magnitude of humoral (antibody) or cellular response depends upon the chemical composition of the antigen, along with its mode of presentation. Experimental evidence suggests that T (thymus-derived) lymphocytes are directly responsible for tumor rejection. Tumor-specific antibodies are also produced; however, uncontrolled humoral responses may potentiate tumor growth.

1. **Tumor-specific transplantation antigens (TSTA)** (Fig. 54-5). In viral or carcinogen-induced tumors, antigens produced may be modified transplantation antigens and can be detected using serologic methods. In humans, the existence of TSTA is not established. Tumors produced by viruses share common antigens (T antigens). These are coded by the viral genome and are found on

---

Figure 54-5

Tumor antigens. (From J. H. Coggin et al., Proposed mechanisms by which autochthonous neoplasms escape immune rejection. Cancer Res 34:2093, 1974. By permission of J. H. Coggin and the publisher, Cancer Research, Inc.)

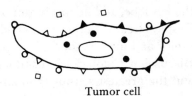

Antigens

△ Organ specific
▲ Tumor specific
○ Fetal (embryonic)
● Cytoplasmic
□ Soluble

Tumor cell

Figure 54-6

In vitro mechanisms of tumor killing; tumors may be lysed by lymphocytes containing large granules (LGL) called natural killer (NK) cells. Both macrophages and specific lymphocytes have receptors for the Fc fragment of immunoglobulin and may lyse tumor cells following binding to antibody (antibody-dependent cellular cytotoxicity, or ADCC).

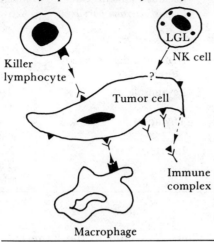

tumors of different histologic type and species. In contrast, chemically induced tumors have antigens that are unique to each tumor.

2. **Oncofetal antigens.** Several tumor antigens in man are found on fetal, but not adult, tissues. These include alpha-fetoprotein, which is specific for hepatomas and testicular cancer, and carcinoembryonic antigen (CEA), present in gastrointestinal tumors. CEA is elevated in 70 percent of colon cancer patients and 90 percent of persons with pancreatic cancer. It is also present in a lower percentage of other tumors. Unlike TSTA, oncofetal antigens are not immunogenic; they are useful, however, as markers for predicting disease status.

C. **Immune mechanisms against cancer**

1. **In vivo evidence.** Characterizing in vivo responses to tumor-specific antigens in man has been difficult because experiments similar to those used in animals are difficult to carry out. However, there is indirect evidence to suggest immunologic responses to human tumors.

   a. Fluorescence techniques have demonstrated the presence, in serum, of circulating antibodies against tumors.

   b. Patients with immunodeficiency disorders, as well as those on immunosuppressive therapy, have a higher incidence of spontaneous cancers.

   c. Persons who are skin tested with extracts of their own tumors often develop a delayed hypersensitivity reaction.

   d. There have been a few documented cases in which metastatic foci disappear following removal of a large primary tumor mass.

2. **In vitro mechanisms** (Fig. 54-6). Several types of immunocompetent cells are capable of killing tumor cells in vitro. In both animals and man a specific cell called a natural killer (NK) cell will lyse virally infected tumor targets. The degree of tumor kill or cytotoxicity can be determined by laboratory techniques. The specificity of this reaction is unclear. In addition, both T lymphocytes and macrophages are capable of lysing tumor cells coated with anti-tumor antibodies (antibody-dependent cellular cytotoxicity [ADCC]).

Table 54-3

Immunotherapy

Type	Agents	Mechanism	Tumors
Nonspecific	Bacillus Calmette-Guérin *Corynebacterium parvum*	Macrophage Activation	Melanoma Leukemia Lung cancer Breast cancer
Specific	Neuraminidase-treated tumor cells	↑ Antigen-specific cellular immunity	Acute leukemia
Immuno-potentiators	Levamisole	↑ T-cell cytotoxicity	Lung cancer
	Thymosin	↑ T-cell maturation	Lung cancer
	Interferon	↑ Natural killer (T cells) cells effect	Multiple myeloma Breast cancer

↑ = increased.

These cells bind to the large end of the antibody (Fc fragment) through special Fc receptors.

3. **Relation between tumors and defense mechanisms.** The identification of host immune responses with malignancies has raised the question of how tumors escape this defense mechanism. Several explanations are offered:

   a. A tumor lacking antigen exposure or with weak exposure may not elicit an immune response.

   b. Tumors may shed antigens or antigen-antibody complexes (Fig. 54-6) that effectively block lymphocyte Fc receptors, preventing ADCC. In man, a direct relation between the presence of immune complexes in serum and progressive tumor growth has been suggested.

   c. During an ongoing humoral and cellular immune response, immunoregulatory lymphocytes or macrophages develop, which suppress further immunoreactivity. These suppressor cells have been noted in patients with advanced disease, although a cause-and-effect relationship between these cells and tumor growth has not been definitely established.

D. **Immunotherapy.** An ideal goal would be the capability to vaccinate people against their own tumors. In practice, this has been a difficult task, in view of the technical problems of isolating tumor-specific antigens. Current forms of immunotherapy are listed in Table 54-3.

   1. **Bacterial adjuvants.** Immunity to certain animal tumors has been nonspecifically enhanced by several bacterial preparations, notably bacillus Calmette-Guérin (BCG) or *Corynebacterium parvum*. In humans these adjuvants have been applied as vaccines or directly injected into superficial tumors. They cause an intense inflammatory reaction by activating macrophages. In a person previously sensitized to BCG, a strong delayed hypersensitivity reaction occurs and tumor cells are indirectly killed in the process. To date, evidence suggesting an anti-tumor effect, other than through direct tumor inoculation with these agents, is scanty.

   2. Irradiated, enzyme-treated tumor cells have been given as vaccines to patients in hopes of eliciting a tumor-specific immune response. There is minimal evidence to suggest that immunizations may be of some benefit in prolonging survival in leukemia and lung cancer.

3. **Immunopotentiators.** Certain drugs directly stimulate cellular immunity through unique mechanisms.

    a. **Levamisole.** This drug was originally used as an anthelminthic. It causes an increase in T-cell cytotoxicity and macrophage migration toward tumors. Trials in lung cancer and other solid tumors are under way.

    b. **Thymosin.** Thymosin, a hormone produced in the thymus gland, is important for T-lymphocyte development and maturation. Evidence suggests it may be effective, when used with drug therapy, in prolonging survival in certain lung cancer patients.

    c. **Interferon.** Interferon is produced by the macrophage. Along with an antiviral effect, it stimulates natural killer cells and may be effective in controlling malignancies such as acute leukemia. Extensive clinical trials with this agent are under way in major centers.

    It is important to realize that immunotherapy has been shown in experimental systems to be effective only if the tumor burden is low. Hence, it is currently used for studies as an adjunct to radiation and chemotherapy.

E. **Clinical examples of tumor antigens and immunologic treatment**

    1. **Clinical example of adenocarcinoma of the cecum**

        a. **Description.** A 45-year-old man had guaiac-positive stools. CEA measurement was 20 units (normal, <5). Barium enema revealed a polypoid lesion in the cecum. A 5-cm adenocarcinoma that infiltrated the cecum was surgically removed. His CEA level fell to 5 units postoperatively. He was followed at 3-month intervals; 18 months later his CEA had increased to 30 units (from a baseline of 5). Liver/spleen scan and barium enema were negative, but computed tomography revealed an abdominal mass. At surgery a large mass was found adjacent to the original resection. Frozen section again revealed adenocarcinoma, and the mass was removed. He remains well approximately a year after surgery.

        b. **Discussion.** The CEA is a useful marker in detecting recurrent disease. Unfortunately, only 20 percent of patients develop recurrence solely adjacent to a previous resection. More often, a rising CEA titer indicates spread to distant organs, such as liver or lung.

    2. **Clinical example of malignant melanoma**

        a. **Description.** A 20-year-old white female noticed an enlarging black mole on her left calf. Biopsy revealed malignant melanoma, and a wide excision, with skin grafting, was made. Three years later, recurrent subcutaneous tumors appeared near the area of original surgery. Following informed consent, she was given BCG injections directly into the tumor nodules, with complete disappearance of the injected lesions. In addition, 30 percent of contiguous uninjected nodules spontaneously regressed.

        b. **Discussion.** Malignant melanoma is a highly immunogenic skin cancer. Direct intratumoral BCG injections will cause 60 percent of injected nodules to regress, along with 10 to 30 percent of uninjected lesions. This treatment is not without side effects. Many persons experience fever and chills, along with ulceration of injected nodules. Rarely, disseminated BCG disease occurs with granuloma formation in distant organs.

More than one answer may be correct.

1. Select a correct statement or statements concerning viral and chemical carcinogenesis:
   a. Burkitt's lymphoma is the only tumor in man in which a DNA virus can be directly implicated.
   b. Interferon acts by blocking reverse transcriptase in the host cell.
   c. Viral-induced malignancies, unlike those induced by carcinogens, may have antigens that are cross-reactive between different tumors.
   d. Most carcinogens are direct acting and do not require metabolic activation by the host.
   e. Lung cancer is an example of two different classes of carcinogens that may act synergistically.

2. Which of the following statements are true concerning differences among immune adjuvants, immunopotentiators, and specific immunotherapy?
   a. Adjuvant therapy (i.e., BCG) is nonspecific, as opposed to therapy with tumor antigen.
   b. Specific immunotherapy has been more commonly used.
   c. Interferon acts by inhibiting natural killer cells and increasing macrophage ADCC.
   d. All of the above.
   e. None of the above.

Extraneoplastic Manifestations of Malignancies

I. **Introduction.** Often the most devastating clinical effects of malignancies are produced not by the tumor masses themselves but by the systemic disorders with which they are associated. This chapter will deal with some of these tumor-induced systemic problems, with emphasis on nutrition, the paraneoplastic syndromes, and hematologic complications of neoplasia.

II. **Nutritional effects of cancer and cancer treatment.** No systemic manifestation of malignant disease is more debilitating or less well understood than malnutrition leading to cachexia. Patients with a wide variety of tumors suffer progressive weight loss and weakness during the course of their illness, along with associated phenomena such as anemia and impaired cellular immune responses. Although anorexia and poor nutritional intake play a major role in the process, cachexia in these patients bears no simple relation to caloric deficits. There is, likewise, no close correlation with tumor burden, histology, or location. Nevertheless, cachexia occurs with staggering frequency. One recent study indicated that 88 percent of hospitalized cancer patients had some degree of protein-calorie undernutrition. Severe malnutrition in that study was associated with sharply curtailed survival.

Three potential mechanisms for the development of cachexia are discussed below.

A. **Decreased nutrient intake or absorption**

1. **Anorexia** is a common (though not universal) symptom of malignancy and often leads to decreased caloric intake and cachexia. The pathogenesis of this phenomenon in cancer patients can perhaps be understood by considering the two major determinants of normal food intake control: first, the chemoreceptors in the mouth and nose (taste and smell), which provide both a motivational or excitatory role and a gating function to select nutritive substances and to reject injurious ones, and second, the inhibitory receptors, which are stimulated by accumulated ingested substances within the gastrointestinal (GI) tract. Stimuli from both these receptors are integrated by the central nervous system, which then regulates the type and amount of food ingested.

Cancer patients often have changes in taste and smell sensation, which decrease the normal excitatory stimulation from ingested food. These changes may be related to the altered glucose metabolism and amino acid profiles that these patients sometimes demonstrate. Another mechanism by which anorexia may be mediated is increased inhibitory signals from accumulated substances in the GI tract. These may be mediated by decreased gastric secretions, mucosal atrophy, or muscle atrophy of the upper GI tract, all of which lead to impaired nutrient absorption and prolonged intraluminal accumulated substances. Of course, tumors of the upper GI tract itself may lead to impaired absorption and increased luminal volume, both of which trigger inhibitory stimuli.

   2. **Neoplastic invasion of the gastrointestinal tract,** by either primary GI or metastatic tumors, provides a second important mechanism of simple malnutrition. As noted above, these tumors may produce anorexia by causing increased inhibitory signals. Since these stimuli result from impaired nutrient absorption as well as prolonged retention, it is obvious that malnutrition may be a direct result.

B. **Metabolic effects of cancer leading to cachexia.** Chemically identifiable toxic mediators have been hypothesized to be released by some tumors and to produce cachexia. These substances presumably would act by interfering with intermediary metabolism in host tissue. However, no such toxins have been isolated, even though the rationale for their existence is fairly strong. Conceivably, the tumor itself may parasitize host tissue to satisfy its own nutritional needs, without involving chemical mediators. By whatever mechanism, many cancer patients have weight loss far too rapid or cachexia too severe to be explained by deficient intake or malabsorption alone.

C. **Malnutrition secondary to cancer treatment**

   1. **Surgery.** Both curative and palliative surgical procedures may be associated with serious malnutrition. Immediate postoperative morbidity in cancer patients may be prolonged, sometimes leading to several weeks of decreased caloric intake. Certain procedures permanently alter normal routes of nutritional ingestion or absorption.

   2. **Radiotherapy.** Nearly 90 percent of patients who receive high-dose radiation to some part of the GI tract experience weight loss during treatment. Gastrointestinal mucosal epithelium is quite radiosensitive, and mucosal lesions induced by radiotherapy may lead to nutritional deficiency. For example, radiation to the head and neck often leads to stomatitis and pharyngitis, which impair appetite, mastication, and deglutition. Gastroduodenal irradiation is usually accompanied by nausea and vomiting, while pelvic irradiation may lead to proctitis and diarrhea.

   3. **Chemotherapy.** Most chemotherapeutic agents cause some degree of anorexia, and many produce significant nausea and vomiting. These effects are usually of brief duration, however, and it is often difficult to distinguish the malnutrition induced by the chemotherapy from that caused by the tumor itself.

III. **Paraneoplastic syndromes.** Malignant diseases can produce a variety of remote effects on the host, including the nutritional defects discussed above. Some of the so-called paraneoplastic syndromes can be traced to a chemically identifiable mediator or hormone produced by the tumor; in other instances, the pathophysiology of the process can only be hypothesized.

A. **Ectopic hormone syndromes in non-endocrine tumors**

   1. **Hypercorticism (Cushing's syndrome).** The association of primary lung carcinoma with the clinical syndrome of truncal obesity, hirsutism, hypertension, hyperpigmentation, hyperglycemia, and weakness was first described over 50 years ago. This syndrome is due to the ectopic production of adrenocorticotropic hormone (ACTH) or (rarely) corticotropin-releasing hormone (CRH), leading to increased adrenal production of glucocorticoids, mineralocorticoids, and androgens. ACTH secretion in these patients is usu-

ally not suppressible with high-dose dexamethasone, confirming its independence from the normal pituitary-adrenal axis.

Lung carcinomas (primarily small-cell type) account for about 50 percent of reported cases, but thymomas, carcinoid tumors, bronchial adenomas, medullary thyroid carcinomas, and other tumors may also be associated with the syndrome. Interestingly, it has been shown that virtually all carcinomas are capable of producing a peptide, thought to be a precursor of ACTH, called pro-ACTH. This substance is nonfunctional, however, and only a few tumors elaborate active ACTH. Clinically, the ectopic ACTH syndrome often differs somewhat from the classic Cushing's syndrome caused by pituitary or adrenal adenomas. For example, patients with ectopic ACTH production generally do not show the characteristic cushingoid fat redistribution, perhaps because of their cachexia. The metabolic alkalosis from mineralocorticoid excess tends to be unusually severe and sometimes is life threatening. Hyperpigmentation may also be more marked than expected, perhaps due to the concomitant production of beta-lipotropin, a substance which, like ACTH, has melanin granule-dispersing activity.

2. **Hypercalcemia.** Neoplasia is the most common cause of hypercalcemia in the general population. Although the pathophysiologic consequences of increased serum calcium are similar regardless of etiology, there are multiple mechanisms mediating its occurrence in malignancies.

   a. **Hypercalcemia without bone metastases**

      (1) **Prostaglandin (PG) secretion.** Recent evidence indicates that some cases of tumor-induced hypercalcemia in the absence of bone metastases may be related to excess production of prostaglandin E_2 (PGE_2), probably by the tumor itself. Although mechanisms have not been precisely defined, PGE_2 appears to cause elevations of serum calcium by increasing osteoclastic bone resorption. Significantly, the hypercalcemia in some of these patients has been ameliorated with the use of prostaglandin inhibitors, such as indomethacin.

      (2) **Pseudohyperparathyroidism.** Some tumors, especially squamous cell carcinoma of the lung and renal cell carcinoma, apparently produce substances functionally similar to parathyroid hormone. The resulting hypercalcemic syndrome is termed pseudohyperparathyroidism and may be extremely difficult to distinguish from primary hyperparathyroidism in patients with occult carcinomas.

   b. **Hypercalcemia with bone metastases.** Hypercalcemia may be produced simply by direct bone invasion and destruction by tumor. However, in many tumors which invade bone, additional mechanisms are contributory. Increased PGE_2 synthesis, by increasing osteoclastic activity, may actually promote bone metastasis. The malignant plasma cells in multiple myeloma may produce a non-prostaglandin osteolytic substance called osteoclast activating factor (OAF). What relative contribution to bony invasion by tumor can be ascribed to one or more of these humoral substances is unclear. However, preliminary studies suggest that, while there is no simple relation between amount of bony tumor and degree of hypercalcemia, there seems to be an association between the likelihood of developing bone metastases and the presence of some humoral osteolytic factor.

3. **Inappropriate secretion of antidiuretic hormone (SIADH).** This syndrome, defined clinically as the unexplained excretion of less-than-maximally dilute urine in the presence of hypo-osmolar serum, results from the inappropriate secretion of vasopressin. Both benign and malignant disorders may be associated with SIADH, but it is perhaps most commonly found in small-cell carcinoma of the lung. Production of a vasopressin-like substance by the tumor itself has been repeatedly demonstrated in vitro. The syndrome may result in severe hyponatremia, which in turn can lead to depressed mentation, seizures, and death. Fortunately, however, while perhaps 40 percent of lung cancer patients have excessive vasopressin secretion, the clinical manifestations often remain insignificant.

4. **Hypoglycemia.** The production of insulin has long been recognized to occur in the beta cells of the pancreatic islets. Not surprisingly, tumors arising in these cells (insulinomas) may result in excessive insulin secretion and hypoglycemia. The more than 200 reported cases of hypoglycemia associated with non-islet-cell neoplasms, especially soft-tissue sarcomas, are also interesting. Most of these tumors produce high levels of substances that are functionally insulin-like but structurally distinct from insulin, referred to as nonsuppressible insulin-like activity. These substances are present in low levels in normal persons, and apparently produce hypoglycemia only when secreted in large amounts by certain tumors. Recent data have implicated the somatomedins, a family of hepatic peptides, in the pathogenesis of hypoglycemia in some patients with tumors.

5. **Gynecomastia.** Gynecomastia is sometimes seen in patients with non-seminomatous testicular tumors or lung carcinomas; it may be related to the secretion of chorionic gonadotropin (CG) or related compounds. However, since many patients have dramatic CG elevations without gynecomastia, the actual mechanism by which gynecomastia occurs remains obscure. In females, ectopic CG production by tumor may produce amenorrhea or metromenorrhagia and, if levels are high enough, a falsely positive pregnancy test. Recent studies indicate that virtually all carcinomas can elaborate a CG-like material, though usually in small, subclinical amounts.

6. **Other hormone-related syndromes.** The above-mentioned ectopic hormone disorders are the most commonly encountered. However, many others have been reported in clinical practice. Rare tumors have been shown to produce a variety of hormone or hormone-like compounds, including thyroid stimulating hormone (TSH), prolactin, growth hormone, vasoactive intestinal polypeptide, gastrin, secretin, and glucagon. Associated clinical syndromes in these patients often but not always reflect the measured ectopic hormone. Erythropoietin production has been demonstrated in several different tumors and will be discussed below. Certain tumors, especially those arising in neural crest-derived tissue, can produce multiple hormones, though usually in subclinical amounts. Some investigators believe that small-cell carcinoma of the lung, perhaps the most prolific ectopic hormone-producing neoplasm, is actually a tumor of neural crest origin.

B. Selected neuromuscular syndromes

1. **Myasthenic syndromes: Eaton-Lambert syndrome and myasthenia gravis.** The association of myasthenia gravis and thymoma has been recognized for many years; it is mediated by complex, poorly understood immunologic mechanisms. Myasthenic patients develop progressive weakness, particularly of the respiratory muscles and those of the head and neck, which is partially relieved by rest and anticholinesterase drugs.

   A similar syndrome occurs in some patients with non-thymic neoplasms, particularly small-cell carcinoma of the lung. This Eaton-Lambert syndrome differs from myasthenia gravis in that respiratory muscle weakness rarely occurs, repeated muscular contraction causes increased rather than decreased strength (demonstrable by electromyogram), and improvement does not occur with anticholinesterase drugs but may with administration of guanidine. A humoral mediator has not been identified in this disorder.

2. **Degenerative neurologic syndromes**

   a. **Peripheral neuropathies** are probably the most common remote neurologic complications of cancer, occurring in perhaps 15 percent of patients. Manifestations may reflect purely sensory, both sensory and motor, or only motor dysfunction. Pain may occasionally be the only presenting symptom. For the most part, mechanisms remain obscure, but in some patients, antibodies reacting with neural tissue have been identified. In others, amyloid infiltrates the peripheral nerves. Since many antineoplastic drugs may cause peripheral neuropathies, it is often difficult to distinguish whether the symptoms are due to the disease or its treatment.

   b. **Cerebellar degeneration** has been reported in patients with a variety of neoplasms. Its pathogenesis is unclear, but the clinical course tends not to parallel that of the neoplasm. This suggests that the cerebellar degeneration may be only indirectly related to the tumor and may in fact be due to an associated infection or to the antineoplastic therapy.

IV. **Hematologic disorders associated with non-hematologic tumors**

   A. **Red cell abnormalities**

   1. **Erythrocytosis.** Since the normal source of erythropoietin (Ep) is the kidney, it comes as little surprise that 1 to 5 percent of renal cell carcinomas elaborate large amounts of Ep, leading to the development of erythrocytosis. However, several other benign and malignant neoplasms can also be associated with increased Ep production. These include cerebellar hemangioblastomas, uterine fibromas, adrenocortical tumors, hepatic tumors, ovarian carcinomas, and pheochromocytomas. The cerebellar tumors have been shown to produce a substance that is structurally and functionally identical with normal Ep, but actual Ep production by the other tumors listed above has not been definitively demonstrated.

      Ectopic Ep-induced erythrocytosis can usually be differentiated from polycythemia vera (PV) by the absence of splenomegaly, leukocytosis, and thrombocytosis, which are often found in PV.

   2. **Anemia**

      a. **Hemolytic anemias**

         (1) **Immune-mediated hemolysis,** common in the lymphoid malignancies, has also been associated with a variety of other

tumors, including lung, breast, gastrointestinal, and genitourinary carcinomas. It has been proposed that shared antigens on the tumor cell and red cell surface result in cross-reactive antibody production. Firm evidence for this hypothesis is lacking, however.

(2) **Microangiopathic hemolytic anemia,** resulting from mechanical red cell membrane damage, is sometimes seen in metastatic carcinoma of the prostate and occasionally with other tumors. The pathogenesis of this clinical syndrome involves the deposition of microvascular fibrin in areas of tumor infiltration, so that erythrocytes are unable to traverse the vessel lumen without suffering membrane damage. Characteristically, red cell fragments called schistocytes are found in the peripheral blood smear.

b. **Hypoproliferative anemias**

(1) **The anemia of chronic disorders,** discussed in more detail in Section V, Hematology, is a common concomitant of malignant diseases. Etiologic mechanisms remain poorly defined.

(2) **Iron-deficiency anemia** is also commonly found in neoplasms and can nearly always be traced to blood loss.

(3) **Nutritional anemia,** especially folic acid deficiency, sometimes occurs in severely malnourished patients with advanced cancer.

c. **Myelophthisic anemia.** This anemia is not really a remote effect of neoplasia but, rather, results from the replacement of large amounts of marrow by tumor. Characteristically, these patients are pancytopenic and have both schistocytes and nucleated red cells in the peripheral blood. When early granulocyte precursors are also seen, the term *leukoerythroblastic phenomenon* is used. These abnormal cell forms result from the disruption of medullary sinusoids by tumor, leading to both early release and mechanical damage of hematopoietic precursors.

3. **Red cell aplasia.** Approximately 5 percent of patients with thymoma develop an IgG-mediated syndrome in which the bone marrow becomes devoid of red cell precursors. This IgG antibody appears to be directed against erythroblast nuclei. Similar erythroid aplasia syndromes have rarely been reported in association with other tumors, including lung, thyroid, and gastric carcinomas.

B. **White cell abnormalities**

1. **Leukocytosis.** The control of leukocyte production and release is incompletely understood in normal man (see Chap. 28, Neutrophil Disorders). For reasons that remain obscure, some tumors are associated with persistent leukocytosis, often with a predominance of eosinophils or monocytes.

2. **Leukopenia.** Decreased levels of circulating white cells usually signify marrow replacement by tumor, resulting in decreased effective granulopoiesis.

C. **Platelet abnormalities: thrombocytosis.** Elevated platelet counts, usually of a moderate degree, are commonly found in association with various tumors, especially those with metastatic involvement of marrow. Surprisingly, even with platelet counts exceeding one million per cubic millimeter, thrombotic or hemorrhagic phenomena are unusual.

Although a humoral mediator for platelet production in these tumors is suspected, none has thus far been isolated.

D. Coagulopathies

1. **Hypercoagulability.** Some patients with malignancies develop recurrent thromboembolic phenomena, which often prove refractory to standard therapy. Although a number of mechanisms for this syndrome have been postulated, none have been proved. Unfortunately, there is no reliable in vitro assay for a so-called hypercoagulable state.

2. **Disseminated intravascular coagulation (DIC).** The DIC syndrome, usually of the chronic type, has been associated with a variety of metastatic tumors, particularly the mucin-producing adenocarcinomas. DIC in these patients may be triggered by mucin-induced activation of factor X.

3. **Factor deficiencies or dysfunction.** Isolated coagulation factor deficiencies have been reported in several malignancies, but in many cases were not associated with clinical bleeding. Both impaired production and increased destruction have been implicated. For example, rare lymphomas are associated with antibodies directed against certain factors. Factor X deficiency may result from adsorption onto amyloid, a material which may be associated with several tumors. Defective fibrinogen may be produced by some patients with hepatic carcinomas.

V. Clinical example

A. Hilar mass in a middle-aged man

1. **Description.** A 45-year-old heavy smoker presented with a 3-month history of anorexia, weight loss, increased skin pigmentation, and easy fatigability. Examination revealed generalized hyperpigmentation and mild cachexia, but was otherwise unrevealing. Laboratory studies demonstrated a moderate hypokalemic alkalosis and mild normochromic normocytic anemia. Chest x-ray showed a small right hilar mass, which proved at biopsy to be small-cell carcinoma. Subsequent evaluation disclosed no tumor outside the chest. Serum ACTH levels were strikingly elevated and did not suppress with high-dose dexamethasone. Antineoplastic therapy was given and the alkalosis resolved. Hyperpigmentation slowly improved, but anorexia, weight loss, and fatigue persisted so that the patient was unable to work. Three months after the initiation of therapy, the chest x-ray had become entirely normal, with complete resolution of the mass. Nutritional supplements were given, and gradual weight gain occurred over the next several months. Six months after his original diagnosis the patient returned to work, although therapy was continued on an outpatient basis. One year later he noticed recurrent anorexia, fatigue, and new mid-back pain. Examination was unchanged, but laboratory evaluation revealed moderate anemia with schistocytes and nucleated red cells, leukocytosis with a few early myeloid forms in the peripheral blood, and mild thrombocytosis. Bone marrow biopsy confirmed the presence of metastatic tumor.

2. **Discussion**

   a. Although this patient's tumor originated in the lung, his presentation and course were virtually devoid of pulmonary symptoms.

   b. The ectopic ACTH production, although producing significant hyperpigmentation and alkalosis, did not cause the classic cushingoid facies or fat redistribution.

c. The clinical course in this patient was dominated by malnutrition, demonstrating that even successful antineoplastic therapy may not substantially improve symptomatology until nutritional deficiencies are corrected.

d. The presenting anemia was most likely that associated with chronic disease, whereas late in the course, it was myelophthistic in nature. Bone marrow metastases are common in small-cell carcinoma, and the leukoerythroblastic phenomenon found in this patient was an important clue to that development.

Questions

Select the single best answer.

1. Neoplasms may induce cachexia by multiple mechanisms. Evidence has been presented for each of the following mechanisms, *except:*
   a. Alteration of chemoreceptors, leading to decreased excitatory stimuli.
   b. Increased inhibitory stimuli due to impaired nutrient absorption.
   c. Increased inhibitory stimuli due to the mass effect and replacement of absorptive surface by a primary gastric carcinoma.
   d. Chemically identifiable toxic mediators.

2. Hypercalcemia in malignancy may be mediated by all the following mechanisms, *except:*
   a. Ectopic calcitonin secretion.
   b. Ectopic prostaglandin secretion.
   c. Production of osteoclast activating factor.
   d. Ectopic secretion of a PTH-like substance.

Neoplasms of the Immune System

I. **Introduction.** Until recently, understanding of the malignancies of the immune system relied upon morphologic categorizations that bore no relation to physiology. Only in the past few years has it become possible to separate those diseases originating in the lymphoid system (malignant lymphomas, plasma cell dyscrasias, etc.) from those arising from the reticuloendothelial or monocyte-macrophage system (Hodgkin's disease, monocytic leukemias, etc.). As knowledge of the function of the primary (lymphocyte) and accessory (monocyte-macrophage) cells of the immune system in normal man has expanded, so has insight into the pathophysiology of the malignancies arising from them.

II. **Normal physiology of the immune system**

A. **Lymphocyte ontogeny.** Both lymphocytes and hematopoietic precursors arise from a common stem cell, although such a cell has not been isolated in man. As shown in Figure 56-1, pluripotential cells committed to lymphoid differentiation evolve early, certainly before the development of distinguishable myeloid precursors. These immature lymphoid cells can be identified by the presence of various markers, such as the enzyme terminal desoxynucleotidyl transferase, discussed under section III, A, below.

Further differentiation of these primitive lymphoid cells leads to the development of the various functionally discrete lymphocyte subsets (T cells, B cells, etc.). Monocytes and granulocytes appear to be derived from a common cell, which can be identified by cell culture studies. Monocytes then travel through the peripheral blood to various organs and tissues, where they reside as fixed tissue macrophages.

Thus, while lymphocytes and monocytes originate from a common stem cell, their differentiation pathways are quite distinct. Nevertheless, the functions of lymphocytes and monocyte-macrophages in the immune response are closely interrelated.

B. **The immune response and antigen-stimulated lymphoid differentiation.** The normal sequence of events from antigen recognition to specific immune response is only beginning to be understood. The concept of T and B lymphocytes controlling cellular and humoral responses, respectively, although broadly correct, is an oversimplification of complex mechanisms. It is clear that different subsets of lymphocytes play regulatory as well as effector roles. Macrophages, previously considered to function only as phagocytic cells, are now believed to be important for antigen processing and presentation and for modulation of certain effector responses.

Since the majority of malignant lymphomas arise from B lymphocytes, antigen-stimulated B-cell differentiation is discussed here. Once lymphoid maturation is complete, mature (but unstimulated) B cells bear intrinsically synthesized surface membrane immunoglobulin (smIg), usually of the IgM and IgD heavy-chain classes. These cells, which morphologically are small lymphocytes, circulate in the peripheral blood and lymphatics. Before stimulation, they can also be found in the interfollicular spaces of the lymph nodes. Upon activation by an

Figure 56-1   *Schematic representation of hematopoiesis.*

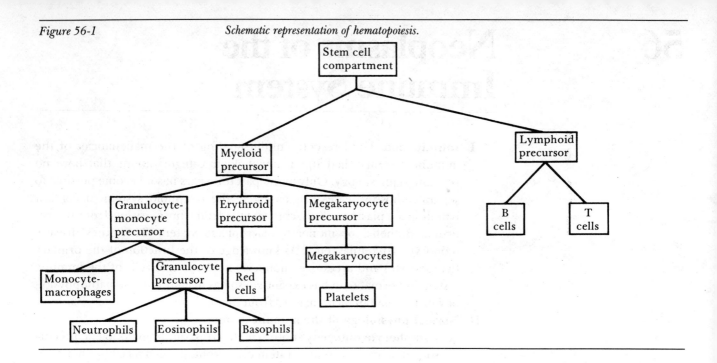

Figure 56-2   *Model for antigen-stimulated B-cell differentiation. (Modified from R. J. Lukes and R. D. Collins, Immunologic characterization of human malignant lymphomas. Cancer 34 (Suppl.):1491, 1974. By permission of R. J. Lukes and the publisher.)*

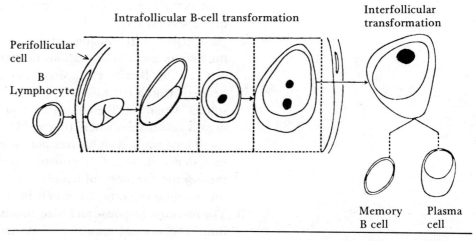

antigen-processing perifollicular cell or immunoregulatory T cell, the B lymphocyte enters a lymphoid follicle and undergoes a series of morphologic transformations, as shown schematically in Figure 56-2. As these changes occur, the B cell proliferates, evolving from an indolent cell with a slow turnover rate to a rapidly dividing follicular center cell. As further differentiation occurs, the clonal expansion diminishes, and the activated B lymphocytes eventually become either immunoglobulin-secreting plasma cells or memory B cells that can be rapidly reactivated upon reexposure to the same antigen. Unlike unstimulated or memory B cells, which are found in peripheral blood, marrow, spleen, and lymph nodes, plasma cells tend to reside in the perivascular areas of the bone marrow and other organs (i.e., gut and spleen).

Hence, there is a clear distinction between the ontogenic differentiation (maturation) of lymphocytes and the differentiation that occurs as a result of antigen stimulation. This concept is critical to the current hypothesis of the pathogenesis of lymphoid neoplasms.

III. Pathophysiology of lymphoid and monocyte-macrophage malignancies

A. Acute lymphoblastic leukemia (ALL). This disease, usually seen in childhood, appears to represent the malignant transformation of cells early in lymphoid maturation and thus is to be contrasted with the malignant lymphomas described below.

The malignant cells in ALL, termed lymphoblasts, usually bear none of the surface membrane markers which identify normal T cells or B cells, although cells from about 25 percent of cases demonstrate sheep erythrocyte receptors, indicating T-cell origin. A smaller percentage have cells with intracytoplasmic IgM, which is the earliest easily recognizable marker of B-cell differentiation (pre-B cells), and rare cases demonstrate immunoglobulins on the lymphoblast surface. Over 90 percent of patients with ALL, however, have cells which contain the DNA synthetic nuclear enzyme terminal desoxynucleotidyl transferase (TdT). This enzyme is found normally in primitive lymphocytes, persists to the pre-B cell and early thymocyte stages of maturation, and is not found in circulating B or T lymphocytes. Therefore, TdT is a marker of early lymphoid maturation, and its presence in ALL lymphoblast nuclei indicates that ALL is a disease of immature cells. Other early differentiation antigens have been found on ALL cells, helping to confirm this hypothesis. The clinical consequences of ALL are similar to those of acute myeloblastic leukemia, described with granulocyte disorders.

B. Malignant lymphomas, non-Hodgkin's type

1. Lymphomas of B-cell origin. The majority of non-Hodgkin's lymphomas arise from B lymphocytes; nearly all of them represent the malignant transformation of a single cell at some stage in the pathway of antigen-stimulated differentiation. Thus, most B-cell lymphomas are clonal diseases. The resulting cell clone generally bears the morphologic, surface marker, and kinetic features of the original progenitor from which it arose (see Fig. 56-2).

a. Chronic lymphocytic leukemia (CLL). If an unstimulated B lymphocyte becomes malignant, its progeny would be likely to be small, mature-appearing lymphocytes, with a slow turnover rate and smIg of the same isotype. Since the progenitor was unstimulated at the time of malignant transformation, it would not have entered a lymphoid follicle, and its progeny would not have follicle-forming tendencies. Biopsies of involved nodes would therefore reveal a diffuse rather than a nodular pattern. Since normal unstimulated B cells are found in bone marrow and peripheral blood, it is not surprising that the progeny of a malignant unstimulated B cell also have this distribution. Thus, this disease commonly involves the marrow, peripheral blood, nodes, spleen, and liver at presentation, yet has an indolent course because of the slow cell turnover rate. Although patients may develop high blood lymphocyte counts and uncomfortably large nodes and spleen, these problems can usually be easily managed. Morbidity and mortality relate primarily to an increased propensity for infection, due in part to low effective antibody levels. Also, some patients may develop symptomatic anemia or thrombocytopenia secondary to marrow replacement by CLL or to abnormal immune destruction. These patients have a particularly short median survival (18–24 mo) whereas those with less aggressive CLL generally live 7 to 10 years or longer.

   b. **Nodular lymphomas.** When a B cell becomes malignant after it has been activated and has entered a lymphoid follicle, its progeny, like normal follicular center cells, are morphologically more primitive in appearance (see Fig. 56-2) than dormant B lymphocytes. These cells also have a tendency to form nodules when infiltrating tissue. By conventional classification, these tumors would be identified as poorly differentiated or histiocytic, even though it is now clear that they represent a more advanced stage of antigen-stimulated differentiation than CLL and that the malignant cells are lymphocytes, not histiocytes. The kinetic behavior of the nodular lymphomas tends to reflect that of their normal follicular center cell morphologic counterparts. Thus, a lymphoma of small, cleaved cells displays the same relatively slow turnover rate as a normal B cell early in transformation (Fig. 56-2), whereas the more aggressive tumor of large, noncleaved cells reflects the rapidly dividing behavior of maximally transformed B cells. The latter type seldom retains nodular characteristics, and in general the nodular lymphomas, all of which are of B-cell derivation, are more indolent than the diffuse lymphomas. Patients with nodular lymphomas, like those with CLL, usually have marrow infiltration early in their course, but despite this have a long median survival (7–9 yr). Cure is not a realistic expectation at this time.

   c. **Diffuse lymphomas (excluding CLL).** When a malignant lymphoma infiltrates a node without forming nodules, it is termed diffuse. These tumors are usually but not always of B-cell origin and behave more aggressively than the nodular lymphomas. They have either lost or never had the tendency to form nodules in infiltrated nodes. Morphologically, most consist of large cells with primitive nuclei and prominent nucleoli, similar to maximally activated normal B cells. Cell kinetics of these lymphomas also parallel that of the normal metabolically active B lymphocyte, with high growth fractions and rapid turnover rates. Since a large fraction of these cells are in the cell cycle at a given time, and since cytotoxic chemotherapy is usually most active against cycling cells, therapy often produces rapid and dramatic remissions, as well as some cures.

2. **T-cell lymphomas.** Malignant lymphomas of T-cell origin are unusual tumors that vary in their clinical presentation from a relatively indolent CLL variant to the rapidly fatal lymphoblastic lymphoma. While it seems likely that the T-cell lymphomas, like B-cell tumors, are of clonal origin, formal proof is lacking. However, recent data indicate that they arise from single subsets of T cells, supporting the theory of clonality. All T-cell tumors have diffuse histologies, and many have a curious predilection for skin infiltration. This phenomenon has been hypothesized to reflect the skin homing of certain T cells and is most characteristic of the Sézary syndrome, which is a leukemic proliferation of helper T cells associated with erythroderma. The most aggressive of the T-cell tumors, the lymphoblastic lymphomas, may well represent the malignant transformation of truly immature T lymphocytes rather

Figure 56-3   *Comparison of normal serum and urine protein electrophoresis with the pattern commonly seen in multiple myeloma. (From V. L. Dickson and E. R. Eichner, Clinical aspects of multiple myeloma. Resident and Staff Physician, August 1975. By permission of E. R. Eichner and the publisher.)*

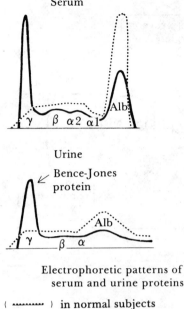

Serum

Urine

Bence-Jones protein

Electrophoretic patterns of serum and urine proteins

(............) in normal subjects
(————) in patients with multiple myeloma

than T cells after antigen-stimulated differentiation. Their clinical and morphologic similarity to the T-cell variant of ALL supports this hypothesis, as well as the presence of the early differentiation marker TdT.

C. **Plasma cell disorders.** The plasma cell disorders range from the apparently benign to the rapidly lethal and have in common the unbalanced proliferation of a single clone of plasma cells or their B-lymphocyte precursors. These disorders are also termed monoclonal gammopathies, since, with very few exceptions, the expanded clone of plasma cells produces a homogeneous, monoclonal protein that can be found in serum, urine, or both (Fig. 56-3). The three most common plasma cell disorders are multiple myeloma, Waldenström's macroglobulinemia, and benign monoclonal gammopathy.

1. **Multiple myeloma** (literally, many marrow–tumors) is a neoplastic proliferation of plasma cells manifested primarily by widespread bony destruction and frequently accompanied by anemia, hypercalcemia, renal failure, and recurrent infections. The classic presenting triad is back pain, anemia, and renal disease, but these may appear in any combination, and there are other presenting features as shown in the Venn diagram (Fig. 56-4).

The major pathophysiologic complications of multiple myeloma are shown in a flow chart in Figure 56-5. The mass of plasma cells expanding in the marrow secretes excessive monoclonal immunoglobulins into the serum. This causes a rouleau of the red blood cells, increases the viscosity of the serum, and coats the platelets. Marrow replacement leads to anemia, leukopenia, and thrombocytopenia. The abnormal plasma cell clone somehow suppresses normal clones, leading to hypogammaglobulinemia. The combination of leukopenia, hypogammaglobulinemia, and a re-

Figure 56-4

Venn diagram of the classical symptomatic triad of multiple myeloma along with some of the other possible presenting features. (From V. L. Dickson and E. R. Eichner, Clinical aspects of multiple myeloma. Resident and Staff Physician, *August 1975. By permission of E. R. Eichner and the publisher.)*

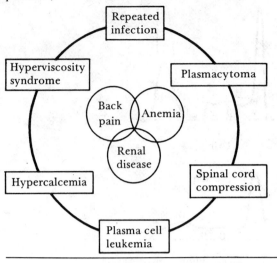

Figure 56-5

Flow chart depicting the major pathophysiology of multiple myeloma. (From V. L. Dickson and E. R. Eichner, Clinical aspects of multiple myeloma. Resident and Staff Physician, *August 1975. By permission of E. R. Eichner and the publisher.)*

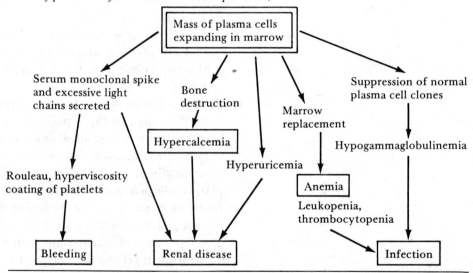

cently described defect in leukocyte chemotaxis increases the vulnerability to infections, which are often from gram-positive bacteria if community-acquired and from gram-negative bacteria if hospital-acquired. The hyperviscosity, coating of platelets, and thrombocytopenia cause abnormal bleeding.

Other major pathophysiologic manifestations are bone destruction and renal disease. Severe bone pain, especially in the lower back and ribs, is the presenting symptom in many patients. The central skeleton, the site of hematopoiesis, is most frequently affected. Osteolytic lesions (punched out circular defects) and osteoporosis are the most common; when present, they signify a body burden of more than 10^{12} tumorous plasma cells. The severe bone pain, increasing demineralization, pathologic fractures, and hyper-

Major diagnostic criteria
     Bone marrow plasmacytosis >30% or multiple plasmacytomas
     Serum monoclonal spike >4 g/dl for IgG or >2 g/dl for IgA, or Bence Jones proteinuria >0.5 g/day

Minor diagnostic criteria
     Lesser degrees of marrow plasmacytosis and serum spike
     Lytic bone lesions or hypogammaglobulinemia

Ancillary features
     Anemia
     Hypercalcemia
     Azotemia
     Hypoalbuminemia
     Osteoporosis

Source: Reproduced with permission from E. R. Eichner, The plasma cell dyscrasias, *Postgrad Med* 67:44, 1980.

calcemia are all attributable mainly to the expanding mass of plasma cells, but part of the bony destruction is caused by the secretion of an osteoclast activating factor by the abnormal clone of plasma cells. The bony destruction of myeloma, then, is partly mechanical and partly humoral.

Renal failure is common in myeloma. The pathogenesis is multifactorial, but chronic urinary excretion of light chains (Bence Jones proteinuria) is probably the dominant factor. Light chains are partly absorbed and processed by the renal tubules and are capable of producing proximal tubular defects (acquired Fanconi syndrome), distal tubular defects (diabetes insipidus or renal tubular acidosis), glomerulopathies, and combined defects. The type and degree of renal damage seem to vary with the type, concentration, and solubility of light chain involved. Hypercalcemia also contributes substantially to renal failure. Biopsy of classical myeloma kidney shows tubular atrophy and degeneration, fibrosis, calcinosis, and large tubular casts with giant cells. Other factors contributing to renal failure in individual myeloma patients are hyperuricemia, pyelonephritis, infiltration of the kidney with plasma cells, amyloidosis, dehydration, and hyperviscosity.

Table 56-1 lists the cardinal clinical features of myeloma, divided into the major criteria needed for a definitive diagnosis, the minor criteria needed for a provisional diagnosis, and the common ancillary features. The bone marrow in an advanced case is often heavily infiltrated with immature or abnormal plasma cells, but there are no morphologic criteria that invariably distinguish the plasma cell of myeloma from the normal plasma cell. It must be emphasized that 20 percent of patients with multiple myeloma secrete only light chains, which, because of their small size, are readily filtered across the renal glomeruli. These patients, then, lack the telltale serum spike, and the correct diagnosis can be missed unless urine electrophoresis is done.

2. **Waldenström's macroglobulinemia.** Macroglobulinemia, originally described by Waldenström, is the name given the plasma cell disorder in which monoclonal IgM is secreted. This disorder is less common than multiple myeloma and has a different pathophysiology. In macroglobulinemia, the abnormal cells have a lymphoplas-

macytoid morphology and there is generally less bony and renal disease. Instead, patients with macroglobulinemia often resemble patients with chronic lymphocytic leukemia in having generalized lymphadenopathy and hepatosplenomegaly. Although some patients are asymptomatic at diagnosis, at least 50 percent have the hyperviscosity syndrome, which largely dominates the early course of macroglobulinemia.

The underlying pathophysiology for the hyperviscosity syndrome is that IgM circulates in the plasma as a large, asymmetric pentamer of high intrinsic viscosity, so that plasma viscosity rises logarithmically with rising concentrations of IgM. The resultant circulatory impairment compromises primarily four target organs: the *fundi*, with visual changes, markedly distended veins, hemorrhages, and exudates; the *nervous system*, with headaches, tinnitus, vertigo, and diverse focal central and peripheral neuropathies; the *heart*, with congestive failure; and the *hematologic system*, with bleeding due to the coating of platelets and the binding of coagulation factors and with a multifactorial anemia that has a large dilutional component. Fortunately, the hyperviscosity syndrome is rather easily treated with plasmapheresis, which is especially effective in macroglobulinemia because 80 percent of the IgM is intravascular, compared with 40 to 50 percent for IgG and IgA.

3. **Benign monoclonal gammopathy.** Small serum monoclonal spikes are occasionally found in asymptomatic, apparently healthy persons. Indeed, benign monoclonal gammopathy is the most common plasma cell disorder. Such benign gammopathies are apparently the result of a controlled proliferation of a single clone of plasma cells scattered widely through the marrow. The clone expands until it reaches a size (about 5×10^{11} cells) at which monoclonal protein can be detected by serum electrophoresis, and then, for unknown reasons, remains stable for many years.

D. **Monocyte-macrophage neoplasms**

1. **Acute monoblastic and myelomonoblastic leukemias.** These malignant disorders are proliferations of cells that represent an early stage in monocyte-macrophage development. The association of both myeloblasts and monoblasts in many cases of acute leukemia supports the hypothesis that these cells are derived from a common progenitor cell. The pathophysiology of these diseases is similar to acute granulocytic leukemia, which is discussed in the section on granulocyte disorders.

2. **Hodgkin's disease.** Until recently, Hodgkin's disease (HD) was considered a subtype of malignant lymphoma. Indeed, a great deal of circumstantial evidence supported this view: lymphoid organs (nodes and spleen) are usually involved and functionally abnormal lymphocytes generally are the predominant cell type in involved tissue. However, recent data suggest that the so-called Reed-Sternberg cell, the large, usually binucleate cell that is an essential diagnostic feature of HD, is the true malignant cell. Furthermore, there is now compelling evidence that the Reed-Sternberg cell is of monocyte-macrophage origin. These cells have been shown to be phagocytic and, under certain culture conditions, to produce the macrophage enzyme lysozyme. Therefore, it now appears that HD is a malignancy of macrophages, perhaps relatively late in their differentiation pathway, and that the surrounding lymphocytes (as

well as plasma cells and eosinophils) in involved tissues are non-malignant reactive cells.

Several histologic subtypes of HD have been identified, but for the most part influence neither prognosis nor therapeutic approach. In sharp contrast with the non-Hodgkin's lymphomas, the outcome in HD generally does not depend upon histology, but upon the extent of disease (or stage) at presentation. Unlike the lymphomas, which often spread hematogenously, HD characteristically spreads from node group to contiguous node group through the lymphatics. If careful clinical evaluation discloses disease in only one or two node groups, then localized treatment (i.e., radiation therapy) is likely to be curative. HD nearly always begins in node groups above the diaphragm, usually in those of the axial skeleton (cervical, supraclavicular, axillary, or mediastinal nodes). Spread is then generally caudad, and when nodes below the diaphragm become involved, the prognosis is less favorable. When spread to other organs (liver, bone marrow, etc.) has occurred, local therapy is no longer sufficient. Systemic symptoms of fever, night sweats, and weight loss are common in advanced disease, although mechanisms by which these symptoms occur are poorly understood. Like the true malignant lymphomas, HD may also impair function of the immune system, resulting in a propensity for infection.

IV. **Clinical examples of neoplasms of the immune system**
   A. **Bone pain and anemia in an elderly female**
      1. **Description.** A 76-year-old female was admitted to the orthopedics service for severe debilitating low back pain. Her initial evaluation disclosed vertebral osteoporosis with compression fracture of lumbar 4 and L5, anemia, elevated total serum protein, and trace proteinuria. Medicine consultation was requested, and subsequent workup revealed a monoclonal IgG λ spike of 7 gm/dl with depression of other Igs; heavy Bence Jones (light chain) proteinuria; serum creatinine of 2.5 mg/dl (normal, 0.6–1.4); marrow plasmocytosis of 27 percent (normal, 0–5%); and lytic lesions of the skull and ribs. The diagnosis of multiple myeloma was made, and both systemic chemotherapy and local radiation therapy to the lumbar spine were initiated. Pain relief was prompt but incomplete. After six cycles of chemotherapy, the paraprotein had decreased to 1.4 gm/dl and Bence Jones protein had disappeared from the urine. Bone marrow plasma cells had dropped to 5 percent of nucleated elements. No further decrement in the paraprotein had occurred after six more cycles, so therapy was stopped. The patient remained clinically stable for 8 months, then developed a fulminant febrile illness and died within 48 hours of its onset. Blood and spinal fluid cultures grew *Streptococcus pneumoniae*.
      2. **Discussion**
         a. Generalized osteoporosis is seen as the initial manifestation of bony disease in about one-third of patients with multiple myeloma.
         b. The discrepancy between the trace proteinuria on initial screening urinalysis and the heavy Bence Jones proteinuria is explained by the fact that routine tests for urine protein primarily detect albumin and are insensitive to Ig light chains.
         c. The development of pneumococcal sepsis is a common terminal

event in patients with multiple myeloma, whose deficiency of normal Igs make them particularly susceptible to infection by encapsulated organisms.

B. Cervical adenopathy in a young man

1. **Description.** A 24-year-old male complained of a painless swelling in his neck of 2 months' duration. He denied all other symptoms. Examination disclosed 2- to 3-cm rubbery, nontender nodes in the right cervical and supraclavicular regions. Routine blood chemistries were normal except for a Wintrobe sedimentation rate of 38 mm per hour (normal, 5–15). Chest x-ray revealed a small anterior mediastinal mass. Hodgkin's disease was found on node biopsy.

   Thorough staging evaluation including exploratory laparotomy was negative. The patient was treated with extended-field irradiation in standard doses. All evidence of active disease disappeared and the patient felt well until 18 months later, when he began to lose weight and have intermittent fevers and night sweats. Examination at that time showed pallor but no adenopathy, although chest film revealed a recurrent mediastinal mass. Lab evaluation demonstrated moderate anemia, leukocytosis, and elevated sedimentation rate. Bone marrow biopsy was positive for Hodgkin's disease and combination chemotherapy was begun. After six cycles of therapy, complete remission was again documented. The patient remained well for the next 4 years, but then complained of recurrent fatigue and malaise. Blood count demonstrated pancytopenia and bone marrow was hypercellular with 90 percent myeloblasts. The diagnosis of acute myeloblastic leukemia was made, and the patient died during attempted induction chemotherapy.

2. **Discussion**

   a. This patient exemplifies the relatively small number of HD patients with initially limited disease who suffer relapse and require systemic chemotherapy for control.

   b. At the time of relapse, only the patient's symptoms suggested recurrent disease, and only x-ray and invasive diagnostic studies provided confirmation. Anemia, leukocytosis, and increased sedimentation rate are commonly seen in HD, but of course are not specific for this diagnosis.

   c. The development of acute leukemia in long-term survivors of HD has become a major problem, especially in those patients who have received both radiation and chemotherapy. Recent data indicate that up to 10 percent of these patients will eventually develop a second malignancy, the most common of which is acute leukemia.

Questions

Select the single best answer.

1. The majority of non-Hodgkin's lymphomas arise from clones of:
   a. B lymphocytes at an early stage of lymphoid maturation (ontogeny).
   b. T lymphocytes late in antigen-stimulated differentiation.
   c. B lymphocytes during antigen-stimulated differentiation.
   d. Stem cells prior to development of lymphoid and monocyte-committed precursors.

2. An 81-year-old man who has been in good health sees his doctor because of a minor upper-respiratory infection. The workup shows an elevated total

serum protein, and subsequent serum electrophoresis shows a small spike, which is identified as monoclonal IgG. The patient has no bone pain and has not had frequent infections. Hemoglobin is 14 gm/100 ml, white blood cell count and differential are normal, and platelet count is normal. Peripheral blood smear shows no abnormalities. There is no proteinuria, and renal function is normal. X-rays of the bones show no lesions. Bone marrow aspiration shows that plasma cells are at the upper limit of normal in number but are normal morphologically. From the data at this point, what is the *single most likely* diagnosis?

a. Waldenström's macroglobulinemia.
b. Chronic lymphocytic leukemia.
c. Multiple myeloma.
d. Benign monoclonal gammopathy.

57 Cancer of the Breast

I. **Introduction.** Cancer of the breast will affect about one of eleven American women. Most of the 100,000 victims in whom a diagnosis was made last year will die of their disease, making this form of cancer a major killer among females aged 40 to 60. Perhaps no other malignancy has been studied with more intensity and dedication, and yet answers to critical questions regarding its pathophysiology and appropriate medical management remain unanswered. Nonetheless, breast cancer can be considered a prototype for other solid tumors not discussed. Figure 57-1 presents a general framework for considering this disease. As in most pathologic states, information concerning predisposing factors, etiologic agents, and course of events without medical intervention form a basis for prophylactic, diagnostic, and therapeutic maneuvers. Unfortunately, the biologic regulation of tumor induction and progression is largely unknown, and important practical issues of primary and secondary therapy controversial. Figure 57-1 attempts to convey the fact that boundaries between phases of natural history and medical interventions have significant transition periods.

II. **Predisposing factors.** A considerable effort has been made to define groups of women at particularly high risk for developing breast cancer. Table 57-1 indicates some of the factors studied. Women who have had cancer of one breast have a significant rate of a second primary cancer occurring in the other breast (approximately 1–3% per year). Increased risks have also been reported when benign breast disease is present, but because of the common clinical and pathologic occurrence of fibrocystic disease, conclusions are difficult. As discussed below, certain specific pathologic findings do appear to be premalignant in character. A number of unusual genetic syndromes have been defined in which a high incidence of breast cancer occurs, suggesting Mendelian dominant inheritance. Features often include early onset of disease, bilaterality, mucocutaneous benign tumors, and other malignancies of the genital or gastrointestinal (GI) tract. For the majority of breast tumors, genetic factors are more difficult to define and risk figures controversial.

Because the breast is a target tissue for the sex hormones undergoing cyclic proliferative responses during menstruation and pregnancy, attempts have been made to relate neoplastic changes to patterns of endocrine regulation. An increased risk for cancer seems to exist in those women with early onset of menarche, a late menopause, and when pregnancy has never occurred. On the other hand, pregnancy before the age of 20 and multiparity appear to have some protective influence. Precise explanations for these effects are speculative. Other associations of breast cancer with environmental or racial characteristics have been put forward. Excessive radiation to the thorax (e.g., patients undergoing repeated fluoroscopy) has been shown to be carcinogenic. Dietary factors have been suggested to explain differences between breast cancer incidences in the Orient and the West. Although Oriental women have a lower incidence of breast cancer, risks increase upon emigration and integration into Western lifestyles.

The epidemiologic study of breast cancer to define women at high risk is important when considering the cost effectiveness and possible adverse effects of mass-screening efforts (e.g., mammography). At the

Figure 57-1

Natural history and therapeutic considerations of cancer of the breast. Solid bars represent transitional periods.

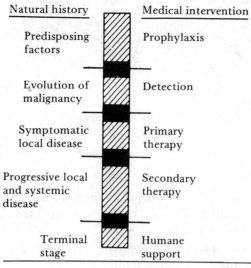

Table 57-1

Factors Related to the Risk of Breast Cancer

Factor	Comment
Preexisting disease	Increased risk when previous cancer or benign dysplastic lesions are present
Genetic	Increased risk for first-degree relatives; dominant transmission in occasional cancer syndromes
Endocrine	Incidence higher when menarche is early, menopause late, or nulliparity is present; pregnancy before 20 and multiparity protects
Environmental	Risk increased by exposure to irradiation, perhaps dietary factors
Racial	Incidence lower in Oriental cultures

moment, known risk factors are so pervasive that for practical purposes all women must be considered potential victims of this malignancy. With the exception of those rare situations of apparent dominantly inherited familial breast cancer syndromes, in which prophylactic mastectomy may be offered, the relative importance of risk factors in determining specific medical interventions remains uncertain.

III. **Evolution of malignancy.** Concepts of the histogenesis of malignant lesions of the breast are based on known endocrine responsiveness inherent to breast tissue. Rudimentary ductal structures present before puberty undergo extensive proliferation due to the influence of estrogens in the pubertal girl. Marked progestational effects during pregnancy and less pronounced effects during the menstrual cycle lead to terminal ductule and alveolar hyperplasia. Anatomically, the breast may be considered to consist of about 25 lobar units, each associated with a major lactiferous duct. The lobes consist of ramifications of the ducts ending in multiple functional microscopic units termed lobules (see Fig. 57-2). Although there are exceptions, most cancers are thought to arise from the terminal ductal epithelium, with histologic evidence of infiltration of surrounding adipose and fibrous tissue. With increasing emphasis on early diagnosis, a spectrum of changes of the terminal ductal epithelium has been defined,

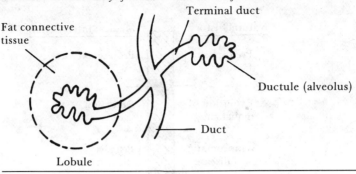

Figure 57-2 *Schematic microanatomy of the lobular structure of the breast.*

short of invasive carcinoma. These findings range from atypia of the epithelium to the cellular morphology of cancer (lobular carcinoma in situ). The incidence, or time to progression of these pathologic premalignant lesions to invasive cancer is uncertain and provide obvious problems for proper management.

The physiology of normal breast tissue is integrally related to responsiveness to the sex hormones. The study of mechanisms of hormonal action at the cellular level is an exciting area of current research focused on the breast cancer problem. Receptors for steroid sex hormones are known to exist in the cytoplasm of target organs. Estrogens, for example, rapidly enter cells and combine with a specific cytoplasmic receptor molecule. The complex then enters the nucleus and interacts with chromosomal deoxyribonucleic acid (DNA) and protein components modulating transcription and cell function. Both activation and inhibitory effects have been described for steroid hormones. It might be expected that tumors arising in target tissue would be heterogeneous or aberrant in terms of the presence of hormone receptors. For breast cancers, evaluation of estrogen receptor status has been most intensively studied. In approximately 50 percent of tumors, significant levels of estrogen receptors can be identified. For many years it has been an empiric observation that a minority of patients respond dramatically to various endocrine manipulations during the course of their disease. It has become apparent that such responses depend on the presence of estrogen receptors. Thus, evaluation of tumors for receptor status is an important part of initial diagnosis.

The pathophysiologic changes occurring with malignancy of the breast declare themselves clinically as a lump, detected in 90 percent of cases by the patient. Palpation is the physician's as well as the patient's major tool for early detection. Details of breast examination should be reviewed and performed monthly by the patient and when seen by her physician. Radiologic examination of the breast (mammography) designed to reveal soft tissue detail has proved to be an excellent diagnostic aid, particularly in examination of the postmenopausal breast and in instances where clinical findings are ambiguous. Considerable discussion is currently directed at defining indications, frequency, and applications of mammography for screening purposes. Potential hazards of radiation exposure are being reduced by improved techniques. Most lesions are found by all methods of detection—self-examination, physician's examination, and mammography. However, occasional tumors are detected only radiologically or clinically. For obvious reasons, monthly self-examination must remain the mainstay of early detection. From time to time questions are raised as to the lack of documentation of early detection as an important determinant of long-term survival. Although direct proof is lacking, there is no doubt that larger lesions (greater than 2 cm in diameter) are associated with a higher incidence of regional and systemic spread of disease. Early detection continues to be the most practical goal for reducing mortality.

Once the lump has been detected, histologic examination of biopsied tissue is the traditional method for making the diagnosis. Alternatively, cytologic examination of aspirated material from the lesion is highly accurate in expert hands. As mentioned earlier, problems may arise in interpreting the significance of minimal noninvasive lobular lesions with dysplastic features.

Primary therapy is based on the concept of an initial period of localized tumor followed by regional spread to lymph node areas and subsequent systemic dissemination. Recent concepts support the view that nodal disease is an indicator of systemic dissemination. Extensive local therapy is therefore unjustified. Modified radical mastectomy techniques are utilized, in which lymph nodes are removed primarily for diagnostic rather than therapeutic reasons. At the time of initial surgery, tumor tissue is assessed for estrogen-receptor status. The prospects for recurrence following surgery best relate to findings in the regional nodes. About 80 percent of patients can expect to remain free of disease when nodes are negative for tumor, while less than 20 percent of patients survive their disease when four or more nodes are positive. Poor survival for node-positive patients is thought to be due to systemic disease present at the time of surgery. The use of adjuvant chemotherapy in such cases is being studied at the present time. Although theoretically attractive, modest long-term benefits have been well documented only for premenopausal women with fewer than four positive nodes.

IV. **Progressive disease.** Despite efforts at early detection and therapy, many women ultimately succumb to the malignancy. Usually the effects of widespread metastatic disease account for this grim picture. The principles governing local invasiveness, entry of tumor cells into lymphatic and vascular channels, and successful seeding of target tissue continue to be studied. The loss of contact inhibition enhances tumor cell shedding. Both platelets and fibrin are thought to be important in the arrest of tumor emboli at sites distant from the primary lesion. Establishment of the cells in the interstitium probably depends on enzyme activity in the local microenvironment. Subsequent cellular proliferation requires vascularization stimulated by angiogenic factor. The question of why certain tumors tend to home to specific metastatic sites is unclear. For example, the tendency for metastatic breast carcinoma to involve bone may depend on microenvironmental influences inherent in the interaction of bony tissue with the cancer cell or upon less subtle considerations of venous and lymphatic pathways associated with the primary tumor. In any case, neither the pattern nor the kinetics of metastatic disease lend themselves to easy explanations. From the clinical standpoint, metastatic disease is not curable. Therapy probably prolongs life, but this has been surprisingly difficult to prove. There is no doubt that treatment can significantly reduce the morbidity arising from local and systemic complications of the tumor.

The unexplained heterogenous course of metastatic breast cancer needs to be emphasized. Historic observations of the natural history of this tumor without treatment are illuminating. While the average survival appeared to be about three years, survivals of 10 to 20 years in untreated cases are well documented. Doubling times for breast tumor lesions vary so greatly that conceptual and kinetic models adapted from rodent systems are far removed from the reality of the patient.

Clinical goals are palliative, directed at the three levels of symptoms and their underlying pathophysiology: (a) locally defined impairment of function (e.g., spinal cord compression due to a metastasis), (b) diffuse metastatic effects (e.g., widespread bone pain), and (c) paraneoplastic phenomenon (e.g., anemia). Parallel medical interventions are local (e.g., x-ray), systemic (e.g., chemotherapy), or supportive (e.g., transfusion), as individual circumstances require. The rational basis for employing hormonal manipulation is somewhat less obscure than in the past but is still far from clear. Deprivation of estrogens may be accomplished by surgical ablative procedures, chemical inhibitors of estrogen action, or agents that inhibit estrogen synthesis. Significant antitumor effects are noted in most estrogen receptor-positive patients. Paradoxically, pharmacologic amounts of estrogen are also used for endocrine therapy, as are other steroid hormones. Menstrual status, duration of disease, and distribution of metastasis are some considerations involved in selecting hormonal therapy. It must be admitted, however, that except for the prerequisite of receptor status, choices are often empiric.

For patients lacking estrogen receptors, with rapidly progressive disease, or with disease refractory to hormonal therapy, responses to combinations of cytotoxic drugs can be obtained in most instances. With current treatment methods, most women can remain active and often symptom-free for years after tumor dissemination has occurred.

The onset of terminal illness encompasses those pathophysiologic features common to the spectrum of end-stage diseases. Specific organ failures related to anatomic incursions by tumor, intercurrent infections, and complications of increasingly difficult attempts at therapy are part of the picture. The recognition of this time in the natural history of cancer of the breast and the role of the physician are issues of current wide discussion. The physical and psychologic burden carried by women struggling with breast cancer is enormous. Throughout the frequently protracted illness, the physician's skill and compassion must be a constant source of relief for the patient and her family. The intense commitment of the profession to unraveling the pathophysiology of this malignancy may help to make the future better.

V. Clinical examples of cancer of the breast

A. Breast lump in a young woman

1. **Description.** A 32-year-old menstruating female noticed a mass in her left breast. She was otherwise asymptomatic. Examination disclosed a 2- by 3-cm hard mass in the upper outer quadrant of the left breast as well as a 2- by 2-cm firm, movable node in the left axilla. Biopsy revealed infiltrating ductal carcinoma, and at modified radical mastectomy 14 of 20 axillary nodes were found to contain tumor. An assay of the tumor tissue for estrogen receptors was negative. The patient was treated with adjuvant combination chemotherapy for one year, but 18 months after her mastectomy she began to notice fatigue, anorexia, and weight loss. A firm, fixed left supraclavicular node was palpated, and a 1.5-cm solitary nodule was noted in the right mid-lung field on chest x-ray. Node biopsy

revealed recurrent breast carcinoma, and further evaluation disclosed subclinical metastases in liver and bone. Chemotherapy with other cytotoxic agents was begun, and after two cycles of treatment there was dramatic reduction (>50%) in the size of all measurable metastases. The patient regained her premorbid body weight, and she felt essentially well for the next 8 months. However, despite continued chemotherapy, she then developed recurrent symptoms of fatigue and weight loss. Progressive metastatic lesions were demonstrated in liver and lungs, which proved refractory to further therapy. The patient died 4 months later from disseminated malignancy.

2. **Discussion**

   a. Premenopausal, estrogen receptor-negative ductal carcinoma is one of the most aggressive, rapidly dividing subtypes of breast cancer. This patient's tumor, apparently confined to regional lymph nodes at presentation, in fact had spread to numerous other sites by hematogenous routes.

   b. Although effective in some groups of patients in preventing the development of clinical metastases or at least in prolonging the disease-free interval after mastectomy, adjuvant chemotherapy was not beneficial in this case. Unfortunately, many if not most receptor-negative patients with four or more positive axillary nodes at mastectomy will eventually develop recurrent disease, whether or not adjuvant therapy is used.

   c. Resumption of chemotherapy when metastases became evident resulted in a gratifying, though transient, partial remission. Over 50 percent of patients with metastatic breast cancer will respond to cytotoxic drugs, but cure is not a realistic expectation.

   d. Since fewer than 10 percent of receptor-negative breast cancer patients respond to hormonal manipulation, none was utilized in this case.

B. **Shoulder pain in an elderly female**

   1. **Description.** A 72-year-old woman complained to her physician of progressive right shoulder pain, limiting the movement of her right arm for the previous 2 months. Pain was progressive and unrelieved by aspirin. Examination disclosed mild tenderness over the head of the right humerus and a small hard mass in the left breast. Bone scan revealed multiple areas of increased uptake consistent with metastases, and excisional biopsy of the breast mass demonstrated estrogen-receptor positive duct carcinoma. A hormonal agent was prescribed and within 6 weeks the patient's symptoms had completely resolved. Six months later the bone scan was markedly improved. The patient remains symptom-free with no evidence of recurrent disease 2 years after her original examination.

   2. **Discussion**

      a. Despite multiple bony metastases at the time of diagnosis, hormonal therapy can often produce long-term remissions in patients with receptor-positive tumors.

      b. When recurrent disease eventually develops, other hormonal agents or cytotoxic chemotherapy can be utilized.

      c. Kinetically, estrogen receptor-positive tumors often seem to be more indolent than their receptor-negative counterparts.

Select the single best answer.

1. A premenopausal woman with metastatic estrogen-receptor–positive breast cancer was initially treated by oophorectomy with a good response lasting for 18 months. She then developed generalized, slowly progressive bone and soft tissue disease. A reasonable approach to therapy would be to:
   a. Surgically remove her adrenal glands.
   b. Support her with pain medication until vital functions are compromised.
   c. Begin cytotoxic chemotherapy.
   d. Systematically irradiate lesions found on physical and radiologic examination.

2. Why is it recommended that breast examination take place shortly after a menstrual period?
   a. The patient is less tense.
   b. The influences of progesterone on breast tissue are avoided.
   c. The breast is largest at this time.
   d. No particular reason other than giving the patient a routine time for self-examination.

XII   Pulmonary Disease

Ralph C. Beckett
Alfred F. Connors
Ann L. DeHart
Barry A. Gray
David C. Levin
D. Robert McCaffree
Thomas L. Murphy
Sami I. Said

58

Pulmonary Gas Exchange

I. **Review of basic physiology.** The lung is unique in that the entire cardiac output flows through its capillaries and is exposed to atmospheric air over a large surface area. Thus, the lung is ideally suited for gas exchange.

Air moves through the larger airways by bulk flow and through very small gas exchange areas by diffusion. Oxygen moves into the capillaries and carbon dioxide into the alveoli by diffusion. The PO_2 in capillary blood leaving the alveolus ($Pc'O_2$) is equal to the PO_2 in the alveolus (PAO_2), which is usually around 100 mm Hg at sea level. From that point, there is a decline in the PO_2 in the arterial blood (PaO_2 is normally about 90 mm Hg at sea level), to the intracellular PO_2 (about 20 mm Hg), to the mitochondrial PO_2 (about 1–3 mm Hg) (Fig. 58-1).

A. **The ideal alveolar gas equation.** A value for PAO_2 is necessary to determine the alveolar-arterial PO_2 gradient (which is useful in assessing the gas exchange function of the lung), but it cannot be directly measured. However, the PAO_2 in an average or "ideal" alveolus can be calculated easily. The general equation is:

$$PAO_2 = PIO_2 - PACO_2 \left(FIO_2 + \frac{1 - FIO_2}{R} \right)$$

where the PIO_2 is the PO_2 of inspired gas, $PACO_2$ is the alveolar PCO_2 (which is essentially the same as the arterial PCO_2 [$PaCO_2$]), FIO_2 is the fraction of inspired oxygen (which is 0.21 in room air), and R is the gas exchange ratio (which is the same as the metabolic respiratory quotient in the steady state). Remember that the metabolic respiratory quotient ($\dot{V}CO_2/\dot{V}O_2$) ranges between 0.7 and 1.0 but averages around 0.8. The PIO_2 is the product of the FIO_2 and the barometric pressure minus water vapor pressure or, at sea level, $PIO_2 = 0.21 \times (760$ mm Hg $- 47$ mm Hg$) = 150$ mm Hg.

In room air, $FIO_2 + (1 - FIO_2)/R = 1.2$, which is about the same as the reciprocal of R. Therefore, a simplified form of the equation is:

$$PAO_2 = PIO_2 - PaCO_2/R$$

(notice that $PaCO_2$ has been substituted for $PACO_2$). This form is less accurate when R varies from 0.8 or when FIO_2 approaches 1.0.

B. **The alveolar-arterial oxygen difference** ($P[A - a]O_2 = PAO_2 - PaO_2$). Calculating the difference between the alveolar PO_2 and arterial PO_2 gives useful information about the efficiency with which the lung functions as a gas exchange organ. In the ideal situation, the entire cardiac output comes in contact with ventilated alveoli and, since the blood leaving the alveolus has the same PO_2 as alveolar gas, the $P(A - a)O_2$ is zero. In reality, 2 to 4 percent of the cardiac output bypasses the lung as a right-to-left shunt, and there is also some mismatching of ventilation and perfusion in the normal lung. Consequently, the normal $P(A - a)O_2$ is usually about 10 mm Hg, and it increases with age and with FIO_2. Because of the latter, the measurement is of little use if the person is not breathing room air. The normal $P(A - a)O_2$ can be estimated using this equation:

Figure 58-1

Representation of the decrease in partial pressure of oxygen from inspired air (PɪO₂) to the alveolus (PᴀO₂) and pulmonary capillary (Pc'O₂) to the arterial blood (PaO₂) and finally to the tissues and mitochondria.

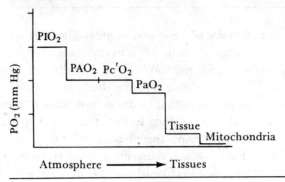

$$P(A - a)O_2 = 2.5 + 0.21 \text{ (age in years)}$$

A good rule of thumb is that a $P(A - a)O_2$ of greater than 20 mm Hg on room air is abnormal.

An abnormal $P(A - a)O_2$ indicates that there is significant impairment of gas exchange, which is probably due to a disorder of the lung itself.

C. Oxygen content and the oxyhemoglobin dissociation curve. The total oxygen content of blood includes that oxygen bound to hemoglobin (oxyhemoglobin) and the small amount dissolved in plasma. Oxygen content in arterial blood (CaO_2) is calculated as follows:

$$CaO_2 = O_2 \text{ bound to hemoglobin} + O_2 \text{ dissolved in plasma}$$
$$CaO_2 = \text{Hb gm/100 ml} \times 1.39 \text{ ml } O_2/\text{g Hb} \times SaO_2/100$$
$$+ .0031 \text{ ml } O_2/100 \text{ ml/mm Hg} \times PaO_2 \text{ mm Hg}$$

where Hb is hemoglobin, 1.39 is the oxygen-carrying capacity of hemoglobin, SaO_2 is the saturation of the hemoglobin with O_2, and .0031 is the solubility of O_2 in plasma.

The oxyhemoglobin dissociation curve describes how the oxygen content of blood (and saturation of hemoglobin with oxygen) is related in a predictable way to the PO_2 of the blood. The sigmoid shape of this curve (Fig. 58-2) is important physiologically. The curve is steep below a PO_2 of 60 mm Hg and flattens above a PO_2 of 60 mm Hg. For example, if the PO_2 increases 40 mm Hg from a PO_2 of 20 mm Hg to a value of 60 mm Hg, the saturation increases 60 percent, from 30 percent to about 90 percent. However, a further 40 mm Hg increase in PO_2 to 100 mm Hg results in only a 5 percent increase in saturation, to about 95 percent. The steep part of the curve is important physiologically because when venous blood arrives at the alveolus with a low PO_2, a large amount of oxygen can be loaded onto the hemoglobin with a small increase in PO_2. When the blood gets to the tissues, with each small drop in PO_2 a great deal of oxygen is released from the hemoglobin. The flat portion of the curve is important clinically since as lung disease progresses and the arterial PO_2 falls, there is not a significant change in the saturation of hemoglobin until the PO_2 falls below 55 or 60 mm Hg. Thus, the shape of the oxyhemoglobin dissociation curve facilitates the loading of oxygen to hemoglobin in the alveolus, eases the release of oxygen to the tissues, and provides a buffer against the effects of the decreasing PaO_2 associated with lung disease.

Figure 58-2

The oxyhemoglobin dissociation curve. Consideration of the shape of the curve is important in clinical decisions. If the partial pressure of oxygen (PO_2) is 60 mm Hg or greater, increasing the PO_2 will not greatly affect hemoglobin saturation (SO_2). On the other hand, any decrement of the PO_2 below 60 mm Hg will cause marked decrease in hemoglobin saturation.

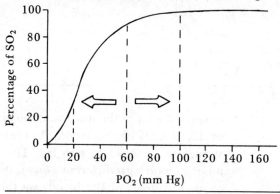

Figure 58-3

Relation between the partial pressure of oxygen (PO_2), the hemoglobin saturation in the blood ($SO_2\%$), and the content of oxygen in blood with a hemoglobin concentration of 15 gm/100 ml.

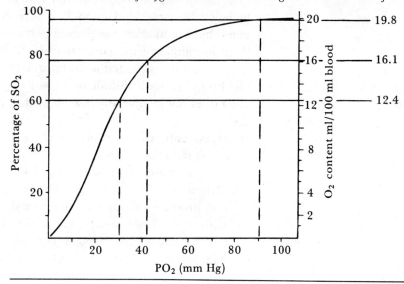

Increases in temperature and in hydrogen-ion concentration (lower pH) shift the dissociation curve to the right, while colder temperatures and higher pH shift the curve to the left. These shifts serve useful adaptive purposes, by enhancing O_2 delivery to the tissues in the presence of fever or acidosis and by promoting O_2 uptake by the pulmonary capillary blood after unloading of CO_2 in the lung.

Another major influence on the dissociation curve is the level of 2,3-diphosphoglycerate (2,3-DPG), with higher levels resulting in a rightward shift.

The concept of oxygen content is important in understanding abnormalities of gas exchange. For example, if a flask with 100 ml of blood having a PO_2 of 30 mm Hg is emptied into a flask with 100 ml of blood having the same hemoglobin concentration of 15 gm/100 ml and a PO_2 of 96 mm Hg, what is the PO_2 of the resulting 200 ml of blood? The answer 63 mm Hg is wrong (Fig. 58-3). The oxygen content of the blood in the first flask is 12.4 ml O_2/100 ml blood, and the oxygen content of the blood in the second flask is 19.8 ml O_2/100 ml. The

Figure 58-4

The effect of hypoventilation on PaO_2, assuming a $P(A - a)O_2$ of 10 mm Hg.

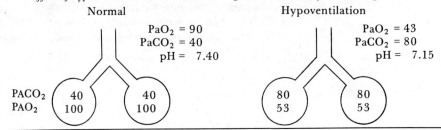

oxygen content of the mixture is the average of the two $(12.4 + 19.8)/2$ or 16.1 ml O_2/100 ml blood. A content of 16.1 ml O_2/100 ml corresponds to a PO_2 of 42 mm Hg. The PO_2 of blood that results from mixing blood with different PO_2s is determined by the average of the oxygen contents of the blood, *not* the average of the PO_2s (see Fig. 58-3).

II. **Pathophysiology: the causes of hypoxemia.** Hypoxemia is defined as an arterial blood PO_2 below the normal range of 80 to 90 mm Hg. As the PO_2 falls, the hemoglobin O_2 saturation also falls, especially with PO_2 values at or below 60 mm Hg (Fig. 58-3). There are four main causes of hypoxemia: hypoventilation, ventilation-perfusion $(\dot{V}/\dot{Q})$ mismatch, shunt, and diffusion impairment. There is also a fifth cause of hypoxemia, which is not necessarily associated with abnormalities of gas exchange: breathing a low PIO_2, i.e., high altitude or a low-FIO_2 gas. Since this cause of hypoxemia does not involve any disease of the respiratory system, it will not be discussed.

A. **Hypoventilation.** Alveolar PCO_2 is inversely related to alveolar ventilation (and directly related to CO_2 production). If alveolar ventilation $(\dot{V}A)$ decreases, then less oxygen is delivered to the alveoli and less carbon dioxide is removed. The tissues will continue to consume O_2 and produce CO_2 at the same rate despite the change in ventilation. Ultimately, a new steady state will result with a higher $PACO_2$ and a lower PAO_2. If the alveolar ventilation falls sufficiently to cause an increase in $PACO_2$ to 80, PAO_2 would fall to 53 mm Hg as calculated from the alveolar gas equation. Even if the $P(A - a)O_2$ is normal (e.g., 10 mm Hg), this would cause severe arterial hypoxemia (Fig. 58-4).

$$PaO_2 = PAO_2 - P(A - a)O_2 = 53 - 10 = 43$$

The change in $PACO_2$ (and thus, the $PaCO_2$) with a change in alveolar ventilation is quite predictable and is described in the equation:

$$PACO_2 = PaCO_2 = K(\dot{V}CO_2/\dot{V}A)$$

where K is a constant and $\dot{V}CO_2$ is CO_2 production. Thus, as alveolar ventilation doubles (assuming $\dot{V}CO_2$ is constant), PCO_2 is halved, and if alveolar ventilation decreases by one half, PCO_2 doubles. Clinically, hypoventilation is said to be present when the $PaCO_2$ is higher than normal (i.e., more than 46 mm Hg). Conversely, a diagnosis of hypoventilation cannot be made in the presence of a normal $PaCO_2$.

Hypoventilation can occur with or without lung disease. When hypoventilation occurs without lung disease, it is usually associated with one of the following: drug intoxications, central nervous system disorders, neuromuscular disorders, or chest wall injuries. When hypoventilation occurs without parenchymal lung disease, the $P(A - a)O_2$ is normal. Hypoventilation is commonly seen with chronic obstructive lung disease, and is then associated with an elevated $P(A - a)O_2$.

An increased FIO_2 will correct the hypoxemia of hypoventilation. The hypoxemia that occurs in hypoventilation is caused by the increased $PACO_2$, which results in a decreased PAO_2. By reviewing the alveolar gas equation, one can see that simply increasing the PIO_2 sufficiently can increase the PAO_2 and cause a subsequent rise in PaO_2 (see note below).

In summary, hypoventilation: (1) causes an increased $PACO_2$ and $PaCO_2$; (2) causes a decreased PAO_2 and PaO_2; (3) is associated with a normal $P(A - a)O_2$ when it occurs acutely; and (4) PAO_2 and PaO_2 (but not the hypoventilation) can be corrected by raising FIO_2.

Note that while an increase in FIO_2 will correct the hypoxemia of hypoventilation, patients with acute hypoventilation may progress to apnea. Therefore, the treatment for acute hypoventilation is endotracheal intubation and mechanical ventilation.

B. **Shunt.** Shunting occurs when blood passes from the right side of the heart to the left side of the heart without contacting a ventilated alveolus. Normally 2 to 4 percent of the cardiac output bypasses the alveoli, primarily through the bronchial circulation and thebesian veins. Pathologic shunting occurs with anatomical shunts, such as congenital heart diseases and AV malformations (atrial and ventricular septal defects), and with pulmonary diseases, such as pneumonia, pulmonary edema, and atelectasis. Hypoxemia occurs with shunting because the shunted blood, which has the low oxygen content of mixed venous blood, mixes with oxygenated blood leaving the alveoli, resulting in an abnormally low arterial oxygen content.

Figure 58-5 is a model of shunting. $\dot{Q}_T$ is the total cardiac output and $\dot{Q}s$ is the portion of the cardiac output that bypasses the ventilated alveolus as shunt. The blood leaving the shunt has the oxygen content of mixed venous blood ($C\bar{v}O_2$), which mixes with the blood leaving the capillaries with a high oxygen content ($Cc'O_2$). The mean oxygen content that results from this blend (CaO_2) will determine the PaO_2. If, for example, half of the cardiac output goes to normally ventilated alveoli and half goes to alveoli that are unventilated due to atelectasis or alveolar flooding with exudate or edema fluid, given a $C\bar{v}O_2$ of 12 ml $O_2/100$ ml blood and a $Cc'O_2$ of 20 ml $O_2/100$ ml blood, then the CaO_2 is the average of the two contents: $(12 + 20)/2$ or 16 ml $O_2/100$ ml blood. This oxygen content corresponds to a PaO_2 of 42 mm Hg. One should be aware that the $P(A - a)O_2$ is increased in shunt. In addition, the $PaCO_2$ is usually normal or low, since ventilation can be increased to normally functioning alveoli, making up for the nonventilating alveoli. Shunt responds poorly to an increase in FIO_2. This is because of the sigmoid shape of the oxyhemoglobin dissociation curve. Blood leaving the ventilated alveolus in Figure 58-5 has a saturation of about 98 percent, with an FIO_2 of .21. Increasing the FIO_2 can increase the saturation by only about 2 percent. Since mixed venous blood does not contact ventilated alveoli, it varies little with change in FIO_2. Thus, increases in FIO_2 have only a small effect on PaO_2 in patients with shunt and cause only a fraction of the increase in PaO_2 that would be expected with the other causes of hypoxemia.

Figure 58-5

A model of shunting. Vol% = ml O_2 per 100 ml blood; $C\bar{v}O_2$ = mixed venous oxygen content.

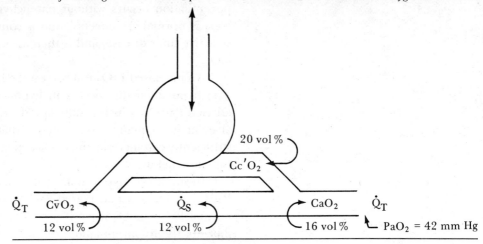

Shunt is measured clinically by determining the $P(A - a)O_2$ on 100 percent oxygen. Breathing 100 percent oxygen completely obliterates the effects of hypoventilation, ventilation-perfusion mismatch, and diffusion impairment; therefore, the $P(A - a)O_2$ on 100 percent oxygen is due entirely to shunt.

In summary, shunt (1) causes a fall in PaO_2; (2) is associated with a normal or decreased $PaCO_2$; (3) results in an increased $P(A - a)O_2$; (4) responds poorly to an increased FIO_2; and (5) is measured clinically on 100 percent oxygen.

C. Low ventilation-perfusion ($\dot{V}/\dot{Q}$) ratios. A low ventilation-perfusion ($\dot{V}/\dot{Q}$) ratio is the most common cause of hypoxemia. In the normal lung, ventilation and perfusion are fairly well matched, with the lower lobes being better perfused and better ventilated than the upper lobes. However, some $\dot{V}/\dot{Q}$ mismatch does occur in normals. $\dot{V}/\dot{Q}$ ratios of about 3.0 occur at the apices, and ratios of about 0.6 at the bases in normal upright subjects.

$\dot{V}/\dot{Q}$ mismatch covers a continuum from an infinitely high $\dot{V}/\dot{Q}$ ratio, which is dead space (space that is ventilated but not perfused), to a $\dot{V}/\dot{Q}$ ratio of zero, which is shunt (space that is perfused but not ventilated) (Fig. 58-6). A normal $\dot{V}/\dot{Q}$ ratio is about 0.8 to 1.0. High $\dot{V}/\dot{Q}$ ratios are associated with a reduced $PaCO_2$ and do not contribute to hypoxemia. The hypoxemia caused by $\dot{V}/\dot{Q}$ mismatch is due to low $\dot{V}/\dot{Q}$ alveoli.

Figure 58-7 depicts a lung with two alveoli. One has a normal $\dot{V}/\dot{Q}$ ratio, and the other has a low $\dot{V}/\dot{Q}$ ratio. The low $\dot{V}/\dot{Q}$ alveolus is essentially a hypoventilated alveolus; the difference is that the PCO_2 in a low $\dot{V}/\dot{Q}$ alveolus cannot increase above the level of the mixed venous PCO_2. However, oxygen consumption continues and the PaO_2 in the low $\dot{V}/\dot{Q}$ alveolus is markedly decreased. The low PaO_2 in the low $\dot{V}/\dot{Q}$ alveolus causes a correspondingly low content in the blood as it leaves the alveolus; thus, CaO_2 and PaO_2 are abnormally low. Notice that $PaCO_2$ is normal and $P(A - a)O_2$ is increased.

The hypoxemia caused by low $\dot{V}/\dot{Q}$ alveoli responds very well to even small increases in FIO_2. Figure 58-8A depicts the effect of an FIO_2 of .24 on PaO_2 in the patient in Figure 58-7. The small increase in FIO_2 increases the PaO_2 from 52 to 89 mm Hg. On 100 percent oxygen the PaO_2 in low $\dot{V}/\dot{Q}$ alveoli is normal. Thus, the effect of low

Figure 58-6

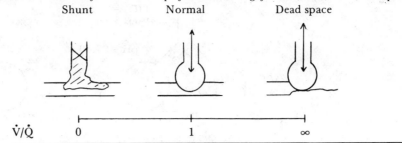

The continuum of ventilation-to-perfusion matching, from 0 (shunt) to ∞ (dead space).

Figure 58-7

A two-compartment model of the effect of low $\dot{V}/\dot{Q}$ areas on oxygen content and PaO_2. Vol% = ml O_2 per 100 ml blood.

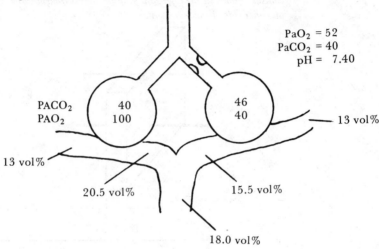

$\dot{V}/\dot{Q}$ alveoli on PaO_2 is completely eliminated by 100 percent oxygen (Fig. 58-8B).

In summary, ventilation-perfusion ($\dot{V}/\dot{Q}$) mismatch: (1) causes a decreased PaO_2 due to low $\dot{V}/\dot{Q}$ alveoli; (2) is usually associated with a normal $PaCO_2$; (3) is associated with an increased $P(A - a)O_2$; (4) characteristically responds well to even small increases in FIO_2; and (5) is completely corrected by 100 percent oxygen.

D. **Diffusion impairment.** As shown in Figure 58-9, the flow of a gas through a membrane by diffusion ($\dot{V}_{gas}$) is inversely proportional to the thickness of the membrane (T) and directly proportional to the surface area of the membrane (A), the diffusion constant (D), and the pressure gradient of that gas across the membrane ($P_1 - P_2$). This is represented in the following formula:

$$\dot{V}_{gas} \propto \frac{A}{T} \cdot D(P_1 - P_2)$$

The diffusion constant (D) is proportional to the solubility divided by the square root of the molecular weight. Carbon dioxide diffuses through tissue 20 times more rapidly than oxygen because of its high solubility; thus, its diffusion is not affected by diseases that impair diffusion. These diseases are thought to impair diffusion by thickening the alveolar membrane or by decreasing the surface area available for diffusion, or both.

When diffusion impairment is present, the PaO_2 is normal, but it

Figure 58-8

The effect of enriched oxygen on low $\dot{V}/\dot{Q}$ areas and PaO_2. Vol% = ml O_2 per 100 ml blood.

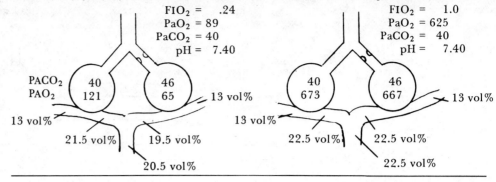

Figure 58-9

Considerations in the diffusion of a gas across a membrane. P_1 and P_2 = partial pressures of gas on either side of the membrane.

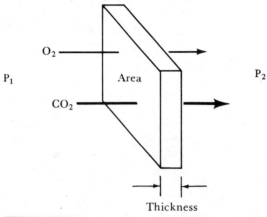

takes longer for capillary blood to come into equilibrium with the alveolar gas. As seen in Figure 58-10, the capillary PO_2 is normally equal to the PAO_2 after 0.25 second of exposure to alveolar gas, one-third of the time available. In the presence of moderately abnormal diffusion, equilibration may not occur until just before the blood leaves the alveolus, but the PaO_2 is still normal. However, on exercise, cardiac output increases and transit time decreases, leaving inadequate time for equilibration and causing a fall in PaO_2. A precipitous fall in PaO_2 during exercise is felt to be characteristic of diffusion impairment. A patient with grossly abnormal diffusion has a low PaO_2 even at rest and suffers a further fall in PaO_2 with exercise.

The hypoxemia of diffusion impairment can be corrected by providing an increased FIO_2. As PAO_2 increases, the pressure gradient from alveolus to capillary increases, increasing diffusion. It is said that any decrease in PaO_2 due to impaired diffusion will largely be corrected by an FIO_2 greater than 0.40. In some instances, however, as in alveolar filling with edema or exudate, or severe thickening of the alveolar-capillary membrane, it is difficult to distinguish between poor diffusion and shunt.

It should be noted that the role of diffusion impairment in hypoxemia is controversial. Certainly, most experts would agree that diffusion impairment is rarely the sole cause of hypoxemia. Indeed, the hypoxemia of many disease states, thought to be due to diffusion impairment, is now known to be due to $\dot{V}/\dot{Q}$ mismatch. However, there is evidence to suggest that diffusion impairment may contribute to the hypoxemia seen in some of these diseases.

Figure 58-10

How exercise might accentuate hypoxemia in the presence of a diffusion abnormality.

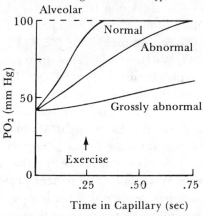

In summary, diffusion impairment: (1) causes a decreased PaO_2 and a normal PAO_2; (2) is associated with a normal or low $PaCO_2$; (3) causes an increased $P(A - a)O_2$; (4) responds well to an increased FIO_2; and (5) is rarely the sole cause of hypoxemia.

E. **Key points**

1. The four abnormal states associated with hypoxemia are hypoventilation, shunt, low $\dot{V}/\dot{Q}$ ratios, and diffusion.
2. Of these, only pure hypoventilation is associated with a normal $P(A - a)O_2$.
3. Of these, only shunt is not corrected by 100 percent oxygen.
4. Of these, the hypoxemia due to low $\dot{V}/\dot{Q}$ ratios responds best to small increases in FIO_2.

III. **Clinical examples of gas exchange.** All patients live in Oklahoma City, where $PIO_2 = 143$ mm Hg.

A. **Hypoxemia and hypoventilation**

1. **Description.** A 21-year-old female plumber was found unconscious next to an empty bottle of barbiturates. In the emergency room, she was comatose and cyanotic. Her arterial blood gases revealed a PaO_2 of 40 mm Hg and a $PaCO_2$ of 80 mm Hg on room air.
2. **Discussion.** The first question that should be asked in evaluating this patient is, Why is she hypoxemic? Specifically, we know from her $PaCO_2$ that she is hypoventilating, but is all of her hypoxemia due to her hypoventilation? A quick calculation of her $P(A - a)O_2$ will give that answer. $PAO_2 = 143$ mm Hg $- (80 \times 1.2) = 47$ mm Hg. Measured PaO_2 is 40 mm Hg. Therefore, $P(A - a)O_2$ ($PAO_2 - PaO_2$) is 7 mm Hg. Thus, the $P(A - a)O_2$ is normal, suggesting that there is no significant abnormality of the pulmonary parenchyma. Therefore, her hypoxemia is due completely to her hypoventilation, which in turn is probably due to an overdose of barbiturates. However, no matter what the cause of her hypoxemia, the most important thing to do first is to place her on supplemental oxygen. This will raise the PaO_2 even in hypoventilation. The patient will, however, if she continues to hypoventilate, develop other problems; therefore, the attending physician should move quickly to endotracheal intubation and mechanical ventilation.

B. **Hypoxemia due to shunt**

1. **Description.** A 42-year-old male truck driver gagged and became short of breath while eating olives. In the emergency room, no breath sounds were heard over the right lung and the chest x-ray

revealed atelectasis of the right lung. Arterial blood gases revealed a PaO_2 of 41 mm Hg, a $PaCO_2$ of 32 mm Hg, and pH of 7.47.

2. **Discussion.** A quick calculation of his $P(A - a)O_2$ reveals that his $PAO_2 = 143$ mm Hg $- (32 \times 1.2) = 105$ mm Hg. His measured PaO_2 is 41 mm Hg. Therefore his $A - a$ gradient is 105 mm Hg minus 41 mm Hg, or 64 mm Hg. Thus, his $A - a$ gradient is markedly increased, and his chest radiograph reveals that he does have pulmonary parenchymal problems. In fact, his hypoxemia is probably due primarily to shunt secondary to the atelectasis. The patient was placed on a 28 percent Venturi mask. Unfortunately, the physicians did not realize that the cause of his hypoxemia was primarily shunt. (The patient's PaO_2 came up only to 45 mm Hg.) Had they realized that the hypoxemia secondary to shunt does not respond readily to oxygen, they would have placed the patient on a non-rebreathing mask to obtain the highest possible FIO_2 and then moved to correct the cause of the shunt.

C. **Hypoxemia due to chronic lung disease**

1. **Description.** A 63-year-old man who had smoked two packs of cigarettes a day for the past 45 years complained of chronic shortness of breath. Arterial blood gases revealed a PaO_2 of 50 mm Hg and a $PaCO_2$ of 39 mm Hg.

2. **Discussion.** Again, if one asks the cause of the hypoxemia, we can quickly calculate that this man's $P(A - a)O_2$ is $96 - 50 = 46$ mm Hg [$PAO_2 = 143 - (39 \times 1.2) = 96$ mm Hg, and the measured $PaO_2 = 50$ mm Hg]; thus, he does have a parenchymal pulmonary problem. However, the only thing that can be determined from the blood gases is the fact that he is not hypoventilating. The history suggests that this man has chronic lung disease and that the most likely cause of his hypoxemia is a low ventilation-to-perfusion ratio. In contrast with the previous patient, this patient was placed on 28 percent oxygen and responded well, his PaO_2 going up to 78 mm Hg. This illustrates that hypoxemia due to low $\dot{V}/\dot{Q}$ responds nicely to enriched oxygen administration, and small amounts of oxygen can be beneficial.

Questions

Select the single best answer.

1. One hundred ml of blood containing 15 g of hemoglobin and having a PO_2 of 25 mm Hg is mixed with 100 ml of blood with the same hemoglobin concentration and a PO_2 of 135 mm Hg. The PO_2 of the resulting mixture would be closest to:
   a. 40
   b. 60
   c. 80
   d. 100
   e. None of these.

2. The hypoxemia associated with $\dot{V}/\dot{Q}$ mismatch is caused by:
   a. Hyperventilation of shunt alveoli.
   b. Hyperventilation of dead space.
   c. Increased numbers of high $\dot{V}/\dot{Q}$ alveoli.
   d. Increased numbers of low $\dot{V}/\dot{Q}$ alveoli.
   e. None of these.

59

Pulmonary Mechanics

I. **Overview of mechanics.** Pulmonary mechanics is the study of factors that influence the movement of air into and out of the lungs. Among other things, it encompasses the forces exerted by the chest wall, the elastic properties of the lung parenchyma, impediments to gas flow, and classification of lung disease based on physical parameters. Diseases of the lung frequently manifest themselves by altering the normal mechanical properties of the lung. Clinical problems such as the following require knowledge and understanding in this area of respiratory pathophysiology: (a) A patient on a ventilator suddenly requires more pressure than usual to deliver a constant volume. What changes in the respiratory system might account for this finding? (b) An asthmatic patient receives an inhaled bronchodilator medication. Is there an objective way of comparing the response to such a medication with that of a new bronchodilator? (c) A patient who smokes has undergone chemotherapy for cancer and complains of shortness of breath. Have the therapeutic agents impaired lung function?

Answers to the clinical questions above would, of course, require more information than is given, but a physician's assessment and therapeutic plans would be based on considerations of pulmonary mechanics.

II. **Static lung volumes.** Figure 59-1 is a spirometric tracing that demonstrates the various subdivisions of lung volume. The subject's breathing is recorded from left to right. The initial sinusoidal excursions represent quiet breathing. They are followed by a maximal inspiration, a maximal expiration, and a return to tidal respiration. The spirometer provides a convenient measurement of tidal volume, expiratory reserve volume, and vital capacity. The amount of gas that cannot be expired from the lungs is defined as the residual volume. The residual volume cannot be determined by simply measuring expired gas volumes but requires other techniques. These techniques include the following:

A. **Plethysmography.** This technique involves placing the subject inside a closed container (the body plethysmograph or box) and measuring pressures at the mouth and inside the box during certain maneuvers. By using simple gas laws it is possible to determine the volume of gas in the chest. Since the determination is made after expiration of a tidal breath, the volume measured is the functional residual capacity. By subtracting the expiratory reserve volume from the functional residual capacity, the residual volume can be determined.

B. **Inert gas dilution.** This technique involves the inhalation of a minute amount of an inert gas such as helium. If the inspired and the expired concentrations of helium are measured, it is possible to calculate the volume of distribution of that gas. The volume corresponds to the functional residual capacity if the helium is introduced at the end of a tidal breath and if the helium is evenly distributed throughout the lung.

III. **Pressure-volume relationships**

A. **P-V curve of the chest wall.** The chest-wall-alone curve (Fig. 59-2) could be experimentally obtained by removal of the thoracic contents and closure of the incision. The horizontal axis represents pressure, either above or below atmospheric pressure, measured in the empty thoracic space. The vertical axis corresponds to the volume of gas

Figure 59-1   *Subdivisions of lung volume.*

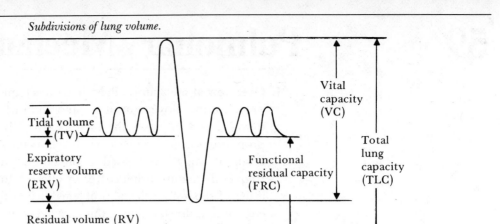

Figure 59-2

Pressure-volume relationships. FRC = functional reserve capacity; RV = residual volume; TLC = total lung capacity.

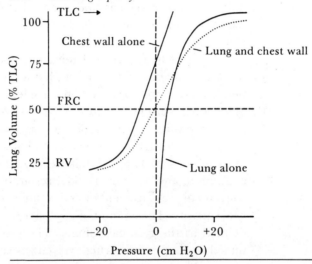

contained in the thorax. Certain qualities of this curve should be appreciated. First, if the pressure in the thorax is equal to atmospheric, then the chest wall assumes a position to contain about 70 percent of total lung capacity. Second, when negative pressure is applied, the chest wall resists deformation and manifests a flattening of the curve at about 30 percent of total lung capacity.

B. P-V curve of the lung. The lung-alone curve (Fig. 59-2) could be experimentally obtained by measurements made on lungs that have been removed from the chest. The pressure in the airway is adjusted either to increase or to decrease lung volume. Negative pressures are not needed, since the elastic properties of the lung cause it to collapse spontaneously if the airway is opened to atmospheric pressure. Notice how this curve becomes flat with increasing pressure—similar to a balloon just before breaking.

C. Compliance. The relative steepness or flatness of these curves is best described by the concept of compliance. Compliance is defined as the slope of a volume-pressure curve at any point. Mathematically, $C = dV/dP$, where C is compliance, dV is the derivative of volume, and dP is the derivative of pressure. Thus, the chest wall has decreased

Figure 59-3

Typical changes in lung-volume subdivisions with disease. ERV = expiratory reserve volume; FRC = functional residual capacity; RV = residual volume; TLC = total lung capacity; VC = vital capacity.

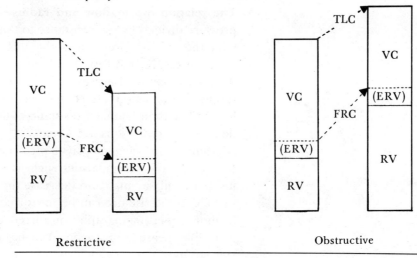

compliance near residual volume, and the lung has decreased compliance near total lung capacity.

D. **The normal determinants of lung volumes.** The lung-plus-chest-wall curve (Fig. 59-2) represents the volume-pressure curve that is obtained with the chest wall and lungs in their usual position. The combined curve is a result of the hydraulic coupling (with pleural fluid) of the chest wall and lung. At a given volume it mathematically represents the sum of pressures from the chest-wall curve and the lung-alone curve. If the airway is open and no muscular forces are applied, the balance of the chest wall and lung forces will cause the system to come to rest at functional residual capacity (FRC). *Residual volume* is determined primarily by the shape of the chest-wall curve, whereas the *total lung capacity* (TLC) is primarily determined by the shape of the lung-alone curve.

Consider the mechanics of President Reagan's lung and chest-wall injury. The bullet allowed air at atmospheric pressure to enter the pleural space and break the hydraulic bond between chest wall and lung. The lung collapsed along its pressure volume curve, and the chest wall sprang outward to about 70 percent of total lung capacity.

E. **The determinants of lung volumes with disease states.** In the intact animal, muscular effort creates the force needed to change lung volume. Weakness, neuromuscular disease, or malingering can be determinants of maximum or minimum lung volumes despite normal compliance of the chest and lungs. Lung volumes represent a static situation and are not theoretically influenced by obstructions to air flow. However, diseases that cause obstruction to air flow, such as emphysema, are frequently associated with increased lung compliance and air trapping within the chest. Restrictive lung defects often reduce or limit the volume of the lung and its compliance. Therefore, two basic patterns of lung volumes emerge (Fig. 59-3). The restrictive category of defects is mostly typified by a reduction in total lung capacity. Obstructive disease, on the other hand, may have an elevation in total lung capacity with an increase in residual volume. A common abnormality of most lung diseases of both types is a reduction in vital capacity. In restrictive defects due to neuromuscular disease, residual volume may be normal or increased.

IV. **Air flow**

A. **The relationship of flow and radius.** Flow is equal to the driving pressure divided by the resistance to that flow. In the respiratory system, the driving pressure is the difference between alveolar and mouth pressure, and resistance is a quantity inversely proportional to the fourth power of airway radius. This means that small changes in radius have a marked effect on flow. Furthermore, if air flow is turbulent rather than laminar, resistance will increase to an even greater degree with reductions in radius.

Smooth muscle tone plays a pivotal role in determining the caliber of the airways. Irregularities such as secretions, edema, or tumors inside the airway may also decrease the cross-sectional area or cause turbulence. Resistance can be measured directly by several methods, including plethysmography or forced oscillation. However, a more accessible measure of air flow can be obtained from the expiratory spirogram.

B. **Dynamic lung volumes and flows.** Figure 59-4 depicts the volume-time curve of the expiratory spirogram in three conditions. The volume-time curve proceeds from left to right. It starts at total lung capacity (TLC) and follows the course of a forced expiration to residual volume. Its curvilinear shape is partly due to the fact that resistance increases as lung volume decreases. To understand how this might occur, imagine that the airway is like a hole in a nylon stocking. As the stocking is stretched, the hole increases in size and as the fabric of the stocking is relaxed, the hole decreases in size. Similarly, when the meshwork of lung elastic and collagen fibers is stretched at TLC, the airways are tethered open. When the lung volume decreases, the tethering of the airways relaxes and the diameter of bronchi decreases. The decreases in caliber of airways with expiration results in an increasing resistance.

Many indices of flow have been advocated for use with the expiratory spirogram. The forced expiratory volume over 1 second (FEV_1) and the forced expiratory flow between the 25 percent and 75 percent points in the vital capacity (FEF25–75%) are two such indices. Other parameters of flow of varying sensitivity and specificity are occasionally used ($FEV_{0.5}$, FEV_2, FEV_3, FEF75–85, etc.). Since flow is affected by lung volume as described above, it has been empirically found that the ratio of forced expiratory volume in 1 second to forced vital capac-

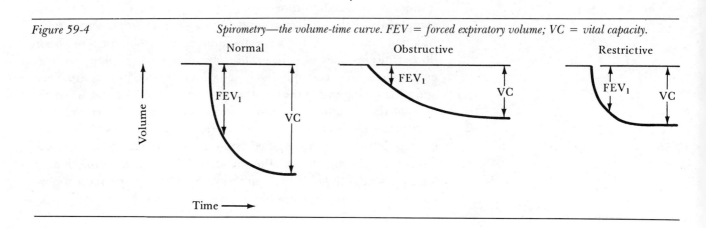

Figure 59-4   *Spirometry—the volume-time curve. FEV = forced expiratory volume; VC = vital capacity.*

Normal   Obstructive   Restrictive

FEV_1 VC FEV_1 VC FEV_1 VC

Volume

Time ⟶

Figure 59-5

Interpretation of spirometry. The question marks indicate that lung volume testing would be needed to verify restriction (low total lung capacity) since forced vital capacity (FVC) may be reduced solely by an obstructive process causing air trapping (high residual volume). FEV = forced expiratory volume; LN = lower limit of normal range; FEF = forced expiratory flow.

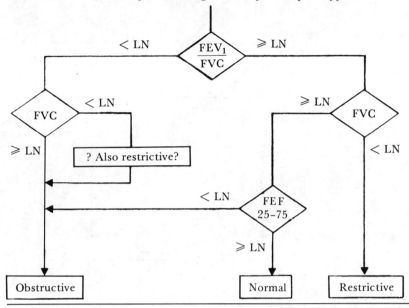

ity (FEV_1/FVC) is helpful in differentiating subjects with air flow limitation (an obstructive defect).

C. **Interpretation of spirometry.** Figure 59-5 schematically describes how many physicians interpret measurements obtained from spirometry. The diagram is by no means all-inclusive but at least gives perspective to the tests thus far described. The lower limit of normal for each of the tests has been determined from large populations of normal, nonsmoking subjects.

D. **The flow-volume loop.** Another presentation of the same data contained within a volume-time curve can be seen by plotting the derivative of the volume-time curve against lung volume (Fig. 59-6). The flow-volume loop in Figure 59-7 reflects various levels of effort during expiratory and inspiratory maneuvers in an otherwise normal respiratory system. The confluence of the curves toward the end of expiration should be noted in Figure 59-7. This region of the curve is referred to as the effort-independent portion. One may infer that a flow-volume line exists, toward the end of expiration, which cannot be exceeded no matter how hard a subject tries. This phenomenon is best explained by the concept of the equal-pressure point.

During a forced expiration, muscular contraction raises the pleural pressure in an attempt to increase the flow above that generated by the elastic recoil of the lungs. There is a gradient of pressure between the alveoli, where the pressure is high, and the mouth, where pressure is zero or atmospheric. If the pleural pressure is raised to a degree such that it exceeds the intraluminal pressure at some point along the gradient, then airway collapse will occur. This point is called the equal pressure point (EPP) (Fig. 59-8). The forces at the EPP have a tendency to limit the flow; furthermore, and not quite so intuitively, the equal pressure point will occur in the same place for a given lung volume no matter what the elevation of pleural pressure is. The equal pressure point probably occurs in the lobar or segmental

Figure 59-6

Spirometry—the flow-volume loop. Dotted lines indicate the response to bronchodilators.

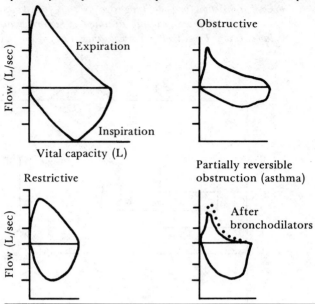

Figure 59-7

The flow-volume loop with various degrees of effort. Dotted lines indicate submaximal effort.

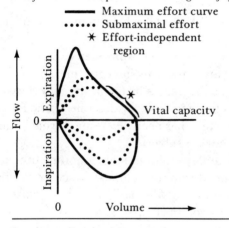

Figure 59-8

Concept of the equal pressure point.

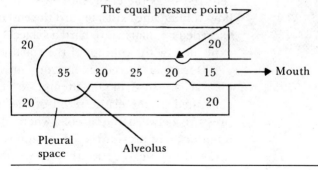

bronchi, but in disease states it may migrate, due to loss of support structures of the airway and turbulence of flow.

E. The silent zone. In normal people 80 to 90 percent of total airway resistance resides in the airways larger than 2 mm in diameter and 10 to 20 percent in the small airways. Consequently, destruction of 50 percent of the small airways would cause less than a 10 percent increase in total lung resistance and virtually no change in the spirogram. Because of this difficulty in detecting changes in small airway resistance, the small airways are referred to as the silent zone of the lung.

V. Surface tension and alveolar surfactant. One of the possible forces resisting lung inflation is surface tension at the alveolar air-liquid (tissue-fluid) interface. Surface forces in the alveoli equal $2T/R$, where T is the tension in the alveolar wall and R is the alveolar radius. Since R decreases with expiration, there is a tendency for surface forces to exceed the forces distending the alveoli. If unopposed, this tendency could lead to alveolar atelectasis (and possibly also to pulmonary edema). The presence of alveolar surfactant, however, guards against these complications, by equalizing surface forces among different alveoli and keeping these forces low, even at small lung volumes (by reducing T).

Chemically, alveolar surfactant is mainly a saturated lecithin present with an apoprotein. Surfactant is formed in alveolar type II cells (large pneumonocytes), where it is stored in, and secreted by, unique lamellar bodies. Surfactant deficiency may result from decreased formation (as in lungs of premature babies or following interruption of pulmonary perfusion) or from inactivation (as by serum in the alveolar space). The consequences of surfactant deficiency include atelectasis, pulmonary edema, noncompliant (stiff) lungs, reduced functional residual capacity, and arterial hypoxemia. The main clinical states associated with surfactant deficiency (and increased alveolar surface forces) are the respiratory distress syndrome of the newborn (hyaline membrane disease) and the adult respiratory distress syndrome.

Instillation of surfactant into the airways has recently been found successful in reversing the pathophysiologic effects of reduced surfactant in animals and human babies with premature lungs. This therapy has not yet been tried in adults with the respiratory distress syndrome. Corticosteroids and thyroid hormone can accelerate the maturation of alveolar type II cells and increase the production of surfactant by premature lungs.

VI. Clinical example of cor pulmonale due to skeletal deformity

A. Description. A middle-aged woman complained of swelling of the ankles, shortness of breath, and cough. She had had Pott's disease as a child with resultant kyphoscoliosis. Examination revealed a thin female with severe kyphoscoliosis of the dorsal spine. The jugular veins were distended to the angle of the jaw, and there was 3^+ pitting edema present over the lower extremities. Treatment with bed rest, low-salt diet, digoxin, and diuretics reduced the edema. Pulmonary function testing revealed an increased ratio of FEV_1/FVC, a decreased FVC, and a markedly decreased TLC.

B. Discussion

1. The patient illustrates the severe restrictive type of pattern that pulmonary function testing will show with thoracic deformity.

2. The right heart failure (cor pulmonale) is due to chronic respiratory insufficiency.

Select the single best answer.

1. At what lung volume would compliance of the chest wall be lowest?
   a. At total lung capacity.
   b. At functional residual capacity minus expiratory reserve volume.
   c. At residual volume plus functional residual capacity.
   d. At total lung capacity minus residual volume.
2. A patient who has had one lung removed has spirometry testing performed. The ratio of forced expiratory volume in 1 second divided by the vital capacity is lower than would be expected for a normal person. Indicate which of the following statements is true.
   a. Because the remaining lung must expand to larger than its normal size, the airways will generally be smaller in size, causing the FEV_1/FVC to fall.
   b. The patient probably has some type of obstructive lung disease.
   c. The remaining lung is normal.
   d. None of the above.

I. **Pathophysiology of hypocapnia, hypercapnia, and dyspnea**
A. **Carbon dioxide elimination by the lungs—basic physiology.** Carbon dioxide is eliminated by the process of alveolar ventilation. Carbon dioxide is present in the pulmonary alveoli, and its concentration in the alveolar gas may be expressed by either its partial pressure, P_ACO_2, or fractional concentration, F_ACO_2.

Alveolar ventilation, $\dot{V}_A$, is the quantity of air that is expired from the alveoli each minute and is equal to the difference between the total quantity of air expired ($\dot{V}_E$) and the quantity of air that is expired from dead space ($\dot{V}_D$). $\dot{V}_D$ includes conducting airways, trachea, bronchi, and alveoli, which are ventilated but not perfused.

$$\dot{V}_A = \dot{V}_E - \dot{V}_D$$

The quantity of carbon dioxide eliminated by the lung each minute ($\dot{V}CO_2$) is equal to the volume of gas expired from the alveoli ($\dot{V}_A$) multiplied by the fractional concentration of carbon dioxide in the alveolar gas (F_ACO_2).

$$\dot{V}CO_2 = \dot{V}_A \times F_ACO_2$$

Since F_ACO_2 is equal to the partial pressure of CO_2 in alveolar gas divided by the total pressure of all gases, excluding water vapor, and since the partial pressure of carbon dioxide is equal in alveolar gas and arterial blood, this equation can be rearranged to relate $PaCO_2$ to alveolar ventilation and metabolic rate or CO_2 production, where 0.863 is simply a constant that includes barometric pressure, water vapor pressure, and a temperature correction factor.

$$PaCO_2 = P_ACO_2 = 0.863 \times \dot{V}CO_2/\dot{V}_A$$

B. **Hypocapnia and respiratory alkalosis.** By definition, hypocapnia indicates alveolar hyperventilation, i.e., in excess of metabolic requirements. The recognition of respiratory alkalosis is of importance primarily because respiratory alkalosis may indicate the existence of a life-threatening medical problem. The treatment of respiratory alkalosis varies with its cause; basically, it is the treatment of the underlying medical problem (Table 60-1).

C. **Hypercapnia and respiratory acidosis**
1. **Spectrum of disease-causing hypercapnia.** By definition, hypercapnia indicates alveolar hypoventilation, i.e., insufficient to meet metabolic requirements. Respiratory acidosis is often a primary feature of acute respiratory failure in patients with lung disease. In patients with severe chronic bronchitis, hypercapnia may also be present during periods of relative compensation and well-being. Respiratory acidosis may also occur as the result of upper airway obstruction; this represents a medical emergency requiring tracheal intubation or tracheostomy. The exception is in children with enlarged tonsils and adenoids, in whom the gradual onset of hypercapnia allows for compensation, and the surgical management is

Table 60-1

Causes and Complications of Respiratory Alkalosis

Causes	Complications
Hypoxemia ($PO_2 < 55$ mm Hg)	Tetany
Septicemia	Seizures
Salicylate toxicity	Cardiovascular collapse (shock)
Asthma	Decreased cerebral blood flow
Congestive heart failure	Decreased ionized calcium
Myocardial infarction	Hypophosphatemia
Pulmonary embolism	
Peritonitis	
Pneumonitis	
Pulmonary fibrosis	
Hepatic encephalopathy	
Central neurogenic hyperventilation	
Anxiety—pain	

Table 60-2

Causes of Hypercapnia

I. Respiratory causes of hypercapnia
  A. Airway obstruction
    1. Chronic obstructive lung disease
    2. Upper airway obstruction
    3. Pulmonary edema
    4. Asthma (rare, but carries poor prognosis)
  B. Wasted ventilation
    1. Chronic obstructive lung disease
    2. Pulmonary embolism (rare)
    3. Adult respiratory distress syndrome (rare)
II. Neurologic causes of hypercapnia
  A. Central nervous system disorders
    1. Narcotics or opiates
    2. Cerebrovascular accident
    3. Head injury
  B. Neuromuscular dysfunction
    1. Guillain-Barré syndrome
    2. Myasthenia gravis
    3. Toxic neuropathy (arsenic)
    4. Botulism
    5. Insecticide poisoning
  C. Abnormal respiratory control (primary alveolar hypoventilation)

less urgent. Respiratory acidosis may also occur in the absence of respiratory disease. In these cases respiratory acidosis is purely the result of central nervous system depression, neuromuscular dysfunction, or abnormal respiratory control (Table 60-2).

2. Complications of hypercapnia. The deleterious effects of hypercapnia result primarily from two physiologic effects of increased PCO_2. First, carbon dioxide, like many other gases, exerts an anesthetic effect on the central nervous system. With the development of CO_2 narcosis, the patient becomes obtunded, and his respiratory drive may be suppressed, eventually resulting in apnea and cardiac arrest. These effects of CO_2 on cellular function are reversible, providing the PCO_2 is returned to tolerable levels before cardiac arrest occurs. The second effect of elevated PCO_2 results from a

$PaCO_2$ (mm Hg)	Arterial Blood pH	Signs
38–42	7.42–7.38	Normal
48	7.34	Breaking point of breath holding
70	7.20	Severe acute respiratory failure
70	7.30	Severe chronic respiratory failure
100	7.15	Drowsiness; coma; carbon dioxide narcosis
130	7.0	Compatible with survival only with oxygen supplementation

depression of alveolar and arterial oxygen tensions. At $PaCO_2$ equal to 40 mm Hg, the PaO_2 is 100. In a patient with lung disease, the alveolar-arterial oxygen gradient may increase to 40 mm Hg, and the arterial PO_2 (PaO_2) decrease to 60 mm Hg (oxygen saturation = 92%). If hypercapnia develops with PCO_2 equal to 60, there will be a decrease in alveolar and arterial PO_2 equal to approximately 20 mm Hg, and the arterial PO_2 will be 40 mm Hg (oxygen saturation = 75%), which represents severe arterial hypoxemia. Table 60-3 shows the relation between the severity of respiratory acidosis, as reflected in arterial PCO_2 and pH, and clinical manifestations of respiratory acidosis.

3. **Hypercapnia in patients with lung disease.** Study of the relation among arterial PCO_2, alveolar ventilation, and CO_2 production contributes to an understanding of hypercapnia in patients with lung disease. Either a decrease in alveolar ventilation or an increase in CO_2 production will result in an elevation of $PaCO_2$.

In patients with emphysema and chronic bronchitis, a decrease in alveolar ventilation occurs for two reasons. First, the dead-space ventilation is increased by the obliteration of pulmonary capillaries and maldistribution of ventilation with respect to blood flow ($\dot{V}/\dot{Q}$). As a result, alveolar ventilation is decreased, even though total minute ventilation may be unchanged or even increased. Second, the airway obstruction in these patients makes breathing more difficult; although alveolar ventilation may be decreased, the work that the patient is exerting to breathe is actually increased.

For a number of years, most workers in this field held the concept that patients with lung disease and hypercapnia had lazy respiratory centers, and the use of respiratory stimulants was advocated. More recently, there has been a change in attitude about the regulation of ventilation. Studies have shown that the respiratory center actually controls the work of breathing rather than the minute ventilation. Healthy subjects show a decreased ventilatory response to increases in PCO_2 if the work of breathing is increased by an external airway resistance (Fig. 60-1). Thus, increased work of breathing appears to blunt the response to increased PCO_2 when expressed as the change in ventilation. Many patients with hypercapnia resulting from lung disease have a normal or increased sensitivity to increases in PCO_2 when the response is measured as the work of breathing.

The increased work of breathing has a second and equally

Figure 60-1

Effect of increased airway resistance on control of breathing in a normal man. Notice that under any conditions an increase in $PaCO_2$ produced by breathing small concentrations of CO_2 leads to an increase in ventilation. However, for any given PCO_2, the ventilation is less and the rate of increase in ventilation is not so steep if the airway resistance is increased, as occurs in asthma and chronic bronchitis. Note also that if inspiratory work rate is plotted for each of these measurements, the data indicate that inspiratory work rate, rather than ventilation rate, is the parameter controlled. Thus, decreased ventilatory response to CO_2 when airway resistance is increased does not indicate abnormal control of breathing. (From J. Milic-Emili, and J. M. Tyler, J Appl Physiol 18:497–504, 1963. By permission of J. Milic-Emili and the American Physiological Association.)

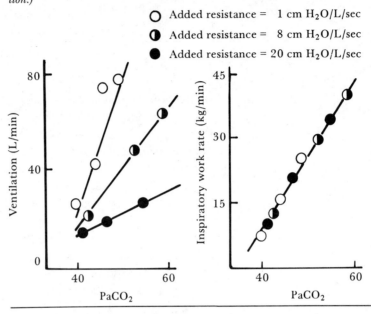

Figure 60-2

Relationship among metabolic rate (CO_2 production), alveolar ventilation, and $PaCO_2$ in a normal subject and a patient with chronic obstructive pulmonary disease (COPD), at rest, and during voluntary hyperventilation. In the normal subject, hyperventilation produces an increase in alveolar ventilation that is much greater than the increase in CO_2 production. Consequently, the $PaCO_2$ decreases. In the patient with COPD, the increase in alveolar ventilation is not so great, and the increase in CO_2 production, which reflects the increased work of the respiratory muscles, is much greater. Consequently, in the patient with COPD during hyperventilation, the PCO_2 may increase, decrease, or remain the same, depending on the relative magnitudes of the increase in alveolar ventilation and the metabolic cost of the increase in ventilation.

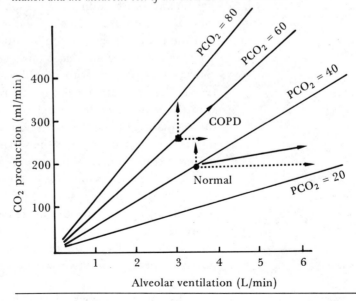

important effect on CO_2 homeostasis. Clearly, if the work of breathing is increased, oxygen consumption and CO_2 production must be increased. Eventually, patients in this situation may reach a point at which increased ventilation results in an increase in CO_2 production by the muscles of respiration greater than the increase in CO_2 elimination by the lungs (Fig. 60-2). With a further increase in pulmonary ventilation, PCO_2 may increase in such patients. Under these conditions the patient with increased work of breathing and inefficient CO_2 elimination must allow the arterial and alveolar PCO_2 to increase in order to improve the efficiency of CO_2 elimination. The total minute ventilation necessary to maintain a PCO_2 equal to 35 mm Hg is twice as great as the minute ventilation necessary to maintain a PCO_2 equal to 70 mm Hg. Further, with the decreased work of breathing necessary to maintain the PCO_2 at 70 mm Hg, more of a patient's maximal rate of respiratory gas exchange becomes available for other, nonventilatory work such as ambulation.

4. **Approach to hypercapnia and respiratory acidosis.** Hypercapnia and respiratory acidosis should be approached in terms of the pathophysiologic mechanisms outlined above. Is there evidence of increased or decreased minute ventilation? Is there evidence of increased work of breathing, i.e., inspiratory stridor (suggesting upper airway obstruction) or rhonchi and wheezes (suggesting airway obstruction within the lung)? If ventilation appears normal or increased, and there is little to suggest upper or lower airway obstruction, one should think of wasted ventilation due to pulmonary vascular abnormalities. If ventilation appears decreased, then one should think of depression of the central nervous system or neuromuscular dysfunction. Finally, a primary defect in respiratory control should be considered after ruling out other possibilities (see Table 60-2).

Hypoventilation and acute respiratory acidosis due to central nervous system depression or neuromuscular dysfunction usually require tracheal intubation and mechanical ventilation because the process may progress to complete apnea. Respiratory acidosis due to primary hypoventilation is usually chronic, stable, and compensated. Emergency treatment is usually not indicated, but the patient should be evaluated for more severe hypoventilation and apnea during sleep.

In patients with chronic obstructive lung disease and hypercapnia, the increase in arterial PCO_2 must be viewed as a physiologic adaptation, rather than simply an abnormal laboratory result. Respiratory stimulants aimed at increasing ventilation only complicate the problem by increasing the work of breathing. Instead, therapy should be directed at decreasing the work of breathing and improving the distribution of ventilation in the lung. Bronchodilators, antibiotics, and clearance of secretions to improve airway function and, in some patients, diuretics to reduce pulmonary vascular congestion should be employed. Of course, since alveolar PCO_2 is increased, alveolar PO_2 is decreased, and the careful administration of oxygen in a controlled fashion is necessary to alleviate the dangerous arterial hypoxemia that usually coexists with hypercapnia in patients with respiratory failure.

D. Pathophysiology of dyspnea. Dyspnea is a commonly encountered symptom for which the pathophysiology is poorly understood. Abnormalities in cardiopulmonary function leading to air hunger and the sensation of smothering are also frequently accompanied by hypoxemia and hypercapnia, and the physician is tempted to attribute all dyspnea to the reduced arterial PO_2 or the increased PCO_2. When the patient is encountered who is dyspneic despite normal or nearly normal arterial blood gas values, the symptom of dyspnea is written off as psychogenic or due to anxiety. Such thinking betrays the physician's incomplete understanding of dyspnea and respiratory drive. True, dyspnea can be caused by decreases in arterial PO_2, but not unless the PO_2 is below 50 to 60 mm Hg, or by smaller increases in PCO_2, but blood gas abnormalities usually play only a minor role in the production of dyspnea. An important insight into the pathophysiology of dyspnea was provided by breath-holding experiments conducted many years ago by W. S. Fowler and his colleagues. Previous investigators, by breathing O_2 and/or hyperventilating prior to beginning the breath hold, demonstrated a precise relationship between PO_2 and PCO_2 at the breaking point of breath holding. From these observations, they argued that changes in PO_2 and PCO_2 completely explained the respiratory drive to resume breathing, which eventually resulted in the breaking point of breath holding. Fowler repeated these experiments with one modification. At the breaking point the subject rebreathed into an empty rubber bag and found that he could continue the breath hold for a longer period of time. Since breathing into and out of an empty bag had absolutely no effect on the PO_2 and PCO_2 in the lungs or arterial blood, this meant that a signal coming from the lungs or chest wall, completely independent of the process of gas exchange, was in part responsible for the respiratory drive to end the breath hold. Somehow, merely expanding the lungs partially satisfies respiratory drive. Diseases that interfere with the movement of air into and out of the lungs can create an abnormal increase in respiratory drive and air hunger, which is totally independent of arterial PO_2 and PCO_2.

Later work demonstrated that the respiratory alkalosis and tachypnea associated with pulmonary fibrosis could not be eliminated by O_2 administration even when this intervention raised the PaO_2 from low levels back to the normal range.

In patients with obstructive disease, it has been found that the level of exertion sufficient to require a minute ventilation greater than one-third of the maximum voluntary ventilation is consistently associated with dyspnea. Thus, in evaluating the patient with dyspnea, although blood gas measurements should be obtained, it is important to remember that they do not provide the full explanation. Abnormalities in lung or chest wall mechanics can play an important role in creating the symptoms of dyspnea.

II. Clinical example of control of breathing

A. Description. A 55-year-old man was admitted to the hospital with a 2-week history of cough, sputum production, and increasing shortness of breath. He had not previously been treated for lung disease, but his wife reported that he had gradually reduced such activities as hunting, fishing, and yard work, due to progressive exertional dyspnea. He had smoked two packs of cigarettes a day since age 18. Examination revealed a middle-aged man in obvious respiratory distress, with labored respirations and use of the accessory muscles of respiration.

    B. Vital signs. Temperature was 37° C; pulse, 116; blood pressure, 110/80; respiratory rate, 28. There was no evidence of heart failure or pneumonia. Diffuse wheezes and rhonchi were heard in all lung fields. The patient was alert, cooperative, and oriented. Blood gases are listed in the following chart. The chest film showed normal heart size, clear lung fields, increased anteroposterior diameter, and depressed diaphragm.

Comment	Insp. O_2	pH	$PaCO_2$	PaO_2	P_AO_2	$P(A - a)O_2$
Admittance to hospital	21	7.26	64	35	67	35
Initial therapy	28	7.23	68	45	?	—
Becoming obtunded	40	7.18	85	55	?	—
If O_2 were discontinued	21	(7.18)	(85)	(10)	40	35

    C. Discussion

      1. The admission blood gases showed severe hypoxemia and combined acute and chronic respiratory acidosis. The evidence of increased respiratory work excluded depressed respiratory drive as a major cause of respiratory acidosis in this patient. Therapy should be directed at reducing the work of breathing with antibiotics, to treat airway infection, and bronchodilators, to reduce bronchospasm.

      2. In response to oxygen therapy the PO_2 had increased, but this was accompanied by a progression of the respiratory acidosis and a change in sensorium suggesting the onset of CO_2 narcosis. If it is assumed that discontinuation of O_2 therapy would return the patient to his status on admission, the last entry in the table would indicate what might happen as the alveolar PO_2 is reduced, with the A − a gradient remaining at 35. These values are not consistent with life. The proper course of management at the time the patient becomes obtunded is to initiate mechanical ventilation to reduce the $PaCO_2$.

Questions

Select the single best answer.

    1. A patient was evaluated (in Cleveland, Ohio, where barometric pressure = 747 mm Hg) for the complaint of dyspnea at rest. The respiratory rate was 35 breaths per minute. Auscultation of the chest revealed no wheezes or rales. Arterial blood was sampled, revealing a pH of 7.42; PCO_2, 25 mm Hg; and PO_2, 60 mm Hg. Which of the following statements about the patient is true?

      a. The hyperventilation and complaint of dyspnea are explained by anxiety, because there is no evidence of lung disease.

      b. The dyspnea and hyperventilation must be explained by something other than blood gas abnormalities, and there is evidence of lung disease.

      c. The dyspnea, tachypnea, and acute respiratory alkalosis are due to arterial hypoxemia.

d. All of the above.

e. None of the above.

2. A patient was evaluated for increased serum bicarbonate noted on routine blood chemistry profile. His arterial blood then revealed a pH of 7.35; PCO_2, 70 mm Hg; PO_2, 55 mm Hg; and HCO_3^-, 37.8 mEq. His arterial blood was sampled again after the patient was instructed to breathe faster and more deeply. The PCO_2 then was 40 mm Hg. Which statement is true?

a. The increased PCO_2 and decreased PO_2 indicate that the patient has chronic obstructive pulmonary disease.

b. The increased PCO_2 and decreased PO_2 in this patient may be due to an intracardiac shunt.

c. The $P(A - a)O_2$ is normal and the response to hyperventilation suggests normal lung function with a primary defect in control of breathing.

d. All of the above.

e. None of the above.

61 Reversible Obstructive Airways Disease (Asthma)

I. **Introduction.** The word *asthma* is derived from the Greek word for panting and for centuries was applied to virtually all respiratory illnesses, serving as a synonym for *breathlessness.* Now, however, it is used to label a specific disease entity characterized by an increased responsiveness of the trachea and bronchi to various stimuli, which is manifested by widespread narrowing of the airways. This narrowing changes in severity spontaneously or as a result of therapy. The two important points of this definition are: (1) people with asthma have irritable airways that respond to various stimuli (that would not affect someone with normal lungs) by developing airway narrowing; and (2) this airway narrowing is reversible (as opposed to the obstruction that occurs in emphysema).

This chapter will review the potential causes of reversible airway obstruction, the actual pathologic changes that have been observed, and various mechanisms by which these pathologic changes may occur. It will also review the effect these changes have on measurements of ventilation and gas exchange. Finally, a brief presentation of the clinical manifestations of and therapy for asthma will be made.

II. **Pathology.** A review of the pathologic changes in the lungs of asthmatics reveals the causes of reversible airway narrowing. Grossly, the lungs are overdistended and fail to collapse. The cause becomes apparent on cut-section, where both large and small airways can be seen to be partially, and occasionally totally, occluded by mucous plugs.

Microscopically, two anatomic areas are involved: the bronchial wall and the bronchial lumen (Fig. 61-1). A third area, the *lung parenchyma,* is unique in asthma because it is normal—free of fibrosis or destruction. However, several changes occur within the *bronchial wall:* mucosal wall edema, an increase in submucosal glands and goblet cells, a decrease in the number of mast cells, apparent smooth-muscle hyperplasia, basement membrane thickening, infiltration by eosinophils, and loss of bronchial epithelial cells. The *bronchial lumen* is partially filled with a heavily cellular infiltrate. The noncellular component of the exudate is composed of mucus, secreted by the goblet cells and the submucosal glands, and a protein-laden transudate exuded from the capillaries in the lung. The cellular components consist primarily of eosinophils and epithelial cells, shed from the bronchial wall. Other components are: (1) creola bodies, aggregates of shed epithelial cells; (2) Charcot-Leyden crystals, collections of free granules from eosinophils; and (3) Curschmann's spirals, which are actual casts of small bronchi formed by the viscous exudate.

The secretions that fill the airways can be coughed up by the patient; this becomes important clinically. This sputum provides the physician with a valuable diagnostic aid. Eosinophils within the sputum denote reversible airway narrowing, while polymorphonuclear cells and bacteria indicate the presence of infection.

III. **Classification.** Numerous types of stimuli have been found to incite acute bronchospasm in different asthmatic individuals. Over the years, multiple classification systems have been developed, based on the principal type of stimulus that seems to be important in a particular patient. The most prevalent classification system is one that divides patients by whether they

Figure 61-1   *Sections of normal airway (left) and an airway from a patient with acute bronchial asthma. (Modified from J. B. West,* Pulmonary Pathophysiology—The Essentials. *Baltimore: Williams & Wilkins, 1977, p. 81. By permission of J. B. West and the publisher; © 1977, The Williams & Wilkins Company, Baltimore.)*

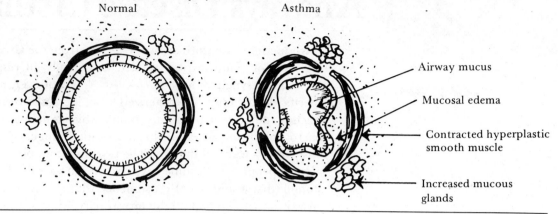

respond to extrinsic or intrinsic stimuli. Extrinsic stimuli operate by a type I (immediate hypersensitivity) reaction and constitute the allergic group. The mechanism through which intrinsic stimuli cause airway narrowing is not well worked out, but an allergic etiology has not been demonstrated. The difference between the two patient groups is that other allergy-associated phenomena occur with higher frequency in the allergic asthmatic; that is, allergic asthma is generally associated with known external allergens (e.g., animal dander, pollens), positive skin tests (i.e., an immediate wheal-and-flare reaction after the injection of extracts of specific allergens), elevated serum immunoglobulin E (IgE) levels in approximately 60 percent of patients, and intermittent, seasonal attacks. This type of asthma occurs more often in children, and is often associated with a personal and family history of diseases such as eczema and rhinitis.

The intrinsic (or nonallergic) asthma group tends to have no known allergens, negative skin tests, normal IgE levels, nonseasonal attacks, and negative personal and family allergic histories.

Many patients do not fit easily into one or the other group. For example, a patient with classic allergic asthma may also develop bronchospasm on exposure to intrinsic types of stimuli (e.g., cold, exercise, anxiety). Also, during an attack, eosinophils may be increased in the blood and sputum of both types of asthma. Thus, eosinophils serve as a marker of reversible airway narrowing and not as an indication of an allergic reaction. The presence of eosinophils is helpful in differentiating someone who smokes and has chronic bronchitis from someone who smokes and has a component of reversible airway narrowing. The former would not have eosinophils in the sputum, although the latter may.

Whether asthmatics are classified as having an extrinsic or intrinsic etiology, the effects of the stimuli are the same. The irritable airways in both groups develop reversible narrowing secondary to smooth-muscle contraction, mucosal edema, and secretions within the lumen.

IV. **Pathogenesis.** For allergic asthma, a pathway responsible for the airway narrowing has been worked out; it involves inhaled allergens, specific IgE, mast cells, and various mediators.

In a type I (immediate hypersensitivity) reaction, an inhaled allergen stimulates plasma cells to produce specific IgE antibodies to that antigen (Fig. 61-2).

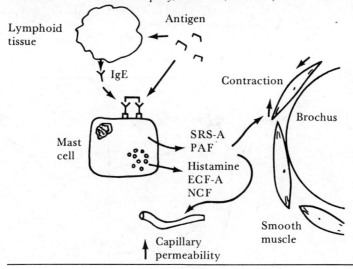

Figure 61-2   *Pathogenesis of asthma. ECF-A = eosinophilic-chemotactic factor of anaphylaxis; PAF = platelet-activating factor; SRS-A = slow-reacting substance of anaphylaxis; NCF = neutrophil-chemotactic factor. (Modified from J. B. West, Pulmonary Pathophysiology—The Essentials. Baltimore: Williams & Wilkins, 1977, p. 82. Reproduced with permission of the author and The Williams & Wilkins Company, Baltimore, © 1977.)*

The IgE enters the circulation and eventually becomes fixed to the Fc receptors on mast cells located in the bronchial submucosa, close to capillaries and smooth muscle. These mast cells are then primed to respond to repeat exposure of that particular antigen. On reexposure, one antigen can attach to and bridge two IgE molecules, thus setting off a series of reactions within the mast cell leading to release of various mediators.

Several mediators have been identified in the lung and are considered to be active in asthma. The primary mediators are released from mast cells, where they are either stored preformed in granules or are synthesized once the mast cell has been stimulated and then released. Histamine, eosinophil-chemotactic factor of anaphylaxis (ECF-A), and neutrophil-chemotactic factor (NCF) compose the group stored in granules. Slow-reacting substance of anaphylaxis (SRS-A) and platelet-activating factor (PAF) are the mediators that are synthesized once the mast cell has been stimulated.

Histamine can cause smooth-muscle contraction, in both large and small airways; an increase in vascular permeability, allowing exudation of fluids and cells; and an increase in mucous secretion. ECF-A attracts eosinophils to the area; NCF attracts neutrophils to the area and may also induce release of lysosomal enzymes from neutrophils. SRS-A has actions that are similar to those of histamine, except that SRS-A causes a prolonged contraction of bronchial smooth muscle in small airways. PAF causes platelet aggregation, which results in release of secondary mediators from the platelets. Among these secondary mediators are serotonin, bradykinin, and various prostaglandins. Serotonin causes smooth muscle contraction. Bradykinin is a potent systemic vasodilator. Prostaglandins of the E series are potent vascular dilators, while prostaglandins of the F series constrict blood vessels and airways.

Mast cells have several other receptors that are important in controlling the release of mediators. Two groups, the guanyl cyclase and adenyl cyclase groups, serve to modulate the mast cell response (Fig. 61-3).

Adenyl cyclase is a membrane-associated enzyme that catalyzes the

Figure 61-3

Factors influencing mast cell degranulation. cGMP = cyclic guanosine monophosphate; PAF = platelet-activating factor; SRS-A = slow-reacting substance of anaphylaxis; ECF-A = eosinophilic-chemotactic factor of anaphylaxis; NCF = neutrophil-chemotactic factor; PGE = prostaglandin E; cAMP = cyclic adenosine monophosphate. (Modified from A. P. Fishman, Pulmonary Diseases and Disorders. New York: McGraw-Hill, 1980, vol. I, p. 570. Copyright © 1980, McGraw-Hill Book Company. Used with the permission of McGraw-Hill Book Company and with consent of the author.)

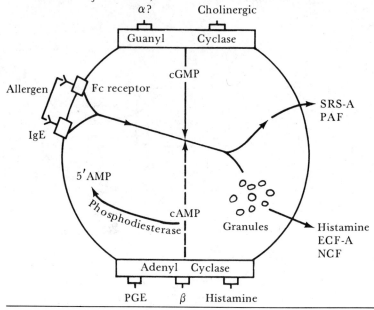

formation of cyclic adenosine monophosphate (AMP) from adenosine triphosphate (ATP). Cyclic AMP is then broken down within the cell by the enzyme phosphodiesterase to 5'AMP, the inactive form. An increase in cAMP blocks mediator release from the mast cell. Adenyl cyclase may be stimulated by beta-adrenergic agonists (part of the sympathetic nervous system). This leads to an increase in cAMP and can block bronchospasm in the asthmatic. On the other hand, beta-adrenergic antagonists may worsen the bronchospasm of an asthmatic. Two other substances, prostaglandin E_2 and histamine, probably operate as part of a negative feedback system. For example, once histamine is released from the mast cell, it feeds back to stimulate adenyl cyclase and increase cAMP, thereby decreasing further histamine release.

Guanyl cyclase is a second membrane-associated enzyme. It enhances the formation of cyclic guanosine monophosphate (GMP), which in turn stimulates the release of mediators. Guanyl cyclase activity is increased through the parasympathetic nervous system (the cholinergic receptor) and perhaps also by an alpha-adrenergic receptor (part of the sympathetic nervous system).

In addition to mediator effects on bronchial smooth muscle, increases in cAMP within the muscle are associated with relaxation and increases in cGMP with contraction.

This model is important in explaining the pathogenesis of reversible airway narrowing and in offering an hypothesis about the beneficial roles of various drugs in therapy for asthma. Epinephrine and metaproterenol (both adrenergic agonists) are helpful therapeutic agents. Methylxanthines, a group of drugs that are competitive inhibitors of phosphodiesterase, block cAMP breakdown and are a mainstay of asthma therapy. Atropine, a cholinergic antagonist, is helpful in treating selected asthmatics, in whom it inhibits guanyl cyclase.

Figure 61-4

Some influences on airway smooth muscle tone. (Modified from A. P. Fishman, Pulmonary Diseases and Disorders. New York: McGraw-Hill, 1980, vol. I, p. 575. Copyright © 1980, McGraw-Hill Book Company. Used with the permission of McGraw-Hill Book Company and with the consent of A. P. Fishman.)

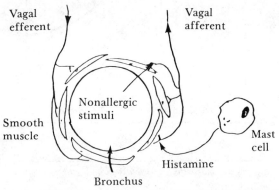

Figure 61-5

The extreme sensitivity of airway resistance to changes in airway radius.

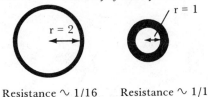

Resistance ∿ 1/16   Resistance ∿ 1/1

In contrast, the beta-adrenergic blocker propranolol can incite acute attacks of asthma.

A third system affects smooth muscle (Fig. 61-4) and may be important in intrinsic asthma. Nerve endings from vagal afferents exist in the subepithelial region of the tracheal-bronchial tree. They are called irritant receptors and appear to respond to various stimuli such as cold, exercise, and smoke. Once stimulated, they feed back to the central nervous system, invoking a neurogenic response that causes stimulation of vagal efferents. These efferents act directly on smooth muscle to cause contraction. Histamine and other mediators may also be able to stimulate the irritant receptors.

V. Measurements of ventilation. The various pathologic changes affect measurements of ventilation. Although measurements of air flow, lung volumes, resistance, and compliance may be totally normal in an asthmatic during a quiescent period, during an attack the measurements change dramatically. Resistance, as defined by Poiseuille's equation, is inversely proportional to the radius to the fourth power:

$$R = K/r^4 \quad (K = \text{a constant}, r = \text{radius})$$

As pointed out, airway narrowing is the major problem during an asthmatic attack and leads to a marked increase in resistance. For example, if the initial radius of an airway was 2, resistance would be $1/2^4$ (or 1/16) (Fig. 61-5). If the airway is narrowed to 50 percent of its initial size, the radius now equals 1, and resistance would now be $1/1^4$, or 1 (a 16-fold increase in resistance).

Spirograms reveal an obstructive pattern with a decreased forced expiratory volume in 1 second (FEV_1), a decreased ratio of FEV_1/FVC, and often, also a decreased forced vital capacity (FVC) (see Fig. 61-6).

Figure 61-6

Comparison of expiratory spirogram in normal subject (A) and in a patient with airway obstructive disease (B).

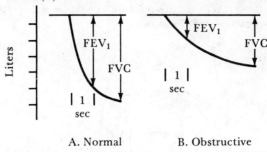

A. Normal   B. Obstructive

Figure 61-7

Changes in flow-volume curve associated with airway obstruction. RV = residual volume; TLC = total lung capacity.

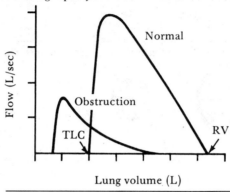

With the increased resistance to air flow, it is harder and takes longer to get the same volume out, thus giving a nonspecific obstructive pattern. This same information can be conveyed in a different form, the expiratory flow volume curve (Fig. 61-7). The same maneuver is used as for the FVC (i.e., a deep breath is taken by the subject and then exhaled as rapidly and completely as possible). However, in this instance instead of plotting volume versus time, flow (vol/time) is plotted against volume. Again, a nonspecific pattern is seen, with lower peak flows.

Lung volumes also change with bronchospasm. Again, the typical pattern is obstructive, with increased total lung capacity (TLC), decreased vital capacity (VC), and increased residual volume (RV) (Fig. 61-8). Clinically, this may be detected as hyperexpanded chest on physical exam and as hyperlucency on chest x-rays.

Compliance (change in volume per unit change in pressure) may increase slightly during an asthma attack.

In summary, the changes that occur in lung mechanics are of a nonspecific obstructive pattern. The finding specific for the reversible airway obstruction of asthma is that all the changes listed in Table 61-1 are potentially reversible.

VI. **Measurement of gas exchange.** Changes can also be seen in measurements of gas exchange. Most commonly, arterial blood gas results are normal; however, during an asthma attack the most common findings are hypoxemia (a lowered PaO_2), hypocapnea (a lowered $PaCO_2$), and acute respiratory alkalosis (raised pH). The hypoxemia occurs because of ventilation-perfusion mismatch (continued perfusion of poorly ventilated regions). This type of hypoxemia responds to therapy with increased inspired oxygen.

Figure 61-8

Changes in lung volumes associated with airway obstructive disease. ERV = expiratory reserve volume; IRV = inspiratory reserve volume; RV = residual volume; TLC = total lung capacity; VC = vital capacity; TV = tidal volume.

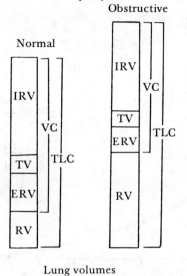

Lung volumes

Table 61-1

Pathophysiologic Changes in Asthma (All Reversible)

Obstructive pattern on spirometry
  Reduced flow rates
  Prolonged exhalation
Obstructive pattern of lung volumes
  Increased residual volume (RV)
  Increased total lung capacity (TLC)
  Reduced vital capacity (VC)
Increased airway resistance
Slightly increased compliance

An important alert is signaled when during an asthma attack a patient has lowered PaO_2 but normal or increased $PaCO_2$. This is an indication that the patient is wearing out, and requires immediate medical intervention; the individual may even require mechanical ventilation.

VII. Clinical manifestations and therapy. Clinically, asthma is manifested by paroxysms of coughing, wheezing, and dyspnea (labored or difficult breathing). Patients tend to be tachypneic (with rapid respiration) and also anxious. The episodes are usually short-lived, but they can become prolonged. Between attacks, asthmatics are asymptomatic.

Preventive therapy consists of avoiding known stimuli whenever possible (e.g., no pets for the child who is allergic to animal danders). When necessary, various drugs may be used. As discussed earlier, the major classes of antiasthma drugs are adrenergic agonists, methylxanthines, and occasionally cholinergic antagonists. A fourth drug, cromolyn, inhibits mast cell degranulation. Corticosteroids are also used and have proved invaluable in treating severe asthma.

VIII. Clinical example of reversible airflow obstruction (asthma)

  A. Description. A 19-year-old man came to the emergency room complaining of being unable to catch his breath and of his chest feeling tight. He had a 10-year history of periodic attacks of dyspnea and marked wheezing, occurring predominantly in the spring and sum-

Figure 61-9

Lung volumes and spirogram in 19-year-old male patient with allergic-type asthma before treat-ment. Height = 68 in.; weight = 135 lb; FEV₁ = forced expired volume in one second; FRC = functional residual capacity; FVC = forced vital capacity; RV = residual volume; TLC = total lung capacity.

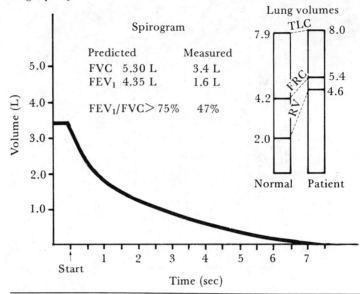

mer. He had had eczema since infancy and hay fever from the age of 7.

On examination there was an increase in the anteroposterior diameter of his chest, which was hyperresonant; on auscultation diffuse, prolonged expiratory wheezes were easily heard. Examination of his sputum revealed numerous eosinophils; the differential white blood cell count had 12 percent eosinophils. Chest x-ray showed full inspiration with very large lung volumes and clear lung fields. Figure 61-9 shows his lung volumes (measured by plethysmography) and spirogram with predicted readings.

Initial spirometry showed: FVC, 3.4 liters (64% of predicted); FEV_1, 1.6 liters (37% of predicted); and FEV_1/FVC, 47%. The patient was treated with a subcutaneous injection of epinephrine and intravenous aminophylline. One hour later, repeat spirometry showed: FVC, 5.2 liters (98% of predicted); FEV_1, 3.6 liters (83% of predicted); and FEV_1/FVC, 69%.

B. Discussion. This was a case of allergic-type asthma with severe ventilatory defect and hyperinflation of the lung at a time of moderately severe bronchospasm. The prompt and dramatic response to bronchodilators (epinephrine and aminophylline) is characteristic of the reversible airflow obstruction of asthma.

Questions

Select the single best answer.

1. The hypoxemia in asthma attacks is usually secondary to:
   a. Low $\dot{V}/\dot{Q}$ areas.
   b. High $\dot{V}/\dot{Q}$ areas.
   c. Shunt.
   d. Diffusion.
   e. Hypoventilation.

2. All the following statements about an acute asthmatic attack are true, except:
   a. Mucosal wall edema contributes to limitation of airflow.
   b. Polymorphonuclear cells in the sputum serve as markers of reversible obstructive airways disease.
   c. Improvement in ventilation can be seen after treatment with methylxanthines.
   d. Resistance to expiratory airflow is increased.

Chronic Airflow Limitation

I. **Terminology.** Over the past 40 years the nomenclature of chronic lung disease has been changed in an effort to better describe the pathologic basis for this problem. Thus, what in the 1940s was called chronic, nonspecific respiratory disease (CNSRD) became chronic obstructive lung disease (COLD) in the 1950s and then chronic obstructive pulmonary disease (COPD) (1960s). In the 1970s the term *chronic airways obstruction* (CAO) was popularized to describe the plight of patients afflicted with what are more commonly referred to as chronic bronchitis and emphysema. Recently, pulmonary physicians and physiologists have suggested that *chronic airflow limitation* (CAL) is the more descriptive name for this group of diseases because a decrease in expiratory airflow associated with airway narrowing is common to nearly all these patients, although actual obstruction of the airway is rarely seen. While CAL is a more descriptive term, COPD is more frequently used in the medical literature at present and will remain so for some time.

II. **Definition.** Diseases included under chronic airflow limitation (primarily chronic bronchitis and emphysema) have two primary characteristics: (1) decrease in *expiratory* airflow rates (as measured by spirometry); (2) airflow *not reversible* to normal after bronchodilators (excludes asthma or reversible airflow limitation).

III. **Basic disease descriptions**

A. **Chronic bronchitis.** Chronic bronchitis is essentially a *clinical* diagnosis characterized by cough and sputum production for at least 3 months in 2 consecutive years, in the absence of another specific diagnosis (tuberculosis, fungal infection, malignancy, foreign body in bronchus, lung abscess, or bronchiectasis). Self-pollution with cigarette smoke is the most common cause, although industrial irritants have been implicated in some cases, as well as recurrent childhood respiratory infection in others. Some may wish to include cystic fibrosis under chronic bronchitis, since the pulmonary manifestations are essentially dyspnea with cough and sputum production.

B. **Emphysema.** Emphysema is basically a pathologic diagnosis requiring examination of lung tissue for documentation. Thus, it is difficult to establish during a patient's lifetime, although certain clinical and radiographic findings are highly suggestive of emphysema (see sections VI and VII below). The pathologic finding in emphysema is an enlargement of distal air spaces plus breakdown of alveolar walls. Simple air-space enlargement was once regarded as an indication (or manifestation) of emphysema; however, this overdistention without tissue loss is now more appropriately referred to as hyperinflation.

IV. **Pathologic features**

A. **Chronic bronchitis.** The excess mucous production in chronic bronchitis is due to an increase in both the number and size of bronchial mucous glands and increased number of goblet cells. In addition to the increase in the amount of mucus produced, the ciliary clearance mechanism is usually impaired by smoking. Thus, warm, moist, glucose-rich puddles of mucus collect in smaller airways, providing an excellent culture medium for bacteria so that local infections cause a

Table 62-1   *Mechanisms of Airflow Limitation*

A. Chronic bronchitis
  1. Airway narrowing
    a. Enlarged mucous glands
    b. Bronchial wall inflammation and edema
    c. Intraluminal mucus or pus
    d. Hypertrophied bronchial support muscles
    e. Loss of alveolar wall support
  2. Airway obstruction
    a. Mucous plug
    b. Fibrosis (with obliteration of lumen)
B. Emphysema
  1. Airway narrowing, due to loss of radial support by alveoli
  2. Reduced driving pressure across large airways, due to decrease in elastic recoil of the parenchyma

further outpouring of purulent secretions that further compromise the bronchial lumen. A course of broad-spectrum antibiotics will usually suffice to break this vicious cycle.

B. Emphysema. Although emphysema has been characterized into a number of types based on to what extent the acinus is involved, the classification has little clinical relevance. *Centrilobular emphysema* is the most common type in chronic airflow limitation. It is seen almost exclusively in cigarette smokers, is more common and more severe in the upper lobes, and as the name implies, is characterized by destruction limited to the central part of the lobule while peripheral alveolar ducts and alveoli are not damaged. In contrast, *panacinar* (or *panlobular*) *emphysema* demonstrates distention and damage to the entire lobule. This type of disease is more common in the lower lobes and encountered in the inherited form of emphysema associated with alpha$_1$-antitrypsin deficiency. Panacinar emphysema is often found in the lower lobes of smokers with extensive upper-lobe centrilobular disease. Finally, mild asymptomatic panacinar disease is fairly common in older patients. Smoking has been implicated in two ways in the development of alveolar wall damage: (1) Smoking leads to inflammation, resulting in an increased number of macrophages and neutrophils in the lung. These cells are metabolically active and contain large amounts of proteases, particularly elastase. (2) Smoking inhibits the natural antiproteolytic activity of alpha$_1$-antitrypsin in the lung, as well as other antiproteases and antielastases in the lung. Thus, there is simultaneously an increased release of proteases into the lung parenchyma while the normal antiproteolytic activity is depressed, resulting in digestion and destruction of lung tissue. Patients with alpha$_1$-antitrypsin deficiency are further compromised by the absence of normal antiprotease activity.

V. Mechanisms of airflow limitation. A comparison of the mechanisms of airflow limitations in chronic bronchitis and emphysema is provided in Table 62-1.

VI. Clinical features. A comparison of typical clinical features of chronic bronchitis and emphysema is given in Table 62-2.

VII. Pulmonary function abnormalities. A comparison of typical pulmonary function abnormalities in chronic bronchitis and emphysema is found in Table 62-3.

Table 62-2

Comparison of Typical Clinical Features of Chronic Airflow Limitation

Feature	Chronic Bronchitis	Emphysema
General appearance	Mesomorphic, overweight, dusky	Thin, purse-lip breathing, use of accessory muscles
Age	40–50	50–75
Onset	Cough	Dyspnea
Cyanosis	Marked	Slight to none
Dyspnea	Moderate	Disabling
Cough	More evident than dyspnea	Less evident than dyspnea
Sputum	Copious	Scanty
Upper respiratory infections	Common	Occasional
Breath sounds	Moderately diminished	Markedly diminished
Cor pulmonale and right-sided heart failure	Common	Only during bouts of respiratory infection and terminally
Radiograph	Normal diaphragm position; cardiomegaly; lungs normal or with increased bronchovascular markings	Small, pendulous heart; low, flat diaphragms; areas of increased radiolucency

Table 62-3

Comparison of Typical Pulmonary Function Abnormalities

Variable	Chronic Bronchitis	Emphysema
FEV_1/FVC	Reduced	Reduced
TLC	Slightly increased	Considerably increased
RV	Moderately increased	Markedly increased
Lung compliance	Normal or low	Normal or low
Airway resistance	Increased	Normal or slightly increased
DLCO	Normal or low	Low
PaO_2	Moderately to severely reduced	Slightly to moderately reduced
Arterial hypercapnia	Chronic	Only during acute respiratory infection
Hematocrit	Generally high and may reach 70%	Normal or slightly high; uncommon to exceed 55%

FEV_1/FVC = ratio of forced vital capacity in 1 second to forced vital capacity; TLC = total lung capacity; RV = residual volume; DLCO = diffusing capacity for carbon monoxide. See Chapter 59 for explanation of terms.
Source: Modified from A. P. Fishman, *Pulmonary Diseases and Disorders*, New York: McGraw-Hill, vol. I, p. 464. Copyright © 1980, McGraw-Hill Book Company. Used with permission of McGraw-Hill Book Company and with the consent of the author.

VIII. Clinical example of chronic airflow limitation

 A. Description. A 66-year-old white male carpenter, who had shortness of breath on mild exertion and chronic cough productive of ¼ cup of white sputum daily, was followed for 3 years in the chest clinic. He had smoked two packs of cigarettes per day for 35 years, but had cut back to one pack per day for the last 2 years. Over the week before the clinic visit he experienced increased dyspnea, increased cough productive of greenish yellow sputum, and persistent ankle edema, but denied hemoptysis, fever, chills, or night sweats. On examination his pulse was 100, respiratory rate 24, blood pressure 105/80, and temperature 36.5° C (rectal). The neck veins were distended while the patient was lying at a 45-degree angle. There were diffuse bilateral rales and rhonchi, and slight end-expiratory wheezing. There was a faint fourth heart sound. The liver was palpable two fingerbreadths below the costal margin, and there was 2^+ pretibial edema.

Room air arterial blood gases showed a pH of 7.34, PCO_2 of 45, and PO_2 of 48. The chest radiograph showed an increased anteroposterior diameter and retrosternal space. The heart size was slightly increased from before; there were no infiltrates or effusion. The ECG showed sinus tachycardia and P-pulmonale, the hematocrit was 56 percent, and the white blood cell count was 8.5×10^3 per cubic millimeter.

The patient improved after hospitalization and treatment with low-flow oxygen, bronchodilators, and antibiotics. A predischarge spirogram showed evidence of moderately severe airways obstruction consistent with the diagnosis of chronic bronchitis and emphysema.

B. Discussion

1. The patient's history of 72 pack/years of smoking and daily sputum production indicate chronic bronchitis, although the chest x-ray suggests some elements of emphysema in this patient with CAL.
2. The recent change in sputum is consistent with an exacerbation of bronchitis with worsening hypoxemia and pulmonary hypertension, leading to cor pulmonale (increased heart size, high venous pressure, and ankle edema).
3. Pneumonia (parenchymal infection) was probably not present (no change on the chest x-ray, normal white blood counts, no fever or chills).
4. Hypoxemia was probably present for some period of time, as indicated by the increased hematocrit.
5. The response to therapy is typical of patients with chronic bronchitis.

Questions

Select the single best answer.

1. What is the most common cause of chronic bronchitis?
   a. Frequent chest infections as a child.
   b. Cigarette smoking.
   c. Industrial pollution.
   d. Prior history of asthma.
   e. None of the above.
2. What is the most likely explanation for the development of alveolar wall damage in emphysema?
   a. Chronic exposure of alveoli to low PO_2.
   b. Alveolar wall necrosis due to decreased minute ventilation.
   c. Compromised circulation due to mucosal edema.
   d. Release of proteases from macrophages and neutrophils in the lung.
   e. None of the above.

63 Interstitial Lung Disease

I. Introduction. There are a large number of diseases that affect the interstitium of the lung. This chapter will describe: (1) the anatomic location of the interstitium, (2) some of the diseases that affect it, and (3) the pathogenesis and pathology of these diseases. Further, it will show how these pathologic changes affect the normal physiology of the lung and how, in turn, an appreciation of the pathophysiology contributes to an understanding of the clinical manifestations and management of interstitial lung disease.

The pulmonary interstitium is the connective tissue of the lung that surrounds blood vessels, alveoli, and the bronchial tree. It is present between the alveolar epithelium and capillary endothelium (Fig. 63-1), as well as surrounding the airways and vessels in the non–gas-exchanging portions of the lung (Fig. 63-2).

There are over 130 diseases that may affect the interstitial space (Table 63-1, top). Some, such as occupational diseases, have known etiologies (Table 63-1, bottom). These may have therapeutic implications: for example, stopping the occupational exposure may stop the disease process. Involvement of the interstitium of the lung may also be secondary to disease in other organ systems. For example, heart disease can lead to chronic pulmonary edema with involvement of the pulmonary interstitium. Overall, the etiology can be determined in around 30 percent of patients presenting with interstitial disease. The rest will have interstitial involvement related to diseases of unknown etiology. The most frequent of these are idiopathic pulmonary fibrosis, pulmonary fibrosis associated with collagen-vascular disorders, and sarcoidosis.

The remarkable thing about all these different diseases is that the pathogenesis of the interstitial involvement tends to be relatively similar. The stimulus can be determined in around 30 percent of the cases; in the others it cannot. The stimulus leads to a *cellular phase* of inflammation in which the interstitium of the lungs is invaded by mononuclear cells, lymphocytes, and macrophages. This cellular phase is potentially reversible; however, if not treated it often leads to *pulmonary fibrosis* and destruction of the normal structure of the lung.

II. Pathology. In the normal lung, the alveolar septa are very thin and contain few cells. Pathophysiologically, the cellular phase in the development of an interstitial lung disease is characterized by cellular infiltrate of these alveolar septa. This tends to destroy the capillaries in the alveolar septa early in the disease process. In addition, the interstitium surrounding the small airways may be involved by this cellular infiltrate. Thus, the small airways can be occluded or partially occluded early in the development of this disease. If left unchecked, fibrosis and disorganization develop, with the almost complete destruction of the normal structures of the lung (end-stage fibrosis).

These pathologic changes are often reflected in the chest x-ray. Early in interstitial lung disease when there is histologic interstitial infiltrate, the chest x-ray may be completely normal. As the disease progresses, more tissue and less air are present in the lung and a reticular, reticulonodular, or sometimes a nodular pattern develops. All these different patterns are seen in interstitial lung disease. End-stage fibrosis is often referred to as honeycomb lung; on the chest x-ray small cystic spaces that resemble a honeycomb are seen.

Figure 63-1

The interstitial space, including a capillary in cross-section with bordering alveoli.

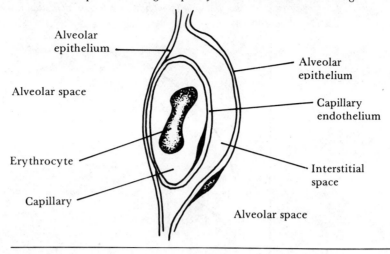

Alveolar epithelium

Alveolar space

Erythrocyte

Capillary

Alveolar epithelium

Capillary endothelium

Interstitial space

Alveolar space

Figure 63-2

The interstitial space, including a bronchiole and alveoli in cross-section.

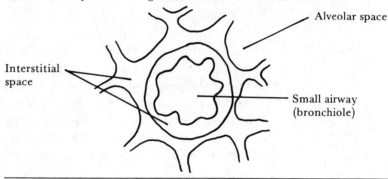

Alveolar space

Interstitial space

Small airway (bronchiole)

Table 63-1

Interstitial Lung Disease

Diseases with unknown etiologies
  Idiopathic pulmonary fibrosis
  Collagen-vascular disorders
  Sarcoidosis
  Eosinophilic granuloma
  Goodpasture's syndrome
  Idiopathic pulmonary hemosiderosis
  Wegener's granulomatosis
  Lymphocytic infiltrative disorders
  Churg-Strauss syndrome
  Hypersensitivity angiitis
  Overlap vasculitides
  Inherited disorders
  Pulmonary veno-occlusive disease
  Ankylosing spondylitis
  Diffuse amyloidosis (lung)
  Chronic eosinophilic pneumonia
  Lymphangioleiomyomatosis
Known etiological agents for interstitial lung diseases
  Occupational and environmental inhalants
  Drugs
  Poisons
  Radiation
  Infectious agents
  Secondary to chronic pulmonary edema
  Secondary to chronic uremia

Figure 63-3

Volume-pressure curves of the respiratory system in normal lungs and lungs with interstitial disease. Note that the slope (compliance) is less in interstitial disease. Volume is a percentage of total lung capacity.

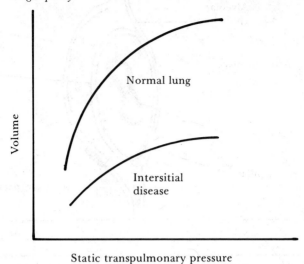

In addition to the destruction and reorganization of normal tissues seen pathologically, there are changes in the constituents of the interstitium. In idiopathic pulmonary fibrosis, the total collagen content of the lung is not increased, but there is a qualitative change in the type of collagen present. Type I collagen tends to be stiffer than type II collagen. The ratio of type I to type II collagen increases in idiopathic pulmonary fibrosis. Such changes remain to be established in the other interstitial lung diseases.

In summary, in interstitial lung disease there is obliteration of normal structures, especially the alveoli and capillaries, and marked alteration of the organization and components of the interstitium. There is destruction of normal alveoli, as well as infiltration of the interstitium of the airways and the alveolar capillary membranes.

III. **Lung mechanics.** These pathologic changes make the lung stiffer (Fig. 63-3). For a relatively small change in the distending pressure of the normal lung, there is normally a large volume change. In interstitial disease, for the same change in pressure there is less of a change in volume: i.e., the lungs are less compliant. This is due to an alteration of the connective tissue present but is also due to destruction of the air-containing structures.

These pathologic changes will also affect the lung volumes. At functional residual capacity (FRC), since airway pressure is equal to alveolar pressure, there is no air movement. The outward forces of the chest wall and the inward forces of the lung are in balance. In interstitial disease, a less compliant lung causes FRC to decrease. In attempting to take a deep breath to total lung capacity (TLC), one's inspiratory muscles will be unable to expand the lung as much as a normal lung. Thus, TLC is decreased. If one exhales down to residual volume (RV), the lung may contain a little less air than normal, due to both the decreased lung compliance and the fact that normal air-containing structures have been destroyed. Usually the decrease in TLC is more than the decrease in RV; thus, the vital capacity (VC) is decreased in severe interstitial lung disease.

One of the other hallmarks of interstitial lung disease is that air flow is

Figure 63-4

Effect of radial tension of the lung on airway diameter in disease.

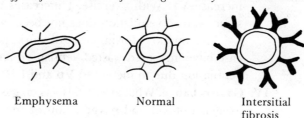

Emphysema   Normal   Interstitial
                                    fibrosis

well maintained despite the fact that lung volumes are decreased. Normally, most of the resistance to air flow is in the large airways. Radial tension of these airways, by the normal lung, tends to keep them open. In emphysema, the radial tension is decreased and the airways tend to collapse during exhalation. A person with interstitial lung disease, breathing at low lung volumes, is able to maintain air flow because the radial tension from the stiff (noncompliant) lungs tends to keep the airways open (Fig. 63-4).

Decreased lung volumes, with maintenance of flow, are evidenced in the *restrictive pattern* of spirometry seen in many people with interstitial lung disease. The vital capacity is often decreased; however, the percentage of air exhaled in 1 second (FEV_1/FVC) is normal (approximately 75% or greater). In advanced obstructive disease, vital capacity may also be decreased; but only a much smaller percentage of air gets out in 1 second ($FEV1/FVC$ is less than normal). Thus, the obstructive and restrictive spirographic patterns are different (see Chap. 59).

Early in the course of interstitial lung disease spirometry may be normal. With progression of the disease the restrictive pattern often develops. It should be remembered that restrictive pattern does not necessarily mean interstitial disease, since this pattern can also be caused by space-occupying lesions, pulmonary resection, pleural disease, chest-wall deformities, neuromuscular disease, and abdominal distention.

To summarize, the changes in lung mechanics are stiff lungs (decreased compliance), as well as decreased lung volumes and maintenance of airflow (FEV_1/FVC ratio is normal).

How do these changes in lung mechanics affect the patient's ventilation? Total ventilation ($\dot{V}E$) is equal to frequency of breathing (f) times the tidal volume ($\dot{V}T$). Each breath ($\dot{V}T$) can be divided into the part that fills the dead space ($\dot{V}D$) and does not undergo gas exchange and the part that goes to the alveoli, where gas exchange occurs ($\dot{V}T - \dot{V}D$). $\dot{V}D$ is increased in interstitial disease; thus, for any given frequency, there is wasted ventilation. In addition, people with interstitial lung disease have an increased frequency. The work of breathing is the sum of nonelastic work and elastic work. Normal patients breathe at a rate requiring the least amount of total work, usually about 15 breaths per minute. In interstitial lung disease the amount of nonelastic work is normal, but the elastic work is increased because of the stiff lungs. The minimum total work done for a given alveolar ventilation ($\dot{V}A$) now tends to occur at a rate of 20 to 30. Despite the increased wasted ventilation (f × $\dot{V}D$) at this rapid respiratory rate, deep slow breathing would require stretching the stiff lung and would greatly increase the work of breathing. Finally, as a normal person exercises, the $\dot{V}T$ increases, the $\dot{V}D$ stays about the same, and consequently more of each breath undergoes gas exchange. One breathes more efficiently during exercise by increasing $\dot{V}T$. In interstitial lung disease, on the other hand, it costs too much, with respect to work of breathing, to increase $\dot{V}_T$. With exercise, f increases and $\dot{V}_T$ and $\dot{V}_D$ stay about the same, and so ventilation does not become more efficient.

In summary, for any rate of work, patients with interstitial lung disease have increased wasted ventilation and, subsequently, increased total ventilation due to increased $\dot{V}_D$ and f.

IV. **Gas exchange.** What are the effects on gas exchange (CO_2 elimination and oxygen uptake) and oxygenation of the arterial blood? Carbon dioxide elimination is not a problem in interstitial lung disease; oxygenation of the arterial blood does present a problem. Thickening of the alveolar interstitium, leading to a decrease in the rate at which oxygen can diffuse across this membrane into the blood, contributes little to hypoxemia at rest. With exercise, the blood has to go through the capillaries more rapidly, leaving less time for equilibrium with alveolar gas to occur. Thus, with exercise, diffusion limitation may make a small contribution to hypoxemia. Shunting of pulmonary venous blood into the arterial blood may contribute to hypoxemia late in the disease; hypoxemia due to shunting does not correct with O_2 administration. The third and major cause of hypoxemia in interstitial disease is low ventilation/perfusion ($\dot{V}/\dot{Q}$) areas in which perfused portions of the lung are poorly ventilated. This has clinical significance, since hypoxemia due to low $\dot{V}/\dot{Q}$ areas responds to a small increase in inspired oxygen (low-flow oxygen).

In summary, low $\dot{V}/\dot{Q}$ areas are the number one cause of hypoxemia in people with interstitial lung disease. Shunt may be a late problem, and diffusion limitation makes a small contribution to hypoxemia during exercise. CO_2 elimination is not a problem except preterminally, when CO_2 retention may occur.

V. **Hemodynamics.** Oxygenated blood must be delivered to the periphery. O_2 delivery is equal to cardiac output times O_2 content of blood. O_2 delivery may be low in interstitial disease because O_2 content may be decreased due to hypoxemia and, in addition, cardiac output is often limited due to destruction of the pulmonary vascular bed with an increase in pulmonary vascular resistance. Early involvement of the capillaries decreases the cross-sectional area of the vascular bed. As a normal person exercises, the pulmonary artery pressure increases little. In severe interstitial lung disease, the restricted capillary bed leads to marked increase in the pressure in the pulmonary artery during exercise as the cardiac output increases. Due to this afterload, the right side of the heart is unable to attain a normal increase in cardiac output in response to exercise (Fig. 63-5). Thus, destruction of the pulmonary vascular bed limits the cardiac output, limiting O_2 delivery.

VI. **Clinical manifestations.** Most patients with interstitial lung disease will usually complain of dyspnea, a disease manifestation marked by wasted ventilation, increased work of breathing, stimulation of the juxta-capillary receptors, and hypoxemia (Table 63-2). In addition, patients quite commonly have a dry (nonproductive) cough due to stimulation of the irritant receptors that lie just under the bronchial epithelium in the large airways. The inflammation in the interstitium and traction due to abnormal mechanics of the lung can stimulate these receptors. Later in the disease, patients develop impaired clearance of bronchial secretions, leading to chronic bronchitis. Pneumonia is a common problem late in the course of this disease and is a frequent cause of death. Tachypnea is the most frequent clinical sign; the patient minimizes respiratory work by breathing rapidly. In addition, crackles in the dependent portion of the lung are

Figure 63-5

Effect of interstitial lung disease on pulmonary artery pressure in response to exercise.

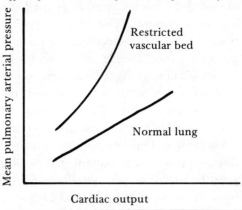

Table 63-2

Clinical and Laboratory Manifestations of Interstitial Lung Disease

I. Clinical manifestations
   A. Symptoms
      1. Dyspnea
      2. Cough
   B. Signs
      1. Tachypnea
      2. Crackles
      3. Clubbing
      4. Cyanosis
      5. Cor pulmonale
II. Laboratory data
   A. Arterial blood gases
      1. Increased alveolar-arterial PO_2 difference (worse with exercise)
      2. Normal to low $PaCO_2$ (may increase late)
   B. ECG—Cor pulmonale
   C. Chest x-ray—interstitial pattern
   D. Spirometry—restrictive pattern
      1. Decreased vital capacity (VC)
      2. Normal FEV_1/FVC
   E. Decreased DLCO (diffusing capacity of the lung for carbon monoxide)

probably related to the involvement of the small airways by the interstitial inflammation. Clubbing is often seen; cyanosis is not a particularly good indicator of arterial hypoxemia but it is frequently seen. The right heart is under increased strain, since it must pump against increased pulmonary vascular resistance. As a result, it tends toward hypertrophy. Often, one can palpate a left parasternal heave and hear an increase in the intensity of the second heart sound. These are signs of cor pulmonale (pulmonary heart disease), which is hypertrophy or dilatation of the right ventricle from pulmonary disease.

Arterial blood gases often show an increased alveolar-arterial PO_2 difference early in the disease process, even before there is a restrictive pattern by spirometry or x-ray changes. The $PaCO_2$ may be normal or low, but just before death it may increase. Patients with interstitial disease generally do not have trouble eliminating CO_2; when given oxygen, they usually do not retain carbon dioxide readily. On the chest x-ray there is often an interstitial pattern. Spirometry often reveals a restrictive pattern, that is, a decreased vital capacity (VC) with a normal FEV_1/FVC ratio. Another of the earliest changes to occur in people with interstitial lung disease is a decrease in DLCO (diffusing capacity of the lung for carbon monoxide). This is a commonly used clinical test that is helpful in following these patients. The DLCO may be decreased in a wide variety of diseases and is not specific at all for interstitial lung disease. Why would interstitial lung disease affect this test? First, there is destruction of the capillaries of the lung, which decreases the surface area over which carbon monoxide can be taken up. Second, there is a decrease in the capillary blood volume in the lung, which would also decrease the amount of carbon monoxide that can be taken up into the red cells during the test.

VII. **Management.** One should always try to determine the type of interstitial disease present. The patient may be able to stop exposure and thus prevent the progression of the disease. In addition, there is specific therapy for certain types of interstitial lung disease. Since low $\dot{V}/\dot{Q}$ is the major cause of hypoxemia and tends to respond to low-flow oxygen, one can often help the patient's symptoms and perhaps increase exercise tolerance by giving oxygen therapy. There is usually little danger of retaining carbon dioxide and developing CO_2 narcosis in response to oxygen (except in far-advanced, preterminal stages of the disorder).

VIII. **Clinical example of interstitial lung disease**

  A. **Description.** A 45-year-old man with idiopathic pulmonary fibrosis complained of progressive dyspnea on exertion over the past 6 months. He had a nonproductive chronic cough. Respiratory rate was 35 breaths per minute. His nails were clubbed, but not cyanotic. Chest examination revealed fine crackles, greater in the dependent portion of the lung. Cardiac examination revealed a parasternal heave and an increased intensity of P_2. He had jugular venous distention.

  Chest x-ray showed he had small lungs with increased interstitial markings. Spirogram results were: FEV, 2.8 liters (55% of predicted); FEV_1, 2.1 liters (60% of predicted); and FEV_1/FVC, 75 percent (normal). Arterial blood gases:

Room air		Nasal O_2	
PaO_2	45	PaO_2	60
$PaCO_2$	30	$PaCO_2$	30
pH	7.43	pH	7.44

  B. **Discussion**

  1. The patient had the typical restrictive pattern of spirometry seen in interstitial pulmonary disease with decreased FVC and FEV_1, but a normal FEV_1/FVC ratio, indicating that there was no obstruction to airflow.

  2. On physical examination the patient had evidence of cor pulmonale with right ventricular heart failure. The increased pulmonary vascular resistance leads to pulmonary hypertension (increased P_2), which contributes to hypertrophy of the right ventricle (parasternal heave). Eventually, the systemic venous pressure increases as the right ventricle fails (jugular venous distention). Note also that cyanosis is not a reliable indicator of hypoxemia.

  3. The patient's hypoxemia responds to low-flow oxygen, since most of the hypoxemia is due to ventilation-perfusion mismatching. Chronic oxygen therapy may improve the patient's dyspnea on exertion by increasing the O_2 content of the arterial blood and the cor pulmonale by partially reversing the hypoxic component of the increased pulmonary vascular resistance.

Select the single best answer.

1. A patient with severe dyspnea has the following physiologic abnormalities: DLCO (diffusing capacity of the lung for carbon monoxide) is 50 percent of predicted; dead space/tidal volume is 50 percent (increased). Lung volumes are: total lung capacity (TLC), 50 percent of predicted; functional residual capacity (FRC), 50 percent of predicted; and residual volume (RV), 50 percent of predicted. Which disease could explain these findings?
   a. Pulmonary embolus occluding the right pulmonary artery.
   b. Emphysema.
   c. Spinal cord tumor with paralysis.
   d. Idiopathic pulmonary fibrosis.
   e. A lung tumor blocking his right main stem bronchus.

2. In patients with interstitial lung disease, which of the following makes the largest contribution to hypoxemia at rest?
   a. Diffusion abnormality.
   b. Low ventilation/perfusion ($\dot{V}/\dot{Q}$) areas.
   c. Shunt.
   d. Increased dead space.
   e. High ventilation/perfusion ($\dot{V}/\dot{Q}$) areas.

Pulmonary Edema

I. **Introduction.** We are born with pulmonary edema and, if we live long enough, we shall probably die with pulmonary edema. The purpose of this discussion is to review the pathophysiology of pulmonary edema and, more importantly, the physiologic mechanisms that keep the lungs dry. Any treatment of water balance in the lung has to take into consideration the factors listed in Table 64-1.

The Starling equation is useful for understanding water balance in any tissue:

$$F = K_f [(Pcap - Pis) - \sigma(\pi cap - \pi is)]$$

where F is the rate of fluid filtration; K_f is the hydraulic filtration coefficient; Pcap and Pis are the hydrostatic pressures in the capillary and interstitial space; σ is the oncotic reflection coefficient of the endothelium, a function of endothelial permeability to protein (equal to 1 if the endothelium is perfectly semipermeable—i.e., impermeable to protein molecules—and 0 if the endothelium exerts no restraint on the diffusion of proteins in relation to H_2O); and πcap and πis are the oncotic pressures in the plasma and interstitial fluid that depend on protein comcentrations in the two compartments.

In 1959, Guyton and Lindsey addressed the problem and formulated concepts that served as the basis for understanding lung water balance until recent times. In a series of experiments in which left atrial pressure (Pla) and plasma protein concentration were varied, and changes in lung water content were measured, they demonstrated that there was no increase in lung water so long as Pla was less than πcap (Fig. 64-1). In terms of the Starling equation this meant that F was 0, σ was equal to 1, and the extravascular forces, Pis and πis, could be ignored. In other words, there was a threshold left atrial pressure (equal to oncotic pressure) at which pulmonary edema began, and below that pressure the lungs were dry and without net transcapillary fluid filtration.

Since that time a number of observations, combined with physiologic insights, have led to a clearer understanding of the mechanisms that control lung water.

First, the concept of a threshold left atrial pressure has questionable physiologic meaning for two reasons: (a) It has been shown that pulmonary arterioles and venules up to 100 microns in diameter play a role in fluid filtration in the lung; thus, pulmonary arterial hypertension at normal left atrial pressure may promote the development of pulmonary edema. (b) There is a vertical hydrostatic pressure gradient in the lung; thus, when the capillary pressure is equal to oncotic pressure in upper lung regions, capillary pressure must exceed oncotic pressure in lower lung regions. Second, to be discussed later in more detail, there is a continuous flow of lymph from pulmonary lymphatics at normal pulmonary vascular pressures, indicating that F in the Starling equation is not zero. Third, pulmonary lymph contains plasma proteins, indicating that πis is not 0, and that σ is probably less than 1.

II. **Role of interstitial fluid pressures.** One of the major conceptual advances is a clearer understanding of interstitial fluid pressures in all tissues and in

Table 64-1   *Factors Determining Fluid Balance in the Lung*

Intravascular forces
    Microvascular hydrostatic pressure
    Plasma oncotic pressure
Extravascular forces
    Interstitial fluid pressure
    Interstitial fluid oncotic pressure
Vascular permeability
    To small molecules, H_2O, Na, etc.—hydraulic filtration coefficient
    To proteins—oncotic reflection coefficient
Lymphatic drainage
    Flow
    Pressures

Figure 64-1   *Parameters for lung water balance. (Drawn from data in A. C. Guyton and A. W. Lindsey, Effect of elevated left atrial pressure and decreased plasma protein concentration on the development of pulmonary edema. Circ Res 7:649–657, 1959.)*

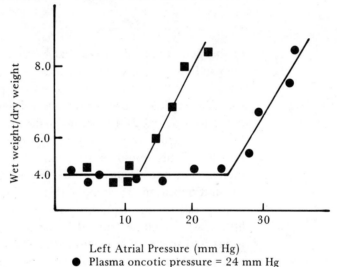

Left Atrial Pressure (mm Hg)
● Plasma oncotic pressure = 24 mm Hg
■ Plasma oncotic pressure = 12 mm Hg

the lung in particular. Guyton has contributed most to our understanding of interstitial fluid pressure. While needles, cannulae, and balloons inserted into subcutaneous tissues always record a slightly positive interstitial pressure, measurements of interstitial fluid pressure using a chronically implanted perforated capsule or a cotton wick have recorded negative interstitial fluid pressure, which becomes more negative with a reduction in vascular pressure or an increase in plasma colloid oncotic pressure; the pressure becomes less negative with a decrease in plasma colloid oncotic pressure. Starting with a totally edematous tissue, fluid separates all the solids so that there is no solid-solid contact and no forces causing the compression or deformation of solid structures. Under this condition, tissue pressure is equal to interstitial fluid pressure. When the tissue is perfused with plasma in which oncotic pressure exceeds hydrostatic pressure, fluid will be resorbed. As this occurs, solid structures will be pulled together to fill the space previously occupied by fluid. Since the surfaces of cells, collagen fibers, and other solids are neither smooth nor congruent, this removal of tissue fluid and compaction of solids will result

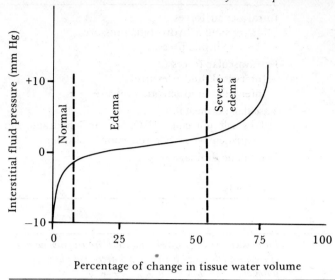

in the generation of forces that resist further compaction of solid elements. This force also resists the resorption of tissue fluid into the capillary, creating a negative interstitial fluid pressure.

This creates a special pressure-volume curve for fluid in the interstitial space (Fig. 64-2). Under normal conditions, total pressure is 0, and if Pcap is 20 while πcap is 28 mm Hg, interstitial fluid pressure will be −8 mm Hg. (This would be true only if πis were 0.) If capillary pressure increases or oncotic pressure decreases, fluid will be filtered into the tissue, but only a small volume of fluid will result in a steep rise in interstitial fluid pressure, and equilibrium with intravascular forces will occur with little loss of volume from the vascular space or gain in volume of the interstitial space. In edematous states, reductions in plasma oncotic pressure or increases in capillary hydrostatic pressure cause further increases in interstitial volume and pressure. At some point interstitial fluid volume is sufficient to eliminate all solid-solid contact. At this point, further increase in tissue fluid volume and pressure is determined only by the pressure-volume characteristics of limiting membranes, i.e., the skin in the case of subcutaneous edema. The pressure-volume relationship is much flatter, i.e., more compliant, and the important homeostatic mechanism that exists with negative fluid pressure has been lost. Only with gross edema leading to increases in tissue pressure, vascular compression, and mechanical dysfunction does tissue fluid pressure begin to increase sufficiently to resist further edema formation. Recent studies have used measurements of hydrostatic pressure in fluid-filled alveoli. The data indicate a negative value for interstitial fluid pressure, which varies from −5 mm Hg at the base of the lung to −20 mm Hg at the top of the lung, with a vertical gradient equal to approximately 1 cm H_2O per centimeter vertical distance down the lung. This is in keeping with the already mentioned vertical gradient for capillary hydrostatic pressure. The data also indicate a pressure-volume curve similar to that in other tissues (Fig. 64-2); i.e., when Pis is negative it changes steeply for small changes in lung water. At an interstitial pressure equal to approximately zero, the curve changes abruptly, and beyond this point large increments in lung water produce relatively small increases in Pis. This may be the pulmonary edema threshold, where lung water increase occurs with little increase in interstitial pressure.

The pulmonary interstitial fluid pressure may be the central issue for ventilatory therapy aimed at the treatment of pulmonary edema. How does it relate to airway pressure and lung volume? To begin with, the interstitium of the lung consists of two compartments, the alveolar compartment located in the alveolar septae and the extra-alveolar compartment located in the bronchovascular sheath. The pressure in the alveolar compartment is equal to about -4 cm H_2O and varies directly with changes in airway pressure. The pressure in the extra-alveolar compartment is more complex. Studies have shown that it is normally more negative than pleural pressure, i.e., about -10 cm H_2O when pleural pressure is -5 cm H_2O. With an increase in lung volume the tethering effect of expanding alveoli causes this pressure to fall even lower. In general, therapy that increases airway pressure and lung volume does not decrease the rate of edema formation in experimental animals, but there is evidence that it does cause a redistribution of edema fluid out of the alveoli into the peribronchial compartment, thereby producing an improvement in respiratory gas exchange.

III. **Importance of interstitial fluid oncotic pressure.** Interstitial oncotic pressure is not zero. Measurement of protein in pulmonary edema and samples of pulmonary lymph both indicate that πis is not zero. The presence of protein in the interstitial fluid is well established and forms the basis for additional insight into lung water balance. In studies on sheep with chronic cannulation of the pulmonary lymphatics, the lymph contains protein at a concentration 50 to 70 percent of that in plasma.

With an increase in capillary filtration pressure, lymph flow increases and, at the same time, lymph protein concentration falls as the plasma ultrafiltrate appearing in the pulmonary interstitium dilutes the existing protein. This washout of interstitial protein decreases πis and decreases the balance of forces favoring edema formation. In other words, there is a negative feedback mechanism involving interstitial protein concentration and oncotic pressure, which tends to retard the rate of fluid filtration in edematogenic states. This will be true, however, only if endothelial permeability is unaltered and water is filtered faster than protein. This defense mechanism is lost when edema is caused by an increase in capillary permeability.

IV. **Lymphatic drainage.** Lymphatic drainage also plays an important role in protecting the lung from pulmonary edema. Studies in sheep have shown that (a) lymph flow is always present in the normal lung; (b) it is facilitated by respiratory movements; (c) lymphatic pumps can generate pressure gradients of at least 10 cm H_2O; (d) an acute increase in capillary filtration is accompanied by an increase in lymph flow; and (e) lymphatic hypertrophy occurs in states of chronic pulmonary vascular pressure elevation. This may be the explanation for the observation that patients with chronic valvular heart disease or congestive cardiomyopathy may be relatively free of pulmonary symptoms at levels of left atrial pressure that would be expected to produce pulmonary edema in acute cardiac decompensation. According to one point of view, pulmonary edema with alveolar flooding occurs only when the rate of fluid filtration exceeds the pumping capacity of the pulmonary lymphatics. Although this may be an oversimplification, there are conditions in which alterations in lymphatic function promote

Table 64-2   *The Two Types of Pulmonary Edema*

Item	Cardiogenic	High Permeability
Mechanism	Heart failure Mitral stenosis	Injury to the capillary endothelium
Pulmonary capillary pressure	Elevated (>25 mm Hg)	Normal (<12 mm Hg)
Edema protein/plasma protein	<50%	>50%
Therapy	Reduce capillary pressure	Reduce capillary pressure

the development of pulmonary edema. These include: (a) immediately following lung transplantation (as demonstrated by autologous transplantation in experimental animals); (b) radiation pneumonitis; (c) (perhaps) mechanical ventilation, which is known to be associated with an unexplained increase in lung water in the absence of heart failure; and (d) (perhaps) right ventricular failure, in which increased right atrial and venous pressures may impede the emptying of pulmonary lymphatics into intrathoracic veins.

V. **Vascular impermeability.** This is an important determinant of pulmonary edema formation. An increase in vascular permeability can produce pulmonary edema at normal or reduced vascular pressures. The demonstration of continuous lymph flow indicates a balance of forces favoring fluid filtration in the lung under normal conditions, and any increase in the hydraulic filtration coefficient could conceivably cause pulmonary edema. Further, if protein permeability increases at the same time, the oncotic pressure of plasma proteins exerts little effect across the capillary endothelium.

In man, high-permeability edema is most easily demonstrated by an increase in the protein concentration of airway fluid. In high-pressure pulmonary edema, the edema fluid protein concentration is always less than 50 percent of the plasma protein concentration. In edema due to increased permeability, the protein concentration is greater than 50 percent, usually about 80 percent of the plasma protein concentration. Edema with a normal pulmonary capillary pressure also suggests altered permeability, but it may be difficult to exclude a period of increased left atrial pressure at the time of edema formation.

Measurement of pulmonary capillary pressure is important in the management of any patient with unexplained pulmonary edema. When the edema is the result of increased permeability rather than increased pressure, the hydraulic filtration coefficient (K_f) is increased, and the rate of fluid filtration is more sensitive to changes in capillary pressure than in the presence of high-pressure, cardiogenic pulmonary edema.

Pulmonary edema can be classified into two major types, based on whether or not vascular permeability is altered (Table 64-2). Both types of pulmonary edema should respond to therapy that leads to a reduction in capillary pressure in the lung. Edema due to heart failure or fluid overload with normal or low plasma protein concentration should also respond to therapy that increases plasma oncotic pressure, because the endothelial protein permeability is low. Edema due to capillary injury, with high endothelial protein permeability, would not be expected to respond to the infusion of plasma protein or other colloids. In both types of edema, general supportive therapy, including oxygen and, in some cases, mechanical ventilation, are necessary to keep the patient alive until the edema resolves.

VI. Summary. There is no threshold pulmonary capillary pressure at which filtration of fluid out of the pulmonary capillary begins abruptly. Rather, the balance of forces favors continuous filtration of fluid into the interstitial space of the lung. Under normal conditions the lung is maintained in a state of relative dryness by lymphatic clearance equal to the filtration rate. When filtration rate exceeds lymphatic clearance due to an increase in capillary pressure or a decrease in protein concentration, several things happen simultaneously that act to retard the rate of filtration: (a) because of the low compliance of the interstitial space, a small increase in interstitial fluid volume produces a sharp increase in interstitial fluid pressure, which opposes fluid filtration; (b) at the same time the increase in interstitial fluid pressure increases the driving pressure for lymph flow; and (c) the increased flow of a plasma ultrafiltrate reduces interstitial fluid protein concentration, which also acts to reduce the net fluid filtration pressure. When filtration increases as the result of an increase in vascular permeability, this last defense mechanism is lost because the filtrate contains protein in a concentration that is equal to or higher than that in the interstitial space.

Although there is no threshold at which filtration begins, there probably is a threshold condition at which pulmonary edema with alveolar flooding occurs. The exact determinants of this condition probably involve: (a) the interstitial fluid volume at which the compliance of the interstitium changes abruptly, accommodating large increases in volume with little increase in pressure; (b) the interstitial pressure at which the alveolar surface breaks down, allowing free access of edema fluid into the alveolar space; and (c) the filtration rate at which the pumping capacity of the lymphatics is overwhelmed.

Thus, the observations of Guyton and Lindsey nearly 20 years ago, which led to a basic understanding of water balance in the lung, are still valid, but we now have a better understanding of the phenomenon; future research will probably uncover new therapies to alter the pulmonary edema threshold.

VII. Clinical example of pulmonary edema

A. Description. A 53-year-old man sustained multiple soft-tissue injuries in an automobile accident and required an emergency splenectomy. In the first 12 hours of hospitalization, he required fluid resuscitation, including four units of packed red blood cells, two units of plasma, and seven liters of Ringer's lactate solution. Surgery was without complication, and the patient appeared to be doing well until the second hospital day, when he became progressively short of breath. Past medical history includes a myocardial infarction.

Examination revealed a temperature of 37.8° C; blood pressure, 130/70; respiratory rate, 48; and inspiratory rales in all lung fields, but no gallop on cardiac exam. A chest film revealed diffuse alveolar infiltrates in all lung fields. Blood gas results are listed in the accompanying tabulation. Mechanical ventilation was required, eventually with positive end-expiratory pressure (PEEP). A Swan-Ganz pulmonary artery catheter was inserted.

Blood gas measures	pH	PaCO$_2$	PaO$_2$
Nasal prongs, 3 L/min	7.52	28	42
High-flow O$_2$ by mask, 20 L/min	7.51	27	46
Mechanical ventilation, 100% O$_2$	7.48	32	55
100% O$_2$, 10 cm H$_2$O PEEP	7.46	36	80
60% O$_2$, 10 cm H$_2$O PEEP	7.47	35	60

Hemodynamic data off respirator were: pulmonary artery pressure (S/D), 20/14; wedge (indirect left atrial pressure), 11 mm Hg; and cardiac index, 4 L/m^2/min.

B. Discussion. This patient has developed adult respiratory distress syndrome. The pathophysiologic mechanism is low-pressure, high-permeability pulmonary edema with a normal (0–12 mm Hg) wedge pressure and cardiac index (3.2 ± 0.5 L/m^2/min). Given the past history of myocardial infarction, and the large amount of fluid administered, cardiogenic pulmonary edema due to volume overload and left ventricular failure could also explain the clinical picture, but the normal hemodynamic data exclude this as the primary mechanism. Despite the normal value for wedge pressure, it will be important to employ fluid restriction and diuretics. With injury to the pulmonary capillary endothelium and increased permeability, lung water balance is highly sensitive to small changes in capillary pressure. The poor response of arterial PO$_2$ to oxygen therapy is typical of the patient with shunting due to alveolar edema and atelectasis. The improved oxygenation with positive end-expiratory pressure is due to reversal of atelectasis and perhaps to redistribution of edema fluid from the alveolar to the interstitial space of the lung. There is no evidence that PEEP reduces lung water.

Questions   Select the single best answer.

1. Two patients are found to have pulmonary edema. *Patient A* has total serum protein equal to 7 g/dl, airway fluid protein equal to 2.5 g/dl, and pulmonary capillary pressure equal to 32 mm Hg. *Patient B* has total serum protein equal to 4 g/dl, airway fluid protein equal to 2.5 g/dl, and pulmonary capillary pressure equal to 10 mm Hg.

    Indicate, by circling the letter *a, b, c,* or *d,* which patient would be expected to benefit from the following proposed therapeutic interventions (*a* = patient A, *b* = patient B, *c* = both patients, *d* = neither patient).

    a b c d   1. Oxygen by face mask 10 liters per minute.

    a b c d   2. The administration of a diuretic to reduce pulmonary capillary pressure.

    a b c d   3. The infusion of plasma (protein = 6.5 g/dl) to increase oncotic pressure.

2. Filtration of fluid from the pulmonary capillary to the interstitium of the lung:
    a. Probably occurs all the time in healthy individuals.
    b. Occurs only when pulmonary capillary pressure is greater than 25 mm Hg.
    c. Occurs only when pulmonary capillary pressure is greater than plasma protein oncotic pressure.
    d. Is prevented by positive pressure breathing.
    e. None of the above is true.

I. Review of basic physiology

A. Function of the lung's circulatory systems

1. **Pulmonary circulation.** The pulmonary circulation normally receives 98 to 99 percent of the cardiac output (with 1–2% going through anatomic shunts, such as the thebesian veins) and serves several key functions.

   a. **Gas exchange.** Its role in gas exchange is the most important function of the pulmonary circulation.

   b. **Filter.** The filter system removes the aggregated platelets, red cells, and fibrin that are normally present from the circulation, thus protecting other organ systems from microemboli. It also filters out larger pathologic emboli.

   c. **Nonrespiratory metabolic functions.** The endothelial cells are the probable sites of biotransformation and uptake of certain substances such as angiotensin I, bradykinin, prostaglandins, and serotonin.

   d. **Nutrient delivery** to terminal bronchioles and alveoli.

   e. **Lung defense participation.**

   f. **Water and protein exchange.**

   g. **Fibrinolysis and anticoagulation.**

2. **Bronchial circulation.** In adults, the bronchial circulation receives 1 to 2 percent of the cardiac output and serves as the nutrient supply to all structures in the lung except the terminal bronchioles and the alveoli. It plays an important role in the fetus, in congenital cardiac abnormalities, and in some chronic pulmonary lesions, such as bronchiectasis.

3. **Lymphatics** function as conduits for water and protein removal and participate in lung defense.

B. Factors influencing blood flow through pulmonary circulation

1. **Intravascular pressures.** All flow is down a pressure gradient. The pulmonary circulation is a low-pressure system in comparison with the systemic circulation, with mean right atrial pressures around 0 to 5 mm Hg, right ventricular pressure around 25/0 mm Hg, pulmonary arterial pressure 25/8 (mean around 15 mm Hg), and mean left atrial pressure around 5 mm Hg. Any alteration in these pressure relationships can affect flow.

2. **Extravascular pressures.** In addition to the intravascular pressures, there are extravascular pressures that influence the degree of distention of the pulmonary vessels. Not all vessels are exposed to the same pressures, however. Functionally, there are alveolar vessels that are exposed to *alveolar pressure* and extra-alveolar vessels that are exposed to *interstitial* and *pleural pressures*.

3. **Gravity.** Because the lung is a low-pressure system, the distribution of blood flow is uneven and partly dependent on gravity. West has postulated four zones for blood flow, describing the relation among alveolar pressure (P_{ALV}), arterial pressure (P_{ART}), venous pressure (P_{VEN}), and, in zone 4, interstitial pressure (P_{IS}). This model requires that the vessels themselves offer no resistance to collapse and that the vessels are exposed to alveolar pressure (Fig. 65-1).

   a. **Zone 1** ($P_{ALV} > P_{ART} > P_{VEN}$). In zone 1, the alveolar pressure will

Figure 65-1

Model of blood flow zones in the lung. (Modified from J. M. B. Hughes, J. B. Glazier, J. E. Maloney, and J. B. West. Respir Physiol 4:58–72, 1968. Reprinted with permission of the author and the publisher.)

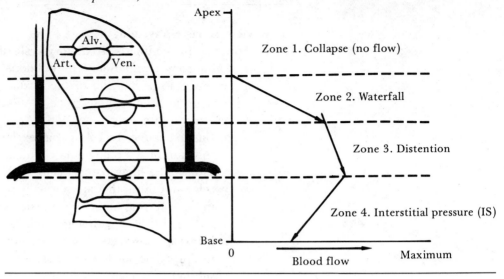

occlude the blood vessels and no flow will exist. Normally, in the upright position, the apical part of the lung is in zone 1.

b. Zone 2 ($P_{ART}>P_{ALV}>P_{VEN}$). In zone 2, flow is dependent on the arterial-alveolar pressure gradient. Therefore, gravity creates a waterfall effect with increasing flow as one goes toward the more dependent portion of the zone. In this zone, alveolar pressure forms a Starling resistor.

c. Zone 3 ($P_{ART}>P_{VEN}>P_{ALV}$). In zone 3, flow is dependent on the arteriovenous pressure gradient (as is generally the case in the systemic circulation).

d. Zone 4 ($P_{ART}>P_{IS}>P_{VEN}>P_{ALV}$). Zone 4 adds another factor, the interstitial pressure. In this zone, flow is dependent on the interstitial-arterial pressure gradient and may be reduced in comparison with zone 3.

4. Pulmonary vascular resistance (PVR). The general formula for frictional resistance (based on Poiseuille's law) is:

$$\text{Frictional resistance} = \frac{8(\text{length of the conduit})\,(\text{viscosity of the fluid})}{\pi(\text{radius})^4}$$

The PVR can also be calculated from the relationship of the change in pressure across the pulmonary vascular bed divided by the flow:

$$\text{PVR} = \frac{(\text{pulmonary artery pressure} - \text{left atrial pressure})}{\text{cardiac output}}$$

The pulmonary circuit is a highly compliant circuit that can accommodate large increases in flow without much change in pressure, indicating large decreases in the PVR.

a. Site of resistance. The major site of resistance probably lies in the pulmonary capillaries, although this has yet to be proved in humans. The capillaries might decrease resistance either by *distention* of capillaries, leading to increased cross-sectional area, or by *recruitment* of capillaries that were previously closed.

b. Factors affecting resistance

   (1) Active factors that decrease PVR: acetylcholine, prostaglandin E1, prostacyclin, vasoactive intestinal peptide (VIP).

(2) **Active factors that increase PVR**

    (a) Humoral substances: catecholamines, histamine, angiotensin II, prostaglandin F2α.

    (b) Chemical stimuli: alveolar hypoxia and acidemia.

(3) **Active factors that increase PVR in experimental animals but not man:** Sympathetic nervous system, serotonin, alveolar hypercapnia.

(4) **Passive factors that decrease PVR**

    (a) Increased pulmonary artery pressure.

    (b) Increased left atrial pressure.

    (c) Increased blood volume.

(5) **Passive factors that increase PVR**

    (a) Change in lung volume from functional residual capacity (FRC) (either increases or decreases in volume from FRC).

    (b) Increased interstitial pressure.

    (c) Increased blood viscosity.

II. **Pathophysiology.** Many pathophysiologic mechanisms can lead ultimately to an increased PVR and consequently increased pulmonary artery pressure, and right ventricular failure.

  A. **Three basic mechanisms** can lead to an increased PVR by decreasing the total cross-sectional area (or radius) of the vascular bed. (It should be remembered that resistance is inversely related to radius^4.)

    1. **Destruction of the vascular bed.** The most common examples of this are emphysema and destructive inflammatory processes such as necrotizing pneumonias.

    2. **Constriction of the vessel wall.** This is most commonly due to alveolar hypoxia or acidemia, which can be found in a variety of acute and chronic lung diseases but may also be due to the circulating humoral substances that cause increases in the PVR. In addition, vasculitis can decrease the distensibility of the vessel walls, as well as decrease the cross-sectional area.

    3. **Obstruction of the vascular bed.** This can be seen in pulmonary embolic disease.

  B. **Other mechanisms,** such as an increase in blood viscosity or change in lung volume, can lead to an increased PVR. When associated with one of the three basic mechanisms, the effect becomes additive.

III. **Examples of pathophysiologic processes affecting the pulmonary vascular bed**

  A. **Primary pulmonary hypertension.** This is pulmonary hypertension for which there is no known cause. It usually occurs in young females and progresses, over months to years, to right ventricular failure and death. It has been associated with a number of collagen-vascular diseases, including Raynaud's phenomenon, progressive systemic sclerosis, systemic lupus erythematosus, rheumatoid arthritis, polyarteritis nodosa, and dermatomyositis. In addition, there may be an association with thromboemboli and amniotic fluid emboli to the lung. Familial occurrences have also been reported, but it is not known if genetic transmission is involved. There has also been one epidemic occurrence in Europe, related to an appetite-suppressant, Aminorex, although proof of a cause-and-effect relationship was not fully established. There is also evidence in laboratory animals that dietary substances can lead to pulmonary hypertension.

    Whatever the cause, the result is progressive increase in pulmonary artery pressures, eventually leading to right ventricular failure.

Figure 65-2

Mechanisms involved in events triggered by thromboemboli in the pulmonary circulation. PPA = pressure in the pulmonary artery; PVR = pulmonary vascular resistance; RVEDP = right ventricular end-diastolic pressure.

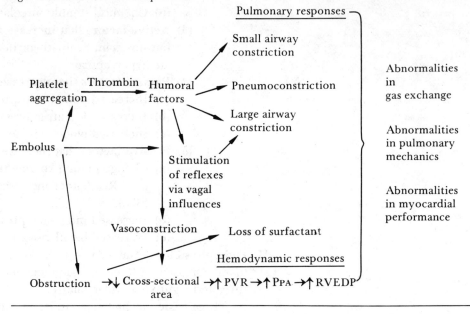

Mild hypoxemia is common, probably due both to ventilation-perfusion mismatching and to myocardial failure, with diminished PO_2 in mixed venous blood being returned to the lung. The mechanical function of the lungs usually remains normal; hyperventilation (a decreased $PaCO_2$) is common.

B. Pulmonary thromboemboli. As a consequence of systemic venous thrombosis, especially in the deep leg veins, a portion of the clot will occasionally break off and become filtered out in the pulmonary circulation. This leads to a series of events affecting lung mechanics, myocardial performance, and gas exchange.

There are three primary mechanisms involved in the changes seen (Fig. 65-2). The most obvious is mechanical obstruction. This not only can increase the PVR (and lead to right ventricular failure if sufficiently severe) but also can be associated with damage to alveolar type II cells and loss of surfactant.

The second mechanism is a neural response mediated by the vagus nerve. This neural mechanism is better demonstrated in laboratory animals than in humans, but could possibly lead to large airway constriction and increases in airflow resistance.

Finally, when the embolus lodges in the pulmonary circulation, platelets adhere to its surface and can release smooth muscle–activating substances such as prostaglandins that can cause vasoconstriction, further aggravating the increased PVR, and bronchoconstriction, leading to loss of lung volume with subsequent loss of compliance and abnormalities in ventilation.

The usual results of these mechanisms are pulmonary hypertension, possible right ventricular failure, hypoxemia due to low ventilation-perfusion ratios and shunting, loss of lung compliance, and an increase in airway resistance.

C. Cor pulmonale. Pulmonary heart disease is the cardiac response to pulmonary hypertension, no matter what the cause, if the hypertension is sufficiently severe or of sufficient duration. The term *cor pulmonale* applies to the right ventricular hypertrophy that results from the increased afterload of the right ventricle. This may result in right ventricular failure, but myocardial failure is not a necessary part of the definition of *cor pulmonale*. Also, while left ventricular dysfunction can accompany cor pulmonale, right ventricular failure secondary to left ventricular failure is *not* cor pulmonale.

While there are multiple causes for pulmonary hypertension, the most common cause is alveolar hypoxia. The keystone of therapy is to reduce the hypertension. In most cases, therefore, amelioration of the alveolar hypoxia by improving ventilatory function or administering oxygen is the most important therapeutic goal.

IV. Clinical example of pulmonary vascular disease

A. Description. A 48-year-old woman reported she had had increased dyspnea for over 6 months. No definite cause was obvious from her history. Her physical examination was remarkable only in an increased pulmonic component of the second heart sound and a grade II/VI systolic murmur.

Her arterial blood gases were: pH 7.36; PCO_2 38 mm Hg; PO_2 57 mm Hg. The DLCO, however, was 56 percent of predicted. The chest radiograph revealed prominent pulmonary arteries centrally, with pruning of the vessels more peripherally. Her complete blood count, differential white count, sedimentation rate, rheumatoid factor, antinuclear antibody assay, and chemical screening profile were all normal or negative.

Subsequently, she underwent right-heart catheterization and a pulmonary arteriogram. The results were:

Pressure	mm Hg
Right atrial pressure	6–8
Right ventricular pressure	56/10 (mean 26)
Pulmonary artery pressure	56/32 (mean 40)
Pulmonary artery wedge pressure	12

There were no unexpected findings in oxygen saturation. The arteriogram revealed multiple filling defects consistent with multiple pulmonary emboli.

B. Discussion. This woman presented with dyspnea, hypoxemia without hypercapnia, reduced diffusing capacity, and evidence of pulmonary hypertension. She had no evidence of abnormal lung mechanics to explain her hypoxemia. In addition, she is older than most patients with primary pulmonary hypertension, although this diagnosis cannot be excluded on that basis alone. Because of the possibility of an intracardiac shunt or pulmonary emboli causing the pulmonary hypertension, cardiac catheterization was performed. Had there been an intracardiac left-to-right shunt, one would have expected to find a step-up in oxygen saturation at the atrial or ventricular level, compared with the value in the vena cava, but this was not present. The pressures confirmed pulmonary hypertension. An arteriogram confirmed that she had had multiple pulmonary emboli as the probable cause of her pulmonary hypertension. The reducton in DLCO was due to the destruction of the pulmonary microvascular bed.

Select the single best answer.

1. Which of the following is the most potent chemical stimulus for pulmonary vasoconstriction in humans?
   a. Increased arterial PCO_2.
   b. Decreased arterial PO_2.
   c. Decreased alveolar PO_2.
   d. Increased pH.
   e. Prostacyclin.

2. In pulmonary embolism the major cause of the hypoxemia is:
   a. Blockage of the pulmonary blood flow with the development of high $\dot{V}/\dot{Q}$ areas.
   b. Diffusion abnormalities.
   c. Secondary changes leading to low $\dot{V}/\dot{Q}$ areas.
   d. Low mixed-venous PO_2.
   e. Both diffusion abnormalities and high $\dot{V}/\dot{Q}$ areas.

66 Pulmonary Neoplastic Disease

I. **Incidence.** Lung cancer was nearly unheard of before the twentieth century, but since the 1930s has increased in incidence until it is now the most common malignancy in males. Men afflicted with this disease outnumber women approximately three to one; however, the incidence in women is increasing rapidly, at approximately the same rate as the increase in smoking among women.

In the United States in 1977 there were 100,000 new cases of lung cancer diagnosed and approximately 80,000 deaths from the disease.

II. **Etiology and epidemiology**
   A. **Smoking.** There is now overwhelming evidence that cigarette smoking is the major cause of bronchial carcinoma.
   1. The rise in deaths from lung cancer reflects the increasing exposure to cigarette smoke over the past 50 years, particularly when the two sexes are studied separately.
   2. The risk of death from bronchogenic carcinoma increases by a factor roughly equal to the number of cigarettes smoked per day. That is to say, an individual smoking 25 cigarettes per day has about 25 times greater chance of dying from the disease than a non-smoker of the same age and sex.
   3. The risk of bronchial carcinoma is greatest in those who inhale cigarette smoke.
   4. The risk of dying from bronchogenic carcinoma lessens dramatically if cigarette smoking stops. The excess risk is approximately halved every 5 years after stopping smoking. Pipe and cigar smokers have a slightly increased risk of bronchogenic carcinoma, much less than that of cigarette smokers.
   B. **Pollution.** The incidence of bronchogenic carcinoma is greater in urban than in rural areas. Atmospheric pollution is regarded as the most likely explanation of this difference, but the relationship is poorly defined.
   C. **Occupation factors.** Occupation appears to play an important part in the causation of the disease in a relatively small number of patients. There is good evidence that industrial exposure to chromates, nickel, arsenic, coal gas, or radioactive gases is associated with an increased risk of bronchogenic carcinoma. The risk of bronchogenic carcinoma is also increased with exposure to asbestos, especially when coupled with cigarette smoking. Asbestos predisposes more to bronchogenic cancer than to mesothelioma.

III. **Pathology**
   A. **Common cell types.** Bronchogenic carcinoma presents as one of four relatively distinct diseases: squamous-cell (or epidermoid) carcinoma, small-cell (oat-cell) carcinoma, adenocarcinoma, and large-cell carcinoma. Variation in the biologic behavior of these cell types accounts for the differences in the mode of presentation, in tendency toward early metastases, and in response to therapy. Squamous- and oat-cell cancers are highly associated with cigarette smoking. There is less convincing evidence that smokers have an increased incidence of the latter two types of bronchial cancer.

1. **Squamous-cell carcinoma** is characterized by the formation of keratin by the tumor cells or the presence of intracellular bridges. The designation may be qualified as highly, moderately well, or poorly differentiated, depending on the amount and type of keratin present. Squamous-cell tumors may metastasize prominently in regional lymph nodes and often recur after resection. They tend to be limited to the thoracic cavity and are definitely related to smoking.

2. **Small-cell carcinomas** are highly malignant tumors that metastasize early and widely by both the lymphatic and the blood vessels. The most common subtype is the lymphocyte-like, or oat-cell, type. Oat-cell carcinomas show little cytoplasm and small, dense, roundish or oval nuclei; they, too, are related to smoking.

3. **Adenocarcinoma.** The basic morphologic feature of adenocarcinoma is the formation of tubules and gland-like structures, which may be accompanied by papillary growth, with or without the presence of mucin. The tumor may be further classified as highly, moderately well, or slightly differentiated. While some adenocarcinomas may originate in the larger bronchi, most seem to arise more peripherally, possibly in an old granuloma; hence, the name *scar carcinoma*. Bronchogenic adenocarcinomas are highly malignant tumors that tend to metastasize widely, predominantly by the blood stream and lymphatics.

4. **Large-cell carcinomas** are, as the name implies, tumors composed of large cells without evidence of keratin or formation of gland-like structures. As a rule, they behave clinically much like bronchogenic adenocarcinoma.

B. **Rarer cell types.** Of the less commonly occurring bronchogenic carcinomas, *bronchioloalveolar carcinomas* are among the most interesting. They are felt by some to be highly differentiated adenocarcinomas, presumably originating in the peripheral part of the lung beyond a grossly recognizable bronchus, and tend to grow upon the walls of preexisting alveoli. The histologic pattern is often papillary, and the alveolar spaces are lined by usually slender, cylindrical cells, often with abundant mucin production. After a varying period of restricted growth, there is a tendency to spread through the air spaces or through the lymphatic vessels. In lymph node metastases, the papillary pattern is often reproduced. Special care must be taken to exclude primary adenocarcinoma in other sites, such as the gastrointestinal tract or the ovaries, before making a definite diagnosis. Half the cases of bronchioloalveolar carcinoma do not metastasize beyond the thoracic cavity, even though they may grow extensively within the lungs.

C. **Relative frequencies of pulmonary malignancies.** The most common type of bronchogenic malignancy is squamous-cell carcinoma. The approximate relative incidence of the other cell types is listed in Table 66-1.

IV. **Clinical features.** The signs and symptoms found in a patient with bronchogenic carcinoma are quite variable and depend on the primary tumor size, location, and cell type as well as the existence and location of any metastases.

Bronchogenic carcinoma may be detected in a few asymptomatic patients by routine chest roentgenograms or sputum cytology examination in high-risk patients (i.e., heavy smokers, certain industrial workers); but the cost-benefit ratio of these procedures may be prohibitive.

Squamous-cell carcinomas	35
Adenocarcinomas	25
Oat-cell carcinomas	25
Large-cell carcinomas	10
Others (alveolar cell, bronchial adenoma)	5

The most common symptoms, when they ultimately develop, are related to thoracic manifestations of the tumor. The primary tumor, even when small, causes bronchial irritation resulting in cough and sputum production in 50 to 75 percent of the patients. Small amounts of hemoptysis are seen in approximately half of the patients. As the tumor grows to fill the bronchial lumen, localized wheeze, dyspnea, and obstructive pneumonitis can develop.

Other thoracic manifestations of lung cancer are related to direct extension of the tumor into adjacent structures or from metastasis to hilar or mediastinal lymph nodes. These extrapulmonary intrathoracic manifestations include hoarseness, diaphragmatic paralysis, arm pain and weakness due to entrapment of the recurrent laryngeal or phrenic nerve or to invasion of the brachial plexus, respectively. Extension to the heart and mediastinal vasculature may result in arrhythmia and cardiac tamponade or, more frequently, face and neck swelling due to superior vena caval obstruction. Stridor or dysphagia may develop in patients with large central tumors due to compression of the trachea or esophagus. Chestwall pain may result from direct extension across the pleuro-parietal space or from osseous metastases. Pleural effusion, significant enough to cause dyspnea, may be related to direct extension of the malignancy to the pleural space or to obstruction of lymphatics by hilar metastases.

Extrathoracic manifestations of pulmonary neoplasia cause a wide variety of symptoms and are the result of either distant metastases or nonmetastatic systemic effects of lung cancer. Common sites of distant metastasis include lymph nodes (commonly cervical) and organ systems with large blood supplies (bone, brain, liver, skin, and the other lung). In addition, bilateral adrenal metastases are common in bronchogenic carcinoma. Anorexia, weight loss, and malaise, though common and worrisome, are nonspecific effects that may resolve following successful surgery. Better understood are the nonmetastatic extrathoracic paraneoplastic syndromes, which appear to be related to tumor secretion of biologically active compounds, including peptide hormones and prostaglandins. A partial list of these syndromes can be found in Table 66-2.

V. Radiography. In patients with bronchogenic carcinoma the chest roentgenogram varies widely depending on the size, location, and secondary manifestations of the tumor and the absence or presence of metastasis to the hilum and mediastinal lymph nodes. The most common findings include round densities ranging from the classic coin lesions (<6 cm in size) to grapefruit-sized lesions that may be cavitary. In addition, atelectasis of a segment or a lobe or the appearance of a new pleural effusion may occur. Lymphangitic carcinomatosis with associated dyspnea is another form of presentation that can be diagnosed by chest x-ray. Occasionally, a normal chest x-ray may be found in a patient with cough, hemoptysis, or chest pain due to lung cancer. In such patients, bronchoscopy usually reveals an endobronchial tumor.

Endocrine
  Cushing's syndrome
  Secretion of inappropriate antidiuretic hormone (SIADH)
  Hypercalcemia
  Gynecomastia
  Hypoglycemia
Neurologic
  Myasthenia-like syndrome (of Eaton-Lambert)
  Polymyositis
  Peripheral neuropathy
Skeletal
  Clubbing of fingers and toes
  Hypertrophic osteoarthropathy
Cardiovascular
  Thrombophlebitis
  Marantic endocarditis
Hematopoietic
  Anemia
  Eosinophilia
  Disseminated intravascular coagulation

VI. **Diagnosis**
  A. **Rationale.** The diagnosis of bronchogenic carcinoma is based on cytologic or histologic studies, or both. These studies are necessary not only to prove the presence of a malignant tumor but also to determine its cell type, in order to estimate the prognosis and plan the treatment.
  B. **Diagnostic studies.** The usual studies include:
    1. **Sputum cytology.** Three deep-cough sputum samples are obtained for examination. A 70 to 90 percent diagnosis rate has been reported with proximal or central endobronchial lesions.
    2. **Bronchoscopy.** With the use of the fiberoptic bronchoscope, there is a 95 percent chance of diagnosing a central tumor (one that can be seen with a bronchoscope). Approximately 65 percent of peripheral tumors can be diagnosed by this technique.
    3. **Pleural cytology and biopsy** are occasionally helpful in making the diagnosis in cases where metastases to the pleural space have already occurred.
VII. **Treatment.** The list of possible treatments for lung cancer is somewhat extensive; in essence, however, these may be divided into two categories—surgery and everything else! If the lesion seems from all available data to be localized and the patient's pulmonary function allows lung resection, then lobectomy, or pneumonectomy, if necessary, gives the best hope for prolonged survival. If the clinical and pathologic evidence documents existing metastasis or if pulmonary function is too poor to permit resection of adequate lung tissue, one must decide whether to use radiation, chemotherapy, or a combination of the two. With a diagnosis of oat-cell carcinoma, even if it seems localized, surgery is contraindicated and a combined protocol of chemotherapy and radiation seems to work best.

For other tumors that are unresectable or inoperable, there is no best treatment. Radiation for palliation of hemoptysis, bone pain, and vena caval or bronchial obstruction occasionally produces remarkable improvement. However, survival is not prolonged. Multiple chemotherapy protocols are currently being tested, but none has proved to be useful for non–oat-cell carcinoma. Occasionally, symptomatic treatment may be the only appropriate action.

VIII. Prognosis. The prognosis for bronchogenic carcinoma is extremely poor. The 5-year survival for all types ranges from 5 to 10 percent, depending on which series one reads. This number is slightly misleading, since some series of oat-cell carcinomas have had essentially no survivors at the end of 2 years, whereas some well-selected patients with localized squamous-cell carcinoma have a 5-year survival rate of 40 percent. Prolonged survival correlates with two factors: cell type and extent of disease at the time of diagnosis.

IX. Clinical example of pulmonary neoplastic disease

A. Description. A 54-year-old white man who had smoked 1½ packs of unfiltered cigarettes per day since age 18, presented with a 2-month history of general malaise and weakness and 10-pound weight loss. During the previous 2 weeks, he noted small amounts of blood in his daily sputum on three occasions. He denied chest pain, nausea, vomiting, or ankle edema.

Physical examination was unremarkable except for mild expiratory wheezing in both lower lobes.

Laboratory results were: hematocrit, 39%; white blood count, $8.1 \times 10^3/mm^3$; platelets, $150 \times 10^3/mm^3$; Na^+, 128 mEq/L; K^+, 3.7 mEq/L; Cl^-, 94 mEq/L; HCO_3^-, 25 mEq/L; serum glutamic oxaloacetic transaminase (SGOT), 85 U/L (normal, 0–30 U/L); alkaline phosphatase, 325 U/L (normal, 30–100 U/L).

Chest x-ray showed a 4-cm mass in right upper lobe approximately 2 cm from hilum.

Sputum cytology was positive for small-cell (oat-cell) carcinoma.

B. Discussion. Since this patient has cytologic evidence for small-cell carcinoma, surgical cure is unlikely. A combination of radiation and chemotherapy would be recommended. Further evaluation should include bone and liver scan and computerized tomography of the head. The elevated SGOT and alkaline phosphatase suggest possible bone and/or liver metastases. In addition, the tumor may be secreting antidiuretic hormone, resulting in hyponatremia.

Questions

Select the single best answer.

1. What is the most useful method of establishing the diagnosis of bronchogenic carcinoma?
   a. Lung scan.
   b. Chest radiography.
   c. Bronchoscopy and biopsy.
   d. Pulmonary function.
   e. None of the above.
2. Which of the following statements is true about lung cancer?
   a. The incidence of bronchogenic carcinoma has been stable for years.
   b. Women are afflicted more than men.
   c. Occupation has not been shown to play a role in the development of lung cancer.
   d. The risk of death from bronchogenic carcinoma increases as the number of cigarettes smoked daily increases.
   e. None of the above.

XIII Surgery and Trauma

Jay P. Cannon

The Metabolic Response to Surgery and Trauma

Following trauma or surgery, coordinated endocrine and metabolic changes occur that seem to have survival value. In general terms, these processes provide glucose to satisfy energy requirements frequently lacking in the diet and supply low molecular weight nitrogen compounds—for collagen synthesis to allow wound healing. These sequential changes compose the biology of convalescence. Surgical convalescence is initiated by the injury itself and is maintained by the action of positive biologic forces. These forces are directed toward restoring homeostasis for the emergency, promoting wound healing, and returning the organism to its normal composition and activity.

I. Metabolic response to starvation and injury

A. Physiologic response to starvation

1. **General.** A knowledge of the physiologic response to starvation, which often accompanies trauma or follows surgery, is important in the understanding of the metabolic response to trauma and surgery itself.

   Early in starvation the physiologic response is mobilization of the body fuel stores to satisfy caloric demands. Cahill demonstrated the limited nature of the body fuel stores. In the hypothetical 70-kg man, energy stores consist primarily of body fat (141,000 calories), protein (24,000 calories), and glycogen (900 calories). Daily caloric requirements may increase fourfold during periods of extreme catabolism; thus, up to 1 kg of muscle-mass per day could be depleted to satisfy this demand. Glucose derived from gluconeogenesis rapidly becomes too expensive, since continued obligatory breakdown of essential body protein is not compatible with survival. The liver, through a sequence of enzymatic alterations, synthesizes glucose from its precursors using fatty acid oxidation as its primary source of energy. The overall effect is to spare body protein and substitute fatty acids as the body's energy source.

2. **Energy requirements**

   a. **General guidelines, sedentary life.** Baseline protein and caloric requirements for individuals leading a sedentary life are approximately 1 g of protein and 35 kcal per kilogram of body weight or approximately 1,400 kcal per square meter of body surface area per day. These requirements are inadequate for patients undergoing surgery or who have suffered trauma.

   b. **Guidelines for surgical patients or patients suffering trauma.** Experimental evidence and clinical experience suggest the following:

      (1) **Following moderate injury.** To maintain weight after moderate injury, an intake of 0.2 gm of nitrogen per kilogram and 50 kcal per kilogram per day are necessary.

      (2) **Acutely ill surgical patients.** An intake of 1,000 to 2,000 kcal per day above baseline expenditures with a calorie-to-nitrogen ratio of about 150 : 1 is appropriate for acutely ill surgical patients.

      (3) **Depleted patient or following major surgery.** The patient undergoing a complicated major surgical procedure or with

Table 67-1

Fuel	Calories
Fat (adipose triglyceride)	141,000
Protein (muscle)	24,000
Glycogen (muscle)	600
Glycogen (liver)	300
Plasma proteins	840
Total	166,740

preexisting nutritional depletion requires between 2,500 and 4,000 kcal, with approximately 12 to 24 g of nitrogen per day. Requirements for nutritional support will vary considerably with the patient's illness. In general, 3,000 kcal per day should be considered the basal need and revised upward when specific indications are present.

3. **Energy metabolism**
   a. **General.** Table 67-1 lists the fuel composition of the typical 70-kg man. Glycogen stored in muscle and liver is combined with water and electrolytes and yields only 1 or 2 kcal per gram instead of the 4 kcal found in 1 g of dry carbohydrate. The body contains essentially no excess protein. Protein fuel stores consist of muscle and enzymes, which are essential for health. Catabolism of body protein to provide energy, even temporarily, costs the body a high price; unchecked, such loss leads to disability and death.

   Lipid is not stored in combination with water; therefore, body fat yields lipid content as high as 90 percent of total weight. A gram of fat provides nearly 9.4 kcal. During starvation, and following trauma, the body attempts to conserve protein by using fat stores to provide energy.

   b. **Glucose metabolism.** In the fasting state, glucose is derived from breakdown of liver glycogen (glycogenolysis), recycled glucose, and gluconeogenesis. Early in starvation, a 70-kg man would derive emergency glucose amounting to approximately 85 g per 24 hours from the breakdown of stored liver glycogen. Glycolytic tissues—such as peripheral nerves, erythrocytes, leukocytes, bone marrow, renal medulla, and to a lesser extent, muscle—metabolize glucose by partial oxidation to lactate and pyruvate. These substances are circulated back through the liver and kidney, where through the Cori cycle they are remade into glucose. This recycled glucose amounts to about 36 g per 24 hours.

   Gluconeogenesis provides new glucose, using as substrate amino acids from muscle and glycerol from body fat. New glucose is provided at a rate of approximately 16 g/24 hr from fat sources and 43 g/24 hr from protein sources. The energy required for these conversions is provided by metabolism of free fatty acids resulting from the breakdown of body fat.

   In prolonged fasting, profound changes in metabolism occur. It is obvious that liver and muscle glycogen are in limited supply, since the total body store is only 224 g. Diminished utili-

Table 67-2

Glucose Available in Starvation State in 70-kg Man

Origin	Amount of Glucose (g/24 hr)	
	Early	Late
Stored or recycled		
Glycogen	85	0
Recycled glucose	36	50
New glucose (gluconeogenesis)		
Fat (glycerol)	16	18
Protein	43	12
Total	180	80

Table 67-3   *Effects of Hormone on Fat, Carbohydrates, and Protein Metabolism*

Hormone	Gluconeogenesis (in Liver, Kidney)	Glycolysis		Glycogenolysis		Lipolysis (Adipose Tissue, Liver, Muscle)
		Muscle	Adipose Tissue	Liver	Muscle	
ACTH-cortisol	+ + +	0	0	0	0	+ +
Epinephrine, norepinephrine	+ +[a]	0	+ +	+ + + +	+ +	+ + + +[a]
Growth hormone	+	0	+ +	0	0	+ +[a]
Glucagon	+ + +[a]	0	0	+ +[b]	0	+ + +[a]

[a]Only in the presence of the adrenal corticosteroids.
[b]By stimulating catecholamine secretion.
ACTH = adrenocorticotropic hormone.

zation of glucose and protein sparing are absolutely essential for survival. Table 67-2 compares the glucose available from different sources in both early and late fasting. The amount of glucose available as an energy source in early fasting is about 180 g/24 hr and decreases to 80 g/24 hr if the starvation state lasts over 3 weeks.

Glycogen breakdown as a source of glucose drops to almost zero (0) in the profound fasting state. Recycled glucose (formed in the liver from lactate and pyruvate) become the major source of glucose, amounting to about 50 g/24 hr.

Two additional changes occur in prolonged fasting. First, all body tissues, including brain, use free fatty acids for energy, thus decreasing glucose requirements. Secondly, the site of gluconeogenesis from protein sources shifts from the liver to the kidney.

B. Metabolic response to trauma

  1. General. In contrast with starvation, injury produces hyperglycemia, marked fatty acid mobilization with elevation of plasma free fatty acids, and a striking catabolism of muscle protein beyond that needed as an energy source. In late starvation, protein conservation is seen. Additionally, there is increased urea synthesis and an increase in serum osmolarity. Table 67-3 summarizes the effect on carbohydrate, fat, and protein metabolism brought about by hormonal changes following trauma.

  2. Carbohydrate metabolism. The elevation in the level of blood glucose that follows most injuries is brought about primarily by catecholamine secretion and to a lesser extent by increases in glucagon,

Table 67-4   *Effects of Hormones on Electrolyte and Water Balance*

Hormone	Sodium Retention	Potassium Loss	Water Retention
ACTH-cortisol	+ +	+ +	+
Renin-aldosterone	+ + +	+ + + +	+ +
Epinephrine, norepinephrine	+	0	
ADH	0	0	+ + + +

ACTH = adrenocorticotropic hormone; ADH = antidiuretic hormone.

cortisol, and growth hormone. Increased glycogenolysis results principally from increases in circulating catecholamines and to a lesser extent from increased glucagon (commonly seen following injury). Increased gluconeogenesis results from increased levels of cortisol, growth hormone, and catecholamines. The resultant hyperglycemia provides not only a ready energy source but also an increase in serum osmolarity that is homeostatic. This homeostasis results from osmotic transfer of fluid into the extracellular space to help maintain circulating blood volume.

3. **Fat metabolism.** Fat is the body's main energy source in trauma as in starvation. Catecholamines, glucagon, adrenocorticotropic hormone (ACTH), and growth hormone all increase cyclic adenosine monophosphate (AMP) in fat, and in the presence of cortisol, lipolysis results. Glycerol provides substrate for gluconeogenesis and free fatty acids from body fat stores replace glucose as the primary energy source.

4. **Protein metabolism.** Healthy young adults take in 80 to 120 g of protein or 13 to 20 g of nitrogen per day. Of this quantity, about 11 to 17 g of nitrogen is lost in the urine each day—nearly all in the form of urea nitrogen.

Following trauma, urinary nitrogen excretion greatly increases, rising to as much as 30 to 50 g per day. ACTH and cortisol are responsible for the increased proteolysis seen following injury. The increase in nitrogen excretion starts shortly after injury, reaches a peak during the first week, and continues for 3 to 7 weeks. After elective operative procedures, negative nitrogen balance is rapidly reversed; however, after severe trauma such as thermal burn, the negative nitrogen balance may remain for a considerable period of time. However, protein catabolism contributes less than 20 percent of caloric requirements. The protein lost following injury does not result from impaired protein synthesis. There is evidence that increased nitrogen metabolism following injury may be related to the need for carbohydrate intermediates for synthesis of glucose. Deamination of amino acids is the primary endogenous source of these intermediates.

C. **Water and electrolyte metabolism**

1. **General.** Maintenance of circulating blood volume following trauma is accomplished in general terms by water retention, sodium retention, and potassium excretion. This homeostasis results (in varying degrees) from increased secretion of ACTH-cortisol, renin-aldosterone, and vasopressin (antidiuretic hormone [ADH]). Table 67-4 summarizes the effects of these hormones on electrolyte and water balance. The mechanisms will be described by

considering changes in sodium and potassium and then by considering changes in water balance.

2. **Sodium and potassium metabolism**

   a. **General.** In the steady state, urinary sodium excretion matches intake and may range from 60 to 200 mEq per day. Following injury, sodium excretion falls abruptly, often to nearly zero. Increased levels of cortisol and aldosterone and other mechanisms responsive to depletion of blood volume cause this sodium retention following surgery.

   b. **Aldosterone.** Most sodium and chloride reabsorption takes place in the proximal tubules and the loop of Henle, whereas potassium and hydrogen excretion occurs in the distal tubules. Increased levels of aldosterone seen in the traumatized patient act on the distal nephrons to increase reabsorption of sodium and the excretion of potassium and hydrogen ion. This is the primary mechanism by which the kidney may excrete potassium and hydrogen ion that build up following trauma. If insufficient sodium is delivered to this site, accumulated potassium and hydrogen ion cannot be adequately excreted, resulting in hyperkalemia and acidosis.

   The increased secretion of aldosterone seen following trauma results from the stimulation of the zona granulosa of the adrenal cortex by increased levels of ACTH, angiotensin II, and potassium ion. The renin–angiotensin II system provides the most potent stimulus to aldosterone production.

   (1) **Renin.** Injury leads to increased secretion of renin from the juxtaglomerular (JG) cells of the renal afferent arterioles. The primary factors leading to increased renin secretion are: increased sympathetic stimulation of the JG cells, decreased arteriolar pressure, and decreased delivery of sodium to the macula densa. Increased circulating renin participates in the conversion of angiotensinogen to angiotensin II, which is a potent stimulus for aldosterone production.

   (2) **ACTH and potassium** cause increased secretion of aldosterone following trauma, though not to the same degree as angiotensin II.

3. **Water balance following trauma**

   a. **General.** Water retention following surgery and trauma is a constant occurrence that is adaptive, since it contributes to the maintenance of circulating blood volume. The major mechanisms are related to vasopressin release and to the impaired renal perfusion that invariably accompanies injury (see Chap. 39).

   b. **Antidiuretic hormone.** Following trauma, both neural stimulation of the hypothalamus and hypovolemia lead to the release of ADH from the posterior pituitary. Vasopressin acts on the distal tubules and collecting ducts to increase water reabsorption. ADH is also important in affecting splanchnic vasoconstriction. In the postoperative state, because of the presence of ADH, the administration of water without salt often leads to hyponatremia and, in the extremes, to water intoxication.

D. **Body cell mass concept.** Francis Moore defined the body cell mass as that component of body composition that is rich in potassium, consumes oxygen, produces carbon dioxide, and performs work. Thus, the body cell mass is the living portion of body composition. It has been demonstrated that body cell mass is linearly related to intracellular water volume and total exchangeable potassium. In catabolic states seen after injury and trauma, the total intracellular water volume and total exchangeable potassium are decreased. On the other hand, in catabolic states, the extracellular water volume and total exchangeable sodium are increased. The mechanisms leading to these changes have been discussed above.

II. Four phases of convalescence

A. **General.** Four phases of convalescence regularly appear in distinct sequence in normal posttrauma patients: phase I, the adrenergic-corticoid phase; phase II, the corticoid withdrawal phase; phase III, the spontaneous anabolic phase; and phase IV, the fat gain phase.

These phases have been given names descriptive of the clinical and metabolic picture. The duration of each of these four phases varies with the magnitude of the trauma and the previous metabolic and nutritional state of the patient. Although this discussion assumes the normal course of events in a previously healthy person, preexisting abnormalities are of great importance in modifying the normal convalescence for any particular patient.

B. **Phase I—adrenergic-corticoid phase**

1. **Clinical.** Clinical signs in this phase stem from increased sympathoadrenal activity. These include increased pulse rate, narrowing of the pulse pressure, peripheral vasoconstriction, and a rise in the blood sugar. A slight increase in rectal temperature and a relative oliguria of less than 700 cc per day on the day of trauma are commonly seen. Clinical symptoms in this phase include loss of appetite, listlessness, inactivity, and lack of interest in conversation or reading. The clinical picture may be summarized as that of a patient whose vascular response has been stimulated but who has no ambition, strength, or appetite. This phase lasts from 3 to 5 days, depending on the magnitude of the trauma.

2. **Metabolic.** Weight drops quickly secondary to rapid utilization of body fat stores. If nitrogen intake and excretion are measured, a negative nitrogen balance is evident. Increased nitrogen excretion is characteristic of the response to extensive trauma but may be minimal after less severe injury.

A negative potassium balance of around 70 milliequivalents (mEq) per day is characteristic of the operative day. Thereafter, net potassium losses are about 40 mEq per day for several days, followed by a gradual change to no net loss if usual replacement is provided.

Sodium excretion is negligible on the day of operation, an adaptation by the body to maintain the extracellular fluid volume. A reduction of the normal serum sodium level from 140 to 143 mEq per liter to 137 to 139 mEq per liter is the expected response to moderate trauma. This drop occurs in the face of sodium retention by the kidney and a potassium loss of 125 to 150 mEq in the first 3 days after trauma. In the normal patient there is no rise in serum potassium concentration in spite of apparent mobilization of potassium from the cells into the extracellular fluid.

Blood and urinary corticosteroids show a sharp rise on the day of operation. Thereafter, these return to a normal level within a few days following surgery.

C. Phase II—the corticoid withdrawal phase

1. **Clinical.** This phase begins around the fourth day after injury and lasts 2 or 3 days. The patient develops increasing peristalsis and passes flatus; appetite improves, and activities return. Water diuresis occurs and it is not uncommon to see urinary output exceed water intake.

2. **Metabolic.** Further weight loss occurs but it is thought to be due to water and lean-tissue changes rather than to fat utilization as in phase I. A marked decrease in nitrogen excretion occurs. This conservation is due to a relative cessation of lean-tissue destruction and a readiness of the organism to begin anabolism.

   Since potassium intake continues and the urinary potassium excretion drops sharply, a modest positive potassium balance is restored.

   A brisk sodium-and-water diuresis typically occurs. The extent of this diuresis depends on the previous sodium-and-water loading during phase I. Because of the concomitant water diuresis, the serum sodium concentration returns to normal in spite of negative sodium balance. The cessation of rapid potassium excretion and sodium diuresis indicates the end of phase II.

D. Phase III—spontaneous anabolic phase

1. **Clinical.** This phase is initiated by and cannot occur without adequate intake of calories. After major peritoneal injury it commences about the seventh to the tenth day. This phase continues for several weeks and is characterized by increased appetite. The patient becomes ambitious and is interested in his surroundings.

2. **Metabolic.** Weight gains generally parallel nitrogen balance in this phase and fat gain is minimum. The characteristic feature of this phase is positive nitrogen balance that is sustained in the range of 3 to 5 g of nitrogen per day in the 70-kg man. Caloric intake must be maintained at a high level in order to provide energy for utilization of the nitrogen provided. A calorie-nitrogen ratio of 150 : 1 is generally accepted as minimum requirement to accomplish rebuilding of the body's stores and healing of wounds. Sodium balance is characteristically zero, and there are no characteristic changes in the serum chemistries in this phase. Total body water increases commensurate with the amount of lean tissue being synthesized. However, fat is not deposited during this phase.

E. Phase IV—fat gain phase

1. **Clinical.** The patient is now eating a normal diet, returns home, and resumes normal activity. This phase may last weeks or months while fat stores are gradually replaced.

2. **Metabolic.** Nitrogen, potassium, and sodium balances are zero. This is an indication that protein, intracellular electrolyte, and extracellular electrolytes remain unchanged. It is characteristic of this phase that total body water remains unchanged in the face of weight gain (fat has little water content).

III. Stimulus response patterns

A. **General.** After trauma, stimuli may occur, eliciting responses that alter the phases of convalescence. Each one produces a particular bias in convalescence. Five fundamental stimulus-response patterns may be identified:

1. **Tissue injury.** The response to tissue injury increases proportionately with the magnitude of the tissue injured. Metabolic effects

include breakdown of body cell mass with net loss of body protein and nitrogen. There are increased levels of catecholamine and ACTH as a result of tissue destruction.

2. **Volume reduction.** The response to a reduced blood volume is roughly proportional to the extent and duration of the reduction. Attempts to maintain extracellular volume include sodium-and-water retention and production of large amounts of antidiuretic hormone. It is likely that most of the changes in sodium-and-water homeostasis seen after tissue injury, low flow states, and infection are entirely mediated by reductions in effective circulating blood volume.

3. **Low-flow states.** A profound reduction in effective circulating blood volume may result from loss of blood and extracellular fluid into the operation site (so-called third-space losses). Additional factors, including impairment of cardiac performance from anesthetic agents or hypoxia, may contribute to a state of inadequate tissue perfusion, with profound consequences (see Chap. 11).

4. **Invasive infection.** There is a tremendous increase in basal energy requirements when infection enters the convalescent sequence. Cardiac output is greatly increased, and if the heart is unable to respond because of underlying cardiac disease, the low-flow vector is greatly accentuated.

5. **Starvation.** Short-term utilization of fatty acids as energy substrate seems to be adaptive for the organism. However, in prolonged starvation the body breaks down protein to provide energy, with loss of both muscle and visceral proteins. If starvation is unchecked, patients commonly die of infection and respiratory failure.

IV. **Clinical examples**
   A. **Adrenergic-corticoid response to trauma**
      1. **Description.** A 24-year-old white male college student was brought to the emergency room in Aspen, Colorado. One hour earlier, he had fallen while skiing. He had an obvious fracture of the right femur, which was substantiated by x-ray. The patient's leg had been splinted by the ski patrol before he was brought in. Physical examination showed the skin to be cool and clammy. His pulse was 100 per minute and regular; blood pressure was 120/94. Serum electrolytes and blood urea nitrogen (BUN) were within normal limits but the serum glucose was 170 mg/dl. Urinalysis revealed a specific gravity of 1.030.
      2. **Discussion**
         a. The clinical appearance of this patient showed evidence of increased sympathoadrenal activity, tachycardia, a narrowing of the pulse pressure, peripheral vasoconstriction, and increased blood glucose.
         b. Increased secretion of ACTH and cortisol results from stimuli arising in the injured area as well as in higher centers. This initial response is directed toward maintenance of circulating blood volume and cardiac output.
         c. If measurements were made in such a patient, increased catecholamine and cortisol levels could be documented.
   B. **Hyponatremia with hyperkalemia**
      1. **Description.** A 70-year-old white female had a hemicolectomy for carcinoma of the right colon 24 hours before being seen. Urinary output following surgery had been in the range of 20 to 30 cc per

hour. The patient had been taking nothing by mouth and had received 125 cc of 5% dextrose and water intravenously every hour. The BUN and electrolytes prior to surgery were within normal limits. Electrolytes 24 hours after surgery were: sodium, 130 mEq/L; potassium, 6.0 mEq/L; HCO_3^-, 15 mEq/L; and chloride, 100 mEq/L.

2. **Discussion**

    a. Hyponatremia is frequently seen in postoperative patients.

    b. Hyponatremia is primarily brought about by ADH secretion associated with the surgical trauma, plus overhydration with non–salt-containing fluids.

    c. Postoperative hyperkalemia probably occurred because of movement of potassium out of the injured cells, breakdown of red blood cells in the wound, or administration of old blood.

    d. Infusion of water without salt, coupled with losses of extracellular fluid volume probably caused avid reabsorption of sodium by the proximal renal tubule. The resulting limitation of distal sodium delivery limited the ability of the distal tubules to excrete potassium and hydrogen ion. This augmented the hyperkalemia and acidosis.

    e. This response would be much worse if the trauma was severe or prolonged. Other factors, such as preexisting renal disease, might make this abnormality much more severe.

Questions

Select the single best answer.

1. Select from the following the fuel store that provides the majority of calories to satisfy the body's acute energy requirements following trauma or injury:
   a. Fat (adipose triglycerides).
   b. Protein (muscle).
   c. Glycogen (liver).
   d. Glycogen (muscle).
   e. None of the above.

2. Gluconeogenesis and catabolism following injury are stimulated by increased levels of each of the following hormones except:
   a. ACTH.
   b. Growth hormone.
   c. Insulin.
   d. Cortisol.
   e. None of the above.

XIV Toxemias of Pregnancy

James A. Merrill

68 Hypertensive Disorders (Toxemia) of Pregnancy

I. **Classification.** Hypertensive disorders, which complicate 2 to 20 percent of pregnancies, are major causes of maternal and perinatal mortality and morbidity. Since some degree of confusion exists in the distinction between preexisting and pregnancy-induced hypertension, a classification is helpful for diagnosis and management: preeclampsia and eclampsia; chronic hypertension with superimposed preeclampsia and eclampsia; chronic hypertension of any etiology; and unclassified.

II. **Definitions**

A. **Preeclampsia** is defined as hypertension associated with edema and proteinuria after 20-week gestation. If this occurs before 20 weeks, one should consider hydatidiform mole or preexisting disease. *Hypertension* is defined as a blood pressure of 140/90 or an increase of 30 or more mm Hg in systolic pressure or a rise of at least 15 mm Hg in diastolic pressure. Edema usually occurs in the upper half of the body. Complaints of facial swelling, tightness of rings, or a weight gain greater than 1 kg in a week may be the first clinical sign(s). *Proteinuria* is defined as 1^+ or 500 mg/24 hr.

B. **Severe preeclampsia.** Preeclampsia is classified as severe if one or more of the following is present:

1. Blood pressure greater than 160/110 on two or more occasions 6 hours apart.
2. Proteinuria of 5 g/24 hr or 4^+.
3. Oliguria—less than 500 ml/24 hr.
4. Visual or cerebral symptoms such as headache, scotoma, blurred vision, or unconsciousness.
5. Epigastric or liver pain or tenderness.
6. Pulmonary edema or cyanosis.
7. Thrombocytopenia or impaired liver function, as reflected in increased serum liver enzymes.

C. **Mild preeclampsia.** Preeclampsia not meeting the definition of severe preeclampsia is classified as mild.

D. **Eclampsia.** Eclampsia is diagnosed in patients with the criteria of preeclampsia who also have convulsions not attributed to identifiable causes such as epilepsy and water intoxication. Eclampsia generally represents progression of preeclampsia without adequate management. However, some have suggested that eclampsia is influenced by preexisting cerebral dysfunction. This is a controversial issue.

E. **Postpartum toxemia** is diagnosed when the first signs or symptoms develop following delivery.

F. **Chronic hypertension with superimposed preeclampsia** is diagnosed in patients with documented chronic hypertension who develop an elevation of greater than 30 mm Hg systolic pressure or 15 mm Hg diastolic pressure above baseline level with the development *or increase* of proteinuria or the development *or increase* of edema in the upper half of the body. The factors to be considered in the documentation of chronic hypertension include: hypertension (140/90) antedating the pregnancy; hypertension recorded on two or more occasions prior to the twentieth week of gestation; hypertension persisting indefinitely following delivery; and preexisting or indefinitely persisting renal disease.

The pathophysiology of preeclampsia/eclampsia superimposed on chronic hypertension is the same as that for the acute pregnancy-induced disorder. It is often difficult to distinguish between the two entities, and diagnostic error may occur in greater than 50 percent of cases. Superimposed preeclampsia/eclampsia occurs more often in multiparous and older patients and is more often recurrent during subsequent pregnancies. Chronic hypertension may be a contraindication to pregnancy. This is especially true in patients with evidence of renal damage and with the severe eye changes secondary to hypertension.

III. **Relevant physiologic changes during normal pregnancy.** A knowledge of the normal physiologic changes during pregnancy is essential to diagnosis, evaluation, and management of patients with hypertensive disorders in pregnancy.

A. **Cardiovascular**

1. The blood volume increases progressively by approximately 30 to 40 percent to term. This primarily represents increased plasma volume with a lesser increase in red cell mass. It results in a so-called dilutional anemia of pregnancy. However, the major cause of anemia during pregnancy is iron deficiency.

2. The interstitial space is also expanded so that both components of the extracellular fluid compartment are significantly increased. Dependent edema may be manifest sometime during pregnancy in 60 to 80 percent of normal gravidas.

3. Cardiac output increases progressively to term.

B. **Hemodynamic**

1. Peripheral resistance is decreased. This is thought to be primarily a progesterone-influenced effect, possibly by modulation of local prostaglandin activity.

2. Blood pressure decreases slightly during the second trimester, with a widening of the pulse pressure, but returns to prior levels during the third trimester as term approaches. This may account for the erroneous diagnosis of preeclampsia near term in patients with chronic hypertension whose mean blood pressure decreases to seemingly normal levels during the second trimester, with return to preexisting hypertensive levels toward term.

3. During pregnancy there are elevated levels of renin, angiotensin II, aldosterone, and antidiuretic hormone. However, pregnancy constitutes a relatively pressor-resistant state. Vascular response to angiotensin II is decreased during normal pregnancy. Response to epinephrine and norepinephrine remains unchanged. This vascular refractoriness is due to altered vascular muscle responsiveness and not to altered blood volume or plasma concentration of angiotensin II.

C. **Renal**

1. Normal pregnancy is accompanied by some degree of hydroureter and hydronephrosis. This is principally a mechanical pressure phenomenon, although hormonal factors may diminish ureteral tone.

2. During normal pregnancy, renal plasma flow (RPF) increases by approximately 50 percent; the glomerular filtration rate (GFR) also increases. This is observed by the second trimester. Thus, blood levels of urea nitrogen and creatinine are decreased, and creatinine

clearance is increased progressively to term. Therefore, levels of blood urea nitrogen (BUN), creatinine, and creatinine clearance, which are normal in the nonpregnant woman, represent diminished renal function in pregnancy. Evaluation of a patient with preeclampsia/eclampsia requires that the physiologic changes of renal function be considered.

IV. **Pathology.** Information concerning the pathology of preeclampsia/eclampsia has been determined, for the most part, from autopsy observation in patients with eclampsia. Therefore, many of the lesions described are not characteristic of mild or even severe preeclampsia.

A. **The primary lesion is arteriolitis** of precapillary arterioles, produced by generalized vasospasm with subsequent fibrin deposition. The gross and microscopic lesions include edema, hemorrhage, and fibrin thrombi in brain, lungs, liver, kidney, and heart. A relatively specific lesion is periportal hepatic necrosis.

B. **The most specific lesion** of preeclampsia has been described in the *kidney* as glomerular capillary endotheliosis. It consists of endothelial cell swelling and subendothelial fibrin deposition. This lesion is considered to be reversible. A much less characteristic renal lesion is arteriolar fibrin thrombi and cortical necrosis.

C. **The decidua** may reveal atherosis and narrowing of sinusoids, and the *placenta* shows evidence of premature aging, with syncytial degeneration, infarction, and premature separation from the uterus.

D. On rare occasions, histologic evidence of *disseminated intravascular coagulation* has been seen in patients with severe preeclampsia or eclampsia. The question of how often this occurs or its relation to the pathogenesis of preeclampsia is controversial at this time.

V. **Pathophysiology of preeclampsia/eclampsia**

A. **Increased vascular reactivity.** The vascular refractoriness to pressors that characterizes normal pregnancy is lost in patients with preeclampsia/eclampsia. This occurs also when preeclampsia/eclampsia is superimposed on chronic hypertension. Further, the change begins prior to the clinical features and occurs despite the fact that plasma concentrations of pressors are decreased in hypertensive pregnancies from the elevated levels seen in normal pregnancy. Vascular reactivity is not altered by the lower plasma concentration of pressors. This differs from the nonpregnant woman, in whom vascular reactivity is inversely proportional to plasma concentration of renin and angiotensin II. Preeclampsia/eclampsia is characterized by increased vascular responsiveness to angiotensin II, compared with both normal pregnancy and the nonpregnant state. This increased vascular reactivity can be demonstrated many weeks before the development of hypertension. There is some evidence of decreased localized vascular prostaglandin activity and evidence that progesterone modulates local prostaglandin synthesis and metabolism. In preeclampsia/eclampsia there is increased sodium concentration in vessel walls, which also may be steroid modulated.

B. **Generalized vasoconstriction** results in hypertension, reduced uteroplacental perfusion (which precedes the hypertension), and reduced perfusion to other vital organs, including kidney and liver. There is unaltered blood flow to the brain, but an increase in vascular resistance and a decrease in oxygen consumption have been reported.

C. **Renal function.** The characteristic lesion of glomerular capillary endotheliosis has been described. There is leakage of protein through glomerular capillaries, resulting in proteinuria. There is reduction in renal plasma flow (RPF) and glomerular filtration rate (GFR); there is also a reduction in renal tubular excretion of uric acid with resultant increase in blood uric acid levels, which correlate with the severity of the disease.

D. Sodium- and water-retention may occur in the normal gravida, but is more pronounced in the patient with preeclampsia/eclampsia. This is not related to sodium intake.

E. Hemodynamics. During preeclamptic pregnancy, cardiac output is unchanged from the increase occurring in normal pregnancy. There is increased capillary permeability and increased peripheral resistance. The hypervolemia of normal pregnancy is not present, but rather, there is reduced plasma volume, which makes these patients more susceptible to acute blood loss. Although there is reduced intravascular volume, the intravascular compartment is not underfilled. Hemoconcentration reflects the severity of the disease. Thus, an increase in hematocrit is indicative of worsening and a decrease in hematocrit may reflect improvement. These hemodynamic changes result in reduced organ perfusion.

F. Placental function. Of great importance is the reduced uteroplacental blood flow and the associated reduced exchange and placental steroidogenesis that occur with preeclampsia/eclampsia. Decreases in uteroplacental blood flow and in placental function are major reasons for the increased incidence of intrauterine fetal growth retardation, small-for-date infants, and perinatal loss. Unfortunately, clinically reliable methods of measuring uteroplacental blood flow are not available.

VI. Etiology. The etiology of preeclampsia/eclampsia is unknown.

A. Factors that predispose to preeclampsia/eclampsia, however, are identifiable. They include:

1. **Social stress**
2. **First pregnancy;** 75 percent of cases of preeclampsia occur in patients who are pregnant for the first time.
3. **Youth**
4. **Poverty**
5. **Preexisting vascular disease,** including hypertension, diabetes, and chronic renal disease.
6. **Multiple gestation**—twins and triplets.
7. **Polyhydramnios**—excess amniotic fluid.
8. **Hydatidiform mole**

  The last three factors are associated with uterine overdistention.

B. Clinical observations. True preeclampsia/eclampsia, as opposed to chronic hypertensive disease or superimposed preeclampsia, is rarely recurrent. There is a familial tendency to preeclampsia. The disease occurs only in the pregnant *human* and can be cured only by delivery.

C. Pathogenesis. These factors and observations support, to varying degrees, the many theories of pathogenesis. Current concepts include:

1. **Placental (trophoblast) excess.**
2. **Immunologic factor(s),** including immunologic deficiency or undesirable response to a challenge with excess trophoblast antigen.
3. **Decreased local prostaglandin synthesis and activity;** this can be of nutritional or hormonal origin. There is experimental evidence that inhibition of prostaglandin synthesis results in increased vascular sensitivity to pressors.
4. **Slow or sudden disseminated intravascular coagulation (DIC).** Although the clinical and pathophysiologic changes can be explained

by such a theory, clinical studies have failed to reveal evidence of DIC in more than a few cases of preeclampsia/eclampsia.

    5. **Other hormonal factors.** Etiologic roles for prolactin, vasopressin, and catecholamines have been suggested without good supporting evidence.

    6. **Other theories.** Early popular theories implicated uterine ischemia as well as sodium retention as the initiating factors. In both instances, these events appear to be the result of the disease and not the cause.

VII. Effect on fetus and mother. The incidence of preeclampsia is 4 to 6 percent in late pregnancies and varies enormously with the nature of the patient population.

    A. **Maternal mortality** still occurs with patients who develop eclampsia. Reported rates vary from 0 to 5 percent. Causes of death include:

      1. **Cerebral hemorrhage**

      2. **Renal failure**

      3. **Pulmonary edema.** In the past, this sometimes has been contributed to by overzealous fluid administration, resulting from the mistaken assumption that the vascular space was underfilled, which it is not.

      4. **Hemorrhage,** associated with disseminated intravascular coagulation.

    B. **Perinatal mortality** rates are reported to vary from 5 to 50 percent. Frequent causes of perinatal loss are prematurity, growth retardation with small-for-dates infants, and intrauterine death resulting from hypoxia. Perinatal mortality is greater when preeclampsia is superimposed on preexisting hypertension.

VIII. Management

    A. **Prevention** is a desirable goal, which may not be possible. It is clear, however, that early recognition and management with modified bed rest can reduce the frequency of severe disease and markedly improve perinatal outcome. Methods of prevention that have been suggested include:

      1. **Elimination of stress**

      2. **Elimination of poverty**

      3. **Adequate nutrition.** Specific suggestions, in addition to adequate protein intake, include supplemental essential fatty acids because of their role in prostaglandin synthesis.

      4. **Early prenatal care**

      5. **Diagnosis and treatment of complicating disease(s)**

      6. **Bed rest or hospitalization** for incipient cases. Carefully controlled studies have demonstrated that this significantly reduces perinatal morbidity and mortality and progression of the severity of the disease. It has not reduced the incidence of preeclampsia.

      7. **Long-term diuretic administration** is contraindicated as a means of prevention. Diuretics further reduce the intravascular space and have been shown to diminish placental perfusion; they are rarely indicated, even in the management of the acute phase of the disease.

      8. **Pregnancy may be contraindicated** in patients with chronic cardiovascular renal disease, depending upon the severity of the disease and the involvement of organs.

    B. **Treatment** is designed to prevent life-threatening maternal consequences and to maximize the opportunity for delivery of a healthy and surviving infant.

1. **Basic principles** of treatment are:
   a. **Observation and bed rest.**
   b. **Evaluate the fetus.** This includes assessment of fetal growth, pulmonary maturity, metabolic well-being, and nervous system reactivity by the several methods available.
   c. **Evaluate the mother.** In addition to monitoring blood pressure and fluid balance, evaluation of renal function and the degree of hemoconcentration are valuable indicators of changing severity of the disease.
   d. **Delivery.** The appropriate time for this will be based on the evaluations of fetus and mother.

2. **Specific measures** in the treatment of hypertensive disorders in pregnancy will include the following:
   a. **Prevent convulsions.** This is most effectively done by the administration of magnesium sulfate, intravenously or intramuscularly.
   b. **Reduce hypertension.** Hydralazine is the agent of choice. It must be used cautiously to avoid too great a reduction in blood pressure.
   c. **Increase uteroplacental and renal blood flows.** Bed rest is the principal modality, and hydralazine has been reported to be beneficial.
   d. **Avoid diuretics.**
   e. **Deliver patient.** This is often by induction of labor and sometimes by cesarean section. The severity of disease must be balanced against fetal maturity and well-being in making a decision concerning the appropriate time.
   f. **Continued observation** and treatment post partum. Failure to maintain vigil into the postpartum period may result in sudden worsening of the disease with adverse maternal consequences.

IX. **Clinical examples of hypertensive disorders**
   A. **Mild preeclampsia**
      1. **Description.** A 16-year-old primigravida received antepartum care from 16 weeks of gestation. Her antepartum course was uncomplicated until the thirty-seventh week of pregnancy, when her blood pressure was recorded as 150/100. She had gained 3 pounds during the previous week and there was 1+ proteinuria. She was admitted to the hospital for observation and treatment.

      Examination revealed the uterine size to be consistent with the gestational age, and fetal heart tones were normal. Deep tendon reflexes were 4⁺. During the first day of observation, blood pressure ranged from 140/90 to 150/100. Amniocentesis revealed a lecithin/sphingomyelin (L/S) ratio of 3.0—an indication of fetal pulmonary maturity.

      Magnesium sulfate, 10 g, was administered intramuscularly and a 5-g maintenance dose was given every 4 hours. At the end of 48 hours, labor was induced by intravenous infusion of oxytocin. After 12 hours of labor, the patient delivered a healthy 6½-pound female infant without difficulty. The maintenance magnesium sulfate was discontinued 24 hours after delivery. The blood pressure fell gradually and stabilized at 120/80 on the second postpartum day. She was normotensive when seen 6 weeks post partum.

      2. **Discussion.** This is an example of mild preeclampsia occurring in a typical patient—a young woman near term during her first preg-

nancy. The diagnosis was established on the basis of a rise in blood pressure, generalized edema (weight gain), and mild proteinuria. Since the blood pressure never exceeded 150/100, hydralazine was not indicated to lower blood pressure. Prophylactic magnesium sulfate was given because of hyperactive reflexes, although the necessity of this might be questioned. There was prompt stabilization with bed rest. There was no evidence of fetal distress from reduced placental function. Since the data indicated that the fetus was mature, a decision was made to terminate the pregnancy by induction of labor before the preeclampsia progressed. This resulted in delivery of a healthy child. There was no residual hypertension.

B. **Severe preeclampsia**

1. **Description.** A 19-year-old primigravida had received no antepartum care. She was unaware of complications until the twenty-ninth week of gestation when she came to the emergency room complaining of headache and swelling of her face and hands. She denied prior hypertension, epigastric pain, scotoma, or blurring of vision. The blood pressure was 160/110 and there was 3+ proteinuria. She was admitted to the hospital for observation and management.

   In the hospital the headaches subsided, although her hypertension persisted. Deep tendon reflexes were 4+. The proteinuria was 2+, blood urea nitrogen (BUN) was 12 g/100 ml, and creatinine 0.8 g/100 ml. Ultrasonography reported fetal size compatible with only 24-week gestation. During the next several days, the patient was treated with intermittent intravenous hydralazine, when the blood pressure exceeded 160/110. Thereafter, her blood pressure was labile but rarely exceeded 150/100. Magnesium sulfate was administered intravenously and intramuscularly for 48 hours. Creatinine clearance was reported to be 86 ml per minute.

   During the next week in the hospital the blood pressure remained labile, the 24-hour urinary protein varied between 2 g and 5 g, the creatinine clearance was 70 ml per minute, and the BUN increased to 16 g/100 ml. A repeat sonogram revealed a diameter of the fetal head consistent with 25-week gestation. L/S ratio of the amniotic fluid was only 0.75. The hematocrit, which had been 32 on admission, rose to 35 at the end of the week. Blood uric acid was 11 mg/100 ml. An attempt at induction of labor was unsuccessful and was accompanied by deceleration of the fetal heart rate. A 1,500-g female infant was delivered by cesarean section and showed the characteristic features of intrauterine growth retardation. The infant developed respiratory distress and had a prolonged but successful neonatal course. The patient's blood pressure returned to normal by the third postpartum day, proteinuria disappeared, and the patient was discharged asymptomatic. At 6 weeks following delivery, she was normotensive.

2. **Discussion.** This is an example of severe preeclampsia occurring acutely in a patient who was not at term. She had received no antepartum care—a common situation in such patients. Evidence of fetal growth retardation was suggested by the discrepancy between gestational age and fetal size. This can best be attributed to reduced uteroplacental perfusion and placental function. Although the BUN and creatinine clearance were reported within the normal range for nonpregnant individuals, each represented an impairment in levels anticipated in normal pregnancy. Blood uric

acid was elevated. Therefore, there was evidence of impaired renal glomerular and tubular function. The rising hematocrit was the result of hemoconcentration, as the preeclampsia worsened. The blood pressure did respond to bed rest, but remained labile and elevated during two weeks of observation.

Even though the L/S ratio of amniotic fluid did not indicate fetal pulmonary maturity, delivery was indicated because of the worsening course of the disease, evidence of renal impairment, and evidence of impaired placental function with fetal growth retardation. Initiation of uterine contractions resulted in deceleration of the fetal heart rate, which is further evidence of placental dysfunction and probably hypoxia. Further, intrauterine existence could not have been expected to improve with time, in the face of a worsening hypertensive disorder. Added gestational age could be gained only at the expense of hypoxia to an already compromised fetus. The infant survived with skillful neonatal care. The hypertension resolved following delivery. This suggests that the hypertensive disorder was probably pregnancy-induced hypertension (preeclampsia) and not preexisting hypertension.

Questions

Select the single best answer.

1. Which of the following clinical features observed in a patient with preeclampsia represents evidence of decreased organ perfusion?
   a. Decrease in hematocrit.
   b. Facial edema.
   c. Prolonged decrease in fetal heart rate with uterine contractions.
   d. Hypertension.
   e. None of the above.
2. Which of the following is not seen in patients with preeclampsia?
   a. Increased vascular responsiveness to angiotensin II.
   b. Increased plasma concentration of angiotensin II.
   c. Decreased glomerular filtration rate.
   d. Decreased intravascular volume.
   e. Decreased uteroplacental blood flow.

Questions, Answers, and Analyses

Questions, Answers, and Analyses

Chapter 1
Physical Consequences of Aging

1. Which of the following is not functionally impaired by age?
    *a. The middle ear (sound conduction).
    b. The inner ear (analysis of mechanical frequency and stimulus transformation).
    c. The peripheral neuron (conduction and acoustic selectivity).
    d. The central auditory pathway (integration and interpretation).
    The sensory cells of the cochlea are affected first, followed by impairment of the inner ear, manifested by disturbed intelligibility of speech. Finally, there is a persistent loss of ganglion cells in the auditory nerve. The middle ear remains unaffected by age.

2. Which of the following is not true concerning skeletal changes related to aging?
    a. The intervertebral disks thin.
    b. The centrum thins.
    *c. The long bones shorten.
    d. Shoulder and chest size decreases.
    Thinning of the intervertebral disks is the major reason for loss of height in the elderly. Osteoporotic vertebral collapse contributes, particularly in women. Shoulder and chest size decreases with age, but the long bones do not undergo significant shortening.

Chapter 2
Electrophysiologic Basis of Cardiac Arrhythmias

1. In the heart the formation of a reentrant circuit generally does not require:
    *a. Prolonged refractory period.
    b. Barrier.
    c. Unidirectional block.
    d. Slow conduction.
    The model of reentry illustrated in Figure 2-5 includes a barrier (hole in the ring), a site of unidirectional block and slow conduction. Prolonged refractoriness is not essential to the model. Therefore, the correct answer is *a*.

2. Which of the following lesions would result in complete heart block?
    a. Fibrosis in the sinus node.
    *b. Interruption of the His bundle.
    c. Interruption of the left bundle branch.
    d. Necrosis in accessory AV pathway.
    Complete heart block involves interruption of impulse transmission from atria to ventricles. While in the normal heart impulses originate in the sinus node, impulse transmission from atria to ventricles requires the AV node and the His bundle but not the SA node. If only the left bundle branch block were interrupted, the impulse could be transmitted through the right bundle branch. An accessory pathway is an extra mode of transmission in subjects with Wolff-Parkinson-White syndrome but the normal conduction system would ensure transmission even if the accessory pathway were necrotic. Therefore, the only correct answer is *b*.

Chapter 3
Myocardial Contraction and Cardiac Performance

1. In a normal heart, increased cardiac output (CO) can be achieved by:
    a. Reduction of ventricular afterload—arterial blood pressure or arterial resistance.
    b. Increase in ventricular preload—ventricular end-diastolic pressure (EDP) or volume (EDV).
    c. Increased myocardial contractility.
    d. Increased heart rate.
    *e. All of the above.

    Cardiac output is the product of stroke volume times heart rate. Reduced resistance to ejection (reduced afterload) allows greater muscle shortening and, therefore, larger stroke volume. An increase in preload causes increased muscle shortening and, therefore, larger stroke volume. Increased contractility causes greater shortening when preload and afterload are unchanged and also a greater stroke volume. When heart rate is increased, more "stroke volume units" are pumped per minute so output is increased. Thus, all are correct.

2. Ventricular preload can be estimated by:
    a. Arterial pressure.
    *b. End-diastolic pressure.
    c. Ventricular contractility.
    d. Ventricular end-systolic pressure and volume.
    e. Velocity of fiber shortening.

    Preload is the tension or length of the muscle in the resting state; that is, during diastole. In the intact heart this is proportional to either the end-diastolic pressure (which is easiest to measure) or the end-diastolic volume. Arterial pressure, contractility, end-systolic pressure and volume, and velocity of fiber shortening all represent systolic events.

Chapter 4
Common Forms of Volume and Pressure Overload

1. The normal response to an acute volume load is:
    a. Elevated diastolic pressure.
    b. Elevated diastolic volume.
    c. Elevated stroke volume.
    d. None of the above.
    *e. All of the above.

    All are correct. An increased volume load must of necessity increase the diastolic volume. The compliance curve (diastolic pressure/volume relationship) is such that this must result in an increased diastolic pressure. Because of this increased preload the stroke volume increases (Frank-Starling law of the heart).

2. Chronic pressure loading produces:
    a. Ventricular hypertrophy.
    b. Elevated end-diastolic pressure.
    *c. Both.
    d. Neither.

    Both are correct. The response of any muscle to increased work is to hypertrophy. This hypertrophied muscle is stiffer (less compliant) and thus requires a higher end-diastolic pressure to fill to the same stroke volume.

Chapter 5
Atherosclerosis

1. Atherosclerosis with the development of coronary disease is often associated with which of the following?
    *a. Cigarette smoking.
    *b. High blood pressure.

*c. Elevated LDL cholesterol levels.
  d. Elevated serum high-density lipoprotein (HDL) levels.
  e. All of the above.
  The first three answers are true. Answer *d* is false. The HDL fraction is low in cholesterol content and appears to be protective by binding cell surface receptors.

2. Select the true statements regarding the relationship between regular aerobic exercise and the progression of coronary atherosclerosis (CAD):
  a. Long-distance runners never experience coronary disease.
  b. Long-distance runners may have coronary disease but do not die from myocardial infarctions.
  *c. Epidemiologic studies demonstrate an inverse relationship between regular exercise and CAD.
  *d. Physical exercise to improve cardiorespiratory function will increase the HDL/LDL ratio.
  e. None of the above.
  Answer *a* is incorrect even though marathon athletes have a significantly lower incidence. There are documented cases with autopsy evidence for myocardial infarction in long distance runners. Answer *c* is true. Answer *d* is true. Also, since HDL protects and LDL is atherogenic, the increased ratio may provide a mechanism for the beneficial effects of exercise.

Chapter 6
Biochemical,
Physiologic, and
Pathologic Consequences
of Ischemia

1. A 45-year-old man was admitted to the hospital with severe chest pain. The cardiac rhythm was regular at 90 beats per minute and blood pressure was 150/80 mm Hg. Bilateral basal rales were audible, and chest x-ray showed cardiomegaly and pulmonary edema. Which of the following statements is false?
  a. History is compatible with acute myocardial ischemia.
  b. Basal rales and pulmonary edema indicate severe left ventricular failure.
  *c. Pulmonary capillary wedge pressure will be low.
  d. Left ventricular end-diastolic pressure will be elevated.
  Myocardial ischemia often results in anginal chest pain and, if prolonged, can severely impair left ventricular function with resultant increase in left ventricular end-diastolic, left atrial, and pulmonary capillary wedge pressures, which may lead to exudation of fluid in the alveoli and pulmonary edema. The correct answer is *c*, since pulmonary capillary pressure will be elevated and not low.

2. Which situations are associated with an increase in myocardial oxygen demand (MVO_2)?
  *a. Tachycardia.
  b. Bradycardia.
  *c. Elevated systolic blood pressure.
  d. Reduced myocardial contractility.
  *e. Cardiomegaly.
  Tachycardia increases MVO_2 because heart rate is an important determinant of MVO_2; and tachycardia also increases myocardial contractility, which further increases MVO_2. Bradycardia has the opposite effect of tachycardia—i.e., reduces MVO_2. Systolic blood pressure is an important determinant of MVO_2 and hence elevation in systolic pressure will result in increased MVO_2. Reduced myocardial contractility will lower MVO_2. Cardiomegaly increases wall tension and hence MVO_2.

**Chapter 7
Clinical Manifestations
of Coronary Artery
Disease**

1. Which of the following is not considered a major isolated manifestation of coronary artery disease?
   a. Sudden death.
   b. Acute myocardial infarction.
   *c. Hypotension.
   d. Angina pectoris.
   e. None of the above.

   Sudden death, acute myocardial infarction, and angina pectoris are all major manifestations of coronary artery disease. Hypotension can accompany acute myocardial infarction or severe anginal attacks but is not an isolated or primary manifestation of coronary disease and therefore is the correct answer.

2. Which of the following is the most common cause of sudden coronary death?
   a. Complete (third-degree) heart block.
   b. Cardiogenic shock.
   *c. Ventricular fibrillation.
   d. Sinus node arrest.
   e. Ruptured left ventricle.

   Certainly third-degree heart block and rupture of the left ventricle (the latter usually after an acute myocardial infarction) can cause sudden death. However these are much less common than ventricular fibrillation (the correct answer, *c*) as a cause of sudden death. Cardiogenic shock is a relatively uncommon cause of sudden death and occurs predominantly in the setting of acute myocardial infarction. Sinus node arrest is also an uncommon cause of sudden death (though not an uncommon cause of syncope or near syncope) because some type of life-sustaining "escape" rhythm usually occurs.

**Chapter 8
Valvular Heart Disease**

1. Which statement does not apply to the left ventricular pressure curve?
   a. At the time of mitral valve closure, the left atrial pressure equals the pressure in the left ventricle.
   b. At the time of aortic valve closure, the aortic pressure equals the pressure in the left ventricle.
   *c. In a normal heart during systole there is always a measurable difference in pressure between the left ventricle and aorta.
   d. In the normal heart during diastole the left atrial pressure never measurably exceeds the pressure in the left ventricle.
   e. All of the above.

   The valves are opened and closed by pressure differences across the valve orifices (see Fig. 8-1). With no stenosis, there is no measurable pressure difference across the AV valves in diastole or across the aortic or pulmonic valves in systole.

2. Which of the following is false concerning the jugular venous pulsation?
   a. The *a* wave is produced by atrial contraction.
   b. The X descent occurs between the *a* and *v* waves and is associated with atrial relaxation.
   c. In pulmonary hypertension, the *a* wave is accentuated.
   d. In pulmonary stenosis, the *a* wave is accentuated.
   *e. In atrial fibrillation, the *a* wave is always present and well seen but diminished in size.

   Answers *a* and *b* are true by definition. The *a* wave is increased in pulmonary hypertension and pulmonary stenosis because the increase in right ventricular pressure causes the right atrium to contract more vigorously in order to fill the right ventricular chamber adequately. The *a* wave is due to atrial contraction; thus, in atrial fibrillation it is absent.

Chapter 9
Intracardiac Shunts

1. Which of the following is not a *direct* determinant of the direction and magnitude of an intracardiac shunt?
   a. Difference in pressure between the communicating chambers.
   *b. The difference in oxygenation of the right- and left-sided blood.
   c. The size of the communications.
   d. The outflow resistance from the communication chambers.

   The major *direct* determinants of the direction and magnitude of an intracardiac shunt are related to the size of the communications and differences in pressures and resistances as described by the hemodynamic application of Ohm's law: Flow = pressure difference/resistance. Oxygenation of blood can also influence the direction and magnitude of shunts, since hypoxemia causes pulmonary vascoconstriction, which can, in turn, cause an increase in pulmonary vascular resistance. However, this is an *indirect* effect. Therefore, statement *b* is the preferred answer.

2. After birth, most intracardiac shunts are initially which of these?
   a. Right-to-left shunts.
   *b. Left-to-right shunts.
   c. Bidirectional shunts.
   d. None of the above.

   After birth, an abnormal communication between the right and left sides of the circulation results in a left-to-right shunt in most instances because the outflow resistance on the right is around one-tenth that on the left and because the pressures on the right are one-fifth that on the left. Both of these contribute to the left-to-right direction of flow. Therefore, *b* is the correct answer.

Chapter 10
Congestive Heart Failure

1. Which statement does not apply to congestive heart failure secondary to mitral valvular stenosis?
   a. The left atrial pressure is elevated.
   b. The pulmonary arterial pressure is elevated.
   *c. The heart failure is due to left ventricular failure.
   d. All of the above.

   In mitral stenosis, congestive heart failure is secondary to obstruction of flow across the stenotic mitral valve. This leads to elevation of left atrial and pulmonary arterial pressures and, eventually, to an increase in right ventricular pressure and volume. Left ventricular function is normal in these patients. Therefore, statement *c* does not apply to heart failure secondary to mitral stenosis.

2. When pulmonary edema results from chronic aortic valvular regurgitation, all but one of the following statements should apply. Select the *one* incorrect statement.
   a. The left atrial pressure, pulmonary arterial pressure, and right atrial pressure are elevated.
   b. Enlarged left ventricular and left atrial volume is present.
   *c. Ventricular hypertrophy is the primary compensatory mechanism of this type of heart failure.
   d. Decreased aortic blood pressure (left ventricular afterload) will increase forward aortic blood flow, decrease regurgitation of blood to the left ventricle, and decrease left ventricular volume.

   In chronic aortic valvular regurgitation, the left ventricle dilates due to increased volume load, with resultant increase in left ventricular, left atrial, pulmonary arterial, and right-sided pressures once heart failure sets in. The primary compensatory mechanism is ventricular dilatation (increased preload), although cardiac muscle does eventually hypertrophy. Afterload reduction reduces the degree of aortic regurgitation and facilitates forward cardiac output, reduces left ventricular dimensions, and is often beneficial in the management of such patients. Therefore, the incorrect statement is *c*.

Chapter 11 Mechanisms of Shock	

Chapter 11
Mechanisms of Shock

1. Which statement or statements do not apply to the pathophysiology of circulatory shock?
   a. Compensatory responses to hypovolemia include tachycardia, tachypnea, vasoconstriction, and reduced urine excretion.
   b. Maldistribution of cardiac output, coagulopathy, and capillary leakage are features of severe sepsis due to gram-negative organisms.
   *c. In the course of shock due to acute myocardial infarction, ventricular filling pressure will always be elevated; therefore intravenous fluids are contraindicated.
   *d. Cardiogenic shock is rarely due to acute myocardial infarction.
   e. All of the above.
   Statement *a* is true. Statement *b* is true. However, these events may also occur in other advanced shock states, including shock associated with pancreatitis and severe trauma. Statement *c* is false. In about 25 percent of patients with a shock state related to myocardial infarction, the left ventricular filling pressure is suboptimal. Cardiac output can be substantially improved in these patients by careful expansion of the extracellular fluid volume with intravenous fluids (saline). Statement *d* is false. Cardiogenic shock is usually due to acute myocardial infarction.

2. Select the correct statement or statements regarding the pathophysiology of shock.
   *a. Circulatory shock and a new cardiac murmur developing after myocardial infarction suggest a ruptured septum or papillary muscle.
   *b. The intraaortic balloon pump (IABP) assists both cardiac output and coronary blood flow.
   *c. In shock due to barbiturate overdose, plasma volume expansion is an important part of the treatment.
   d. In a septic patient with a normal cardiac output we can safely assume that critical tissue perfusion is preserved.
   Statement *a* is true. The most common mechanism of cardiogenic shock is related to loss of functioning myocardium (>40% of left ventricular mass). However, a ruptured interventricular septum or papillary muscle may cause a similar clinical picture which is potentially reversible. Statement *b* is true. Statement *c* is true. This is a distributive type of shock that usually responds to expansion of extracellular fluid volume. Statement *d* is false. A gross maldistribution of cardiac output may occur in septic shock. Hence, blood flow may be diverted from certain tissues despite a normal cardiac output.

Chapter 12
Hormone Action

1. The following statements concerning peptide hormones are all true except:
   a. The peptide hormones include insulin, parathyroid hormone, and all of the pituitary hormones.
   b. Catecholamine hormones are similar to peptide hormones with regard to physicochemical characteristics and receptors.
   *c. Peptide hormones act by binding initially to a cytoplasmic receptor, which is then translocated to a nuclear receptor site.

d. In general, peptide hormones work through activation of a protein kinase, which in turn phosphorylates a protein substrate, yielding an activated enzyme.

Peptide hormones act by binding to a cell membrane receptor where they activate adenylate cyclase, which in turn produces cAMP. It is the cAMP that acts as a second messenger and activates a protein kinase, leading to formation of an activated enzyme. By contrast, steroid hormones bind initially to a cytoplasmic receptor, which is then translocated to a nuclear receptor site.

2. Endocrine disease may result from which of the following disturbances of a hormone-receptor system?

   a. Increased hormone-mediated activity due to autonomous production of the hormone by an adenoma.
   b. Increased hormone-mediated activity due to ectopic production of the hormone by a malignancy.
   c. Decreased hormone-mediated activity due to production of an abnormal, biologically inactive hormone.
   d. Decreased hormone-mediated activity due to a defect or absence of the hormone receptor.
   *e. All of the above mechanisms may result in endocrine disease.

All of the disturbances of the hormone-receptor system described may lead to clinically significant endocrine diseases characterized by either increased or decreased hormone-mediated metabolic activity. Specific examples of the resulting clinical disease for each described defect are provided under section IV, Endocrine disease due to disorders of hormone-receptor systems, in this chapter.

Chapter 13
Anterior and Posterior
Pituitary

1. If the connection between the hypothalamus and pituitary is destroyed, which one of the following will occur?

   *a. Increase in prolactin.
   b. Increase in prolactin and growth hormone secretion.
   c. Increase in the secretion of all anterior pituitary hormones.
   d. Decrease in the secretion of all anterior pituitary hormones.
   e. Increase in ACTH secretion if the adrenals are intact.

Since the predominant effect of hypothalamic hormones appears to be stimulatory to pituitary production of hormones, the vast majority will decrease with destruction of the pituitary stalk. The one exception appears to be prolactin. Since hypothalamic dopamine inhibits prolactin secretion, interference of this pathway leads to excessive prolactin release. Thus, *a* is the correct answer.

2. Which is the incorrect statement regarding control of vasopressin secretion?

   a. A rise in serum osmolality, such as that caused by hypernatremia, stimulates vasopressin release.
   b. Osmotic factors are the principal regulators of vasopressin release under physiologic conditions.
   c. Decreased effective blood volume stimulates vasopressin release.
   d. Severe hypovolemia can override osmoregulation and result in vasopressin release in a patient with hyponatremia.
   *e. Pain and stress inhibit vasopressin release.

Statements *a* through *d* are all true. Pain and stress stimulate vasopressin release; they do not inhibit it as stated in *e*. Therefore, *e* is false, making this the correct response.

Chapter 14
Adrenal-ACTH

1. Adrenal insufficiency is usually associated with:
   a. Hyperglycemia.
   b. Decreased serum sodium and potassium.
   *c. Normal or low aldosterone.
   d. Need for catecholamine replacement therapy.
   e. All of the above.

   Answer *a* is false because hypoglycemia, rather than hyperglycemia, occurs in adrenal insufficiency due to the lack of cortisol effect of carbohydrate metabolism. Answer *b* is false. Serum sodium is often low, but serum potassium is normal in secondary adrenal insufficiency and is characteristically increased in primary adrenal insufficiency. Statement *c* is correct. Aldosterone is low in primary adrenal insufficiency secondary to the destruction of the *zona glomerulosa,* but is usually normal in secondary adrenal insufficiency since ACTH is not the dominant regulator of aldosterone secretion. Answer *d* is false. Catecholamines from the adrenal medulla are not essential for normal health; therefore, replacement therapy is not needed. Answer *e* is incorrect because *a, b,* and *d* are false.

2. Patients with Cushing's disease (hypercortisolism due to excess pituitary ACTH) usually have:
   a. Resistance to the ACTH-suppressive effects of exogenous glucocorticoids.
   b. Loss of the diurnal rhythm of ACTH secretion.
   c. A failure of ACTH secretion to respond to hypoglycemic stress.
   d. Normal plasma aldosterone.
   *e. All of the above.

   A relative resistance to the effect of glucocorticoids on ACTH secretion is characteristic of patients with Cushing's disease and forms the basis of the dexamethasone suppression test. There is little change in plasma ACTH and cortisol levels in patients with Cushing's disease throughout a 24-hour period. Lowering of the blood sugar to less than 40 mg/dl does not increase ACTH secretion in Cushing's disease, whereas in normal people hypoglycemia causes a brisk increase in ACTH. Since ACTH is not the major regulator of aldosterone secretion, the vast majority of patients have normal aldosterone. Answer *e* is the correct one, since *a, b, c,* and *d* all accompany Cushing's disease.

Chapter 15
Thyroid and TSH

1. Hyperthyroidism may be characterized by all of the following except:
   a. Weight loss.
   *b. Cold intolerance.
   c. Tremor.
   d. Tachycardia.

   Hyperthyroidism is characterized by increased metabolic and adrenergic activity and is thus associated with heat intolerance, as well as weight loss, tremor, and tachycardia. Hypothyroidism is characterized by decreased metabolic activity and adrenergic activity and is therefore usually associated with cold intolerance.

2. The most common cause of hypothyroidism is:
   a. Pituitary destruction.
   b. A congenital defect in thyroid hormone synthesis.
   *c. Autoimmune thyroid disease.
   d. Ingestion of thyroid-inhibiting drugs.

   While all of the causes listed may lead to hypothyroidism, autoimmune thyroid disease is the most common cause and may be the end result of Graves' disease, Hashimoto's or chronic lymphocytic thyroiditis, or some other less well-characterized autoimmune phenomenon.

Chapter 16 **Hypertension**	1. Which of the following cause exacerbation of previously well-controlled long-standing essential hypertension? a. Damage to the renal vasculature. b. Increased sodium intake. c. Acceleration of atherosclerosis. d. Superimposed secondary forms of hypertension. *e. All of the above.

Prolonged hypertension, even when mild, causes renal arteriolar sclerosis with resultant hyalinization of glomeruli and tubular atrophy and a decrease in renal function. In some patients, this may become clinically significant and exacerbate their essential hypertension. Excess sodium intake may overwhelm the effect of diuretics on sodium excretion and exacerbate previously well-controlled essential hypertension. Hypertension is a major risk factor for the development of atherosclerosis. Atherosclerosis, in turn, increases peripheral resistance, thereby increasing blood pressure. Renal artery stenosis due to atherosclerosis of a main renal artery is one of the most common types of secondary hypertension, which may worsen hypertension. Other forms of secondary hypertension (pheochromocytoma, estrogen-induced, etc.) may also worsen longstanding and well-controlled hypertension. Answer *e* is correct, since answers *a* through *d* are right.

2. Select the correct statement concerning essential hypertension.
   a. The etiology and pathophysiology are known.
   b. Sodium intake of patients with essential hypertension exceeds that of normotensive patients and is the cause of essential hypertension.
   c. The sympathetic nervous system is overactive in all patients with essential hypertension.
   *d. Total peripheral resistance may be normal or increased.
   e. None of the above are correct.

Answer *a* is wrong. There are likely to be multiple causes of what we call essential hypertension, but they have eluded us despite intensive research for decades. Answer *b* is wrong. Although societies with the highest ingestion of sodium have the highest average blood pressures within any given society studied to date, there has been no correlation between sodium intake and blood pressure, i.e., hypertensive patients have sodium intakes that are similar to normotensive persons. Answer *c* is wrong. A current major hypothesis of the etiology of essential hypertension is an abnormality in the sympathetic neural control of blood pressure. However, evidence of excess sympathetic activity is not demonstrable in many hypertensive patients, and some recent studies have not confirmed the presence of higher catecholamine levels or greater responsiveness to sympathetic inhibition among hypertensive patients. While abnormalities in the sympathetic nervous system undoubtedly exist in many hypertensives and may be causal in some, there is no evidence that all essential hypertension is of neurogenic origin. Answer *d* is a true statement, based upon direct observation.

Chapter 17 **Diabetes Mellitus and** **Glucose Metabolism**	1. Choose the *least* appropriate statement regarding the pathophysiology of non–insulin-dependent mellitus. a. A decrease in the number of insulin receptors contributes to the insulin resistance seen in this type of diabetes.

*b. Patients will have no measurable blood levels of connecting peptide.
c. Patients inherit a susceptibility for this type of diabetes even though the disease may not be manifested until after the age of 40.
d. Basal insulin secretion may be normal or increased, but there is often a subnormal or delayed rise in insulin after meals.
e. This type of diabetes can occur at any age.

Statement *a* is correct. Statement *b* is incorrect. Since these patients generally have elevated insulin release and since C-peptide is secreted concurrently, measurable levels will be present. Thus, *b* is the answer for this question. There is a strong familial tendency for inheriting this condition. Statement *d* is a true observation. Although it is generally found in older individuals, a significant number of young patients are found to have this condition.

2. Which one of the following is *not* a part of the pathophysiology of diabetic ketoacidosis?
a. Lipolysis with liberation of free fatty acids into the circulation.
*b. Oxidation of glucose to ketone bodies in the liver.
c. Osmotic diuresis resulting in sodium and water depletion.
d. Enhanced gluconeogenesis.
e. Failure of glucose to be transported inside cells.

Answer *a* is a correct statement. The correct answer is *b*, since it is not a true statement. Free fatty acids are metabolized to ketone bodies in the liver. Answer *c* is true. Answer *d* is a prominent finding, leading to increased plasma levels of glucose. Answer *e* is a fundamental defect in diabetes.

**Chapter 18
Reproductive
Endocrinology**

1. Infertility in the female due to anovulation may be the result of which of the following?
a. Decreased pituitary production of FSH and LH.
b. Increased pituitary production of prolactin.
c. Decreased ovarian production of estrogens.
d. Increased ovarian production of androgens.
*e. All of the above.

Any event which impairs the midcycle surge in LH and FSH may result in anovulation. Thus, a pituitary defect resulting in decreased production of FSH and LH might result in a blunted or absent midcycle surge of the gonadotropins. An elevated prolactin can inhibit both secretion and action of gonadotropins. Decreased ovarian estrogen production may result in disappearance of the midcycle gonadotropin surge, since its occurrence is triggered by follicular estrogen production. Finally, increased androgen production may directly inhibit FSH secretion by the pituitary. The correct answer is therefore *e*.

2. Androgen deficiency in the male results in a loss of normal secondary sexual characteristics and may be due to all of the following except:
a. Decreased pituitary production of LH.
b. A destructive lesion of the Leydig cells.
*c. Congenital absence of spermatogonia (Sertoli-cell-only syndrome).
d. A defect in testosterone receptors (partial androgen insensitivity).

A defect in pituitary LH production, testicular Leydig cells, or testosterone receptors may all lead to loss of normal secondary male sexual characteristics. However, in the Sertoli-cell-only syndrome, there is a congenital absence of spermatogonia resulting in absence of spermatogenesis and infertility, but the Leydig cells are normal and testosterone production is not impaired so secondary male sexual characteristics are normal, making *c* the answer.

Chapter 19
The Esophagus

1. Dysphagia noted in achalasia patients is probably caused by:
   a. Inability of the esophagus to contract.
   *b. Inability of the LES to relax.
   c. Inflammation within the esophagus.
   d. Cricopharyngeal incoordination.
   The correct answer is *b*, inability of the LES to relax. This causes food to "hang up," which is the mechanism of the dysphagia. Although the esophagus does not contract properly, food can still traverse its length. Without a tight LES area, dysphagia would probably not result. Inflammation can be seen within the esophagus, but does not cause the dysphagia. Cricopharyngeal incoordination is not a part of achalasia.

2. Which of the following can be symptoms of reflux esophagitis?
   a. Waterbrash.
   b. Coughing.
   c. Odynophagia.
   *d. All of the above.
   The correct answer is *d*. All can be symptoms of reflux esophagitis. Waterbrash can be caused by regurgitation, coughing by regurgitation and aspiration, and odynophagia by severe inflammation or ulceration.

Chapter 20
Peptic Ulcer Diseases of the Stomach and Duodenum

1. Regarding *gastric* ulcer formation, which of the following are true?
   *a. Acid secretion from the stomach is normal or below normal.
   b. Acid is not required for ulcer formation.
   *c. Alcohol can increase gastric cell permeability to H^+.
   *d. Stress can play some role in ulcer formation.
   Of the above, answer *b* is the only one that is incorrect. Acid is required for ulcer formation, although in gastric ulcers acid secretion from the stomach is often below normal. Alcohol will increase the permeability of gastric mucosa to H^+. Multiple lines of evidence indicate that stress can contribute to gastric ulcer formation.

2. Major determinant(s) of acid secretion include(s):
   a. Gastrin.
   b. Acetylcholine.
   c. Histamine.
   *d. All the above.
   The correct answer is *d,* all the above. Gastrin, acetylcholine from vagal stimulation, and histamine all interact at a final pathway for H^+ secretion by the parietal cell.

Chapter 21
The Pancreas

1. Regarding gallstones as a cause of pancreatitis, the only connection known with any certainty is that most patients with pancreatitis and gallstones:
   a. Reflux bile into the pancreatic duct.
   *b. Pass gallstones into the duodenum.
   c. Have gallstones impact at the sphincter of Oddi.
   d. Have lymphatic spread of infection from the gallbladder to the pancreas.
   The answer to the above question is *b*, patients pass gallstones into the duodenum. Why this causes pancreatitis is not known. Both answers *a* and *c* may be related, but are not proved causes.

2. The first step in alcohol causing chronic relapsing pancreatitis appears to be:
   a. Protein precipitates within the ductuals.
   b. Acinar cell destruction.

*c. Increased protein in the pancreatic secretions.
d. Stenosis of the main pancreatic duct.
e. Periductular inflammation.

The correct answer is *c*. Increased protein in the pancreatic secretions occurs first and the rest of the events listed above follow this.

Chapter 22
The Gallbladder and
Biliary Tract

1. Which of the following is the most important factor in gallstone formation?
   a. The concentration of cholesterol in the bile.
   b. The concentration of bile salts found in the bile.
   *c. The relative percentage of cholesterol in comparison to the percentage of bile salts and lecithin.
   d. The age of the patient.
   e. None of the above.

   The correct answer is *c*. The relative percentage of cholesterol in comparison to the percentage of bile salts and lecithin is the most important determinant of gallstone formation. Normally, the concentration of cholesterol increases as the gallbladder removes water from the bile, but the concentration of bile salts and lecithin also increases and stones do not result.

2. If a gallstone were impacted in the distal common bile duct as opposed to the cystic duct, which statement is correct?
   a. The patient would be more likely to have fever.
   b. The patient would be more likely to have pain.
   c. The patient would be more likely to have nausea and vomiting.
   *d. The patient would be more likely to be jaundiced.

   The correct answer is *d*. Obstruction of the cystic duct will not lead to jaundice. It can lead to the other things listed, as can obstruction of the common bile duct.

Chapter 23
The Liver

1. An alcoholic man with histologically proved cirrhosis had not drunk alcohol in 2 years. He and his wife had an argument and he went to the local bar, where he drank three beers. Along with the beer, he ate three large packages of potato chips, an unspecified number of pretzels, and two salty ham sandwiches. That evening his pants were tight, and the next day he could not button them. On physical examination he had obvious ascites. Which of the following are true?
   *a. He had been in a fragile balance of hepatic compensation.
   b. The alcohol in the three beers caused his ascites.
   *c. The salt was a bigger load than his kidneys could excrete.
   *d. He should have a diagnostic paracentesis.
   e. The amount of fluid in the three beers caused his ascites.

   Statement *a* is true. He decompensated rapidly, with only a limited external (salt) insult. Statement *b* is false. This is an inadequate amount of alcohol. Statement *c* is true. High sodium intake is the only factor identified in history that could worsen his ascites. Statement *d* is true. One must always consider spontaneous peritonitis in a patient with cirrhosis and ascites. Statement *e* is false. The ascites is due to his liver disease. It could be worsened by sodium retention but not by drinking three beers (inadequate amount of fluid).

2. A 24-year-old nurse who had been receiving treatment for chronic active hepatitis for 4 years was referred by her supervisor, who complained that

recently the patient had begun confusing medications, writing rambling notes, and napping on duty. When seen in the office, the patient was slightly confused and had asterixis. Which statement(s) are true?

*a. The patient probably has hepatic encephalopathy.

b. Her liver chemistries will be more abnormal than before.

c. If a blood ammonia test is obtained and it is normal, the diagnosis of hepatic encephalopathy may be ruled out.

d. Recently she had been on a high-carbohydrate diet to increase her weight, and this was probably the cause of her problem.

*e. A careful search should be made for all possible causes of her problem.

Statement *a* is true. This is a good clinical picture for hepatic encephalopathy. Statement *b* is false. Hepatic encephalopathy can develop without worsening of liver chemistries. Statement *c* is false. Blood ammonia is not elevated in all cases of hepatic encephalopathy. Statement *d* is false. Increased protein ingestion, and not increased carbohydrate ingestion, can precipitate encephalopathy. Statement *e* is true. The diagnosis of hepatic encephalopathy is based in part on the clinical picture and in part on ruling out other possible causes.

Chapter 24 Maldigestion, Malabsorption, and Diarrhea	

1. A 72-year-old woman complained of increasing weakness. She had felt tired for the last few years, but during the last 2 months the weakness had worsened. Recently she had also noted shortness of breath and swelling of her ankles. There was no history of other disease or prior surgery. She was sallow and had signs of congestive heart failure. Initial laboratory studies were essentially normal, except for a marked macrocytic anemia (Hgb of 3.1 g/dl) and a very low serum level of vitamin B_{12}. Which of the following are true?

*a. A maximum stimulated gastric analysis for the presence of acid would probably give abnormal results.

*b. Addition of intrinsic factor to oral radioactive vitamin B_{12} would demonstrate normal B_{12} absorption, if the patient has pernicious anemia.

c. She probably absorbs dietary vitamin B_{12} normally.

d. A biopsy of her gastric mucosa would be normal.

Statement *a* is true. If she has true pernicious anemia secondary to lack of gastric secretion of intrinsic factor, she should have achlorhydria. The test for this is cheap and easy to obtain. Statement *b* is true. Lack of intrinsic factor secretion is the cause of pernicious anemia. Statement *c* is false. She has no intrinsic factor and therefore cannot absorb vitamin B_{12}. Statement *d* is false. If she has pernicious anemia, it would show atrophic gastritis.

2. An alcoholic man is diagnosed as having chronic pancreatitis with pancreatic insufficiency, based on findings of calcification of the pancreas and increased stool fat. Studies for other causes for the steatorrhea were negative. Which of the following are probably true?

*a. The patient secretes inadequate amounts of lipase.

*b. This represented a digestive defect.

c. Pancreatic lipase is a stable enzyme and not influenced by acid.

d. His diarrhea is due to an osmotic load.

Statement *a* is true. Steatorrhea in chronic pancreatitis is due to the loss of over 90 percent of lipase secretion. Statement *b* is true. Lacking lipase, the patient is unable to hydrolyze dietary fat. Statement *c* is false. Lipase is inactivated in an acid pH. Statement *d* is false. Bacterial lipase hydrolyzes the malabsorbed fat in the colon and produces fatty acids, which stimulate colonic secretion, causing the diarrhea.

**Chapter 25
Gastrointestinal
Malignancies**

1. Based on the assumption that the tumor size is the same, symptoms of partial obstruction would occur earliest with carcinoma of the:
   *a. Esophagus.
   b. Stomach.
   c. Right colon.
   d. Sigmoid colon.

   The correct answer is *a*, the esophagus. Dysphagia or difficulty in swallowing is a symptom of partial obstruction. The diameter of the esophagus is smaller than the diameter of the three other structures named; therefore, symptoms of partial obstruction would occur earlier with esophageal carcinoma.

2. The steatorrhea that can be seen with pancreatic carcinoma can be caused by:
   a. Malabsorption secondary to jejunal abnormalities.
   *b. Inadequate micelle formation from obstruction to the flow of bile.
   *c. Inadequate amounts of lipase entering the duodenum from the pancreas.
   d. Malnutrition.
   e. Inadequate mixing of food, pancreatic enzymes, and bile salts.

   Answers *b* and *c* are both correct. Inadequate amounts of lipase and bile may enter the duodenum because of cell destruction (lipase) or obstruction of the main pancreatic duct in the head of the pancreas (bile and lipase).

   The jejunal mucosa is not affected by pancreatic carcinoma. Also, inadequate mixing of food, enzymes, and bile salts has not been identified in carcinoma of the pancreas.

**Chapter 27
Disorders of the
Erythron**

1. Leukopenia and thrombocytopenia would be expected to occur along with anemia if the anemia is due to:
   a. A cytoplasmic maturation defect (e.g., iron deficiency).
   *b. A nuclear maturation defect (e.g., pernicious anemia).
   *c. A stem-cell defect (e.g., aplastic anemia).
   d. Hemolysis (e.g., hereditary spherocytosis).

   Answer *a* is incorrect, since cytoplasmic maturation defects are confined to impaired hemoglobin synthesis. Iron is not a major building block for the development of leukocytes and platelets as it is for erythropoiesis in the production of hemoglobin. Nuclear maturation defects refer to impaired nucleic acid synthesis. All three hemopoietic cell lines are continuously replicating and depend upon intact nucleic acid synthesis for cell division. Therefore, all three cell elements may be reduced in the circulation. Defects at the level of pluripotent or totipotent stem cells, as in aplastic anemia, would preclude differentiation and proliferation of all three hemopoietic cell lines in contrast to defects at the level of the committed stem cells. Therefore, answer *c* is correct. Hemolysis refers to destruction of erythrocytes, not leukocytes or platelets. In an uncomplicated disease such as hereditary spherocytosis, leukopenia and thrombocytopenia would not be expected.

2. Measurement of the arterial oxygen saturation distinguishes:
   a. Polycythemia rubra vera from polycythemia caused by a kidney tumor.
   *b. Polycythemia rubra vera from polycythemia caused by chronic lung disease.
   c. Polycythemia rubra vera from relative polycythemia.
   d. Polycythemia due to right-to-left intracardiac shunt from polycythemia caused by emphysema.

   Polycythemia rubra vera is an autonomous proliferation of the erythroid marrow, while kidney tumors may be the site of ectopic erythropoietin secretion. In neither case would altered arterial oxygen saturation be expected. Chronic lung disease impairs oxygen delivery to the pulmonary circulation and hence reduces arterial oxygen saturation. Therefore, answer *b* is correct. In relative polycythemia the red-cell volume is normal but the plasma volume is reduced. This state does not alter blood oxygenation and would not be distinguished from polycythemia rubra vera by an arterial oxygen saturation determination. Like emphysema, a right-to-left shunt would reduce maximal reoxygenation of systemic venous blood and desaturate arterial blood hemoglobin.

Chapter 28
Neutrophil Disorders

1. A patient has developed agranulocytosis from a drug and there is loss of all granulocyte precursor cells in the bone marrow. After the drug is stopped the blood neutrophil count would be expected to increase at the earliest after:
   a. 6 hours.
   b. 24 hours.
   *c. 7–9 days.
   d. 3 weeks.
   The absence of granulocyte precursors in the bone marrow indicates that recovery of the blood neutrophil count is not possible before new granulocytes can differentiate, proliferate, and mature. The latter events take place over a period of 6 to 7 days. Therefore, *c* is the correct answer.

2. Acute leukemia predisposes to infection because it is accompanied by:
   a. A lack of opsonins (immunoglobulins and complement).
   b. A lack of NADPH-dependent oxidase in neutrophils.
   *c. Decreased neutrophil production.
   d. Increased neutrophil destruction.
   Acute leukemia is generally not associated with lack of immunoglobulins or defects in the complement system. Neutrophil NADPH-dependent oxidase is normal in acute leukemia unless the patient has this genetic abnormality independently. The acute leukemia clone impairs the development of normal neutrophil precursors into neutrophils through inhibition of normal stem cell differentiation and nutritional and mechanical crowding of the marrow microenvironment. Therefore, *c* is correct. Neutrophil destruction is not known to be enhanced in acute leukemia unless complicated by severe bacterial infection.

Chapter 29
Platelets

Match each item in A with an appropriate one from B. You may use items in B more than once or not at all.

A	B
(1) Thrombocytopenia of B_{12} or folate deficiency	(a) Inhibits platelet aggregation
(2) Immune thrombocytopenia	(b) Normal number of megakaryocytes
(3) Petechial bleeding in a patient with normal platelet count	(c) Increased marrow megakaryocytes
(4) Prostacyclin	(d) Promotes vasoconstriction
(5) Hypersplenic thrombocytopenia	(e) Platelet dysfunction
(6) Thromboxane A_2	(f) Absent megakaryocytes

(1) = (b) Thrombocytopenia of B_{12} or folate deficiency is the result of ineffective thrombopoiesis so that the megakaryocytes are normal, but are unable to mature.

(2) = (c) Rapid destruction of platelets leads to reduction in the total platelet mass. This stimulates thrombopoietin secretion, which in turn causes megakaryocytic hyperplasia.

(3) = (e) Petechial bleeding generally does not occur with platelet counts over $50 \times 10^3/mm^3$ unless the platelets are defective.

(4) = (a) Prostacyclin, a prostaglandin, is a strong inhibitor of platelet aggregation, unlike thromboxane A_2, which promotes platelet aggregation.

(5) = (b) In hypersplenism, a greater than normal proportion of circulating platelets is pooled in the enlarged spleen, but the total platelet mass is normal. Thrombopoiesis is therefore not stimulated despite thrombocytopenia.

(6) = (d) Thromboxane A_2 is a potent vasoconstrictor as well as a platelet aggregant.

Chapter 30
Disorders of Blood
Coagulation

1. An individual is discovered who lacks the enzyme necessary to carboxylate the glutamic acid groups on the vitamin K–dependent clotting factors. When this person begins to bleed, effective treatment might include:
   a. Infusion of phospholipid intravenously.
   b. Administration of large doses of vitamin K.
   *c. Infusion of plasma from a normal donor.
   d. Administration of aspirin to prevent platelet aggregation, followed by intravenous calcium.

   Options *a*, *b*, and *d* would not correct the defect in the production of the vitamin K–dependent clotting factors because none of these would provide either the enzyme or functioning clotting factors. The only possible solution would be the administration of normal clotting factors found in normal plasma, *c*.

2. Warfarin works as an anticoagulant because it:
   a. Increases the rate of destruction of prothrombin, factors VIII, IX, and X in the liver and thus lowers their circulating levels.
   b. Blocks platelet participation in the formation of a hemostatic plug.
   c. Blocks the synthesis of all amino acid peptides that make up the clotting factors.
   *d. Results in the formation of clotting factors, which lack dicarboxylglutamic acid groups.

   Warfarin affects the production but not the destruction of vitamin K–dependent clotting factors. Warfarin does not affect platelet function. Warfarin does not affect peptide synthesis. Answer *d* is true. The specific action of warfarin is to interfere with vitamin K–dependent addition of the extra carboxyl group to certain clotting factors (V, VII, IX, X).

Chapter 31
Immediate
Hypersensitivity Disease

1. Which of the following is/are true?
   a. Anaphylactic reactions to penicillin will not occur in patients without prior hay fever, asthma, or other allergic disease.
   b. Most cases of chronic urticaria are caused by food or drug allergy.
   c. IgE is required for histamine release.
   *d. Immediate hypersensitivity reactions may be nonimmunologic.

   Anaphylactic drug reactions are not confined to persons with other allergies. Most cases of chronic urticaria are idiopathic. An allergic cause is found only occasionally. Histamine release and immediate hypersensitivity can involve IgE, IgG plus complement, or nonimmunologic mechanisms.

2. Death from anaphylaxis usually is *not* caused by:
   a. Shock.
   b. Angioedema of the upper airway.
   c. Asthma.
   *d. Gastrointestinal bleeding.

   Shock, upper airway angioedema, asthma, or some combination is the usual cause of death from anaphylaxis. Gastrointestinal bleeding is a rare manifestation.

Chapter 32
Allergic Respiratory
Diseases

1. Which of the following is/are seen only in severe asthma?
   a. Arterial hypoxemia.
   *b. Arterial hypercapnea.
   *c. Elevated right heart pressures.
   *d. Lack of response to bronchodilators.

   Arterial hypoxemia typically occurs even in mild asthma. The other occurrences reflect the profoundly disordered physiology of severe asthma.

2. The pathophysiology of bronchial asthma does not necessarily include:
   a. Mediator release.
   b. Respiratory eosinophilia.
   c. Bronchial smooth muscle constriction.
   *d. IgE.

   Bronchial asthma may or may not involve allergy and IgE. Regardless, the mechanism does involve mediator release, as evidenced by the respiratory eosinophilia that is a consequence of the mediator ECF-A. Demonstration of the reversible airway obstruction that is due to smooth muscle constriction is one of the diagnostic criteria for asthma.

Chapter 33
Immunologically
Mediated Disease

1. Which microorganism has been implicated in the etiology of polyarteritis nodosa (by demonstration in circulation and in the immune deposits in involved arteries)?
   a. *Plasmodium falciparum.*
   b. *Streptococcus pneumoniae.*
   *c. Hepatitis B.
   d. *Cryptococcus neoformans.*
   e. Varicella-zoster virus.

   Plasma hepatitis B surface antigen (HBsAg) or antibody to HBsAg (anti HBs) has been identified in 35 to 70 percent of persons with polyarteritis nodosa. Several authors have also identified HBsAg in involved vessel walls, along with antibody and complement components, as part of an immune complex vasculitis.

   Older children with polyarteritis nodosa have frequently been noted to have elevated titers of antistreptolysin O (ASO), implicating hemolytic streptococci in the etiology of the disease. The pneumococcus has not been implicated in polyarteritis nodosa, nor has malaria, *Cryptococcus,* or varicella-zoster virus.

2. Which one of the following statements is *incorrect*?
   *a. If immune complexes are present in the circulation, symptoms of immune complex disease will invariably exist.

b. Immune complexes may occur in tissues and be associated with disease in patients who fail to show immune complexes in circulation.

c. Circulating immune complexes primarily cause disease by involvement of blood vessels (vasculitis or glomerulitis).

d. The antigen present in immune complexes may be exogenous (such as bacterial antigens) or endogenous (such as DNA).

e. Certain autoimmune diseases are mediated by immune complexes; however, this mechanism does not explain all autoimmune disorders or all disorders with an immunologic component.

Circulating immune complexes may be found in a variety of nonimmunologic diseases (i.e., cancer) and in some apparently normal individuals. Therefore, statement *a* is incorrect. Statement *b* is correct, presumably because immune complexes may be rapidly removed from the circulation or may be formed in situ. Statement *c* is correct, although other organs and tissues may be injured by immune complexes occasionally. Statement *d* is correct (see Table 33-1). Statement *e* is correct; type II and type IV reactions may also be involved in autoimmune disorders.

Chapter 34
Inflammatory Rheumatic
Diseases (Noninfectious):
Mediation by
Immunologic
Mechanisms

1. The direct cause of destruction of bone and cartilage in rheumatoid arthritis is most likely to be:
   a. Lymphokines.
   b. The complement system.
   c. A type III immunologic reaction.
   *d. Proteolytic enzymes.
   e. An infectious agent.

   Destruction of bone and cartilage requires degradation of structural macromolecules, such as collagen. Of the possible answers listed, only proteolytic enzymes, such as collagenase, would have this ability.

2. Autoantibody formation to various cellular constituents is common in the inflammatory rheumatic disease. The presence of such autoantibodies:
   a. Establishes a role for autoimmunity in the etiology of these diseases.
   b. Excludes an infectious etiology for these diseases.
   c. Is most likely to be a result of the widespread distribution of the lesions in these diseases in the connective tissues of the body.
   *d. May be a result of defective suppressor function of T lymphocytes.
   e. Excludes the possibility that these diseases may result from an ingested chemical.

   The immunological hyperactivity and extensive autoantibody formation that occurs in some of these diseases is believed to be related, at least in part, to defective suppressor function of T lymphocytes. The correct answer, therefore, is *d*. The presence of autoantibodies does not establish a pathogenic role for them, since in some instances they are clearly the result of, rather than the cause of, tissue injury. Rheumatic fever is caused by an infection and yet is associated with autoantibody formation. There are no experimental data to support the idea that widely distributed chronic inflammation in the connective tissues of the body could entirely account for the autoantibody formation seen in these diseases. A form of lupus erythematosus is caused by the ingestion of certain drugs.

Chapter 35
Degenerative Joint
Diseases and Gout

1. All of the following are features of osteoarthritis except:
   a. Subchondral bone sclerosis.
   b. Subchondral bone cysts.
   *c. Marginal erosions.

d. Osteophyte formation.

e. Joint space narrowing.

Marginal erosions of bone are characteristic of rheumatoid arthritis. The synovial membrane is converted into an inflammatory mass, and destructive changes of bone first occur where the synovial membrane attaches to bone at the joint margins. The four other possible answers are all characteristic features of osteoarthritis.

2. The hyperuricemia in gouty patients may be related to any of the following except:

a. An enzymatic defect leading to overproduction of purines.

b. Increased turnover of nucleic acid purines.

c. Administration of a thiazide diuretic.

d. Chronic lead poisoning.

*e. Increased absorption of purines from a normal diet.

Hyperuricemia in gout is caused by overproduction of uric acid and underexcretion of uric acid by the kidney. Enzymatic defects leading to overproduction of uric acid have been demonstrated in a small minority of gouty patients. The cellular proliferation that occurs in certain diseases such as polycythemia vera leads to increased formation and subsequent degradation of nucleoproteins. Hyperuricemia and gout are well-known associations. Thiazide diuretics cause urate retention. Patients with gout have frequently had their initial attack after they were started on a diuretic drug for hypertension. The kidney lesion of chronic lead poisoning frequently leads to hyperuricemia and gout. Increased dietary purine intake is a possible cause of hyperuricemia. However, placing gouty patients on a purine-free diet lowers their serum urate levels only slightly. They remain hyperuricemic and continue to have gouty attacks.

Increased absorption of purines from a normal diet is not considered to be a factor in the hyperuricemia of gout. The correct response is *e*.

Chapter 36
Immunodeficiency

1. Match the following infections (A) with the immune defect (B).

A	B
(1) Disseminated *Neisseria* infections	(a) Defective humoral immunity
(2) Fatal pneumococcal bacteremia	(b) Defective cellular immunity
(3) Recurrent pneumococcal pneumonia	(c) Splenectomy
(4) Recurrent staphylococcal pneumonia	(d) Absence of C6
(5) Chronic *Candida* infections	(e) Defective granulocyte function

(1) = (d) Disseminated *Neisseria* infections have been reported in patients with deficiencies of C6, C7, and C8. Complement-mediated lysis of *Neisseria gonorrhoeae* and *Neisseria meningitidis* (with involvement of the late components of the complement pathway) is probably necessary, in part, for the efficient destruction of these microorganisms.

(2) = (c) Early in life the spleen serves as a source of antibody formation, complement components, and fixed phagocytic cells. Splenectomy (or functional splenectomy as seen in sickle cell disease) impairs handling of particulate antigens and especially the pneumococcus. This is especially true where splenectomy is done in the face of other immune deficiency mechanisms, such as in Hodgkin's disease.

(3) = (a) Pneumococci are among the pyogenic-encapsulated microorganisms that resist phagocytosis unless opsonized by antibodies. For this reason, patients with Bruton's agammaglobulinemia or acquired defects of humoral immunity have recurrent pneumococcal pneumonias.

(4) = (e) Staphylococci are handled primarily by phagocytosis and intracellular lysis. Antibodies facilitate phagocytosis but are not essential for the process. Once ingested, degradation of staphylococci requires oxygen radicals and halides. Catalase-positive microorganisms such as pathogenic staphylococci are significant problems in patients whose granulocytes are deficient in the generation of hydrogen peroxide and other free oxygen radicals (e.g., chronic granulomatous disease).

(5) = (b) Chronic mucocutaneous candidiasis is seen in patients with specific defects of cellular immunity to *Candida* or in persons with broader defects of cellular immunity. Occasionally patients with chronic mucocutaneous candidiasis have systemic dissemination of *Candida* or other fungal infections. Patients with combined humoral and cellular immunity often have overwhelming bacterial, viral, fungal, and protozoal infections.

2. Identify the *incorrect* statement.
   a. Antibody production to thymus-dependent antigens requires that B lymphocytes interact with helper T cells.
  *b. K cells need to be primed (sensitized) to the specific target cell antigen before they can interact with the antibody for the particular cell target.
   c. T cells release lymphokines on exposure to the specific antigen to which they are sensitized.
   d. The complement system can be activated by mechanisms that do not involve antigen-antibody complexes.
   e. Suppressor cells for T and B lymphocytes have been identified in many primary and secondary immune deficiency disorders.

   Statement *b* is incorrect because K cells are not primed to specific antigens. (Do not confuse these cells with killer T lymphocytes which *do* require priming.) K cells, by virtue of their high-affinity receptor for the Fc portion of IgG (and perhaps other immunoglobulin isotypes), can bind to IgG fixed on cells or tissues. The other statements are all correct.

**Chapter 37
Inflammation**

1. In the microvasculature, pavementing and emigration of neutrophilic leukocytes during inflammation occur basically along:
   a. Arterioles.
   b. Capillaries.
  *c. Venules.
   d. Closed capillary channels.
   e. None of the above.

   Answers *a* and *b* are wrong. The pavementing, an important early process in inflammation, is most intense on the venular side of the capillary bed. Answer *c* is correct. Direct histologic observation discloses the pavementing in this area. Answer *d* is incorrect for the above-mentioned reasons.

2. The principal perivascular phenomenon associated with acute inflammation is:
   a. Migration of eosinophils.
   b. Activation of Hageman factor.
   c. Increased size of fenestrae in capillaries.
  *d. Accumulation of neutrophils.
   e. None of the above.

Answer *a* is false. Migration of eosinophils usually plays a rather minor part in the process of inflammation. Answer *b* is false. Activation of Hageman factor appears to be basically an intravascular phenomenon. Answer *c* is incorrect. Fenestration of capillaries is a vascular, not perivascular, event. Answer *d* is correct. The outstanding feature of acute inflammation is a tremendous accumulation of neutrophils.

Chapter 38
Hyperthermia and Fever

1. In fever, the set point circuitry:
    a. Is unresponsive to stimuli.
    b. Is activated directly by endotoxin.
    c. Is damaged and therefore unresponsive to stimuli.
   *d. Remains intact but behaves in such a way that body temperature is raised.
    e. Causes a decreased secretion of sodium in sweat.

   Answer *a* is incorrect because, in fever, the set point specifically changes to a *new* point, and does so in response to endogenous pyrogen. Answer *b* is incorrect because the effect of endotoxin is mediated by endogenous pyrogen, which is elaborated from cells, especially leukocytes, in response to endotoxin. Thus, the effect of endotoxin is *indirect*. Answer *c* is incorrect because in fever, as distinguished from malignant hyperpyrexia, the set point is intact but adjusted to a higher level. Answer *d* is correct because a change in the set point moves the dynamic equilibrium of the body in a way that favors a net gain of heat in the body. Answer *e* is incorrect. Following acclimatization to a hot environment, sweat contains less sodium. The mechanism for accomplishing this involves aldosterone but does not appear to be related to changes in the set point.

2. Which one of the following is true?
    a. Only fever associated with exogenous pyrogens may be called hyperthermia.
    b. All hyperthermia is fever.
   *c. Fever is a special kind of hyperthermia that arises from release of endogenous pyrogens.
    d. Hyperthermia is a special aspect of fever in which endogenous pyrogen acts upon bacteria to produce exogenous pyrogen.
    e. None of the above is true.

   Answer *a* is incorrect because fever may be regarded as a form of hyperthermia (of a special kind), but there are other forms of hyperthermia that cannot be considered to be fever—for example, the elevation of body temperature associated with vigorous muscular activity. Answer *b* cannot be true, based upon the same reasons as given for *a*. However, the converse is true: all fever must be hyperthermia. Answer *c* is true because this statement is basically a definition of fever. Answer *d* cannot be true. There is no evidence that endogenous pyrogens act upon bacteria, or that an *exogenous* pyrogen is derived from any such action. The *reverse* is true; that is, exogenous pyrogens (i.e., endotoxin) may be derived from bacteria (or more correctly, are part of the structure of bacteria) and these act upon host cells which then release endogenous pyrogen.

Chapter 39
Disorders of Sodium and
Water Metabolism

1. Sodium depletion is virtually always associated with:
    a. Hyponatremia.
    b. Contraction of the intracellular space.
   *c. Contraction of the extracellular space.

d. Expansion of the extracellular space.

e. None of the above.

Answer *a* is incorrect since a low concentration of sodium (hyponatremia) can be associated with a normal or increased, as well as decreased, total body sodium. Sodium is lost exclusively from the extracellular space. Therefore, the size of the intracellular compartment would change only if the osmolality of body fluids also changed. The sodium content is the major determinant of the volume of the extracellular space. Therefore, *c* is the correct answer. Sodium excess, not sodium depletion, would be associated with expansion of the extracellular space. Answer *e* is incorrect because *c* is correct.

2. What would be the effect of intravenous infusion of 1 liter of isotonic saline in an anuric patient?

   a. Expansion of the interstitial space by about 1 liter.

   b. Expansion of the intracellular space by about 670 cc.

   c. Expansion of the blood volume by about 670 cc.

   *d. Essentially no effect on the size of the intracellular space.

   e. None of the above.

The infusion of 1 liter of isotonic saline would expand the extracellular space by 1 liter. Consequently, the plasma volume would increase by about a quarter of a liter, or 250 ml, and the interstitial compartment would expand by 750 ml. Since no change in osmolality would be expected, intracellular water would not shift. Hence, statement *d* is correct; the others are wrong.

Chapter 40
Potassium Homeostasis

1. Renal potassium secretion is enhanced by all except which *one* of the following?

   a. An increase in intracellular potassium content.

   b. An increased urine flow rate.

   c. Increased concentrations of aldosterone.

   *d. A decrease in distal tubular sodium reabsorption.

   e. An increase in potassium intake.

   Answers *a*, *b*, *c*, and *e* are true. Answer *d* is incorrect. A decrease in distal tubular sodium reabsorption would decrease distal tubular potassium secretion, whereas an increase in sodium reabsorption would increase the cell-to-lumen electrochemical gradient and enhance potassium secretion.

2. Hypokalemia can be associated with all except which *one* of the following?

   a. Cardiac arrhythmias.

   *b. Impairment of urinary diluting ability.

   c. Neuromuscular paralysis.

   d. Impaired glucose tolerance.

   e. Polyuria.

   Answers *a*, *c*, *d*, and *e* are true. Answer *b* is incorrect because urine diluting capacity is usually maintained; however, hypokalemia is associated with a decrease in ability to concentrate the urine.

Chapter 41
Hydrogen Ion
Homeostasis: Metabolic
Acidosis and Alkalosis

1. The following statements are related to the role of the kidney in H^+ homeostasis. Which *one* of the following is false?

   a. The amount of free H^+ in urine is less than 1.0 mEq/L.

   b. The bulk of H^+ secretion is involved in bicarbonate reclamation.

   *c. The kidney is capable of correcting acidemia rapidly (within hours).

   d. The kidney is the major organ for the excretion of nonvolatile acids.

   e. At a pH of 6.0, the amount of HCO_3^- in urine is negligible.

Statement *a* is true. The amount of free hydrogen ion in the urine is quite small; if the urine were acidified to a pH of 4.5, the concentration of hydrogen ion in the urine would be 0.03 mEq/L. Statement *b* is true because of the large amount of bicarbonate that is filtered and reclaimed daily.

While the kidney is the major organ for the excretion of metabolic nonvolatile acids, it responds only *slowly* to changes in acid-base homeostasis and maximum response does not occur until 2 to 5 days after the initiation of the disturbance. Hence, statement *c* is false, and statement *d* is true.

At a pH of 6.0, the amount of bicarbonate present in urine is quite small; this can usually be neglected in any calculation of urinary bicarbonate excretion. Hence, statement *e* is true.

2. A 24-year-old man is brought to the hospital in a confused state with a rapid respiratory rate. Examination demonstrates blindness and hyperemic optic disks. The initial laboratory studies:

Venous blood	Arterial blood
Na^+ 136 mEq/L	pH 6.98
K^+ 5.5 mEq/L	$PaCO_2$ 30 mm Hg
Cl^- 100 mEq/L	
HCO_3^- 4 mEq/L	

BUN is 25 mg/100 ml; Cr, 1.2 mg/100 ml. Which of the following statements is false?

a. The patient has metabolic acidosis.
*b. The respiratory response is appropriate.
c. There is an increased utilization of HCO_3^-.
d. An acid urine pH is anticipated.
e. This represents a life-threatening problem.

The patient has metabolic acidosis because of the ingestion of methyl alcohol. Methyl alcohol is metabolized to formic acid, which causes the utilization of bicarbonate. Clinical signs of methyl alcohol ingestion include the ocular findings and the demonstration that the patient has an increase in the calculated anion gap. The usual method of calculating the anion gap (AG) is to take the sodium concentration and subtract from this the concentrations of bicarbonate plus chloride:

$$AG = Na^+ - (Cl^- + HCO_3^-)$$

The normal unmeasured anion gap is approximately 12 ± 4 mEq/L. Patients with a metabolic acidosis due to the accumulation of nonvolatile acids, other than hydrochloric acid, have an increase in anion gap. Thus, in ketoacidosis, lactic acidosis, uremic acidosis, and certain organic acid intoxications, metabolic acidosis is associated with an increase in anion gap. The only incorrect answer is statement *b;* in this patient, a $PaCO_2$ of 12 to 16 would be anticipated.

$$PaCO_2 = 1.5 (HCO_3^-) + 8$$
$$14 = 1.5 (4) + 8$$

Thus, this patient not only has metabolic acidosis, but also has a concurrent respiratory acidosis because of impaired ventilation. In the presence of both metabolic and respiratory acidosis, an acid urine would be anticipated. A blood pH of 6.98 represents a life-threatening problem. Hence statement *e* is true, as are *a*, *c*, and *d*.

Chapter 42
Calcium, Phosphate, and
Vitamin D

1. The following statements regarding calcium are true except:
   a. Approximately 50 percent of the total serum calcium exists in the ionized form.
   b. The extracellular concentration of calcium depends upon a balance between Ca absorption from the gut, the deposition in bone, and excretion through the kidney and gut.
   c. $1,25(OH)_2D_3$ augments calcium absorption from the gut.
   *d. In parathyroidectomized animals hypocalcemia will increase $1,25(OH)_2D_3$ production.
   e. Acute hypercalcemia may induce acute renal failure.
   Statement *d* is incorrect. Hypocalcemia does not directly stimulate $1,25(OH)_2D_3$ production, but does so only by increasing parathyroid hormone levels. Statements *a, b, c,* and *e* are true.

2. The following statements regarding phosphorus and vitamin D are true except:
   a. Hypophosphatemia is a stimulus for increased $1,25(OH)_2D_3$ production.
   b. Parathyroid hormone increases phosphorous excretion by the kidney.
   *c. More than 50 percent of the plasma phosphorus is protein bound.
   d. Vitamin D is produced in the skin upon exposure to sunlight.
   e. The production of $1,25(OH)_2D_3$ occurs in the renal cortex.
   Answer *c* is incorrect. Since only 12 percent of plasma phosphate is protein bound, the remainder exists as a free ion in association with various cations. Statements *a, b, d,* and *e* are true.

Chapter 43
Glomerulonephritis and
the Acute Nephritic
Syndrome

1. Mediators of glomerular injury include:
   a. Platelets.
   b. Monocytcs and polymorphonuclear leukocytes.
   c. Serotonin and histamine.
   d. Fibrin.
   *e. All of the above.
   In immune-complex glomerular nephritis, the aggregation and consumption of platelets result in the release of serotonin and histamine. These factors can increase capillary permeability and, thus, increase the deposition of immune complexes. Monocytes and polymorphonuclear leukocytes have been implicated by cell-depletion studies, and platelets and fibrin are commonly involved in crescentic glomerular nephritis. Therefore, the correct answer is *e* (all of the above).

2. Which of the following conditions is *not* typically associated with the acute nephritic syndrome?
   a. Red blood cell casts in the urine sediment.
   b. Hypertension.
   *c. Polyuria due to a defect in renal concentrating ability.
   d. Glomerular injury from immune complexes.
   e. Edema.
   The acute nephritic syndrome is characterized by hypertension, edema, and hematuria, frequently with red blood cell casts. Acute glomerulonephritis frequently has an immune-complex pathogenesis. Although a mild concentrating defect may occur in severe cases, oliguria, not polyuria, is characteristically seen. Therefore, *c* is the incorrect statement.

Chapter 44
The Nephrotic Syndrome

1. Which of the following statements is/are true?
   *a. Proteinuria of greater than 4 g per day can result from infection.
   b. In adults, the nephrotic syndrome is easily treated even if the cause is unknown.

c. Most cases of nephrotic syndrome in adults are associated with a systemic disease.

*d. Membranoproliferative glomerulonephritis has a worse prognosis than membranous glomerulopathy.

*e. If a patient has a serum albumin of 4 g/dl and excretes 4 g of protein per 24 hours, he may not have edema.

Answer *a* is true. Proteinuria of this amount is characteristic of the nephrotic syndrome, which can be caused by many bacterial, protozoan, helminthic, and viral infections. Answer *b* is false. If the cause is known, and can be treated, the nephrotic syndrome may disappear with that treatment. This is uncommon, however. In most adults, only symptomatic treatment can be offered. Answer *c* is false. Only 20 percent of adults with nephrotic syndrome have renal disease that is secondary to an underlying systemic condition. Answer *d* is true. Membranoproliferative glomerulonephritis proceeds to end-stage renal disease in 1 to 5 years, while only some of the patients with membranous disease lose all renal function. In addition, membranous nephropathy usually takes 5 to 15 years to effect the loss of all renal function. Answer *e* is true. Since this patient has an albumin level that is normal (even with nephrotic range proteinuria), the colloid osmotic pressure of the blood is normal and Starling's forces should be normal.

2. Which of the following statements is false?

a. Selective proteinuria is more characteristic of lipoid nephrosis than of focal sclerosis.

b. Gamma globulin loss may increase susceptibility to infection in nephrotic patients.

c. Nephrotic patients have an increased tendency to form blood clots.

d. The prognosis of minimal change disease is much better than that of focal sclerosis.

*e. None of the above.

Answer *a* is true. Selective proteinuria (albumin and low molecular weight proteins) is seen with most patients in minimal change (lipoid nephrosis), while nonselective proteinuria (high and low molecular weight proteins) should alert the physician to another disease. Answer *b* is true. Gamma globulins are antibodies. They may be lost in significant quantities, leading to increased susceptibility to infections. Answer *c* is true. The hypercoagulability of patients with nephrotic syndrome may be manifested by both arterial and venous thrombosis. Answer *d* is true. Minimal change disease almost never proceeds to end-stage renal disease; focal sclerosis usually does. Thus, the correct answer is *e*.

Chapter 45
Acute Renal Failure

1. The rate of sodium excretion from a patient with oliguric parenchymal acute renal failure is commonly:

a. 0.1 percent of filtered sodium.

b. 0.5 percent of filtered sodium.

c. 1.0 percent of filtered sodium.

*d. More than 2.0 percent of filtered sodium.

e. None of the above.

Answer *d* is the correct answer. Normally more than 99 percent of the sodium that is filtered at the glomerulus is reabsorbed by the renal tubules. Most patients with acute renal failure have significant tubular damage; this is usually associated with a decrease in tubular reabsorption. Thus, in most patients, more than 2 percent of filtered sodium is excreted, and in certain instances 10 percent of filtered sodium is excreted.

2. If a patient is intermittently anuric, i.e., variable urine volumes with intervals of zero urine, the most likely diagnosis is:

a. Acute tubular necrosis.

b. Prerenal failure.

c. Ureteral obstruction.

d. Renal infarction.

*e. Bladder outlet obstruction.

Intermittent anuria is the classic symptom of urinary tract obstruction. The obstruction is overcome at intervals by the pressure of an increased volume of urine behind the obstruction. (The pressure is actually generated by muscular contraction or peristaltic action of the muscular urinary tract tissue.) Because the normal urinary tract is a paired system to the level of the bladder, bladder-outlet obstruction is the most likely cause of total intermittent obstruction. Obstruction of the bladder outlet would block the entire system, while ureteral obstruction would have to be a bilateral process to cause anuria. Therefore, *e* is the correct response.

**Chapter 46
The Uremic State**

1. Select the true statement(s) regarding the retention of phosphate, magnesium, and uric acid that occurs in chronic renal failure:

   a. Serum levels rise in proportion to the reduction in glomerular filtration rate.

   *b. Retention of these ions is modified by tubular functional adaptation.

   c. These ions are directly responsible for uremic symptoms.

   d. Retention occurs only in the preterminal phase.

   e. Retention is of no pathophysiologic significance.

   Only answer *b* is correct. In contrast with ions excreted mainly by glomerular filtration (which are retained as filtration rates decrease), uric acid excretion is influenced both by renal tubular reabsorption and by secretion. Also, the tubular reabsorption of magnesium and phosphate decreases as glomerular filtration declines. Thus, the serum concentrations of these ions are relatively stable until the glomerular filtration rate is severely reduced.

2. The clinical features of the uremic syndrome may be related to which of the following:

   a. Accumulation of toxic metabolic waste products.

   b. Malnutrition.

   c. Alterations in biosynthesis.

   d. Increased hormone levels.

   *e. All of the above.

   The pathogenesis of the uremic syndrome is poorly understood. However, there is evidence that certain features or aspects of uremia may be related to each of the factors listed. Therefore answer *e* is the correct response.

**Chapter 47
Metabolic Bone Disease**

1. Which of the following is *not* a factor involved in the evolution of renal osteodystrophy?

   a. Phosphate retention.

   b. High PTH levels.

   c. Altered collagen synthesis.

   *d. Increased levels of 24,25-dihydroxycholecalciferol.

   e. Skeletal resistance to the calcemic action of PTH.

   All of the above are involved except *d*, increased levels of 24,25-dihydroxycholecalciferol ($24,25(OH)_2D_3$). As with $1,25(OH)_2D_3$, $24,25(OH)_2D_3$ is produced by the kidney and with severe renal failure levels of both $1,25(OH)_2D_3$ and $24,25(OH)_2D_3$ are decreased. Phosphate retention is believed to be directly involved in the resultant secondary hyperparathyroidism (increased

PTH levels). Altered collagen synthesis has been observed with renal failure and may play a role in the evolution of renal osteodystrophy. In addition, resistance to the calcemic actions of PTH has been shown to occur even with mild renal failure.

2. Which of the following statements about osteoporosis is false?
   a. Osteoporosis is a loss of bone mass with a normal ratio of unmineralized matrix to mineralized bone.
   *b. *Osteopenia* is another name for osteoporosis, and the terms can be used interchangeably.
   c. Osteoporosis is more frequently observed in females than males.
   d. After the third decade there is a decrease in skeletal mass of 8 percent per decade in females.
   e. Menopause results in an accelerated loss of skeletal mass.

   Statement *b* is the only statement that is incorrect. While individuals with osteoporosis have osteopenia, osteoporosis must be differentiated from other causes of osteopenia. Thus, statement *a*, the presence of a normal ratio of unmineralized matrix to mineralized bone, is an important consideration. Other disease processes such as osteitis fibrosa or osteomalacia may present with osteopenia, but there will be a difference in the ratio of unmineralized matrix to mineralized bone and, frequently with osteitis fibrosa, in the extent of cellular activity. Statements *c* through *e* are all true.

Chapter 48
Renal Cell Carcinoma:
Mechanisms of Clinical
Manifestations

1. The most common cause of hypercalcemia in a patient with hypernephroma is:
   a. Immobilization.
   b. Prostaglandin production.
   *c. Bone invasion.
   d. Parathyroid hormone production.
   e. Thyroid hormone production.

   Metastases to bone are common, but prostaglandin or PTH-like hormone production is not. Therefore *c* is the correct answer. Immobilization does not cause hypercalcemia unless the patient is completely immobile. The tumor has not been reported to produce thyroid hormones.

2. Which of the following serum electrolytes would be likely in a patient with renal cell carcinoma?
   a. K^+ 4.0, Cl^- 100, HCO_3^- 25
   b. K^+ 5.7, Cl^- 114, HCO_3^- 15
   c. K^+ 2.8, Cl^- 90, HCO_3^- 35
   d. *a* and *b*
   *e. *a* and *c*

   Answer *a* is a normal electrolyte picture, and this can be seen in patients with renal cell carcinoma. Answer *b* suggests hyperkalemic metabolic acidosis. This is not seen with renal cell cancers. Answer *c* indicates hypokalemic metabolic alkalosis, which may be seen with ACTH production by the tumor. Since *a* and *c* are correct, the single best answer is *e*.

Chapter 49
Pain

1. Select the correct statement(s) regarding acute pain:
   a. It is different from chronic pain, since it involves no psychologic factors.
   *b. Painful muscle injury involves stimulation of nociceptors by released cellular constituents such as K^+ and histamine.
   *c. Tissue levels of bradykinins and prostaglandins are often elevated, which adds to nociceptor stimulation.

d. Sympathetic stimulation of the smooth muscles and blood vessels in the area of injury decreases the pain input to spinal cord.

Answer *a* is incorrect because acute pain perception involves facilitating and inhibiting psychophysiologic mechanisms at all levels of nociceptive transmission from the periphery (sympathetic facilitation), spinal cord and brain stem (descending serotonin and enkephalin inhibition), and hypothalamus and limbic system (autonomic and emotional responsivity). It differs from chronic pain only in the quality and quantity of psychologic factors as shown in Table 49-2. Answer *b* is correct. Potassium is released from all damaged cells, and histamine is released from mast cells and histocytes in inflamed areas. Answer *c* is correct. Bradykinins and prostaglandins are formed in areas of either trauma or disease-producing inflammation; each potentiates the nociceptive effects of the other as well as those of serotonin, histamine, K^+, and the H^+. Answer *d* is incorrect. Efferent stimulation of sympathetic nerves to an injured area potentiates all pain mechanisms by producing vasoconstriction and other smooth-muscle contraction, which increases the elaboration of compounds, which stimulate the nociceptor.

2. In chronic pain:
   a. Strong pain medicines are needed because the pain threshold is lower.
   b. Placebos, if successful, prove that the pain is purely psychologic.
  *c. Enkephalins are inhibitory to pain transmission toward the cortex; they are elevated after acupuncture, transcutaneous nerve stimulation, and even with the belief that a placebo will be effective.
  *d. Depression is a major factor in most, if not all chronic intractable pain states.

Answer *a* is incorrect. Although the pain threshold is lowered, strong pain medicine provides only acute relief and soon becomes ineffective. The lowered threshold of chronic pain has both psychologic and physiologic determinants—hence the futility of intervention with only narcotics. Answer *b* is incorrect. Although the statement was a popular concept in the past, placebo effectiveness has been shown to be associated with a definite increase in met-enkephalin in the spinal fluid. Quite possibly, the psychologic counterpart to this reaction is a suggestible state and a lot of hope that the agent given will successfully relieve the pain. Answer *c* is correct. Enkephalins are involved in nociceptive inhibition at several levels of pain integration from the cord, brain stem, and even in the limbic affective mechanism, where memory and affect influence behavior and autonomic responses. Answer *d* is correct. If there is one thing common to all chronic intractable pain syndromes, it is depression. The amelioration and control of this pain is not possible until depression is reduced.

Chapter 50
Epilepsy

1. The origin of electrical activity detected by the electroencephalogram is most likely to be:
   a. Potentials arising from axonal activity in the cerebral cortex.
   b. Potential arising from the cerebellum.
  *c. Summated synaptic potentials generated by the pyramidal cells of the cerebral cortex.
   d. Potentials arising from electrical activity in the periaqueductal gray matter.

The electroencephalogram is a record of electrical potentials recorded from the scalp. The origin of the activity is felt to be in the superficial layers of the cortex. These potentials appear to be summated synaptic potentials. Axonal activity contributes little, if any, to the surface EEG recording. Therefore, *c* is the correct answer.

2. Partial seizures with complex symptomatology:
   a. Formerly were called Jacksonian seizures.
   b. Are rarely if ever associated with impairment of consciousness.
   c. Are not related to focal cerebral dysfunction.
   *d. Generally are accompanied by impairment of consciousness.

Partial seizures with complex symptomatology are associated with some degree of alteration of consciousness. This may vary from a slight disturbance of either awareness or responsiveness during the attack to loss of both awareness and responsiveness with amnesia for the episode. By contrast, simple or elementary partial seizures have no associated disturbance of consciousness. Hence, *d* is the correct answer.

Chapter 51
Cerebrovascular Disease

1. The internal carotid artery through its branches supplies:
   a. The entire cerebral cortex, including the occipital lobes.
   b. Only the anterior portions of the cerebellum.
   *c. The anterior two-thirds of the brain.
   d. The brain stem and the posterior portions of the cortex.

The carotid artery system supplies approximately the anterior two-thirds of the brain. Since the anterior two-thirds of the brain contains the motor cortex, the somatosensory cortex, and cortical language centers, deficits of function referable to one of these areas are common in carotid artery disease. Therefore, *c* is the correct answer.

2. A patient complains of sudden severe headaches and rapidly loses consciousness. Examination reveals a progressive slowing of the pulse, a rising systolic blood pressure, and a dilated, nonreacting left pupil. Of the following types of cerebrovascular disease, which appears to be the most likely?
   a. Cavernous sinus thrombosis.
   b. Diffuse cortical infarction from hypoglycemia.
   *c. A cerebral hemorrhage with an associated intracerebral hematoma.
   d. Transient cerebral ischemia due to an atheromatous plaque of the internal carotid artery.

The combination of progressive slowing of the pulse, rising systolic blood pressure, and a unilateral dilated pupil in an unconscious patient suggests midbrain and medullary dysfunction due to an expanding supratentorial mass. Since the onset was sudden, a vascular etiology is likely. Cerebral hemorrhage with bleeding into the brain substance with formation of an intracerebral hematoma would best explain this constellation of findings. Therefore, *c* is the correct answer.

Chapter 52
The Upper Motor Neuron System and the Motor Unit

1. Saltatory conduction:
   a. Results in *increased* nerve conduction velocity in *unmyelinated* nerves.
   b. Results in *decreased* nerve conduction velocity in *unmyelinated* nerves.
   *c. Results in *increased* nerve conduction velocity in *myelinated* nerves.
   d. Results in *decreased* nerve conduction velocity in *myelinated* nerves.

The speed of conduction of nerve impulses in unmyelinated nerves is relatively slow. While larger unmyelinated fibers carry impulses faster than smaller ones, even the largest fibers are capable of conducting at the rate of only a few meters per second. In the case of myelinated nerve fibers, conduction is speeded because the nerve impulse jumps from one node of Ranvier to the other. Furthermore, diseases that affect mainly the myelin sheaths of peripheral nerve demonstrate measurable slowing of the nerve conduction velocity. Therefore, *c* is correct.

2. The principle cause of failure of neuromuscular transmission in myasthenia gravis is:
*a. Competitive displacement of acetylcholine from its receptors by antiacetyl-choline receptor antibody.
b. Reduced destruction of acetylcholinesterase.
c. A deficiency of acetylcholinesterase.
d. Impaired release of acetylcholine from the axon terminal.

Myasthenia gravis can be considered an autoimmune disorder affecting the acetylcholine receptors at the myoneural junction. Antibodies occupy acetyl-choline receptor sites so that acetylcholine is prevented from combining with the receptor to produce depolarization of the muscle fiber. Hence, *a* is correct.

Chapter 53
Clinical Malnutrition

1. Which of the following items may be useful in the nutritional assessment of a malnourished patient?
a. History.
b. Serum albumin concentration.
c. Physical examination.
d. Intradermal skin tests, including PPD, mumps, *Candida albicans*.
e. Triceps skin fold.
f. Total lymphocyte count.
g. Mid-arm muscle circumference.
h. History of recent weight loss.
i. Creatinine-height index.
*j. All of the above.

The history (*a*) and physical examination (*c*) are part of the initial assessment of all patients, including the malnourished. Triceps skin fold (*e*) and mid-arm muscle circumference (*g*), together with the creatinine-height index (*i*), assess the fat and somatic muscle protein stores, respectively. Total lymphocyte count (*f*), intradermal skin tests (*d*), and serum albumin concentration (*b*) indicate the status of the visceral protein pool. Therefore, the proper answer is (*j*), encompassing all of the other answers.

2. Calculate nitrogen balance for a patient whose protein intake is 100 g and whose urinary urea nitrogen is 10 g per 24 hours.
a. +90 g
b. +9 g
*c. +3 g
d. −3 mg
e. None of the above

Nitrogen balance is calculated by first converting grams of protein intake into grams of nitrogen. Nitrogen output is estimated from the 24-hour urine urea nitrogen output plus 3 g of nitrogen to account for the extrarenal losses through the skin and gastrointestinal tract. Thus:

$$\text{N balance} = 100 \text{ g } (0.16) - (10 \text{ g} + 3 \text{ g})$$
$$= 16 - 13$$
$$= +3 \text{ g}$$

Chapter 54
Carcinogenesis, Cell Kinetics, and Tumor Immunology

1. Select the correct statement or statements concerning viral and chemical carcinogenesis:
*a. Burkitt's lymphoma is the only tumor in humans in which a DNA virus can be directly implicated.
b. Interferon acts by blocking reverse transcriptase in the host cell.

*c. Viral-induced malignancies, unlike those induced by carcinogens, may have antigens that are cross-reactive between different tumors.

d. Most carcinogens are direct acting and do not require metabolic activation by the host.

*e. Lung cancer is an example of two different classes of carcinogens that may act synergistically.

Correct answers are *a*, *c*, and *e*. Interferon does not block reverse transcriptase but, rather, acts as a signal to adjacent cells, which then become resistant to further viral penetration. Therefore, *b* is incorrect. Also, most carcinogens *do* require metabolic activation by the host; hence, *d* is incorrect.

2. Which of the following statements are true concerning differences among immune adjuvants, immunopotentiators, and specific immunotherapy?

*a. Adjuvant therapy (i.e., BCG) is nonspecific, as opposed to therapy with tumor antigen.

b. Specific immunotherapy has been more commonly used.

c. Interferon acts by inhibiting natural killer cells and increasing macrophage ADCC.

d. All of the above.

e. None of the above.

Of the above, only *a* is true. *Nonspecific* therapy is more commonly used. Interferon acts to increase natural killer cell activity, not to inhibit it.

Chapter 55
Extraneoplastic Manifestations of Malignancies

1. Neoplasms may induce cachexia by multiple mechanisms. Evidence has been presented for each of the following mechanisms, *except:*

a. Alteration of chemoreceptors, leading to decreased excitatory stimuli.

b. Increased inhibitory stimuli due to impaired nutrient absorption.

c. Increased inhibitory stimuli due to the mass effect and replacement of absorptive surface by a primary gastric carcinoma.

*d. Chemically identifiable toxic mediators.

Altered oral chemoreceptors, impaired nutrient absorption, and impaired gastric filling have all been demonstrated in certain cancer patients. Although it seems reasonable that toxic mediators of malnutrition are elaborated by some tumors, none have thus far been identified. Therefore, *d* is the correct answer.

2. Hypercalcemia in malignancy may be mediated by all the following mechanisms, *except:*

*a. Ectopic calcitonin secretion.

b. Ectopic prostaglandin secretion.

c. Production of osteoclast activating factor.

d. Ectopic secretion of a PTH-like substance.

Prostaglandins, OAF, and a PTH-like substance have all been implicated in the hypercalcemias of certain malignancies. Calcitonin, which is occasionally produced in abnormal amounts by medullary thyroid carcinoma, does not produce hypercalcemia physiologically or in pathologic states. Thus, *a* is the correct answer.

Chapter 56
Neoplasms of the Immune System

1. The majority of non-Hodgkin's lymphomas arise from clones of:

a. B lymphocytes at an early stage of lymphoid maturation (ontogeny).

b. T lymphocytes late in antigen-stimulated differentiation.

*c. B lymphocytes during antigen-stimulated differentiation.

d. Stem cells prior to development of lymphoid and monocyte-committed precursors.

Most lymphomas are of B-cell origin, since surface membrane immunoglobulin can be found on the malignant lymphocytes. Investigators now believe that these tumors arise from the clonal proliferation of malignant B cells frozen at some stage of antigen-stimulated differentiation, since these cells morphologically and kinetically resemble normal B cells in various stages of transformation.

2. An 81-year-old man who has been in good health sees his doctor because of a minor upper-respiratory infection. The workup shows an elevated total serum protein, and subsequent serum electrophoresis shows a small spike, which is identified as monoclonal IgG. The patient has no bone pain and has not had frequent infections. Hemoglobin is 14 gm/100 ml, white blood cell count and differential are normal, and platelet count is normal. Peripheral blood smear shows no abnormalities. There is no proteinuria, and renal function is normal. X-rays of the bones show no lesions. Bone marrow aspiration shows that plasma cells are at the upper limit of normal in number but are normal morphologically. From the data at this point, what is the *single most likely* diagnosis?
   a. Waldenström's macroglobulinemia.
   b. Chronic lymphocytic leukemia.
   c. Multiple myeloma.
   *d. Benign monoclonal gammopathy.

Benign spikes are relatively common in the elderly, perhaps up to 5 percent of persons over 80. This man is healthy and has a small IgG spike but absolutely no pathophysiology to suggest multiple myeloma. He fits the strict definition of *benign monoclonal gammopathy,* and it is unlikely that his process will evolve into multiple myeloma.

Chapter 57
Cancer of the Breast

1. A premenopausal woman with metastatic estrogen-receptor–positive breast cancer was initially treated by oophorectomy with a good response lasting for 18 months. She then developed generalized, slowly progressive bone and soft tissue disease. A reasonable approach to therapy would be to:
   *a. Surgically remove her adrenal glands.
   b. Support her with pain medication until vital functions are compromised.
   c. Begin cytotoxic chemotherapy.
   d. Systematically irradiate lesions found on physical and radiologic examination.

Estrogen-receptor positivity correlates well with subsequent response to estrogen deprivation by removal of the ovaries. Since estrogen synthesis occurs in the adrenal gland as well as in peripheral tissue from androgenic steroids, elimination of the adrenal source of estrogens by adrenalectomy would be a logical approach. Indeed, such therapy is followed by good results in most women who have had a previous excellent response to oophorectomy.

2. Why is it recommended that breast examination take place shortly after a menstrual period?
   a. The patient is less tense.
   *b. The influences of progesterone on breast tissue are avoided.
   c. The breast is largest at this time.
   d. No particular reason other than giving the patient a routine time for self-examination.

During the luteal phase of the menstrual cycle, the effects of progesterone on the breast include increased blood flow and proliferation of the terminal ductile system. Fullness, discomfort, and exaggeration of lobular structure or cystic disease may make adequate physical examination difficult at this time.

1. One hundred ml of blood containing 15 g of hemoglobin and having a PO_2 of 25 mm Hg is mixed with 100 ml of blood with the same hemoglobin concentration and a PO_2 of 135 mm Hg. The PO_2 of the resulting mixture would be closest to:

  *a. 40
  b. 60
  c. 80
  d. 100
  e. None of these.

  To answer this question, refer to the oxyhemoglobin dissociation curve (Fig. 58-2). When mixing aliquots of blood, total oxygen contents are averaged and not the small amount of dissolved oxygen reflected by the partial pressure. Therefore, in this example the first aliquot with a pressure of 25 mm Hg has a hemoglobin that is approximately 50 percent saturated with oxygen. The second aliquot with a PO_2 of 135 mm Hg is approaching 100 percent saturation. Since the hemoglobin concentration and volume in each sample are the same, one does not need to calculate the content but can simply average their saturations, which would give a saturation in the mixed sample of 75 percent. When one looks at the oxyhemoglobin dissociation curve, the partial pressure of oxygen that most closely corresponds to 75 percent saturation is a PO_2 of 40 mm Hg.

2. The hypoxemia associated with $\dot{V}/\dot{Q}$ mismatch is caused by:

  a. Hyperventilation of shunt alveoli.
  b. Hyperventilation of dead space.
  c. Increased numbers of high $\dot{V}/\dot{Q}$ alveoli.
  *d. Increased numbers of low $\dot{V}/\dot{Q}$ alveoli.
  e. None of these.

  The answer is d, an increased number of low $\dot{V}/\dot{Q}$ alveoli. Situation a is impossible, since shunt alveoli are not ventilated at all. Hyperventilation of dead space alone would not alter the preexisting arterial blood gases, since there is no perfusion of dead space. Possibility c, increased numbers of high $\dot{V}/\dot{Q}$ alveoli, is simply a less severe form of wasted ventilation (dead space) and will not cause hypoxemia. However, situation d, increased numbers of low $\dot{V}/\dot{Q}$ alveoli, will lead to a decreased PO_2 in the alveolus and, therefore, decreased PO_2 in the blood perfusing that alveolus. This blood, when mixed with blood from other areas of the lung, will tend to reduce the overall content and therefore lower the partial pressure of oxygen in arterial blood.

1. At what lung volume would compliance of the chest wall be lowest?

  a. At total lung capacity.
  *b. At functional residual capacity minus expiratory reserve volume.
  c. At residual volume plus functional residual capacity.
  d. At total lung capacity minus residual volume.

  The compliance of the chest wall would be lowest at residual volume. This can be seen from the pressure-volume curve of the chest alone. The lowest compliance corresponds to the lowest slope of the chest-alone curve, which is at residual volume. The residual volume is calculated as the difference between functional residual capacity and expiratory reserve volume; thus, answer b is correct.

2. A patient who has had one lung removed has spirometry testing performed. The ratio of forced expiratory volume in 1 second divided by the vital capacity is lower than would be expected for a normal person. Indicate which of the following statements is true.

a. Because the remaining lung must expand to larger than its normal size, the airways will generally be smaller in size, causing the FEV1/FVC to fall.

*b. The patient probably has some type of obstructive lung disease.

c. The remaining lung is normal.

d. None of the above.

Answer *a* is incorrect. As the remaining lung is expanded, the airways that are tethered to the parenchyma must also expand (not become smaller). Under these conditions airway resistance should fall and FEV1/FVC increase. Answer *b* is correct. The FEV1/FVC ratio is lower than normal; thus, an obstructive pattern is present. Answers *c* and *d* are incorrect.

Chapter 60
Control of Breathing

1. A patient was evaluated (in Cleveland, Ohio, where barometric pressure = 747 mm Hg) for the complaint of dyspnea at rest. The respiratory rate was 35 breaths per minute. Auscultation of the chest revealed no wheezes or rales. Arterial blood was sampled, revealing a pH of 7.42; PCO_2, 25 mm Hg; and PO_2, 60 mm Hg. Which of the following statements about the patient is true?

   a. The hyperventilation and complaint of dyspnea are explained by anxiety, because there is no evidence of lung disease.

   *b. The dyspnea and hyperventilation must be explained by something other than blood gas abnormalities, and there is evidence of lung disease.

   c. The dyspnea, tachypnea, and acute respiratory alkalosis are due to arterial hypoxemia.

   d. All of the above.

   e. None of the above.

   Answer *a* is not true. The PO_2 of 60 mm Hg when the PCO_2 is 25 indicates a large alveolar-arterial oxygen gradient (approximately 56 mm Hg; normal, 5–15 mm Hg). The pH and PCO_2 indicate chronic compensated respiratory alkalosis combined with metabolic acidosis. The large A − a gradient and the chronic acid-base disorder indicate chronic lung disease or congestive heart failure. Answer *b* is true, for the reasons stated above. Answer *c* is not true. Hypoxemia with PO_2 of 60 mm Hg provides only minimal, if any, chemical stimulus for breathing. This could be demonstrated by administering O_2, which would probably increase the PO_2 above 100 mm Hg without any noticeable change in respiratory rate, PCO_2, or subjective symptomatology. The respiratory drive in patients in this situation arises from receptors in the lungs.

2. A patient was evaluated for increased serum bicarbonate noted on routine blood chemistry profile. His arterial blood then revealed a pH of 7.35; PCO_2, 70 mm Hg; PO_2, 55 mm Hg; and HCO_3^-, 37.8 mEq. His arterial blood was sampled again after the patient was instructed to breathe faster and more deeply. The PCO_2 then was 40 mm Hg. Which statement is true?

   a. The increased PCO_2 and decreased PO_2 indicate that the patient has chronic obstructive pulmonary disease.

   b. The increased PCO_2 and decreased PO_2 in this patient may be due to an intracardiac shunt.

   *c. The P(A − a)O_2 is normal; the response to hyperventilation suggests normal lung function with a primary defect in control of breathing.

   d. All of the above.

   e. None of the above.

   Answer *a* is not true. Patients with hypercapnea secondary to COPD cannot achieve a normal PCO_2 with hyperventilation because alveolar ventilation increases less than the CO_2 produced by the increased work of breathing. Answer *b* is not true. Shunting does not produce increased PCO_2. Answer *c* is true. Alveolar ventilation can be returned to normal voluntarily in these patients. When this is done, the normal alveolar PO_2 produces a normal arterial PO_2.

Chapter 61 **Reversible Obstructive** **Airways Disease** **(Asthma)**	1. The hypoxemia in asthma attacks is usually secondary to: *a. Low $\dot{V}/\dot{Q}$ areas. b. High $\dot{V}/\dot{Q}$ areas. c. Shunt. d. Diffusion. e. Hypoventilation.

1. The hypoxemia in asthma attacks is usually secondary to:
   *a. Low $\dot{V}/\dot{Q}$ areas.
   b. High $\dot{V}/\dot{Q}$ areas.
   c. Shunt.
   d. Diffusion.
   e. Hypoventilation.
   Answer *a* is true. Areas with low $\dot{V}/\dot{Q}$ ratios are characteristic of asthma and are the major reason for hypoxemia in most asthmatic patients. Answer *b* is false. High $\dot{V}/\dot{Q}$ areas occur in asthma but do not contribute unsaturated blood to pulmonary venous flow and therefore do not cause hypoxemia. Answer *c* is false. Shunting occurs in severe asthma but significant shunting is not characteristic of most asthma attacks. Answer *d* is false. Asthma is characterized by a normal alveolar-capillary structure. There is no evidence that a diffusion block contributes to hypoxemia in this or other obstructive airways diseases. Answer *e* is false. Hypoventilation occurs only in severe (life-threatening) asthma.

2. All the following statements about an acute asthmatic attack are true, except:
   a. Mucosal wall edema contributes to limitation of airflow.
   *b. Polymorphonuclear cells in the sputum serve as markers of reversible obstructive airways disease.
   c. Improvement in ventilation can be seen after treatment with methylxanthines.
   d. Resistance to expiratory airflow is increased.
   Answer *a* is true. Answer *b* is false. Eosinophils, not polymorphonuclear leukocytes indicate reversible airways disease. Answer *c* is true. Methylxanthine drugs relax bronchial smooth muscle and therefore can reduce airways resistance and improve ventilation. Answer *d* is true. A high airways resistance is the physiologic hallmark of an asthmatic attack.

Chapter 62
Chronic Airflow
Limitation

1. What is the most common cause of chronic bronchitis?
   a. Frequent chest infections as a child.
   *b. Cigarette smoking.
   c. Industrial pollution.
   d. Prior history of asthma.
   e. None of the above.
   Although individual cases of chronic bronchitis have been reported following *a*, *c*, and *d*, cigarette smoking is by far the primary etiology. Hence the correct answer is *b*.

2. What is the most likely explanation for the development of alveolar wall damage in emphysema?
   a. Chronic exposure of alveoli to low PO_2.
   b. Alveolar wall necrosis due to decreased minute ventilation.
   c. Compromised circulation due to mucosal edema.
   *d. Release of proteases from macrophages and neutrophils in the lung.
   e. None of the above.
   Hypoventilation or alveolar hypoxia have not been implicated in alveolar damage. Mucosal edema does not compromise alveolar circulation. Smoking leads to inflammation resulting in an increased number of macrophages and

neutrophils in the lung. These cells release proteases, especially elastase. Therefore, statement *d* is correct.

Chapter 63 **Interstitial Lung Disease**	1. A patient with severe dyspnea has the following physiologic abnormalities: DLCO (diffusing capacity of the lung for carbon monoxide) is 50 percent of predicted; dead space/tidal volume is 50 percent (increased). Lung volumes are: total lung capacity (TLC), 50 percent of predicted; functional residual capacity (FRC), 50 percent of predicted; and residual volume (RV), 50 percent of predicted. Which disease could explain these findings?

    a. Pulmonary embolus occluding the right pulmonary artery.
    b. Emphysema.
    c. Spinal cord tumor with paralysis.
  *d. Idiopathic pulmonary fibrosis.
    e. A lung tumor blocking his right main stem bronchus.

Answer *a* is incorrect. Such a large reduction in lung volumes would not be expected. Also, since atelectasis may accompany a pulmonary embolus, the dead space/tidal volume ratio does not typically increase to this extent. Answer *b* is incorrect, since RV and TLC tend to rise in emphysema. Answer *c* is incorrect, since RV tends to rise with weakness or paralysis. Answer *d* is correct. The findings described would be consistent with pulmonary fibrosis. Answer *e* is incorrect. Compensatory expansion of the unobstructed lung, vascular redistribution of flow, and recruitment of unperfused vessels all serve to moderate functional deterioration. Dead space/tidal volume may actually decrease.

2. In patients with interstitial lung disease, which of the following makes the largest contribution to hypoxemia at rest?
    a. Diffusion abnormality.
  *b. Low ventilation/perfusion ($\dot{V}/\dot{Q}$) areas.
    c. Shunt.
    d. Increased dead space.
    e. High ventilation/perfusion ($\dot{V}/\dot{Q}$) areas.

Answer *a* is incorrect. Diffusion contributes to hypoxemia mainly with exercise. Answer *b* is correct. Poorly ventilated alveoli with good blood flow make up the major cause of hypoxemia in interstitial disease. Answer *c* is incorrect. Shunt is increased but has less of an effect than low $\dot{V}/\dot{Q}$, as demonstrated by the marked improvement in PaO_2 by administration of oxygen to most patients with interstitial disease. Answer *d* is incorrect. Dead space is increased, but this contributes little to hypoxemia. Answer *e* is incorrect. There are more high $\dot{V}/\dot{Q}$ areas, but they do not contribute to hypoxemia.

Chapter 64 **Pulmonary Edema**	1. Two patients are found to have pulmonary edema. *Patient A* has total serum protein equal to 7 g/dl, airway fluid protein equal to 2.5 g/dl, and pulmonary capillary pressure equal to 32 mm Hg. *Patient B* has total serum protein equal to 4 g/dl, airway fluid protein equal to 2.5 g/dl and pulmonary capillary pressure equal to 10 mm Hg.

    Indicate, by circling the letter *a, b, c,* or *d,* which patient would be expected to benefit from the following proposed therapeutic interventions (*a* = patient A, *b* = patient B, *c* = both patients, *d* = neither patient).
a b *c d 1. Oxygen by face mask 10 liters per minute.
a b *c d 2. The administration of a diuretic to reduce pulmonary capillary pressure.
a b c *d 3. The infusion of plasma (protein = 6.5 g/dl) to increase oncotic pressure.

Patient A has high-pressure pulmonary edema with apparently normal capillary permeability, as evidenced by the low airway-fluid protein/serum-protein ratio. Patient B has high-permeability edema with normal pressure and increased airway fluid protein. Both patients will experience hypoxemia due to alveolar flooding and will benefit from oxygen. Both patients will improve with a reduction in pulmonary capillary pressure—patient A because elevated pressure is the primary cause of his increased filtration and edema; patient B because with increased permeability the rate of fluid filtration into the lung is more sensitive to small changes in capillary pressure. Neither patient will respond to the infusion of plasma. For patient A, this infusion would reduce the plasma protein concentration and increase capillary pressure, leading to an increased rate of edema formation. For patient B, the increase in capillary pressure would be deleterious for the same reason, and the increase in protein concentration would be of little benefit because the injury to the basement membrane has decreased the oncotic reflection coefficient for protein. Hence, even though the plasma oncotic pressure might be increased by the plasma infusion, this would have minimal effect on lung water balance. Eventually, the protein would be filtered into the lung.

2. Filtration of fluid from the pulmonary capillary to the interstitium of the lung:

  *a. Probably occurs all the time in healthy individuals.

  b. Occurs only when pulmonary capillary pressure is greater than 25 mm Hg.

  c. Occurs only when pulmonary capillary pressure is greater than plasma protein oncotic pressure.

  d. Is prevented by positive pressure breathing.

  e. None of the above is true.

Answer *a* is true, as evidenced by lung lymph flow in all animal preparations studied. Answers *b* and *c* are not true, for the above reason. Pulmonary capillary pressure and plasma protein oncotic pressure are only two of four forces that control fluid filtration. The other two, interstitial pressure, which is negative, and interstitial protein osmotic pressure, both operate in favor of fluid filtration. Answer *d* is not true; positive pressure breathing appears to increase fluid filtration, possibly by increasing lung volume and reducing interstitial pressure.

Chapter 65
Pulmonary Vascular
Disease

1. Which of the following is the most potent chemical stimulus for pulmonary vasoconstriction in humans?

  a. Increased arterial PCO_2.

  b. Decreased arterial PO_2.

  *c. Decreased alveolar PO_2.

  d. Increased pH.

  e. Prostacyclin.

Alveolar hypoxia (decreased alveolar PO_2) is the most potent chemical stimulus for pulmonary vasoconstriction, because alveolar hypoxia affects pulmonary arteries and pre-capillary vessels most directly. Decreased arterial PO_2 (hypoxemia) and increased arterial PCO_2 (hypercapnia) also induce pulmonary vasoconstriction; together, their combined effect is additive. Elevated pH does *not* cause pulmonary vasoconstriction. Prostacyclin actually *dilates* pulmonary vessels.

2. In pulmonary embolism the major cause of the hypoxemia is:

  a. Blockage of the pulmonary blood flow with the development of high $\dot{V}/\dot{Q}$ areas.

  b. Diffusion abnormalities.

*c. Secondary changes leading to low $\dot{V}/\dot{Q}$ areas.

d. Low mixed-venous PO_2.

e. Both diffusion abnormalities and high $\dot{V}/\dot{Q}$ areas.

The major cause of arterial hypoxemia is the occurrence of low $\dot{V}/\dot{Q}$ ratios in the unembolized parts of the lung. The embolized lung segments (with high $\dot{V}/\dot{Q}$ ratios) contribute to increased dead space, but not to hypoxemia. Diffusion abnormalities probably occur if embolism is widespread, but are not a major cause of hypoxemia. Low mixed-venous PO_2 can accentuate arterial hypoxemia, but it is not the principal mechanism in pulmonary embolism.

Chapter 66 **Pulmonary Neoplastic** **Disease**	1. What is the most useful method of establishing the diagnosis of bronchogenic carcinoma?

1. What is the most useful method of establishing the diagnosis of bronchogenic carcinoma?

  a. Lung scan.

  b. Chest radiography.

*c. Bronchoscopy and biopsy.

  d. Pulmonary function.

  e. None of the above.

Only cytologic or histologic (biopsy) studies can definitely establish the presence and cell type of a bronchogenic carcinoma. Heavy smokers may have abnormal lung scans, chest radiographs, or pulmonary function, without having lung cancer. Hence, statement *c* is correct.

2. Which of the following statements is true about lung cancer?

  a. The incidence of bronchogenic carcinoma has been stable for years.

  b. Women are afflicted more often than men.

  c. Occupation has not been shown to play a role in the development of lung cancer.

*d. The risk of death from bronchogenic carcinoma increases as the number of cigarettes smoked daily increases.

  e. None of the above.

Answer *a* is incorrect; the incidence of lung cancer has been steadily rising for the past 50 years. Although the incidence in women is increasing rapidly, there are three times as many men as women with lung cancer. Although the role played by occupation is small in comparison with smoking, working with chromates, nickel, and radioactive gases is associated with an increased incidence of bronchogenic carcinoma. Considerable evidence links cigarette smoking to the occurrence of epidermoid (squamous-cell) and small-cell (oat-cell) carcinoma of the lung; thus, *d* is the correct answer.

Chapter 67
The Metabolic Response
to Surgery and Trauma

1. Select from the following the fuel store that provides the majority of calories to satisfy the body's acute energy requirements following trauma or injury:

*a. Fat (adipose triglycerides).

  b. Protein (muscle).

  c. Glycogen (liver).

  d. Glycogen (muscle).

  e. None of the above.

With starvation or trauma, glycogen stores are rapidly depleted and protein is not a major source of energy until fat stores are depleted. Fat stores provide the major source of energy in this situation. Hence, answer *a* is correct.

2. Gluconeogenesis and catabolism following injury are stimulated by increased levels of each of the following hormones except:

  a. ACTH.

  b. Growth hormone.

*c. Insulin.
d. Cortisol.
e. None of the above.

All of these hormones are increased in response to injury. All but insulin are catabolic; therefore, *c* is the correct response.

Chapter 68
Hypertensive Disorders
(Toxemia) of Pregnancy

1. Which of the following clinical features observed in a patient with preeclampsia represents evidence of decreased organ perfusion?
   a. Decrease in hematocrit.
   b. Facial edema.
   *c. Prolonged decrease in fetal heart rate with uterine contractions.
   d. Hypertension.
   e. None of the above.

   Decrease in hematocrit results from increase in the plasma volume with improvement of the disease. Facial edema results from sodium and water retention. Answer *c* is correct. In the face of decreased uteroplacental perfusion, further reduction of blood flow occurring with contractions may produce hypoxia. Hypertension is the result of increased vascular reactivity and vasoconstriction.

2. Which of the following is not seen in patients with preeclampsia?
   a. Increased vascular responsiveness to angiotensin II.
   *b. Increased plasma concentration of angiotensin II.
   c. Decreased glomerular filtration rate.
   d. Decreased intravascular volume.
   e. Decreased uteroplacental blood flow.

   The correct response is *b*. The increase in plasma concentration of pressors seen in normal pregnancy is lost in patients with preeclampsia, although the levels may still be higher than in the nonpregnant individual. Each of the other physiologic changes is characteristic of hypertensive pregnancy.

Index

Index

Abscesses
  pancreatic, 133
  protein malnutrition with, 349
  shock with, 76
Absorption (food), normal, 149–150.
  See also Malabsorption
Acanthosis nigricans, insulin resistance in, 200
Acetoacetic acid (AAA)
  from fat oxidation, 268
  in ketoacidosis, 108
Acetone, in ketoacidosis, 108
Acetylcholine (ACh)
  in asthma, 195
  as hydrochloric acid secretion ago-
    nist, 125
  in myasthenia gravis, 200
  in neuromuscular transmission,
    328, 340, 341–342
  and pulmonary vascular resistance,
    450
Acetylcholinesterase, in neuromuscular junctions, 340–342
Achalasia, 122
  clinical example of, 124
Acid-base disturbances, 269–277
Acidemia, 269
  consequences of, 272
  and pulmonary vascular constric-
    tion, 451
Acidosis
  defined, 269
  hyperkalemic metabolic, from Ad-
    dison's disease, 94
  lactic, 270–271
  metabolic
    causes of, 271
    clinical example of, 274–276
    described, 269, 270–272
    with heat illness, 243
    hyperkalemia from, 265
    and potassium depletion, 262
    from shock, 73
  post-traumatic, 467
  renal tubular
    hypokalemia from, 262
    metabolic acidosis from, 271
    with multiple myeloma, 381
    in Sjögren's syndrome, 210
  respiratory, 269, 413–415, 417
    carbon dioxide and pH values in,
      415
    clinical example, 418–419
    hyperkalemia from, 265
  serum phosphorus in, 281
Acid perfusion studies, in esophagus
  examination, 122
Acids, nonvolatile, 268. *See also specific
  acids*
Acinar agglomerates, 142
Acinus, hepatic, 141–142
Acromegaly, 86
ACTH. *See* Adrenocorticotropic hor-
  mone (ACTH, Corticotropin)

Actin
  in contraction mechanism, 21, 22
  defective, 172
  in myofibrils, 340
Acyl carnitine, in diabetic
  ketoacidosis, 108
Acyl-CoA-carnitine transferase, 41,
  42
Addison's disease
  hyperkalemia with, 265
  hypocortisolism from, 93
  and pituitary hormones, 85–86
Adenocarcinoma, 455, 456
  disseminated intravascular coagula-
    tion with, 373
Adenoma
  bronchial, Cushing's syndrome
    with, 369
  villous, with acidosis and alkalosis,
    273
Adenomatosis, type I multiple endocrine, 128
Adenopathy, cervical, clinical example of, 384
Adenosine diphosphate (ADP), in
  hemostatic plug formation,
    176, 177
Adenosine monophosphate (AMP),
  cyclic
  and body temperature regulation,
    240
  for lipolysis, 466
Adenosine phosphate, source of,
  280
Adenosine triphosphate (ATP)
  and ischemia, 41, 42
  in mast cell degranulation, 424
  and peptide hormones, 81
  in tumor cells, 355
Adenyl cyclase
  in lipolysis, 106
  in mast cell degranulation, 423–
    424
  and peptide hormones, 81
ADH. *See* Antidiuretic hormone,
  (ADH); Vasopressin
Adipose triglyceride, 106
Adjuvant chemotherapy, 360
Adrenal adenoma, aldosteronism
  from, 103
Adrenal cortex
  anatomy of, 90
  and erythropoiesis, 160–161
  hormones from, 90–92
    abnormalities of, 92–95
    in chemotaxis and phagocytosis,
      172
    mechanism of action, 82
  hyperplasia, congenital, hypocor-
    tisolism from, 93
Adrenal medulla, anatomy of, 90
Adrenergic pain mechanisms, 330
Adrenocorticotropic hormone
  (ACTH, Corticotropin)

ACTH—*Continued*
  and aldosterone regulation, 92
  and cortisol regulation, 90–91
  disorders of, 85
  function of, 85
  in hypercortisolism (Cushing's syn-
    drome), 92–93, 368–369
  in hypocortisolism, 93
  post-traumatic metabolism and,
    465, 466
  release of, 85
Adriamycin, for lymphoma, 361
Adult respiratory distress syndrome
  clinical example, 448
  surfactant deficiency, 411
Adventitia, in atherosclerosis, 34–35
Afterload
  cardiac contraction and, 25–26
  cardiac stroke volume and, 25
  defined, in muscle contraction, 21,
    22, 23
  ventricular function and, 27, 30,
    67
Agammaglobulinemia, acquired, 223.
  See also Bruton's
  agammaglobulinemia
Aging
  autoreactive cells and, 223
  and bone diseases, 317
  and cardiovascular system, 6
  and eyes, 4
  and hair, 3
  and hearing, 4
  and immune system, 7–8
  muscle changes with, 4–5
  nervous system changes with, 5–6
  and osteoporosis, 319
  pneumonia and, 8
  pulmonary function and, 7
  and renal function, 6
  and skin, 3–4
  stature changes with, 3
Agranulocytosis, 172
  drug-induced, 171
Airflow
  in asthma, 425–426
  limitation, chronic, 430–433
    clinical example of, 432–433
Airway collapse, point of, 409
Airways obstruction, chronic (CAO),
  defined, 430
Akathisia, with renal failure, 309
Albumin, plasma
  and ascites formation, 144
  bilirubin binding and, 142–143
  calcium binding and, 279
  in kwashiorkor, 348
  in malnutrition assessment, 350
  in nephrotic syndrome, 298, 299
Alcohol
  and gastric ulcers, 127
  and gastritis, 126
  and gout, 217
  and megakaryocyte production, 176

Alcohol—*Continued*
  and vasopressin release, 87
Alcoholism
  hypokalemia with, 262
  hypophosphatemia with, 285
  and leukocyte migration, 236
  malnutrition with, 349
  pancreatitis from, 133, 134, 135
Aldosterone
  deficiency and hyponatremia, 256
  for heat adaptation, 242
  and hyperkalemia, 264
  hypertension from, 101
  and intracellular potassium concentration, 261
  mechanism of action, 82
  in nephrotic syndrome, 299
  normal secretion of, 90, 91–92
  and post-traumatic metabolism, 467
  in pregnancy, 476
  and sodium excretion, 249
  source of, 90
Aldosteronism, 103
Alkalemia, 269. *See also* Alkalosis
  consequences of, 274
Alkalosis, 269
  metabolic, 269, 270, 272–274
    causes, of, 273
    clinical example of, 276–277
    with Cushing's syndrome, 93, 369
    hypokalemia from, 262
    post-hypercapnia, 273
    with renal cell carcinoma, 323
  respiratory, 269, 413
    with asthma, 426
    causes of, 414
    hypokalemia from, 262
    serum phosphorus in, 281, 285
    from shock, 74
Allergens, 189
  in asthma, 422
  nephrotic syndrome from, 300
Allergic diseases. *See* Hypersensitivity diseases
Allergy, 189
  causes of, 196
  urticaria and, 191
Alpha-adrenergic agonists
  and guanyl cyclase activity, 424
  and lower esophageal sphincter pressure, 120
  and serum potassium, 261
Alpha$_1$-antitrypsin deficiency, in emphysema, 431
Alpha cells, pancreatic, 131
Alpha-fetoprotein, 363
Alpha-2 macroglobulin, in nephrotic syndrome, 299
Aluminum, in osteomalacia, 313, 319
Alveolar-arterial oxygen difference, 395–396
Alveolar gas equation, 395
Alveolar surfactant, 411
Alveolitis, allergic (hypersensitivity pneumonitis), 198
Amenorrhea
  and chorionic gonadotropin, 370
  clinical example of, 83, 88–89

Amenorrhea—*Continued*
  and cyclic ovarian function, 113
  with hyperprolactinemia, 86
  infertility and, 114
  with renal failure, 309
Amino acids
  and cholecystokinin-pancreozymin secretion, 149
  in malnutrition, 347
  post-traumatic deamination of, 466
Aminopyrine, neutropenia from, 171
Aminorex, and primary pulmonary hypertension, 451
Ammonia, in hepatic encephalopathy, 145, 146
Ammonium, urinary, 272
Ammonium chloride, and metabolic acidosis, 271
Amniotic fluid emboli, 451
Amphetamines, and polyarteritis nodosa, 205
Amylase
  function of, 149
  and maldigestion, 150
  pancreatic, 131, 132, 149
Amyloid. *See* Amyloidosis
Amyloidosis
  diffuse, interstitial lung disease and, 435
  in malignancies, 373
  with multiple myeloma, 381
  nephrotic syndrome from, 300
  in peripheral neuropathy, 371
Analgesics, for fever, 242
Anaphylactoid reactions, 192
Anaphylatoxins, in allergic sensitization, 189
Anaphylaxis, 189, 190, 192
  eosinophil-chemotactic factor (ECF-A), as mediator, 190–191, 195
  neutrophil chemotactic factor of (NCF-A), as a mediator, 190–191
  slow-reacting substance of (SRS-A), as a mediator, 190–191, 195
Androgens
  Δ_4-androstenediol, secretion of, 90
  androstenedione
    excessive, in female, 113
    in polycystic ovary syndrome, 114
    production of, 111
  in erythropoietin production, 161
Anemia
  aplastic
    cerebral hemorrhage with, 338
    with hypoproliferative marrow, 161
    and thrombocytopenia, 178
  autoimmune hemolytic, 203
  with cancer, 367
    hypoproliferative, 372
    immune-mediated hemolysis and, 371–372
    iron-deficiency, 154, 372
    leukemia, 173, 377
    lung, 458
    microangioplastic hemolytic with, 372
    with multiple myeloma, 379

Anemia, with cancer—*Continued*
    myelophthisic, 372
    nutritional, 372
    with renal cell carcinoma, 323
  clinical example of, 167
  dilutional, of pregnancy, 476
  with gluten-sensitive enteropathy, 152
  heart failure with, 66
  hyperproliferative, 162–163
  hypoproliferative, 161–162
  iron deficiency, 163
    with reflux esophagitis, 123
  macrocytic, 162
  with malnutrition, 349
  mechanisms of, 161–162
  megaloblastic, 162, 174
  microcytic-hypochromic, 163
  and myocardial oxygen demand, 41
  pernicious
    from atrophic gastritis, 126
    gout with, 217
  physiologic effects of, 165
  red cell life span in, 160
  with renal failure, 309, 310
  sickle cell, defective opsonization in, 172
  sideroblastic, 163
  in systemic lupus erythematosus, 203
Anesthesia, hyperthermia from, 242
Aneurysm
  abdominal aortic, clinical example, 30
  arterial, in polyarteritis, 205
  from atherosclerosis, 33, 35
  cerebral, clinical example, 338–339
  left ventricular, with myocardial infarction, 43
Angiitis. *See* Vasculitis
Angina pectoris
  with aortic stenosis, 54
  clinical description of, 46–47
  clinical example of, 48
  electrocardiogram with, 48
  versus esophageal pain, 121
  incidence of, 45
  with mitral regurgitation, 53
  nocturnal, 47
  at rest (decubitus), 47
  as a symptom, 46
  walk-through, 46–47
Angioedema, 189, 191, 192
Angiogenesis factor, in cancer, 355
Angiotensin II
  in acute renal failure, 305
  in aldosterone regulation, 91–92, 467
  conversion in lung, 449
  cortisol effect on, 102
  hypertension from, 101
  in preeclampsia/eclampsia, 477
  in pregnancy, 476
  and pulmonary vascular resistance, 451
  in renal vascular hypertension, 103
Angiotensinogen, 467
Ankylosing spondylitis, 208, 209
  and interstitial lung disease, 435

Anorexia
  with cancer, 367–368, 457
  from hypercalcemia, 283
  nervosa, hypokalemia with, 262
  with renal failure, 309, 311
Anosmia, in Kallman's syndrome,
    112
Anovulation, causes of, 113
Anoxia, tissue, from hypophos-
    phatemia, 285
Antibodies
  lymphocytes and, 221
  in systemic lupus erythematosus,
    210
Antibody-dependent cell-mediated
    cytotoxicity (ADCC), 200
  lymphocyte mediation of, 220
  in tumor killing, 363, 364
Antibody-synthesizing cells, helper
    lymphocytes and, 221
Anticholinergics, and lower esopha-
    geal sphincter pressure, 120
Anticholinesterases. See also Acetyl-
    choline (ACh); Acetylcholines-
    terase, in neuromuscular junc-
    tions
  and lower esophageal sphincter
    pressure, 120
  for myasthenic syndromes, 371
  and neuromuscular transmission,
    342
Anticoagulants, cerebral hemorrhage
    from, 338
Anticonvulsants
  hypocalcemia from, 284
  rickets from, 317
Antidiuretic hormone (ADH). See also
    Vasopressin
  body water and, 249
  inappropriate secretion of (SIADH)
    in cancer, 370, 458
    hyponatremia from, 256, 257
    pathogenesis and clinical aspects
      of, 88
  post-traumatic secretion of, 467
  in pregnancy, 476
  renal concentration and dilution
    and, 252–253
Antidepressants, for pain, 331
Antigen-antibody complexes
  and chronic inflammation, 235
  in glomerulonephritis, 290, 292,
    387
Antigens
  in immune complex disorders,
    201
  oncofetal, 363
  stimulation of B-cell differentiation
    by, 375–377, 378
  tumor-specific transplantation,
    362–363
Anti-glomerular basement membrane
    (anti-GBM) disease, 290–
    292
Antihistamines, and sweating, 242
Antineoplastic drugs, peripheral
    neuropathies from, 371
Antipyretic agents
  action of, 241
  for fever, 242

Antrum, gastric
  function of, 125, 126
  ulcers and, 127
Anxiety. See Stress
Aorta
  aging and the, 3
  atherosclerosis in, 35
  coarctation of, 67
Aorticopulmonary windows, 62
Aortic pressure, stroke volume and,
    25
Aortic stenosis
  clinical example of, 56
  effects of, 67
  hemodynamic changes and, 53–
    54
  and myocardial ischemia, 41
Aortic valve, sound of, 50
Aortic valvular regurgitation
  effects of, 67
  signs and clinical picture of, 54
Apatite crystals in bone, 313
Apex cardiogram, 51
Aphasia, with transient cerebral isch-
    emia, 339
Aplasia, red cell, 161, 372
Apnea, 399, 414
Arachidonic acid, in platelet aggrega-
    tion, 176, 177
Arachnoiditis, chronic pain with, 330
Arcus senilis, 4, 8
Arrhythmia. See Cardiac arrhythmias
Arterial disease, occlusive, in brain,
    337–338
Arterial pressure
  hemodynamics of, 101
  pulmonary versus sytemic, 73
  as ventricle afterload, 26
  systemic
    drugs to support, 75
    in myocardial infarction, 74
Arteries
  atherosclerosis and, 33–38
  structure of, 33–35
Arteriolitis, with preeclampsia/
    eclampsia, 477
Arteriovenous oxygen difference,
    with heart failure, 70
Arthritis
  chronic pain with, 330
  gout, 215–217, 218
  infectious, 206
  juvenile, 208
  in Reiter's syndrome, 209
  rheumatoid, 207–208
    antibodies to nucleoprotein in,
      210
    autoimmunity in, 206–207
    as chronic inflammation, 235
    clinical example of, 211–212
    etiology of, 206
    hypersensitivity in, 203
    peptic ulcers with, 127
    and pulmonary hypertension,
      451
    seropositive versus seronegative,
      208
    with Sjögren's syndrome, 210
    small vessel coronary disease
      with, 40

Ascites
  mechanisms of, 144–145
  with heart failure, 71
  with kwashiorkor, 348
  with liver disease, 144–145
  from metastases, 154–155
  with pancreatitis, 133
Aspergillosis, allergic bronchopulmo-
    nary, 197–198
Aspirin
  and asthma, 197
  and gastritis, 126
  peptic ulcers from, 127
  and prostaglandin synthesis, 179,
    241
Asterixis
  with hepatic encephalopathy, 146
  with renal failure, 309, 310
Asthma, 421–429
  with anaphylaxis, 192
  aspergillosis with, 197–198
  with atopic dermatitis, 192
  classification of, 421–422
  clinical examples of, 198–199, 427–
    428
  clinical manifestations and therapy
    for, 196–197, 427
  differential diagnosis, 197
  gas exchange in, 426–427
  mechanism of, 189, 190, 195–196,
    427
  nonallergic, 422
  pathogenesis of, 422–425
  pathology of, 421
  respiratory alkalosis from, 414
  and slow-reacting substance of
    anaphylaxis, 191
  spirogram in, 426
  status asthmaticus, 197
Asystole, from hyperkalemia, 263
Ataxia telangiectasia, 224
Atelectasis
  shunting with, 399
  from surfactant deficiency, 411
Atheromatous plaque, rupture of,
    337
Atherosclerosis, 33–38. See also Coro-
    nary artery disease; Myocardial
    ischemia
  cerebral, 337
  clinical example of, 37–38
  distribution of, 33
  etiology of, 33
  in myocardial ischemia, 40
  with nephrotic syndrome, 300
  plaque formation in, 35–37, 45
  with polycythemia, 166
  with renal failure, 309
  risk factors, 34
  therapy for, 37
Atrial fibrillation
  cerebral arterial occlusion from, 337
  and coronary embolism, 41
  jugular venous pulsation in, 52
  with mitral regurgitation, 53
  with mitral stenosis, 52
Atrial pressure
  cardiac preload and, 25
  in heart failure, 68
  normal, 30

Atrial septal defects, 62
Atrioventricular (AV) node
    excitation and the, 13, 14
    in reentrant arrhythmia, 15, 16
Atropine
    for asthma, 424
    and lower esophageal sphincter
        pressure, 120
    and sweating, 242
Auditory sensors in brain, 333
Autoantibodies
    in collagen-vascular diseases, 209–
        210
    in Sjögren's syndrome, 211
Autoimmune diseases, 203–204. See
        also Immune entries
    in immunodeficiencies, 222–223
    leukocytes and, 221
    neutrophil autoantibodies, 171
    rheumatic diseases and, 206–
        207
Automaticity, cardiac, 13, 16
Autonomic reflexes, in hypersensitiv-
        ity reaction, 191
AV node. See Atrioventricular (AV)
        node
Axonal function, impairment of, 341
Axons, 333
    impairment of function, 341
    of motor unit, 340
Azoospermia, with Klinefelter's syn-
        drome, 115
Azotemia
    acute, 303, 304, 305
    with leukemia, 173
    with multiple myeloma, 381
    postrenal, 303, 304
    prerenal, 303, 304
        from Addison's disease, 94
        from sodium depletion, 250
    renal parenchymal, 303, 304, 305–
        306

Babinski's sign, 340
Bacterial infections
    diarrhea from, 151
    immunodeficiencies with, 225
    neutropenia in, 171
    neutrophil defense against, 169,
        171, 172
Bacterial overgrowth syndromes, 151
Barbiturate intoxication
    circulatory problems with, 76
    clinical example of, 76–77
    and hypoxemia, 403
Barbiturates, and vasopressin release,
        87
Bacillus Calmette-Guérin, in tumor im-
        munotherapy, 364
Barium contrast radiography, 122
Bartter's syndrome, hypokalemia
        from, 262
Basal energy expenditure, assessment
        of, 350
Basal metabolic rate, age and, 5
Basilar artery system, atherosclerosis
        in, 35
Basophils, and hypersensitivity reac-
        tions, 189
Benztropine, and sweating, 242

Beriberi, heart failure with, 66
Bernstein test, 122
Beta-adrenergic agents
    in asthma, 424
    and lower esophageal sphincter
        pressure, 120
    and serum potassium, 261
Beta cells, pancreatic, 131
Beta-hydroxybutyric acid (BHB)
    in ketoacidosis, 108
    source of, 268
Beta-lipoprotein in nephrotic syn-
        drome, 299
Beta-lipotropin, function of, 85
    in Cushing's syndrome, 369
Beta-melanocyte-stimulating hormone
        (MSH), 85
Bethanechol, and lower esophageal
        sphincter pressure, 120
Bicarbonate
    in acid-base disturbances, 269, 270
    body fluid content of, 247, 248
    kidney regulation of, 271–272
    in metabolic acidosis, 270–272
    in metabolic alkalosis, 272–274
    pancreatic secretion of, 149
    and potassium concentration, 261
    source of, 268
Bicarbonate-carbonic acid buffer sys-
        tem, 268
Bile
    components of, 137, 138
    in gastritis, 126
    and jaundice, 142
    ulcers from, 127
Bile acid
    malabsorption of, 151
    in triglyceride absorption, 150
Bile duct
    anatomy of, 137
    obstruction of
        in cancer, 155
        in pancreatitis, 134
Bile salts
    circulation of, 137
    in normal bile, 137, 138
    in pancreas, 132
Biliary tract, abnormalities of with hy-
        pocalcemia, 284
Biliary tract fistulae
    from cholecystitis, 139
    with duodenal ulcer, 128
Biliary tract, gallstones and the, 138–
        139
Bilirubin
    with cholecystitis, 138
    in gallstones, 138
    from heme, 160
    in jaundice, 142–143
    metabolism of, 142–143
Billroth II, 151
Bismuth, nephrotic syndrome from, 300
Blastic cell line, in leukemia, 173
Bleeding
    and coagulation factor defects, 184
    gastrointestinal
        with cancers, 154
        dialysis effect on, 310–311
        hepatic encephalopathy and, 146
        with renal failure, 309

Bleeding—Continued
    with macroglobulinemia, 382
    with multiple myeloma, 380
    and platelet insufficiency, 175–
        179
    subarachnoid, 3
Blood. See Circulation; Factors, coag-
        ulation; Hemorrhage
Blood cells, production and types of,
        159
Blood flow. See also individual organs
    cerebral, 337
    coronary, 39
    skin and heat regulation, 238
    zones, in lungs, 449, 450
Blood pressure. See Hypertension;
        Arterial pressure; Shock
Blood urea nitrogen (BUN)
    in aging, 8
    in heart failure, 70
    post-trauma, 468
    in pregnancy, 477
    in prerenal azotemia, 250
Blood vessels
    aging and the, 6
    inflammation and, 231–232
Blood volume
    and ascites formation, 145
    and hypernatremia, 254
    and polycythemia, 166
    post-traumatic, 470
    in pregnancy, 476
    and vasopressin secretion, 87
Body cell mass concept, 467–468
Body fluids
    composition of, 247, 248
    distribution of, 251, 252
    metabolism disorders of, 253–257
    sodium and water balance and,
        247–248
    volume disorders, 249–251
Body fuel, normal stores of, 463,
        464
Bohr effect, 109
Bombesin, and LES pressure, 120
Bone
    cells of, 313, 315
    destruction of, with multiple my-
        eloma, 380
    function of, 313
    in hyperparathyroidism, 319
    marrow
        and anemia, 161–162
        damage and stem cells, 161
        and erythrocyte production, 160
        glucose metabolism in, 464
        leukemia in, 173
        multiple myeloma in, 379–381
        neutrophil production in, 169,
            170, 171
        platelets from, 175, 176
    metabolic diseases of, 315–321
    metastases and hypercalcemia, 369–
        370
    minerals in, 313
    normal physiology of, 313
    phosphate in, 280
Botulism, neuromuscular transmis-
        sion in, 341, 342
Bowel, small, atrophy in, 348

Bradyarrhythmias, mechanism of, 16
Bradykinin
    in asthma, 423
    as inflammation mediator, 233, 234,
      236
    in lung, 449
    and pain nociceptors, 327
Brain
    association areas of, 334
    blood flow and aging, 5
    cerebrovascular physiology, 337
    cerebral physiology, 333
    cortex and pain pathways, 328
    in hypertonic states, 255
    in hyponatremia, 257
    immune complex diseases in, 202
    lupus erythematosus in, 204
    motor areas of, 333
    somatosensory area of, 333
    upper motor neuron system of,
      340–343
    in pain transmission, 328–329,
      330–331
Breast
    anatomy of, 387–388
    cancer. See Cancer, breast
Breathing. See also Ventilation
    airway resistance and PCO_2, 415,
      416
    control of, 413–420
Bright's disease, 298
Bright, Richard, 298
Bromocriptine
    for acromegaly, 86
    for infertility, 114
    and prolactin release, 89
    for prolactinoma, 87
Bronchi, described, 194–195
Bronchial lumen, in asthma, 421
Bronchial wall, in asthma, 421
Bronchiectasis, and aspergillosis, 198
Bronchitis, chronic, 430–432
    alveolar ventilation in, 415
    with interstitial lung disease, 438
Bronchoscopy, for lung cancer diag-
    nosis, 458
Bronchospasm
    with asthma, 196
    lung volumes in, 426, 427
Bruit, from renal cell carcinoma, 322
Bruton's agammaglobulinemia
    B lymphocyte absence in, 222
    clinical example of, 225–226
Budd-Chiari syndrome, portal hyper-
    tension from, 143
Bundle branches, excitation and the,
    13, 14
Burns
    malnutrition with, 349
    secondary immunodeficiency from,
      224
Buterophenones, and prolactin re-
    lease, 86

Cachexia, with cancer, 367–368
Caffeine
    and gastric function, 125
    and lower esophageal sphincter
      pressure, 120
Calcification, metastatic, 282–283

Calcium. See also Hypercalcemia; Hy-
    pocalcemia
    absorption of, 279–280
    accumulation in injured tissue,
      42
    and anticoagulants, 183
    in bone, 313
    in clotting cascade, 181
    hormonal regulation of, 281–282
    in myocardial excitation, 12–13
    normal homeostasis, 279–280
    and peptide hormones, 81
    serum phosphate relationship with,
      281
Calcium adenosine triphosphatase
    (ATPase), 280
Calcium-binding protein, 280
Calcium hydroxyapatite, 280
Calcium phosphate, 280
Calcium pyrophosphate, in pseudo-
    gout, 218
Calories
    inadequate intake of, 347
    normal requirements for, 463
Cancer
    antigens in, 362–363
    in bone, hypercalcemia from, 282
    brain, hemorrhage with, 338
    breast, 386–393
      clinical goals in, 390
      clinical examples of, 390–391
      detection of, 388–389
      incidence of, 386
      predisposing factors for, 386–
        387
      prognosis in, 389
    carcinogenesis, 355–357
    cell growth in, 357–360
    cells versus normal cells, 355
    chronic pain with, 330
    clinical examples of, 360–361, 365–
      366
    doubling time and therapy, 360–
      361
    of esophagus, 154
    etiology of, 355–357
    gastrointestinal, 154–156
      clinical example of, 155–156
      malnutrition with, 368
    hematologic disorders with, 371–
      373
    Hilar mass, clinical example of,
      373–374
    hormones in, 370
    immune mechanisms against, 363–
      364
    of immune system, 375–385
    lung
      clinical example of, 459
      clinical features of, 456–457
      with Cushing's syndrome, 368–
        369
      diagnosis of, 458
      etiology and epidemiology of,
        455
      incidence of types, 457
      pathology of, 455–456
      and pituitary hormones, 86
      prognosis in, 459
      radiography in, 457

Cancer, lung—Continued
    small cell carcinoma of, 370
    syndromes associated with, 458
    therapy for, 365, 458
    malnutrition with, 349, 367–368
    membranous nephropathy with,
      300
    monocyte-macrophage neoplasms,
      382–383
    neuromuscular syndromes with,
      371
    peripheral neuropathies with, 371
    plasma cell disorders, 379–383
    renal cell carcinoma, 322–324
    and thrombocytopenia, 178
    treatment of, 359–360
Candida, killing activity and age, 7–8
Candida albicans, in malnutrition as-
    sessment, 350
Candidiasis, chronic mucocutaneous,
    224
Capillary Starling forces, edema and,
    251, 252
Carbohydrates
    intolerance to and dialysis, 310–
      311
    maldigestion of, 150
    nutritional requirement for, 347
    post-trauma metabolism of, 465–
      466
Carbon dioxide (CO_2)
    in acid-base disturbances, 268–
      277
    lung elimination of, 413–420
Carbonate, in bones, 313
Carbonic acid, as source of hydrogen
    ion, 268
Carboxyhemoglobinemia, red cell
    production and, 165, 167
Carboxypeptidase
    A and B, in pancreas, 132
    production of, 149
Carcinoembryonic antigen (CEA),
    363
Carcinogenesis, described, 355–357
Carcinoma. See also Cancer
    bronchioloalveolar cell, 456
    in situ, 355
    large cell, 455, 456
    medullary thyroid, Cushing's syn-
      drome with, 369
    oat-cell, 455, 456
      hormone production from, 82
      syndrome of inappropriate ADH
        from, 88
    ovarian, erythropoietin in, 371
    scar, 456
    squamous cell, 455, 456
    of the stomach, gastritis and, 126
Carcinomatosis, lymphangitic, on X-
    ray, 457
Cardiac anoxia, myocardial contractil-
    ity in, 67
Cardiac arrest, hypercapnia with, 414
Cardiac arrhythmias
    from alkalemia, 274
    bradyarrhythmias, 16
    diagnosis of, 17
    digitalis-induced with hypercal-
      cemia, 283

Cardiac arrhythmias—*Continued*
  electrocardiograms and, 17
  heart block, 19–20
  with lung cancer, 457
  mechanisms for, 14–17
  from myocardial infarction, 47
  reentrant, 15–16
  tachyarrhythmias, 15–16. *See also*
    Tachycardia
  ventricular
    with ischemia, 42
    with myocardial infarction, 43
  Wolff-Parkinson-White syndrome,
    15, 19
Cardiac catheterization, in intracardiac shunts, 63, 64
Cardiac cycle, 51
Cardiac pump function
  failure of, 74
  normal values, 30
  physiology of, 27–28, 29
  volume and pressure overload, 28–32
Cardiac tamponade
  with infarction, 43
  with lung cancer, 457
  mechanism of, 66
  shock with, 76
Cardiomegaly, with high output heart
    failure, 70
Cardiomyopathy, and coronary embolism, 41
Cardiovascular disease. *See also specific
    diseases*
  atherosclerosis, 33–38
  coronary artery disease, 45–49
  electrophysiology of, 11–20
  ischemia, 39–44
  shock, 73–77
  shunts, 58–64
  valvular heart disease, 50–57
  volume and pressure overload, 27–32
Cardiovascular system
  aging and the, 3, 6
  regulation, 73
Carotids, atherosclerosis in, 35
Cartilage, in joint degeneration, 213–214
Cartilaginous interstitial fluid, 213
Cataracts, with aging, 4, 8
Catecholamines
  in acute renal failure, 305
  in heart failure compensation, 65
  mechanism of action, 81
  post-trauma secretion of, 465, 466
  and potassium distribution, 261
  in preeclampsia/eclampsia, 479
  and pulmonary vascular resistance,
    451
Cathepsins, in rheumatoid arthritis,
    207
Catheterization, cardiac, in intracardiac shunts, 63, 64
Causalgia, 330
Celiac disease, malnutrition with, 349
Cells
  anatomy and physiology of, 333
  growth of, 358–359
  normal cycle of, 358

Cell membrane potential
  in hyperkalemia, 263
  in hypokalemia, 264
  potassium and, 260
Celsus, 231
Central nervous system
  disorders and hypoventilation,
    398–399, 417
  infection, differential diagnosis, 8
Cerebellar degeneration, with cancer,
    371
Cerebellar hemangioblastomas, erythropoietin in, 371
Cerebral hypoperfusion, 338
Cerebral infarction
  types of, 337–338
  from vasospasm, 338
  from venous thrombosis, 338
Cerebrovascular disease, 337–339
Ceruloplasmin, in fever, 241
Charcot-Leyden crystals, in asthma,
    421
Chédiak-Higashi syndrome
  as immunodeficiency state, 224
  leukocyte migration and, 236
Chemoreceptors, in cancer, 367
Chemotactic factors, as inflammation
    mediators, 234
Chemotaxis
  defective, 172
  inhibition of, 172
  in malnutrition, 348
  neutrophil capacity of, 169
  stimulation of, 233
Chemotherapy
  efficacy of, 359, 360
  hypocalcemia and hypophosphatemia from, 284
  for lung cancer, 458
  and malnutrition, 368
Chenodeoxycholic acid, in bile, 137
Chest wall, pressure-volume curves
    of, 405–406, 407
Chief cell, in stomach, 125
Chlamydial infections, and Reiter's
    syndrome, 209
Chloramphenicol, and leukocyte production, 236
Chloride
  body fluid content of, 247, 248
  in pancreas, 132
Cholangitis, ascending, 139
Cholecystitis, 138–139
Cholecystokinin-pancreozymin
  gallbladder stimulation by, 137
  inadequate, 150–151
  and lower esophageal sphincter
    pressure, 120
  in pancreas, 131–132
  and pancreatic enzymes, 149
  and triglyceride digestion, 150
Choledochaljejunostomy, 155
Choledocholithiasis, 139
Cholelithiasis, 138
Cholestasis, in jaundice, 143
Cholesterol
  adrenocortical hormones from, 90
  in atherosclerosis, 35–36
  in bile, 137, 138
  digestion of, 150

Cholesterol—*Continued*
  gallstones of, 137, 138
  and lipid disorders, 36, 37
  in nephrotic syndrome, 298, 299
  steroid hormones from, 82
  testosterone from, 111
  in transient cerebral ischemia, 337–338
Cholesterol esterase, in pancreas, 132
Cholic acid, in bile, 137
Cholinergic agents, and lower esophageal sphincter pressure, 120
Cholinergic antagonists, and asthma,
    427
Chondrocalcinosis, 218
Chorionic gonadotropin (CG), in gynecomastia, 370
Chromophobe adenoma, and prolactin release, 86
Chromosome, marker, in leukemia,
    173
Chronic airflow limitation (CAL), 430
Chronic airways obstruction (CAO),
    430
Chronic nonspecific respiratory disease (CNSRD), 430
Chronic obstructive lung disease
    (COLD), 430
Chronic obstructive pulmonary disease (COPD), 413–420, 430
Churg-Strauss syndrome, and interstitial lung disease, 435
Chvostek's sign, 284
Chymotrypsin
  in pancreas, 132
  production of, 149
Chymotrypsinogen, 149
Circadian variation of ACTH, 91
Circulatory volume, and inflammation, 232, 235
Circulation
  fetal, 58–59, 60, 61
  physiology of normal, 73
  postnatal, 59–60, 61
  pulmonary, 59–60
Cirrhosis
  ascites with, 145
  biliary with choledocholithiasis, 139
  and clotting dysfunction, 183
  collateral circulation with, 144
  edema with, 251
  metabolic acidosis with, 271
  hepatic encephalopathy with, 146
  hyponatremia from, 256
  portal blood flow with, 143–144
Citrate
  as anticoagulant, 183
  binding of calcium, 279
  and hypocalcemia, 284
Clinical examples
  adrenergic-corticoid response to
    trauma, 470
  aging, physical consequences of, 8
  allergic rhinitis and asthma, 198–199
  anemia, 167
  asthma, 427–428
  atherosclerosis, 37–38
  breast cancer, 390–391
  cancer (hilar mass), 373–374

Clinical examples—*Continued*
  cardiac failure, high-output, 70–71
  cardiac volume and pressure overload, 30–32
  cerebrovascular disease, 338–339
  chronic air-flow limitation, 432–433
  coagulation abnormality, 184–185
  control of breathing, 418–419
  cor pulmonale due to skeletal deformity, 411
  coronary artery disease, 48
  diabetes, mellitus, non-insulin dependent, 109–110
  diabetic peripheral neuropathy, 343
  distributive shock, 76–77
  enteropathy, gluten-sensitive, 152
  epilepsy, 334–335
  esophageal disease, 124
  galactorrhea and amenorrhea, 88–89
  gallstone disease, 139
  gastrointestinal malignancy, 155–156
  gouty arthritis, 218
  Guillain-Barré syndrome, 342
  heart block, 19–20
  heat stroke, 243–244
  hemorrhagic gastritis, 129
  hypercalcemia, 285–286
  hypercortisolism (Cushing's disease), 94–95
  hyperkalemia, 266–267
  hypernatremia, 257–258
  hypertension, 104–105
    with pregnancy, 480–482
  hyperthyroidism (Graves' disease), 99–100
  hypokalemia, 265–266
  hyponatremia, 258, 470–471
  hypoxemia and hypoventilation, 403–404
  immune complex disease, 204–205
  immune system neoplasm, 383–384
  interstitial lung disease, 440
  intracardiac shunting, 62–64
  Klinefelter's syndrome (hypogonadism), 114–115
  liver disease, 146–147
  lung cancer, 459
  malnutrition, 351–352
  metabolic acidosis, 274–276
  metabolic alkalosis, 276–277
  myocardial ischemia, 43–44
  nephritic syndrome, acute, 297
  nephrotic syndrome, 301–302
  neutropenia, 174
  osteomalacia, 319–321
  pain, chronic, 331–332
  pancreatic insufficiency, 152–153
  pancreatitis, chronic, 135–136
  penicillin allergy, 192–193
  peptic ulcer, 129
  polycythemia, 167–168
  pulmonary edema, 447–448
  pulmonary vascular disease, 453
  renal cell carcinoma, 323–324
  renal failure
    acute, 306–307
    chronic, 311
  rheumatoid arthritis, 211–212

Clinical examples—*Continued*
  testicular feminization, 83
  thrombocytopenia, 179–180
  tumor antigens and immunologic treatment, 365–366
  ulcer, 129
  valvular heart disease, 55–56
  ventricular tachycardia and fibrillation, 17–19
  Wolff-Parkinson-White syndrome, 19
Clomiphene, in fertility therapy, 112, 114
Clonal diseases
  B-cell lymphomas, 377
  T-cell lymphomas, 378
Clostridium botulinum, 341
Clostridium welchii, 164
Clotting. *See also* Coagulation; Factors, coagulation
  and disseminated intravascular coagulation, 183, 235
  process of, 231–233
Clotting factors, 159. *See also specific factors*
  activation of, 181, 182, 183
  defects in, 183–185
  in nephrotic syndrome, 299, 300
Clubbing
  with interstitial lung disease, 439
  with lung cancer, 458
  with patent ductus arteriosus, 63
Coagulation. *See also* Blood; Factors, coagulation
  cascade, 181, 182
  defects in, 181–185
  factors in, 159
Collagen
  aging and, 6
  fibers in collagen-vascular diseases, 209
  in idiopathic pulmonary fibrosis, 436
  parts of, in bones, 313
  source of, 315
Collagen-vascular diseases, 209–210
  with Bruton's agammaglobulinemia, 226
  etiology of, 206
  and interstitial lung disease, 434, 435
  nephrotic syndrome from, 300
Collagenases
  in osteoclasts, 315
  in rheumatoid arthritis, 207
Collateral venous circulation, with portal hypertension, 144
Colon
  cancer of the, 154, 361
  and diarrhea, 152
  function of, 149
Colony-stimulating factor (CSF)
  in leukemia, 173
  in neutrophil production, 169
Coma
  with hypercalcemia, 283
  from hypophosphatemia, 285
  with renal failure, 309
Complement system, 221–222
  activation of, 294, 295

Complement system—*Continued*
  alternative pathway in, 221–222
  classic pathway in, 221
  glomerular injury and the, 294
  and inflammation mediators, 233, 234
Compliance
  of cardiac chambers, 27, 28
  of lung, in asthma, 426
  and pressure-volume curves of lung, 406–407
Congenital diseases. *See also* Genetic diseases; Hereditary diseases
  adrenal hyperplasia and hypocortisolism, 93
  heart, 61–62
Congestive heart failure. *See* Heart failure, congestive
Conjunctivitis, in Reiter's syndrome, 209
Connective-tissue diseases, 222
Contraceptives, oral
  for androgen excess, 114
  pancreatitis from, 133
  and prolactin release, 88
Contractility, cardiac. *See* Myocardial contractility
Convalescence
  metabolic demands of, 463–471
  phases of, 468–469
  stimulus response patterns during, 469–470
Converting enzyme inhibitor, and angiotensin II, 296
Convulsions. *See also* Epilepsy
  with eclampsia, 475
  from hypophosphatemia, 285
Coronary angiography, 45
Coronary arterial spasm, myocardial infarction with, 43, 47
Coronary artery disease. *See also* Atherosclerosis; Myocardial ischemia
  angina pectoris, 46–47
  arteries affected by, 45
  clinical examples of, 48
  incidence of, 45
  myocardial infarction, acute, 47
  nonatherosclerotic, 40
  pathology of, 45–46
  sudden coronary death, 47–48
  symptoms of, 46
Coronary artery spasm, in myocardial ischemia, 40
Coronary death, sudden, 47–48
  clinical example of, 48
  as first symptom, 46
Coronary embolism, 41
Coronary, proximal, atherosclerosis in, 35
Cor pulmonale (pulmonary heart disease), 452–453
  in chronic air-flow limitation, 432
  with interstitial lung disease, 439
Corticosteroids
  for aspergillosis, 198
  for asthma, 197, 427
  Cushing's syndrome from, 204
  for lipoid nephrosis, 300

Corticosteroids—*Continued*
  for nephrotic syndrome, 301
  pancreatitis from, 133
  post-trauma use of, 468
  secondary immunodeficiency from, 224
  for surfactant production, 411
  for systemic lupus erythematosus, 204
Corticotropin releasing factor (CRF)
  and adrenocorticotropic hormone, 85
  in Cushing's syndrome, 368–369
  release of, 90, 91
Cortisol
  chemical structure of, 91
  deficiency and hyponatremia, 256
  hypercortisolism and, 92–94
  hypertension from, 102
  and insulin, 106
  in malnutrition, 349
  mechanism of action, 82
  normal secretion of, 90–91
  post-trauma gluconeogenesis and, 465–466, 467
  source of, 90
  synthesis of, 82
  in uremic syndrome, 310
Corynebacterium parvum, in cancer immunotherapy, 364
Coughing, mechanism of, 195
Coxsackie viruses, and diabetes mellitus, 107
C-peptide, in insulin, 106
C-reactive protein, in fever, 241
Creatine phosphate, in ischemia, 42
Creatinine (serum)
  age and, 6, 8
  in hypertension, 103, 105
Creatinine height index, 350
Creola bodies, in asthma, 421
Cricopharyngeus muscle, pressure of, 119
Crohn's disease, malnutrition with, 349
Cromolyn, for asthma, 427
Crystal-induced inflammation, 217–218
Curare, allergic reactions to, 189
Curschmann's spirals, in asthma, 421
Cushing's syndrome. *See also* Hypercortisolism
  with cancer, 368–369
    of lung, 458
    with renal cell carcinoma, 323
  clinical example of, 94–95, 204–205
  described, 92–93
  and pituitary hormones, 86
Cyanosis
  with interstitial lung disease, 439
  with patent ductus arteriosus, 63
  with preeclampsia, 475
Cyclic adenosine monophosphate (cAMP)
  in mast cell degranulation, 424
  and peptide hormones, 81
  and thyroid regulation, 96
  in vasopressin action, 87

Cyclic guanosine monophosphate (cGMP), and peptide hormones, 81
Cyclophosphamide, for lymphoma, 361
Cystic duct
  anatomy of, 137
  obstruction of, 138
Cystic fibrosis
  and chronic bronchitis, 430
  and pancreatitis, 134
Cysts
  renal, polycythemia from, 166
  subchondral bone, in osteoarthritis, 214
Cytomegalovirus, nephrotic syndrome from, 301
Cytotoxic drugs
  for breast cancer, 390
  secondary immunodeficiency from, 224

Death, coronary. *See* Coronary death, sudden
Decamethonium bromide, and neuromuscular transmission, 341–342
Dehydration. *See also* Water
  with asthma, 196
  with multiple myeloma, 381
7-Dehydrocholesterol, and vitamin D, 282
Dehydroepiandrosterone (DHEA), secretion of, 90, 111
Delta cells, pancreatic, 131
Demeclocycline, diabetes insipidus from, 87–88
Dementia, 8
Demethylchlortetracycline, prerenal azotemia with, 303
Dendrites, from nerve cells, 333
Depolarizing block, 342
Deoxycholic acid, in bile, 137
Deoxyribonucleic acid (DNA)
  antibodies to, in systemic lupus erythematosus, 210
  as antigen, in autoimmune complex diseases, 201
  in cell cycle, 358
  chemical damage to, 357
  DNA/anti-DNA complexes, 207
  synthesis in carcinogenesis, 355, 356
  synthesis impairment, 162
Depression
  and pain, 330, 331
  with renal failure, 309
Dermatitis, atopic, 192
Dermatomyositis (DM)
  pathogenesis of, 209
  and pulmonary hypertension, 451
Dexamethasone suppression test, for hypercortisolism, 92, 94
Dextrose, therapy and malnutrition, 349
Diabetes
  insipidus
    with multiple myeloma, 381
    pathogenesis and clinical aspects of, 87–88

Diabetes—*Continued*
  mellitus
    and atherosclerosus, 33
    and autoimmunity, 203
    chemotaxis inhibition in, 172
    clinical example of, 109–110
    and coronary artery disease, 48
    from hypercortisolism, 93
    hyperkalemia with, 264
    insulin-dependent (type I, IDDM), 106–107
    juvenile, 106–107
    and leukocyte migration, 236
    nephrotic syndrome from, 300
    neuropathy with, 343
    non-insulin-dependent (type II, NIDDM), 107–108
    with pancreatic cancer, 155
    with pancreatitis, 133, 134, 135
    and preeclampsia/eclampsia, 478
    small vessel coronary disease with, 40
Diabetic ketoacidosis
  fat oxidation and, 268
  hypophosphatemia with, 285
  pathophysiology and treatment of, 108–109
Diapedesis, of leukocytes, 232
Diarrhea
  classification of, 151–152
  definition of, 151
  metabolic acidosis from, 274–276
  metabolic alkalosis from, 273
  with protein-calorie malnutrition, 348
Diastolic compliance curve, 28
  in myocardial ischemia, 42
Diastolic depolarization
  enhanced, 16
  normal, 13
Diet
  and breast cancer, 386
  and pulmonary hypertension, 451
Diffusing capacity of the lung for carbon monoxide, 440
Diffusion impairment, pathophysiology of, 401–403
Di George syndrome, 224
Digestion
  of fat, 150
  normal, 149–150
Digitalis, and hyperkalemia, 265
1,25-Dihydroxycholecalciferol
  function of, 308
  mechanism of action, 82
  in osteomalacia, 318
  in rickets, 317
Dilantin, for epilepsy, 335
Diphosphoglycerate, in red blood cells, 66
2,3-Diphosphoglycerate (2,3-DPG), and oxyhemoglobin dissociation curve, 397
Disaccharidases
  action of, 149
  inadequate, 150
  hydrolization by, 149
  maldigestion and, 150
Disks, intervertebral
  anatomy of, 213, 214

Disks, intervertebral—*Continued*
  degenerative changes in, 3, 214–215
  herniated, 214–215
Disseminated intravascular coagulation (DIC), 183, 235
  with cancer, 373, 458
  cerebral hemorrhage from, 338
  with heat stroke, 243
  platelet consumption in, 177
  with preeclampsia/eclampsia, 477, 478–479
  and thrombocytopenia, 178
Distal tubule, and potassium excretion, 261
Diuresis
  hypokalemia from, 262, 266
  solute, prerenal azotemia with, 303
Diuretics
  gout and, 217
  hypophosphatemia from, 285
  loop, prerenal azotemia with, 303
  mercurial, nephrotic syndrome from, 300
  metabolic alkalosis from, 270
  for preeclampsia/eclampsia, 479
  and reduced plasma volume, 166
  and sodium and calcium excretion, 280
  thiazide
    hypercalcemia from, 285
    and megakaryocyte production, 176
    metabolic alkalosis from, 273
    and pancreatitis, 133
    and sodium and calcium excretion, 280
    and thrombocytopenia, 178
DNA. See Deoxyribonucleic acid.
Dopamine
  inhibitors of, 86
  and lower esophageal sphincter pressure, 120
  and prolactin release, 85
  for systemic arterial pressure, 75
Drug addiction
  pancreatitis with, 134
  withdrawal and epilepsy, 334
Drug intoxication, hypoventilation with, 398
Drugs. *See also specific drug names*
  anaphylaxis from, 192
  antiepileptic, 334, 335
  antigens in immune complex diseases, 201
  for asthma, 427
  and cancer, 358–360
  chemotherapeutic and neutrophil production, 171
  for distributive shock, 76
  dosage and age, 5
  enteric-coated, malabsorption of, 152
  for heart failure, 71
  hypothyroidism and, 98
  and immune platelet destruction, 176–177
  and lower esophageal sphincter pressure, 120
  neutropenia and, 171

Drugs—*Continued*
  pancreatitis and, 133
  and platelet aggregation, 36
  and platelet production, 176
  and renal function, 6
  sweat inhibitors, 242
  thrombocytopenia from, 178
  vasodilators, 103
  and vasopressin release, 87
Ductus arteriosus
  closure of, 60
  patent, 62
Duodenal bulb, ulcers in, 127, 128
Duodenal mucosal disease, 150
Duodenum
  cholecystokinin from, 137
  disease of, and ulcers, 127, 128–129
  function of, 126
  pancreatic influence on, 131
Dysphagia
  with achalasia, 122
  in esophageal cancer, 154
  in esophageal diseases, 120–121, 122, 123, 124
  with lung cancer, 451
  oropharyngeal, 120
Dyspnea
  with angina pectoris, 48
  with aortic regurgitation, 54
  with aortic stenosis, 54
  with asthma, 196, 427
  with heart failure, 70
  with interstitial lung disease, 438
  with lung cancer, 457
  with mitral regurgitation, 52
  with mitral stenosis, 52
  with myocardial infarction, 44
  pathophysiology of, 418

Ear, infection and lateral sinus thrombosis, 338
Eaton-Lambert syndrome with lung cancer, 458
Echocardiogram
  of cardiac tamponade, 76
  of mitral stenosis, 56
  of ventricular pressure overload, 31
Eclampsia. *See* Preeclampsia/eclampsia
Ectopic ventricular beat, on electrocardiogram, 18
Eczema, atopic, 192
Edema
  with acute glomerulonephritis, 296
  angioneurotic (hereditary), 222
  causes of, 251
  cerebral, signs of, 338
  with chronic hypertension, 475
  in nephrotic syndrome, 299
  peripheral, with kwashiorkor, 348
  with preeclampsia, 475
  pulmonary. *See* Pulmonary edema
  from renal cell carcinoma, 322
  from sodium excess, 251
Edrophonium, and lower esophageal sphincter pressure, 120
Ehlers-Danlos syndrome, connective tissue in, 209
Eisenmenger physiology, 62
Elastase, in pancreas, 132, 133

Elastic elements, myocardial, 21, 22
Elastin, in bones, 313
Elastomucase, in pancreas, 132
Electrocardiogram
  and age, 6
  in angina pectoris, 48
  of heart block, 19
  of mitral stenosis, 56
  normal, 17, 51
  of premature atrial beat, 19
  P wave in, 17, 19
  related to electrophysiology, 17
  S-T segments in coronary artery disease, 42, 43
  of supraventricular tachycardia, 19
  T wave in, 17
  of ventricular ectopic firing, 18
  of ventricular tachycardia, 18
  in ventricular volume overload, 30–31
  in Wolff-Parkinson-White syndrome, 19
Electroencephalogram
  of epileptic seizures, 334
  origin of electrical activity in, 333
Electrolyte
  absorption of, 150
  imbalance in hepatic encephalopathy, 146
  pancreatic secretion of, 131
  therapy and malnutrition, 349
Electromyography, single-fiber, 342
Electrophoresis, serum and urine protein, 379
Electrophysiology
  abnormal cardiac, 14–17
  normal cardiac, 11–14
Electroshock therapy, epilepsy from, 334
Embolism
  cerebral arterial occlusion from, 337
  with mitral regurgitation, 53
  with mitral stenosis, 52
Emphysema, 430
  alveolar ventilation in, 415
  clinical features of, 432
  inflammation and, 235
  and lung volumes, 407
  pathologic features of, 431
  and pulmonary vascular disease, 451
Empyema, with cholecystitis, 138–139
Encephalopathy
  dialysis effect on, 310–311
  hepatic, 145–147
    with cancer, 155
    with cirrhosis, 144
    clinical example of, 146–147
    respiratory alkalosis from, 414
  from hypernatremia, 255
  metabolic, differential diagnosis, 8
Encrustation, theory of atherogenesis, 35
End-diastolic pressure
  as ventricle preload, 27
  and volume overload, 28
End-diastolic volume, normal, 30

Endocarditis
  bacterial
    with mitral regurgitation, 53
    with mitral stenosis, 52
    mycotic aneurysms from, 338
  and coronary embolism, 41
  marantic, with lung cancer, 458
Endocrine glands. See also specific
    glands
  adrenal cortex, 90–95
  adrenal medulla, 90
  hormones from, 81–83
  hormone-receptor diseases, 82–
    83
  hyperplasia of, 82
Endocrinology, reproductive, 111–
    115
Endomitosis, of megakaryoblast, 175
Endoperoxides, and platelet aggrega-
    tion, 233
Endoplasmic reticulum, in tumor
    cells, 355
Endorphins, in beta-lipotropin, 85
Endoskeleton. See Bone
Endothelial cell
  in atherosclerosis, 36
  function of, in lung, 449
  pavementing by leukocytes, 232
  types of, 232
  and vascular permeability, 231–
    232
Endothelium, leukocyte migration
    through, 232
End-systolic pressure (ventricular), in
    pressure overload, 30
End-systolic pressure-volume relation-
    ship, 27, 28, 29
Enkephalin, and pain receptors, 328
Enterokinase
  action of, 149
  in pancreas, 132
  and trypsin, 131
Enteropathy
  gluten-sensitive, 150, 151, 152
  protein-losing and malnutrition,
    349
  protein-losing and secondary
    immunodeficiency, 224
Entrapment syndrome, and axonal
    function, 341
Enzymes. See also names of specific en-
    zymes
  activation of, 81
  and myocardium oxygen use, 41
  pancreatic, 132, 149
  renin, 91
Eosinophil arylsulfatase, in allergic
    reactions, 191
Eosinophil-chemotactic factor of
    anaphylaxis (ECF-A), in
    asthma, 423, 424
Eosinophilia
  with lung cancer, 458
  with renal cell carcinoma, 322
Eosinophils
  in allergic rhinitis and asthma, 195,
    196, 197, 421, 422
  endogenous pyrogen from, 241
  in type I allergic reactions, 191
Ephapses, 330

Epilepsy, 333–336
  clinical examples of, 334–335
  evaluation and management of, 334
Epinephrine
  for asthma, 424
  and hyperkalemia, 264
  and insulin, 106
  and lower esophageal sphincter
    pressure, 120
  with pheochromocytoma, 102
  post-trauma effect on metabolism
    of, 465
Epithelial cells, in asthma, 421
Epstein-Barr virus
  in cancer, 356–357
  nephrotic syndrome from, 301
Equal pressure point, in air flow, 409,
    410
Erythema nodosum, with vasculitis,
    203
Erythroblasts, 162, 163
Erythrocyte
  anemia and, 161–163
  destruction of (hemolysis), 163–165
  function of, 160
  glucose metabolism in, 464
  increase, 165–166
  normal production and regulation
    of, 159, 160–161
Erythrocytosis
  relative, 166
  with renal cell carcinomas, 371
Erythron, defined, 160
Erythropoiesis
  autonomous, 166
  ineffective, 162
Erythropoietin
  action of, 160, 161
  in cancers, 322, 370, 371
  excessive, 166
  function of, 308
  inadequate and anemia, 161
  in uremic syndrome, 310
Erythropoietin-responsive cells (ERC),
    160
Escherichia coli, in septic shock, 75
Esophageal manometry, 122
Esophageal spasm
  diffuse, 122
  pain from, 121
Esophagoscopy, 122
Esophagus, 119–124
  anatomy and physiology of, 119–
    120
  cancer of, 154
  diseases of, 122–124
  symptoms of problems in, 120–121
  tools to study, 121–122
C1 esterase inhibitor deficiency, 222
Esterase, in pancreas, 132
Estradiol
  mechanism of action, 82
  source of, 90, 113
Estrogen
  deficiency and ovarian failure, 113
  function of, 113
  and hyperprolactinemia, 86
  hypertension, 105
  and lower esophageal sphincter
    pressure, 120

Estrogen—Continued
  and megakaryocyte production, 176
  in ovulation, 112
  and prolactin release, 88
  receptors in breast cancer, 388, 390
  therapy, 114
  and thrombocytopenia, 178
Estrone
  in polycystic ovary syndrome, 114
  source of, 113
Ethanol. See also Alcohol
  and lower esophageal sphincter
    pressure, 120
  and thrombocytopenia, 178
Ethosuximide, for epilepsy, 335
Ethylene glycol, and metabolic
    acidosis, 271
Ethylenediaminetetraacetic acid
    (EDTA)
  and hypocalcemia, 284
  spurious thrombocytopenia and,
    178
Etiocholanalone, and body tempera-
    ture, 241
Eunuchoidism
  in Kallman's syndrome, 112
  in Kleinfelter's syndrome, 111
Excitation, cardiac
  abnormal, 14–17
  normal, 11–14
Exercise
  hypoxemia and, 402, 403
  and lipid disorders, 36, 37
Extensor plantar response, 340
Extracellular fluid
  potassium content of, 260
  sodium influence on, 247–249
  volume contraction, 249–251
  volume expansion, 251–252, 258
  volume and hyponatremia, 256
Eyes
  aging and the, 4
  immune complex diseases and the,
    203
  metastatic calcification in the, 283

Factors, coagulation, 159, 181–185
  in malignancies, 373
  clotting cascade, 181, 182
  VIII
    in atherosclerosis, 36
    in hemophilia, 183
    in von Willebrand's disease, 178–
      179, 184
  IX
    deficiency, 183
  X, and disseminated intravascular
    coagulation, 373
    in clotting mechanism, 181, 182
  XII, as inflammation mediator,
    233–235
Fanconi syndrome
  hypocalcemia with, 284
  hypophosphatemia with, 285
  with multiple myeloma, 381
Farmer's lung, 198
Fasting, metabolism during, 464–
    465

Fats
  depletion of, with malnutrition, 347
  diarrhea from, 151
  incomplete oxidation of, 268
  maldigestion of, 150–151
  normal body store of, 464
  nutritional requirement for, 347
  post-trauma metabolism of, 466
Fatty acids
  and cholecystokinin-pancreozymin, 149
  in diabetic ketoacidosis, 108
  in diarrhea, 152
  in gluconeogenesis, 466
  and hormone release, 85
  insulin and, 106
  myocardium use of, 41
Fatty meal, and lower esophageal sphincter pressure, 120
Felty's syndrome
  and granulocyte production, 171
  shift neutropenia in, 171–172
Feminization, with renal cell carcinoma, 323
Fetus, circulation in the 58–59, 60, 61
Fever
  defined, 239
  mechanisms of, 240–241
  role of, in disease, 241–242
Fever of undetermined origin (FUO), 242
Fibers
  afferent, 328
  myelinated and unmyelinated, 333, 340, 341
Fibrin
  in arrest of tumors, 389
  and glomerular injury, 295
Fibrinogen
  in atherosclerosis, 34
  defective, with cancer, 373
  and platelet aggregation, 233
Fibrinoid necrosis, in collagen-vascular diseases, 209
Fibrinolytic process, 231–233
Fibrinopeptides, in inflammation, 233
Fibroblast, 34–35
Fibromas, uterine, 371
Fibrosis, pulmonary
  with interstitial lung disease, 434
  respiratory alkalosis from, 414
  with rheumatoid arthritis, 208
Filariasis, nephrotic syndrome from, 300
Fistula, protein malnutrition with, 349
Flow-volume loop, 409, 410, 411
  in asthma, 426
Fluid accumulation, with heart failure, 70
Folate deficiency, 178
Foley, E.J., 362
Folic acid deficiency, 162, 178
  with cancer, 372
  with uremic syndrome, 310
Follicle-stimulating hormone (FSH)
  disorders of, 86
  in hypogonadism, 111, 112
  in ovulation, 112, 113

Follicle-stimulating hormone (FSH)—
    Continued
  in polycystic ovary syndrome, 114
  function of, 85
  spermatogenesis and, 111
Foramen ovale, 60
Forebrain, in pain mediation, 329
Frank-Starling curve (mechanism), 24–25, 27, 65
  in coronary occlusion, 42
  in heart failure, 66, 67–68
  in pressure overload, 30
  in volume overload, 28, 29
Frontal lobe, and association, 334
Fundus, gastric, function of, 125, 126
Fungal infections, disseminated, 223
  causing arthritis, 206
  associated with immunodeficiency states, 225
Fungi, as allergens, 198

Galactorrhea
  clinical example of, 88–89
  with prolactin-secreting tumor, 86
  with renal cell carcinoma, 323
Gallbladder, anatomy and physiology of, 137
Gallstones, 137–139
  clinical example of, 139
  and pancreatitis, 132–133, 135
Gamma globulin, for Bruton's agammaglobulinemia, 226
Gammopathy, benign monoclonal, 382
Ganglionic blockade, 76
Gangrene
  with cholecystitis, 139
  with vasculitis, 203
Gas, diffusion through a membrane, 401, 402
Gas exchange
  in asthma attacks, 426–427
  in interstitial lung disease, 438
  pulmonary, 395–404
Gastrectomy, and neutropenia, 174
Gastric alkalinization, 120
Gastric enzyme/acid deficiency, 150
Gastric inhibitory peptide (GIP) hormone, 120
Gastric outlet obstruction, with ulcers, 127, 128
Gastrin
  excess, with uremia, 310
  as hydrochloric acid agonist, 125
  and lower esophageal sphincter pressure, 120
  from tumors, 370
Gastrinoma, 128
Gastrin-producing cells (G-cells), 125, 126
Gastritis
  acute erosive, 126
  chronic atrophic, 126
  hemorrhagic, clinical example, 129
Gastrohepatic ligament, ulcer penetration in, 128
Gastrojejunostomy, 155
Gaucher's disease
  platelet pooling in, 177–178
  and thrombocytopenia, 178

Gell-Coomb's classification, 189, 200–203. See also Hypersensitivity diseases
Genetic diseases. See also Inherited diseases
  breast cancer, 386
  glomerulonephritis, 290
  hemophilia, 183
  leukemia, 172
  rheumatic disease, 207
  vitamin D-resistant rickets, 317
Geodes, in osteoarthritis, 214
Gigantism, from acromegaly, 86
Glands. See names of specific glands
Glaucoma, aging and, 4, 8
Globus hystericus, 121
Glomerular capillary endotheliosis, 477–478
Glomerular filtration rate
  in acute glomerulonephritis, 296
  in acute renal failure, 305
  aging and the, 5
  and calcium filtration, 280
  in hypokalemia, 263
  normal, 303
  in preeclampsia/eclampsia, 478
  in pregnancy, 476
  in renal hypertension, 103
Glomerulonephritis
  acute
    clinical characteristics of, 296
    clinical example of, 297
    with renal parenchymal azotemia, 305
  anti-glomerular basement membrane disease, 290–292
  in Goodpasture's syndrome, 203
  hypertension with, 104
  immunopathogenesis of, 287–292
  in situ immune complex disease, 292
  membranoproliferative, 295, 300
  mechanisms of damage in, 292, 294–295
  from renal cell carcinoma, 323
  in Sjögren's syndrome, 210
Glomerulopathy, with multiple myeloma, 381
Glomerulus
  as calcium filter, 279
  immune complex disease in, 202
  in lupus erythematosus, 204
  phosphate filtration by, 281
Glucagon
  and insulin, 106
  and lower esophageal sphincter pressure, 120
  post-trauma metabolic effect of, 465, 466
  source of, 131
  from tumors, 370
Glucocorticoids
  hypokalemia from, 262
  metabolic effects of, 93
  and thyroid hormones, 96
  and vasopressin release, 87
Gluconeogenesis, 464–465
  insulin and, 106
Glucose
  brain consumption of, 337

Glucose—*Continued*
  in diabetic ketoacidosis, 109
  hormones affecting production, 106
  and hormone release, 85
  insulin and formation of, 106
  metabolism of, 464–465
  oxidation of, 42
  tolerance with hypokalemia, 264
Glucose-6-phosphate dehydrogenase
  deficiency of, 172
  in neutrophil bacterial killing, 170
Glutamine, ammonia from, 272
Glutathione peroxidase
  deficiency, 172
  in neutrophil bacterial killing, 170
Glycine
  in bile, 137
  in bones, 313
Glycogen
  calories from, 464
  depletion of, 347
  digestion of, 149
  in starvation diet, 465
Glycogenolysis
  insulin and, 106
  and ischemia, 41
Glycolysis, anaerobic, in tumor cells, 355
Glycolytic flux, and ischemia, 41
Glycoprotein
  in bones, 313
  in cell communication, 355
Glycosaminoglycans, in joints, 213
Goiter, multinodular, hyperthyroidism with, 97
Golgi apparatus
  in cell, 333
  and peptide hormones, 81
Gompertzian growth, 358
Gonadal steroids, mechanism of, 82
Gonadotropin-releasing hormone, 112
Gonadotropins
  elevated, 113
  human chorionic, 112, 370
  prolactin and, 85
  in spermatogenesis therapy, 112
Gonads, 111–112
Gonococci, in infectious arthritis, 206
Goodpasture's syndrome
  glomerulonephritis in, 292
  and interstitial lung disease, 435
  mechanisms of, 203
Gout, 200, 215–216
  clinical example of, 218
  hyperuricemia with, 216, 217
  with leukemia, 173
  secondary, 217
Gram-negative infections, shock with, 76
Gram-positive infections, shock with, 76
Granulocyte-releasing factor, and neutrophil production, 169
Granulocytes
  endogenous pyrogen from, 241
  in leukemia, 173
  production of, 169
  origin of, 159, 375, 376
  in polycythemia rubra vera, 166
  suppressor T cells and, 171

Granuloma, eosinophilic, 435
Granulomatosis
  Wegener's, 202, 435
Granulomatous disease, chronic, 222
Granulopoiesis, and neutrophil production, 171
Granulopoietin, 169
Graves' disease. *See also* Hyperthyroidism
  antibodies in, 200
  clinical example of, 99–100
  hyperthyroidism from, 96–97, 98
  and pituitary hormones, 86
  type II hypersensitivity in, 203
Growth, impairment with malnutrition, 347
Growth hormone
  disorders of, 85, 86
  function of, 85
  and insulin, 106
  in malnutrition, 349
  post-trauma metabolic effect of, 465, 466
  release of, 85
  from tumors, 370
Growth kinetics in malignancy, 358–359
Guanidine, for Eaton-Lambert syndrome, 371
Guanidinosuccinic acid, and platelet dysfunction, 179
Guanosine monophosphate (GMP), cyclic, in mast cell degranulation, 424
Guanyl cyclase
  in asthma, 424
  in mast cell degranulation, 423, 424
Guillain-Barré syndrome
  and axonal function, 341
  clinical example of, 342
Guyton, Arthur C., 442, 443
Gynecomastia
  with cancer, 370
  with Kallman's syndrome, 112
  in Klinefelter's syndrome, 111
  with lung cancer, 458

Hageman factor. *See* Factors, coagulation, XII
Hair, aging and, 3
Halide, oxidation of, 172
Hallucinations, and hypercalcemia, 283
Haptoglobin, serum, with intravascular hemolysis, 164
Harris-Benedict formula, 350
Hearing, aging and, 4
Heart
  aging and the, 6
  circulation in the fetus, 58–60
  congenital disease of the, 61–62
  contractility, 26. *See also* Myocardial contractility
  defects of the, 62
  electrophysiology of the, 11–20
  muscle contraction of the, 21, 24–26
  normal physiology of the, 39
  shunts in the, 58–64
Heart block
  clinical example, 19–20
  from hypercalcemia, 283

Heart block—*Continued*
  from hyperkalemia, 264
  mechanism of, 16–17
Heartburn, mechanisms and symptoms of, 121, 123
Heart disease. *See also* Cardiovascular disease
  congenital
    and cerebral arterial occlusion, 337
    shunting with, 339
Heart failure, congestive, 65–72
  classification of, 66–67
  clinical examples of, 70–72
  compensatory mechanisms in, 65–66
  from essential hypertension, 104
  with heat stroke, 243
  hemodynamic alterations with, 70–71
  hyponatremia from, 256
  from hypophosphatemia, 285
  with macroglobulinemia, 382
  from myocardial infarction, 47
  pathologic and physiologic correlations of, 71
  physiologic consequences of, 67–70
  with renal cell carcinoma, 322
  with renal failure, 309
  respiratory alkalosis from, 414
  symptoms of, 70–71
  systemic adaptation to, 65–66
Heart failure, right ventricular
  with chronic air-flow limitation, 432
  from cor pulmonale, 453
  lymphatic drainage with, 446
  pathophysiology of, 451
  and portal hypertension, 143
  with primary pulmonary hypertension, 451
  with pulmonary thromboemboli, 452
Heart rate
  influences on, 101
  normal, 30
Heart sounds
  in aortic regurgitation, 54
  in aortic stenosis, 54, 56
  in heart failure, 70
  in interstitial lung disease, 439
  in intracardiac shunting, 62–63
  in mitral regurgitation, 53, 56
  in mitral stenosis, 52–53, 55–56
  normal, 50, 51
  in patent ductus arteriosus, 63
  in pulmonary stenosis, 55
  in pulmonic regurgitation, 55
  in tricuspid regurgitation, 54
  in tricuspid stenosis, 55
Heart valve, prosthetic, and thrombocytopenia, 177
Heat, nociceptors, 327
Heat cramps, 242
Heat exhaustion, 242
Heat illnesses, 239, 242–243
Heat stroke, 240, 242–243
  clinical example of, 243, 244
Heberden, William, 46
Helminths, and immunodeficiency states, 225
Hematemesis
  with cancers, 154
  with reflux esophagitis, 123
Hematochezia, with cancers, 154

Hematoma, intracranial, 338
Hematopoiesis, 159, 375, 376
Hematopoietic precursors, 375, 376
Hematuria
    with acute glomerulonephritis, 296
    from renal cell carcinoma, 322
Heme
    bilirubin from, 142, 160
    in sideroblastic anemias, 163
Hemochromatosis, and pancreatitis,
        134
Hemodialysis, neutropenia from, 172
Hemoglobin
    bilirubin from, 142
    defective synthesis of, 163
    and erythrocytes, 160
    as hydrogen ion buffer, 268
    oxygen-carrying capacity of, 396–
        397
    release into plasma, 164
    synthesis, iron in, 160
Hemoglobin A_{1c}, in diabetes, 107
Hemolysis
    in erythrocyte disorders, 163, 164
    hyperkalemia from, 265
    from hypophosphatemia, 285
    with renal failure, 309
Hemolytic uremic syndrome
    glomerular ischemia with, 296
    platelet consumption in, 177
    and thrombocytopenia, 178
Hemopexin, in intravascular hemoly-
        sis, 164
Hemophilia
    cerebral hemorrhage with, 338
    factor VIII deficiency in, 183
Hemoptysis
    in mitral regurgitation, 53
    in mitral stenosis, 52
Hemorrhage. *See also* Bleeding
    from acute erosive gastritis, 126
    cerebral, causes and symptoms of,
        338
    intracranial, with leukemia, 173
    in macroglobulinemia, 382
    in pancreatitis, 133
    with preeclampsia/eclampsia, 477,
        479
    pulmonary, in Goodpasture's syn-
        drome, 203
    secondary thrombocytosis with, 179
    shock from, 73–74
    subarachnoid, clinical example,
        338–339
    with ulcers, 127, 128
Hemorrhoids, 144
Hemosiderinuria, with intravascular
        hemolysis, 165
Hemostasis
    inflammation and, 235
    platelets and, 175–176
Heparin
    for glomerulonephritis, 295
    and platelet destruction, 177
Hepatic decompensation, with cir-
        rhosis, 144
Hepatic duct, anatomy of, 137
Hepatic glycogen synthesis, insulin
        and, 106
Hepatic failure. *See* Liver

Hepatic vein thrombosis, portal hy-
        pertension from, 143
Hepatitis
    acute fulminant, with hepatic en-
        cephalopathy, 146
    B viral infection
        glomerulonephritis from, 290
        nephrotic syndrome from, 301
        and polyarteritis nodosa, 203, 205
    viral
        with Bruton's agammaglobuline-
            mia, 226
        jaundice in, 143
Hepatomegaly
    with erythrocyte phagocytosis, 163
    with heart failure, 71
Hepatosplenomegaly, with macroglob-
        ulinemia, 382
Hereditary diseases. *See also* Genetic
        diseases
    asthma, 422
    complement system deficiencies,
        222
    defective chemotaxis and opsoniza-
        tion, 172
    diabetes mellitus, 107
    of endocrine glands, 82
    enzyme defects and gout, 217
    hypersensitivity diseases, 190
    immunodeficiencies, 222–223
    Kallman's syndrome (hypogonad-
        ism), 112
    myopathies, 342
    nephritis, 300
    nephrogenic diabetes insipidus, 87
    pancreatitis, 134
    Sjögren's syndrome, 211
    stem cell defects, 171–172
    thrombocytopenia, 176
    Turner's syndrome, 113
Hernia, hiatal, in reflux esophagitis,
        123
Heroin, nephrotic syndrome from,
        300
Herpesvirus, nephrotic syndrome
        from, 301
Hexose monophosphate, in neutro-
        phil bacterial killing, 170
Hip, osteoarthritis in the, 215
Hirsutism
    from androgen excess, 113–114
    from hypercortisolism, 93
His bundles
    excitation and the, 13, 14
    firing rates of, 16–17
Histaminases, in allergic reactions, 191
Histamine
    as allergic reaction mediator, 190–
        191, 195
    in asthma, 423
    and glomerular injury, 294–295
    as hydrochloric acid agonist, 125
    and impaired chemotaxis, 172
    as inflammation mediator, 233, 234
    and irritant receptors, 425
    and lower esophageal sphincter
        pressure, 120
    from mast cells and basophils, 190
    in mast cell degranulation, 424
    and pain nociceptors, 327

Histamine—*Continued*
    and pulmonary vascular resistance,
        451
    and stomach acid regulation, 191
    ulcers and, 127
Histidine, histamine from, 191
Histidine decarboxylase, in mast cells
        and basophils, 190
Histocompatibility antigen
    HLA-B27, in seronegative spondy-
        loarthropathies, 208, 209
    HLA-D/DR, in transplantation,
        220–221
Hives. *See* Urticaria (hives)
Hodgkin's disease, 382–383
    anergy in, 223
    clinical example of, 384
    doubling time in, 360
    nephrotic syndrome from, 300
Hormones. *See also* specific hormones
    adrenocortical, 90–95
    adrenocorticotropic, 82
    blood cell producing, 160
    causing hypertension, 101–102
    diseases of, 82–83
    female sex and immune system, 204
    for glucose homeostasis, 106
    and lower esophageal sphincter
        pressure, 120
    mechanism of action, 81
    pancreatic, 149
    pituitary, 85–87
    reproductive, 111–115
    and breast cancer, 388
    steroid, 82
    testicular feminization, clinical ex-
        ample, 83
    thymic, 7
    thyroid, 96–100
    tumor produced, 370
Human chorionic gonadotropin
        (HCG), 112
Hyaline articular cartilage, 213
Hyaline membrane disease, from sur-
        factant deficiency, 411
Hydatidiform mole, and preeclamp-
        sia, 475, 478
Hydralazine
    for low output heart failure, 71
    for preeclampsia/eclampsia, 480
Hydrocephalus, differential diagnosis, 8
Hydrochloric acid (HCl)
    in chronic atrophic gastritis, 126
    metabolic acidosis from, 271
    normal secretion of, 125
    in ulcers, 126–127, 128
    and vitamin B_{12}, 149
Hydrogen ion
    and pain nociceptors, 327
    and potassium concentration, 261
    in stomach ulcers, 127
Hydrogen ion homeostasis, 268
    disturbances of, 269–277
Hydrogen peroxide, in neutrophil
        bacterial killing, 171
Hydrolysis, in digestion, 150
Hydronephrosis, polycythemia from,
        166
Hydroxyapatite, in bone mineraliza-
        tion, 313

Hydroxyl radicals, in neutrophil bacterial killing, 171
Hydroxyproline, in bones, 313
5-Hydroxytryptamine. See Serotonin
Hymenoptera, anaphylaxis from sting, 190
Hyperadrenergic states, 82
Hyperaldosteronism
  hypokalemia from, 262
  metabolic alkalosis from, 273
Hyperalimentation
  hypokalemia from, 262
  hypophosphatemia with, 285
Hyperbilirubinemia
  familial unconjugated non-hemolytic, 143
  as sign of hemolytic disease, 163
Hypercalcemia, 282–283. See also Calcium
  with cancer, 324, 369–370
  clinical example of, 285–286
  from hyperparathyroidism, 319
  and lung cancer, 458
  metabolic alkalosis from, 273
  with multiple myeloma, 379, 381
  nephrogenic diabetes insipidus from, 87–88
  with renal cell carcinoma, 322, 323
  kidney stones from, 286
Hypercapnia
  alveolar, and pulmonary vascular resistance, 451
  with asthma, 196
  causes of, 414
  complications of, 414–415
  diagnosis of, 417
  with lung disease, 415, 417
  respiratory acidosis with, 413–414, 417
Hypercholesterolemia, in atherosclerosis, 35, 36
Hypercoagulation
  with cancer, 373
  in nephrotic syndrome, 300
Hypercortisolism. See also Cushing's syndrome
  with cancer, 368–369
  clinical example of, 94–95
  effects of, 92
Hyperglobulinemia
  with renal cell carcinoma, 323
  in Sjögren's syndrome, 211
Hyperglycemia, 264–265
  with ketoacidosis, 108
  post-traumatic, 465, 466
  with renal failure, 309
Hyperinflation, defined, 430
Hyperkalemia, 264–265
  with acute renal failure, 307
  clinical example of, 266–267
  dialysis effect on, 310–311
  post-traumatic, 467
Hyperlipoproteinemia, 38
  in nephrotic syndrome, 298
  and pancreatitis, 133
  with renal failure, 309, 310
Hypermetabolism, from pheochromocytoma, 102
Hypernatremia, 253–256
  clinical example of, 257–258
  and vasopressin secretion, 87

Hypernephromas, 322–324. See also Renal cell carcinoma
Hyperosmolality, 253–256
Hyperostosis, and uremic syndrome, 310
Hyperparathyroidism
  clinical example of, 285–286
  hypercalcemia from, 282
  hypophosphatemia with, 285
  with osteomalacia, 318
  and phosphate clearance, 281
  primary, 319
  with renal failure, 309, 310
Hyperphosphatemia, acute, 284
Hyperpigmentation, with Cushing's syndrome, 369
Hyperplasia
  adrenal, aldosteronism with, 103
  lymphoid, antibody production in, 220
Hyperpnea, with shock, 74
Hyperprolactinemia, 86–87
Hyperreflexia, 340
Hypersensitivity
  age and, 7
  angiitis, and interstitial lung disease, 435
  leukocytes and, 221
Hypersensitivity diseases
  anaphylaxis, 192
  type I, immediate, 189–193
    allergic rhinitis, 195–199
    asthma, 195–199, 422–429
    atopic dermatitis or eczema, 192
    as autoimmune disease, 203
    clinical example of, 192–193
    intensity of, 191
    list of diseases, 189
    mechanisms of, 189–191
    urticaria, 191–192
  type II, 200–203
  type III. See Immune complex diseases (type III hypersensitivity)
  type IV, 200, 203
Hypersplenism
  erythrocytes in, 163
  neutrophils pooled in, 171
Hypertension, 101–105
  with acute glomerulonephritis, 296
  with angina pectoris, 48
  with atherosclerosis, 33, 34
  chronic, with superimposed preeclampsia, 475–476
  clinical example of, 104–105
  definition of, 101, 475
  and diabetes, 107
  endocrine models of, 102–104
  essential (idiopathic), 104
  hormones affecting, 101–102
  with hypercalcemia, 283
  from hypercortisolism, 93, 310
  jugular venous pulsation in, 52
  malignant, nephrotic syndrome from, 301
  mechanism of, 67
  with mitral stenosis, 52
  portal
    ascites with, 144
    clinical example of, 147
    with hepatic cancer, 155
    intrahepatic causes, 143–144
    platelet pooling in, 177

Hypertension, portal—Continued
  and thrombocytopenia, 178
  with pregnancy, 475–482. See also Preeclampsia/eclampsia
  pulmonary
    with asthma, 196
    clinical example of, 453
    cor pulmonale from, 452–453
    primary, 451–452
    and pulmonary thromboemboli, 452
  with renal cell carcinoma, 322
  with renal failure, 309
  and ventricular pressure overload, 31
  volume-dependent, and dialysis, 310–311
Hyperthermia, 239
  causes of, 240
Hyperthyroidism. See also Graves' disease
  bones in, 319
  clinical aspects of, 97
  clinical example of, 99–100
  heart failure with, 66
  malnutrition with, 349
  pathogenesis of, 96–97
  treatment of, 98
Hypertrophy
  in heart failure compensation, 65
  with mitral stenosis, 52
  in ventricular pressure overload, 30
  with volume overload, 29, 30
Hyperuricemia, 216
  gout with, 216, 217
  with multiple myeloma, 381
Hyperuricosuria, from salicylates, 217
Hyperventilation
  central neurogenic and respiratory alkalosis, 414
  with pulmonary hypertension, 452
Hyperviscosity
  with multiple myeloma, 381
  syndrome, of macroglobulinemia, 382
Hypnosis, and pain, 331
Hypoalbuminemia
  with acute glomerulonephritis, 296
  with multiple myeloma, 381
  in nephrotic syndrome, 298, 299
  with renal cell carcinoma, 323
Hypoaldosteronism, hyperkalemia with, 265
Hypoaminoacidemia, with uremic syndrome, 310
Hypocalcemia. See also Calcium
  described, 283–284
  epilepsy from, 334
  with leukemia, 173
  in pancreatitis, 133
  and parathyroid hormone, 281
  in renal osteodystrophy, 318
Hypocapnia, 413
  with asthma, 426
Hypocortisolism, clinical manifestations of, 93–94
Hypogammaglobulinemia, with multiple myeloma, 379
Hypoglycemia
  from cancer, 370
  cerebral effects, 338
  epilepsy from, 334
  and hydrochloric acid production, 125
  with lung cancer, 458

Hypogonadism
from acromegaly, 86
ovarian, 113
and pituitary gland, 86
primary, 111–112
with prolactin-secreting tumor, 86
secondary, 112
Hypokalemia, 261–264
causes of, 262
clinical example of, 265–266
with leukemia, 173
nephrogenic diabetes insipidus
from, 87–88
Hypomagnesemia. *See also* Magnesium
hypokalemia with, 262
hypophosphatemia with, 285
Hyponatremia, 256–257
clinical example of, 258
dialysis effect on, 310–311
epilepsy from, 334
with hyperkalemia, clinical example, 470–471
from hypocortisolism, 94
postoperative, 467
from SIADH, 88, 370
from sodium depletion, 251
Hypoosmolality, 256–257. *See also* Hyponatremia
Hypoparathyroidism
and hypocalcemia, 283
metabolic alkalosis from, 273
Hypophosphatemia, 284–285
from hyperparathyroidism, 286, 319
respiratory alkalosis from, 414
with vitamin D-resistant rickets, 317
and vitamin D synthesis, 282
Hypopituitarism
causes of, 85
secondary hypogonadism from, 112
Hypoproteinemia, with uremic syndrome, 310
Hypospadias, in Reifenstein's syndrome, 111
Hypotension
with acidemia, 272
with anaphylaxis, 192
with myocardial infarction, 44
with pancreatitis, 133
with renal cell carcinoma, 323
Hypothalamus
acromegaly and, 86
and body heat regulation, 238, 240
and cortisol regulation, 90
in diabetes insipidus, 87
and gonadotropin-releasing hormone, 112
in hyperprolactinemia, 86
and hypopituitarism, 85
and ovarian failure, 113
and pain pathways, 328
and pituitary hormone secretion, 85
and vasopressin release, 87
Hypothyroidism
and hyperprolactinemia, 88
hyponatremia from, 257
pathogenesis and treatment of, 98–99
from thyroid-stimulating hormone deficiency, 85, 86

Hypouricemia, from salicylates, 217
Hypoventilation, 398–399
clinical examples of, 403–404
effects of, on PaO_2, 398
Hypovolemia
with pancreatitis, 133
and vasopressin release, 87
Hypoxemia
with asthma, 196, 426
clinical examples of, 403–404, 418–419
with interstitial lung disease, 438
with pulmonary hypertension, 452
with pulmonary thromboemboli, 452
respiratory alkalosis from, 414
Hypoxia
alveolar
pulmonary hypertension from, 453
and pulmonary vascular disease, 451
cerebral hypoperfusion with, 338
with inflammation, 235
sensor tissue, 160
Hysteria, chronic pain with, 330

Icterus, scleral, with gallstones, 139
Idiogenic osmoles, in hypernatremia, 255
Ileitis, destruction and vitamin B_{12} deficiency, 167
Ileus, adynamic
from hypokalemia, 263
with pancreatitis, 133
Immune complex diseases (type III hypersensitivity)
antigens in, 201
autoimmunity in, 207
clinical example of, 204–205
glomerulonephritis, 287, 290
in situ, 292
mechanisms in, 201–203
in New Zealand mice, 290
with parasitic disease, 290
studies of, 287, 290
viral-induced, 290
Immune complexes, circulating, 201
Immune mechanisms, type IV cell-mediated, 198
Immune system, 220
aging and the, 7–8
and antigen-stimulated lymphoid differentiation, 375–377
chronic inflammation and, 235
complement system and, 221–222
in Hodgkin's disease, 383
and hypersensitivity, 189–193
lymphocyte function in, 220–221
in myasthenic syndromes, 371
neoplasms of, 375–385
normal physiology of, 375–377
in protein-calorie malnutrition, 348
and tumor growth, 362–366
Immunodeficiencies, 220–224
and cancer incidence, 363
clinical evaluation of, 223
clinical example of, 223, 225–226
congenital, 222–223
list of, 224

Immunodeficiencies—*Continued*
in preeclampsia/eclampsia, 478
severe combined, 224
tests for evaluation of, 226
Immunofluorescent microscopy, 287, 288, 290, 291
Immunoglobulins, general
as B lymphocyte markers, 220
that activate complement, 221–222
inherited deficiencies of, 172
in malnutrition, 348
Immunoglobulin A, deficiency, 223
Immunoglobulin E
and allergens, 189
in aspergillosis, 198
in asthma, 422–423
mediated reactions, 190
in Praustnitz-Küstner procedure, 190
production and function of, 190
Immunoglobulin G
and allergens, 189
in antibody-dependent cell-mediated cytotoxicity, 200
in anti-glomerular basement membrane disease, 290
as antigen in immune complex diseases, 201
in red cell aplasia, 372
rheumatoid factors, in arthritis, 207, 208
Immunoglobulin M
and allergens, 189
intracytoplasmic, in B cell differentiation, 377
monoclonal, in macroglobulinemia, 381–382
rheumatoid factors, and arthritis, 208
Immunologically mediated disease, 200–205. *See also* Hypersensitivity diseases
allergic respiratory, 194–199
immune complex, 200–203
kinds of, 200
rheumatic, 206–212
Immunology, transplantation, 362
Indomethacin
and platelet dysfunction, 179
as prostaglandin inhibitor, 369
Infection. *See also* Inflammation
kinds associated with immunodeficiency states, 225
malnutrition with, 349
with multiple myeloma, 379
post-traumatic, 470
Infertility
female, 113, 114
with hyperprolactinemia, 86
male, 112
with renal failure, 309
Inflammation
blood vessels in, 231–232
chronic, 233–234, 235
clinical example, 236
exaggerated, 235
granulomatous, 234–235
mediators of, 233, 234
swelling from, 231
Influenza, secondary immunodeficiency from, 224

Inherited diseases. *See also* Congenital diseases; Genetic diseases
  chronic granulomatous disease, 172
  panacinar emphysema, 431
  platelet dysfunction, 178–179, 184
  preeclampsia/eclampsia, 478
Inhibin, and spermatogenesis, 111
Injury. *See also* Trauma
  energy requirements after, 463
  metabolic response to, 463–471
Insecticides, and neuromuscular transmission, 342
Insect stings, anaphylaxis from, 190
Insudation theory, of atherosclerotic plaque formation, 35
Insulin
  in diabetic ketoacidosis, 108
  effects of, on metabolism, 106
  in hyperkalemia, 264
  in malnutrition, 349
  as peptide hormone, 81
  and potassium distribution, 261
  resistance in acanthosis nigricans, 200
  resistance and hypersensitivity, 203
  source and mechanism of action, 106, 131
  tumor, and secretion of "insulin-like" material, 370
  increased, in uremia, 310
Integument, in malnutrition, 348
Interferon
  as anti-cancer agent, 356, 364, 365
Interstitial fluid. *See also* Body fluids
  composition of, 247, 248
  in pregnancy, 476
  pressures, 442–445
  volume increased, 251
  volume reduced, 250
Interstitium, lung, 434, 435
Intestine
  large. *See* Colon
  small
    calcium absorption by, 279–280
    cancer of, 154
    and diarrhea, 152
    functions of, 149–150
    malabsorption in, 151
Intima, in atherosclerosis, 34
Intraaortic balloon pump (IABP), 75
Intracranial mass, differential diagnosis, 8
Intraesophageal pH monitoring, 122
Intraluminal acid, and cholecystokinin-pancreozymin, 149
Intramedullary hemolysis, 162
Intrinsic factor
  low secretion of, 126
  in malabsorption, 151
Iodine, radioactive, hypothyroidism from, 98
Iron
  deficiency anemia, 123, 163
  deficiency and thrombocytosis, 179
  in hemoglobin synthesis, 160
Irritant receptors, in asthma, 425
Ischemia
  chronic pain with, 330
  epilepsy from, 334
  glomerular, with acute glomerulonephritis, 296

Ischemia—*Continued*
  myocardial. *See* Myocardial ischemia
  renal, hypertension from, 103
  transient cerebral, 337, 339
Isohydremia, defined, 269
Isometric contraction, of myocardium, 21
Isoproterenol, and lower esophageal sphincter pressure, 120
Isotonic contraction, of myocardium, 21

Jaundice, 142–143
  cholestatic, 143
  with duodenal ulcer, 128
  with gallstones, 139
  hepatic, 143
  with hepatic cancer, 155
  with pancreatic cancer, 155
  with pancreatitis, 133, 135
  prehepatic, 143
Jejunum, phosphate absorption by, 281
Job's syndrome, and cell migration, 236
Joint (diarthroidal), 213, 214
Joints
  acromioclavicular, and osteoarthritis, 215
  crystal deposits in, 216, 217–218
  degenerative diseases of, 213–215
  interphalangeal, and osteoarthritis, 215
  lubrication of, 213
  metatarsophalangeal, and osteoarthritis, 215
Jugular venous distension, from heart failure, 70, 71
Jugular venous pressure
  in aortic stenosis, 54
  in mitral regurgitation, 53
  in mitral stenosis, 52
Jugular venous pulsation
  mechanism of, 50, 51
  in tricuspid stenosis, 55

Kallikrein
  as allergic reaction mediator, 190–191
  in inflammations, 233
Kallman's syndrome, 112
Karotyping, in Klinefelter's syndrome, 115
Keratin, in tumor cells, 456
Keratinization, in malnutrition, 348
Kerato-conjunctivitis sicca, with Sjögren's syndrome, 210
Ketoacidosis, diabetic, 107, 108–109
  metabolic acidosis from, 271
  potassium depletion with, 263
Ketones, in diabetic ketoacidosis, 108
17-Ketosteroids, excretion of, 90
Kidneys. *See also* all *Renal* entries
  in acid-base disorders, 270
  adaptations to renal failure, 308–309
  aging and the, 6
  albumin in, 298
  aldosterone action on, 101

Kidneys—*Continued*
  bicarbonate regulation by, 268, 271–272, 273, 277
  calcium filtering in, 280
  and erythrocyte production, 160–161
  and extracellular fluid volume, 248
  function of, 308
  in hyperkalemia, 264–265
  and hypokalemia, 263
  in nephrotic syndrome, 299
  nonvolatile acid excretion by, 268
  polycystic disease with hypertension, 104
  and potassium excretion, 260–261
  serum creatinine levels and function of, 105
  transplant, focal sclerosis with, 300
  uric acid removal by, 216
  urine concentration and dilution by, 252–253
  vasopressin and, 87–88
  and vitamin D synthesis, 284
  and water balance regulation, 252
Klinefelter's syndrome
  clinical example, 114–115
  hypogonadism from, 111
Knee, osteoarthritis in, 215
Kupffer cells, endogenous pyrogen from, 241
Kwashiorkor, 347–348

Lacrimal glands, in Sjögren's syndrome, 210
Lactate, in glucose metabolism, 464, 465
Lactation, hormone for, 85
Lactase, deficiency, and diarrhea, 151
Lactic acidemia, hyperuricemia from, 217
Lactose, in osmotic diarrhea, 151
Langerhans, islets of, in pancreatitis, 134
Laplace relationship, in volume overload, 29
Lazy leukocyte syndrome, 172
Lead, in bones, 313
Lead poisoning, and gout, 217
Lecithin, in bile, 137, 138
Lesions, mucocutaneous, in Reiter's syndrome, 209
Leukapheresis, thrombocytopenia with, 178
Leukemia, 172
  acute granulocytic, 172, 173
  acute, with Hodgkin's disease, 384
  acute lymphoblastic (ALL), 377
  acute monoblastic, 382
  acute, treatments for, 360
  blastic phase of, 173
  cerebral hemorrhage with, 338
  chronic
    gout with, 217
    granulocytic, 173, 179
    lymphocytic (CLL), 377–378
  immunizations for, 364
  and leukocyte production, 235–236
  myelomonoblastic, 382
  nephrotic syndrome from, 300
  from polycythemia, 166

Leukocytes
decreased migration of, 236
deficient numbers of, 235–236
dialysis effect on, 311
emigration of, through endothelium, 232–233
glucose metabolism of, 464
lazy leukocyte syndrome, 172
in megaloblastic anemia, 162
pavementing of, 232
polymorphonuclear, 7–8
mediators of glomerular injury,
284
pyrogen from, 241
Leukocytosis
with allergic alveolitis, 198
with cancer, 372
with cholecystitis, 138
hyperkalemia from, 265
with renal cell carcinoma, 322
Leukoerythroblastic phenomenon,
372
Leukopenia
with anemia, 161
with cancer, 372
with multiple myeloma, 379
neutropenia with, 171
Leukostasis, with leukemia, 173
Levamisole, in tumor immunity, 364–
365
Levothyroxine, 99
Leydig cells
in hypogonadism, 111
testosterone from, 111
Lindsey, Arthur W., 442
Lipase
and maldigestion, 150, 151
in pancreas, 131, 132, 149, 150
in pancreatitis, 133
Lipids
in bones, 313
disorders of, 37
insulin and synthesis of, 106
Lipofuscin pigment, 5
Lipolysis, insulin and, 106
Lipoproteins
and atherosclerosis, 33
high-density (HDL), 36–37
low-density (LDL), 36–37
in atherosclerosis, 34, 35, 36
in nephrotic syndrome, 299
very low-density (VLDL), 37
Lithium
hypothyroidism from, 98
nephrogenic diabetes insipidus
from, 87–88
prerenal azotemia with, 303
Lithocholic acid, in bile, 137
Liver, 141–148. See also all Hepatic entries
anatomy of, 141
anemia and disease of, 161
ascites with disease of, 144–145
blood flow in, 141–142, 143–144
cancer of, 155
cirrhosis of, 144, 145
clotting factors from, 181, 183
congestion with heart failure, 70–
71
disease, diffuse parenchymal, 284

Liver—Continued
erythropoietin from, 160
glucocorticoid effect on, 93
and granulocytes in leukemia, 173
in heat stroke, 243
hepatic encephalopathy in disease
of, 145–146
and jaundice, 142–143
in nephrotic syndrome, 299
platelet removal in, 175
portal hypertension in, 143–144
in preeclampsia, 475
in renal cell carcinoma, 323
vitamin D conversion in, 282
Livido reticularis, with vasculitis,
203
Lobectomy, 458
Log-kill hypothesis, 359–360
Lower esophageal sphincter (LES)
pressure, 119–120, 122–124
Lung. See also Pulmonary entries; Ventilation, alveolar
aging and the, 7
airflow in, 408–411
cancer. See Cancer, lung
and carbonic acid regulation, 269
circulatory system of, 449–451
diseases of. See Lung diseases
exaggerated inflammations in, 235
filter system, 449
flow/radius relationship in, 408
fluid balance and pressures in, 442–
445, 447
mechanics of, 405–412
in metabolic acidosis, 271
noncompliant, from surfactant
deficiencies, 411
physiology of, 395–398, 413
pressure-volume curve of, 406,
407
residual volume in, 407
static volumes of, 405–408
surface tension and inflation, 411
total capacity of, 407
transplantation and lymphatic function, 445–446
vascular disease of, 449–454
ventilation measurements, 425–427
volume-pressure curves with interstitial disease, 436
volumes with disease states, 407–
408, 426–427
Lung diseases
asthma, 421–429. See also Asthma
chronic airflow limitation, 430–433
chronic
hypoxemia from, 404
peptic ulcers with, 127
chronic obstructive, 430
hypoventilation with, 399, 415,
417
dyspnea, 418
hypercapnia, 413–414, 415, 417
hypocapnia, 413
interstitial, 434–441
chest x-ray of, 434
clinical example of, 440
clinical manifestations of, 438–
440
hypoxemia from, 438

Lung diseases—Continued
management of, 440
mechanics of, 436–438
pathology of, 434–436
spirometry in, 437
Lupus erythematosus, systemic
antibodies in, 210
autoimmunity in, 206–207
autoreactive cells in, 223
complement system deficiencies
with, 222
described, 203–204
hyperkalemia from, 265
nephrotic syndrome from, 300
neutrophils in, 171
pathogenesis of, 209
and pulmonary hypertension, 451
secondary immunodeficiency from,
224
with Sjögren's syndrome, 210
small-vessel coronary disease with,
40
Luteinizing hormone (LH)
disorders of, 86
function of, 85
in hypogonadism, 111, 112
in ovarian function, 112, 113
in ovulation, 112, 113
in polycystic ovary syndrome, 114
in testosterone production, 111
Lymph
formation and ascites, 144
in lung fluid balance, 442, 445, 447
nodes
in breast cancer prognosis, 389
in Hodgkin's disease, 383
and pulmonary edema, 445
Lymphadenopathy
with macroglobulinemia, 382
in Sjögren's syndrome, 210
Lymphangioleiomyomatosis, and interstitial lung disease, 435
Lymphatics, function of, 449
Lymphoblasts, in acute lymphoblastic
leukemia, 377
Lymphocytes
abnormal and stem-cell function,
161
aging and, 7
antigen stimulation of, 375–377
B cells, 220
function of, 221
in glomerulonephritis, 292
markers of, 220–221
membrane receptors, 221
in non-Hodgkin's lymphomas,
377–378
ontogeny of, 375, 376
in plasma cell disorders, 379
production of, 220
subclasses of, 220
source of, 159
T cells, 220
age and, 7
in malnutrition, 348
in non-Hodgkin's lymphomas,
377–378
in rheumatoid arthritis, 208
and tumor rejection, 362, 363–
364

Lymphocytes—*Continued*
total count, in malnutrition assessment, 350
Lymphocytic infiltrative disorders, and interstitial lung disease, 435
Lymphokines, 221
in endogenous pyrogen production, 241
as inflammation mediators, 233, 234
in rheumatoid arthritis, 208
Lymphomas
Burkitt's, clinical example of, 360–361
diffuse, 378
lymphoblastic, 378–379
nodular, 378
nephrotic syndrome from, 300
non-Hodgkin's, 360, 377–379
systemic lupus erythematosus with, 176
T cell, 378–379
Lymphopheresis, for systemic lupus erythematosus, 204
Lysolecithin, ulcers from, 127
Lysosomal enzymes, in asthma, 423
Lysozyme
in leukemia, 173
from Reed-Sternberg cells, 382
Lysozymuria, with leukemia, 173

Macroglobulinemia, Waldenström's, 381–382
Macrophages
and neutrophil destruction, 171
tissue, pyrogen from, 241
in tumor killing, 363–364
Macular degeneration, with age, 4
Magnesium
in bones, 313
depletion and hypokalemia, 262
in intracellular space, 247
Magnesium sulfate, for eclampsia, 480
Malabsorption, 150, 151
osteomalacia from, 318
rickets from, 317
Malaria
glomerulonephritis with, 290
nephrotic syndrome from, 300
Maldigestion, 150–151
Malignancies. *See* Cancer
Malnutrition
assessment of, 349–350
with cancer, 367–368, 373–374
clinical, 347–352
in nephrotic syndrome, 300
protein-calorie, 347
and starvation, 463, 470
support for, 350–351
with uremic syndrome, 310
Maltose, source of, 149
Mammography, 388
Marasmus, 347
Marrow erythroid hyperplasia, and red cell production, 163
Masculinization, with renal cell carcinoma, 323

Mast cells
in asthma, 423–424
degranulation, 424
and hypersensitivity reactions, 189
source of, 190
Mastoid, infection and lateral sinus thrombosis, 338
Measles
and diabetes mellitus, 107
glomerulonephritis from, 290
secondary immunodeficiency from, 224
Media (of artery) and atherosclerosis, 34
Megakaryoblast, 175
Megakaryocytes
in leukemia, 173
in megaloblastic anemia, 162
platelets from, 175
in polycythemia rubra vera, 166
Melena
with cancers, 154
with gastric ulcer, 129
with reflux esophagitis, 123
Membranes
gas diffusion through, 401, 402
potential in excitation, 11–12, 13
abnormal, 14, 16
Meningitis
diagnosis and age, 3
syndrome of inappropriate ADH from, 88
Menopause, 113
Menstrual dysfunction. *See also* Amenorrhea
from hypercortisolism, 93
Mercaptans, in hepatic encephalopathy, 146
6-Mercaptopurine, hypothyroidism from, 98
Mesencephalic periaqueductal gray formation, 328
Metabolic respiratory quotient, 395
Metabolism
during fasting, 464–465
hormones and, 81–83
insulin action on, 106
normal, 464
post-trauma, 464–468
Metaproterenol, for asthma, 424
Metastases, bone, hypercalcemia from, 282. *See also* Cancer
Metchnikoff, Elie, 231
Methanol, and metabolic acidosis, 271
Methemalbuminemia, with intravascular hemolysis, 165
Methimazole, and hypothyroidism, 98
Methoxyflurane, nephrogenic diabetes insipidus from, 87–88
Methyldopa, and prolactin release, 86, 88
Methylxanthines, for asthma, 424
Metoclopramide, and lower esophageal sphincter pressure, 120
Metromenorrhagia, and chorionic gonadotropin excretion, 370
Micellar dispersion, in digestion, 150
Microbial killing, neutrophil capacity for, 169, 171

Mid-arm muscle circumference, to assess malnutrition, 349
Migration inhibition factor, as inflammation mediator, 234
Minerals, nutritional requirement for, 347
Mitochondria, in tumor cells, 355
Mitosis, 358
Mitral valve regurgitation
clinical example of, 56
clinical picture of, 53
mechanism of, 67, 69
Mitral valve, sound of, 50
Mitral valve stenosis
clinical description and signs, 52–53
clinical example of, 55
hemodynamic changes in 50–51, 52
mechanism of, 66–67
Monoblasts, in leukemia, 382
Monoclonal gammopathies, 379–382
Monocyte-macrophage neoplasms, 382–383
Monocytes
endogenous pyrogen from, 241
epithelialization of, inflammations, 234–235
and glomerular injury, 295
in neutrophil production, 169
source of, 159, 220, 375, 376
Mononeuritis multiplex, with vasculitis, 203
Mononucleosis, infectious
Epstein-Barr virus in, 356
secondary immunodeficiency from, 224
nephrotic syndrome from, 301
Monosaccharides, production of, 149
Monosodium urate crystals, in gout, 216
Moore, Francis, 467
Morphine
action of, in brain, 328
and vasopressin release, 87
Motilin, and lower esophageal sphincter pressure, 120
Motor unit
disorders of, 340–342
physiology of, 340
Mucin
in adenocarcinoma, 456
in bronchioloalveolar carcinomas, 456
Mucosal disease, with reflux esophagitis, 123
Multiple gestation, and preeclampsia/eclampsia, 478
Mumps
antigen in malnutrition assessment, 350
and diabetes mellitus, 107
and pancreatitis, 133
testicular failure from, 112
Munchausen syndrome, chronic pain with, 330
Muscle
aging and, 4–5
bridge, 21, 22
contraction (cardiac)
force-velocity relationship in, 23–24

Muscle—*Continued*
    mechanism of, 21–24
      tension-length relationship in, 24
      velocity of, 21, 23
    disorders, and motor unit, 340–342
    glucose metabolism in, 464
    in hyperkalemia, 264
    in hypokalemia, 263
    wasting, with renal failure, 309, 310
Muscular dystrophies, fiber impairment in, 342
Myalgias, chronic pain with, 330
Myasthenia gravis
    acetylcholine and antibodies with, 200
    hypersensitivity in, 203
    neuromuscular transmission in, 341–342
    with thymoma, 371
Myasthenia-like syndrome, with lung cancer, 458
Mycobacteria
    associated with immunodeficiency, 225
    in infectious arthritis, 206
Myelin, and vitamin B_{12} deficiency, 162
Myeloblasts, in acute leukemia, 382
Myeloma, multiple, 379–381
    clinical example of, 383–384
    gout with, 217
    immunodeficiency in, 223
    nephrotic syndrome from, 300
Myeloperoxidase
    deficiency of, 172
    in neutrophil microbial killing, 169, 170
Myocardial cells, necrosis with hypokalemia, 263
Myocardial contractility. *See also* Muscle, contraction
    with acidemia, 272
    definition of terms in, 21
    estimation of, 26, 27
    in heart failure, 65
    measure of, 25
    mechanism of, 21, 24–26
    in myocardial disease, 42, 67
    and stroke volume, 25
    ventricular pressure-volume relationship and, 24–25
Myocardial infarction. *See also* Myocardial ischemia
    atherosclerosis in, 33
    cerebral arterial occlusion from, 337
    clinical example of, 43–44, 47
    damage from, 43
    versus esophageal pain, 121
    with interventricular septum rupture, 62
    with ischemia, 42–43
    respiratory alkalosis from, 414
    shock with, 74
    as a symptom, 46
    therapy for, 74–75
    time course of, 47
    with ventricular tachycardia, 18
Myocardial ischemia, 39–44. *See also* Coronary artery disease; Myocardial infarction

Myocardial ischemia—*Continued*
    and angina pectoris, 46
    from aortic stenosis, 54
    atherosclerosis and, 33, 40
    biological consequences of, 41–42
    clinical examples of, 43–44
    contractility in, 67
    coronary artery spasm and, 40–41
    from coronary embolism, 41
    coronary thrombosis in, 40
    and excitation, 15
    mechanism of, 39–40
    nonatherosclerotic causes, 40
    pathologic consequences of, 42–43
    peripheral vascular response to, 74
    physiologic consequences of, 42
    and platelet hyperactivity, 179
    therapy for, 74–75
    transient, 44
    vasoconstriction and hypokalemia with, 263
Myocardial oxygen consumption
    in heart failure, 65
    in myocardial ischemia, 39–40, 41
    normal, 39
Myocardial rupture, with infarction, 43
Myocarditis, with renal failure, 309
Myocardium
    aging and the, 6
    lupus erythematosus and, 204
    shunts and the, 62
Myofibrils, 340
Myoglobinuria, from hypophosphatemia, 285
Myopathy
    muscle fiber impairment in, 342
    with renal cell carcinoma, 323
Myosin
    in myocardial contraction, 21, 22
    in myofibrils, 340
Myositis, chronic pain with, 330
Myotonia congenita, 342
Myotonic dystrophy
    muscle fiber impairment with, 342
    secondary immunodeficiency from, 224

Naloxone, action of, in brain, 328
Narcotics, action of, in brain, 328
Natriuretic hormone substances, in uremia, 310
Natural killer (NK) cells
    lymphocytes as, 200, 220
    in tumor killing 363–364
Nausea, dialysis effect on, 310–311
Necrosis
    acute tubular, with renal failure, 305
    cortical, with preeclampsia, 477
Neisseria gonorrhoeae
    infection and complement system deficiencies, 222
    temperature and, 241
Neisseria meningitidis, infections and complement system deficiencies, 222
Neoplasia. *See also* Cancer
    and chronic urticaria, 191
    and pituitary hormones, 86

Neostigmine, in neuromuscular transmission, 342
Nephritic syndrome, 296–297
Nephritis. *See also* Glomerulonephritis
    anti-glomerular basement membrane, 290–292
      glomerular injury from, 287
    hereditary, nephrotic syndrome from, 300
    Heymann, 292
    in situ antigen-antibody complex, 292
      glomerular injury from, 287
    interstitial
      hypersensitivity in, 203
      with renal parenchymal azotemia, 305
      with Sjögren's syndrome, 210
Nephropathy, membranous, with nephrotic syndrome, 300
Nephrosclerosis, malignant, glomerular ischemia with, 296
Nephrosis, lipoid, with nephrotic syndrome, 300, 301
Nephrotic syndrome 298–302
    clinical example of, 301
    defined, 298
    osteomalacia from, 318
    renal diseases with, 300
    secondary causes of, 300–301
    secondary immunodeficiency from, 224
Nerves, peripheral, in glucose metabolism, 464
Nervous system
    aging and the, 5–6
    demyelinating diseases and type IV hypersensitivity, 203
Neuralgias, chronic pain with, 330
Neurofibrillary tangles, 5
Neurohypophysis, 87–88
Neuromas, chronic pain with, 330
Neuromuscular disorders, hypoventilation with, 399
Neuromuscular function, and calcium concentration, 279, 283
Neuromuscular junction, 340, 341
Neuromuscular syndromes, with cancer, 371
Neuromuscular transmission, disorders of, 341–342
Neurons
    cortical
      in epilepsy, 334
      structure of, 333
    electrical activity of, 333
    pain inhibitory, 328
    upper motor, 340
Neuropathy
    diabetic, 107
      chronic pain with, 330
      clinical example, 343
      differential diagnosis, 290, 292
    dying back, 341
    with macroglobulinemia, 382
    peripheral
      with cancer, 371
      with lung cancer, 458
      with renal cell carcinoma, 323
    segmental demyelinating, 341
    with uremic syndrome, 310

Neurophysin, carrier for vasopressin, 87
Neuroses, chronic pain with, 330
Neutropenia
  causes of, 235–236
  clinical example of, 174
  with leukemia, 173
  mechanisms of, 171–172
  shift, 171–172
Neutrophil-chemotactic factor (NCF), in asthma, 423
Neutrophilia, neutrophil kinetics in, 170
Neutrophils
  aggregation of, 232, 233
  in asthma, 423
  altered distribution of, 171–172
  disorders of, 169–174
  function of, 169, 171
  production and regulation of, 169, 170
  release of, 233
Nicotinamide adenine dinucleotide phosphate (NADPH)
  defective activation of, 172
  in neutrophil bacterial killing, 169, 170, 171
Nicotine, See also Smoking
  and lower esophageal sphincter pressure, 120
  and vasopressin release, 87
Nissl substance, in brain cell, 333
Nitrates, and lower esophageal sphincter pressure, 120
Nitrites, and lower esophageal sphincter pressure, 120
Nitrogen
  balance calculated, 350–351
  blood urea elevated, 8
  intake of, 466
  post-trauma excretion of, 466, 468
Nitroprusside reaction, 108
Nociceptor system, 327, 328
Nocturia, as symptom of renal disease, 311
Nodes. See also Lymph nodes; Lymphadenopathy
  in Hodgkin's disease, 383
Noradrenalin. See Norepinephrine
Norepinephrine
  and body temperature, 240
  hypertension from, 101
  and lower esophageal sphincter pressure, 120
  in pain transmission, 328
  with pheochromocytoma, 102
  post-trauma metabolic effect of, 465
Nose, structure and function of, 194
Nuclear endoreduplication, of megakaryoblast, 175
Nuclear number, defined, 175
Nucleic acids, phosphate in, 280
Nucleoprotein, antibodies to, 210
Nutrition, See also Malnutrition
  aging and, 5
  requirements of, 347

Obesity
  and coronary artery disease, 38
  from Cushing's syndrome, 93
  and renal cell carcinoma, 322

Occipital lobes, and visual sensors, 333
Occlusive pulmonary disease, 70
Occupational diseases
  lung cancer, 455
  respiratory, 197
Odynophagia
  with diffuse esophageal spasm, 122
  in dysphagia, 121
Ohm's law, 60
Oligomenorrhea, from hyperprolactinemia, 86
Oliguria
  post-trauma, 468
  with preeclampsia, 475
  with shock, 73
Oncogene, formation of, 356
Oncorna viruses, tumors from, 356
Opiates
  action of, in brain, 328
  allergic reactions to, 189
Opsonization, defective, 172
Ophthalmopathy, with Graves' disease, 97
Orchitis, viral, testicular failure from, 112
Orthopnea
  with aortic regurgitation, 54
  with heart failure, 70
  with mitral regurgitation, 53
  with mitral stenosis, 52
Osmolality
  of body fluids, 247
  in hyperosmolality, 253–256
  in hypoosmolality, 256–257
  intracellular and potassium, 260
  sodium influences on, 247–248
  and vasopressin secretion, 87
Osteitis fibrosa, with renal disease, 318
Osteoarthritis, 213–215
Osteoarthropathy, hypertrophic, with lung cancer, 458
Osteoarthrosis, defined, 215
Osteoblasts, 313, 315
Osteoclast-activating factor (OAF)
  in bone metastases, 369
  and hypercalcemia, 282
Osteoclasts, 315, 316
Osteocytes, 315, 316
Osteodystrophy, renal, 272, 309–310, 318–319
Osteogenesis imperfecta, connective tissue in, 209
Osteoid, composition of, 313, 314
Osteolytic lesions, with multiple myeloma, 380
Osteomalacia, 317–318
  from anticonvulsants, 284
  causes of, 318–319
  clinical example of, 319–321
  with uremic syndrome, 310
Osteopenia, 319
  with osteomalacia, 320
Osteophytosis
  with degenerative disk disease, 215
  with osteoarthritis, 214
Osteoporosis, 319
  with multiple myeloma, 380
Osteosarcoma, doubling time in, 360

Ovaries
  dysfunction of, 113–114
  hormones and, 85
  normal function of, 112–113
Overshoot, in cardiac electrophysiology, 11, 12, 14
Oxygen
  alveolar-arterial difference, 395–396
  arteriovenous content of, in heart failure, 68
  brain consumption of, 337
  content in blood, calculated, 396–398
  deficits and erythrocyte production, 165
  demand and ischemia, 39–41, 42
  myocardial supply of, 39
  partial pressure of, versus hemoglobin saturation, 395–398
  supply and red cell production, 160–161
Oxyhemoglobin dissociation curve, 396–398

Pacemaker cells
  in heart block, 19–20
  rate of firing of, 13–14, 16
Paget's disease
  heart failure with, 66
  hypercalcemia with, 282
Pain
  acute, 327–329
  afferent fibers, 327–328
  chronic
    causes of, 330
    clinical example of, 331–332
    defined, 327
    mechanisms of, 329–331
    mediation of, 328
  placebo effect on, 331
  psychophysiologic signs of, 329
  referred, 329
  stimulators of, 233
Palpitations
  with aortic regurgitation, 54
  with mitral regurgitation, 53
  with mitral stenosis, 52
  from pheochromocytoma, 102
Pancreas, 131–136. See also Pancreatitis
  anatomy, physiology and biochemistry of, 131–132
  cancer of, 155
  clinical example of insufficiency, 152–153
  endocrine function of, 131
  exocrine function of, 131
  insulin formation in, 106
  and maldigestion, 150
  in malnutrition, 348, 349
  secretions from, 149
  ulcer penetration in, 127, 128
Pancreatitis
  acute, 132–133
  chronic, 134–136, 151
  classification of, 132
  clinical example of, 135–136
  familial, 134
  gallstones and, 139

Pancreatitis—*Continued*
 and hypercalcemia, 283
 and hypocalcemia, 284
 secondary to ulcer penetration, 128
Pancreozymin. *See* Cholecystokinin-pancreozymin
Panencephalitis, subacute sclerosing (SSPE), 203
Pannus, in rheumatoid arthritis, 207
Paralysis
 diaphragmatic, with lung cancer, 457
 hyperkalemic familial, 262, 265
 periodic, 342
 with renal failure, 309
Paramyotonia, 342
Paramyxoviruses, secondary immunodeficiency from, 224
Parasympathetic cholinergic discharge reflex, in asthma, 195–196
Parathyroid hormone (PTH), 81
 and bone cells, 315
 and calcium homeostasis, 279, 280, 281, 282
 in hypocalcemia, 283
 osteitis fibrosis from, 318
 and phosphate reabsorption, 281
 and renal cell tumor, 323
 in renal osteodystrophy, 318
 in uremia, 310
Paratyphoid, neutropenia with, 171
Paraventricular nuclei, vasopressin and, 87
Paresthesias
 with hyperkalemia, 264
 from hypophosphatemia, 285
 with renal failure, 309
Parietal lobe, and association, 334
Patent ductus arteriosus (PDA), 63–64
Pathways, complement system, 221–222, 294, 295
Penicillamine, nephrotic syndrome from, 300
Penicillin
 allergy to, 192–193
 anaphylaxis from, 190, 192
 as antigen in immune complex diseases, 201
 and platelet dysfunction, 179
 and rheumatic fever, 211
Pentagastrin, and lower esophageal sphincter pressure, 120
Peppermint, and lower esophageal sphincter pressure, 120
Pepsin
 source of, 125
 ulcers and, 127
Pepsinogen, source of, 125
Peptic ulcer. *See* Ulcer, peptic
Peptidases, action of, 149
Peptides. *See also* Hormones
 corticotropin-releasing hormone, 90
 hydrolization of, 149
 in insulin, 106
 mechanism and characteristics of, 81
 and pancreas, 149
Peptones, and cholecystokinin-pancreozymin, 149

Pericardiocentesis, for obstructive shock, 76
Pericarditis
 constrictive, mechanism of, 66
 constrictive, and portal hypertension, 143
 dialysis effect on, 310–311
 with myocardial infarction, 43
 with renal failure, 309
Pericardium, lupus erythematosus and, 204
Peritoneum, and granulocytes in leukemia, 173
Peritonitis
 bacterial, with ascites, 145
 with pancreatitis, 133
 from perforated ulcers, 127
 respiratory alkalosis from, 414
 shock with, 76
Petechiae, from insufficient platelets, 179
Phagocytosis
 erythrocyte, 163
 in fever, 241–242
 inhibition of, 172
 neutrophil capacity of, 169
Phantom limb sensation, 330
Pharyngitis, glomerulonephritis from, 297
Phenothiazines
 and neutropenia, 171, 174
 and pituitary hormones, 86
 and sweating, 242
Phentolamine, and lower esophageal sphincter pressure, 120
Phenylbutazone
 and leukocyte production, 236
 neutropenia from, 171
Phenylephrine, and lower esophageal sphincter pressure, 120
Phenytoin, and vasopressin release, 87
Pheochromocytoma, 102
 erythropoietin in, 371
Philadelphia chromosome, in leukemia, 173
Phosphatase, acid, and osteoclasts, 315
Phosphate. *See also* Hypophosphatemia; Phosphorus
 in diabetic ketoacidosis, 108–109
 normal homeostasis of, 280–281, 282
 retention and renal osteodystrophy, 318
 serum calcium relationship with, 281
Phosphodiesterase, in mast cell degranulation, 424
Phospholipase A, in pancreas, 132
Phospholipids
 in bile, 137
 in clotting cascade, 181
 phosphate in, 280
 and platelet factor III, 176
 from platelets, 175
Phosphoproteins, phosphate in, 280
Phosphorus. *See also* Phosphate
 function of, 280–281
 quantity of, in bone, 313

Phrenoesophageal ligaments, and lower esophageal sphincter, 119
Physostigmine, in neuromuscular transmission, 342
Pinocytosis, 34
Piperazine, as antigen in immune complex diseases, 201
Pituitary
 ACTH release by, 90–91
 anterior hormones, 85–87
 and erythropoiesis, 160–161
 hormones of, 81
 and hypogonadism, 112
 and ovarian failure, 113
 posterior, 87–89
 and reproductive hormones, 111, 112
Placebo effect, 331
Plaques
 formation in atherosclerosis, 35, 45
 senile, 5
Plasma. *See also* Body fluids
 cells
  disorders of, 379–382
  source of, 159
 composition of, 247, 248
Plasmapheresis
 for macroglobulinemia, 382
 for systemic lupus erythematosus, 204
 thrombocytopenia with, 178
Plasmin, activation of, 233
Platelet-activating factor (PAF)
 as allergic reaction mediator, 190–191
 as asthma mediator, 195, 423
 as inflammation mediator, 234
Platelets, 175–180. *See also* Thrombocytopenia
 aggregation of, 176, 232, 233
  in atherosclerosis, 34, 36
  and coronary artery spasm, 40–41
  and ischemia, 40
 altered distribution of, 177–178
 in arrest of tumors, 389
 and coagulation, 159
 decreased production of, 176
 dialysis effect on, 311
 dysfunction of, 178–179
 elevated, in cancer, 372–373
 excessive destruction of, 176–177
 insufficient, 179
 function of, 175–176
 and glomerular damage, 294–295
 in nephrotic syndrome, 299, 300
 and polycythemia, 166
 production and regulation of, 175
 source of, 159
Platelet factor 3 (PF$_3$), in hemostatic plug formation, 176, 177
Plethysmography, to measure lung volumes, 405
Pleura, lupus erythematosus and, 204
Pleural cytology, 458
Ploidy value, 175
Pluripotent myeloid precursor cell, 159

Pluripotent stem cells
  in anemia, 161
  in polycythemia rubra vera, 166
Plutonium, in bones, 313
Pneumococci, in infectious arthritis, 206
Pneumonectomy, 458
Pneumonia. *See also* Pneumonitis
  chronic eosinophilic, and interstitial lung disease, 435
  in elderly, 8
  with interstitial lung disease, 438
  necrotizing, and pulmonary vascular disease, 451
  shock with, 76
  shunting with, 399
  syndrome of inappropriate ADH from, 88
Pneumonitis. *See also* Pneumonia
  aspiration, from reflux esophagitis, 123–124
  hypersensitivity, 198
  radiation, and lymphatic drainage, 446
  respiratory alkalosis from, 414
Poiseuille's equation (law), 425, 450
Polyarteritis nodosa
  diagnosis of, 205
  pathogenesis of, 209
  and pulmonary hypertension, 451
  with Sjögren's syndrome, 210
  small-vessel coronary disease with, 40
  vasculitis in, 203
Polyclonal immunoglobulin deficiency, 223
Polycystic renal disease, 311
Polycystic ovary syndrome, 114
Polycythemia
  classification of, 165
  clinical example of, 167–168
  consequences of, 166
  mechanisms of, 165–166
  from renal cell carcinoma, 322
  rubra vera, 166
    differential diagnosis, 371
    gout with, 217
    thrombocytosis with, 179
Polydipsia
  with diabetes insipidus, 88
  with diabetes mellitus, 107
  with hypokalemia, 264
Polyhydramnios, and preeclampsia/eclampsia, 478
Polymorphonuclear leukocytes (PMNs), in gout, 218
Polymyositis
  antibodies in, 210
  esophagus in, 123
  hypersensitivity in, 203
  with lung cancer, 458
Polymyxin, allergic reactions to, 189
Polyradiculoneuropathy, acute inflammatory motor, 342
Polysaccharides, in bones, 145
Polyuria
  with diabetes insipidus, 88
  with diabetes mellitus, 107
  from hypercalcemia, 283
Portal hypertension. *See* Hypertension, portal

Portal pressure, in liver, 142
Positive pressure ventilation, hyponatremia from, 256, 257
Postpartum toxemia, 475
Potassium
  and aldosterone regulation, 92, 467
  body content of, 260
  in bones, 313
  depletion with heat, 242
  depletion and ischemia, 42
  in diabetic ketoacidosis, 108
  glucocorticoid effect on, 93
  in hyperkalemia, 264–265
  in hypokalemia, 261–264
  in intracellular space, 247
  and myocardial excitation, 11, 12
  in neuron membrane potential, 333
  normal balance of, 260–261
  and pain nociceptors, 327
  post-trauma excretion of, 466, 467, 468, 469
  role of, in body, 260
Prausnitz-Küstner (PK) reaction, 190
Prednisone, for thrombocytopenia, 180
Preeclampsia/eclampsia, 475–482
  clinical example of, 480–482
  defined, 475
  effects of, 479
  etiology of, 478–479
  management of, 479, 480
  and nephrotic syndrome, 301
Pregnancy
  and breast cancer incidence, 386
  hypertensive disorders of, 475–482
  malnutrition with, 349
  neutrophil isoantibodies in, 171
  physiologic changes during, 476–477
  toxemia and nephrotic syndrome, 301
Preload. *See also* Frank-Starling law
  cardiac stroke volume affected by, 25
  defined in intact heart, 25
  and myocardial contraction mechanism, 21, 22, 23
  of ventricle, 27
Premarin, and hypertension, 105
Premature atrial beat, in Wolff-Parkinson-White syndrome, 19
Premature ventricular beat, on electrocardiogram, 18
Presbyopia, with aging, 4
Pressure-volume loop (of ventricle), 27–28, 29
Pretibial myxedema, with Graves' disease, 97
Proadrenocorticotropic hormone, 369
Probenecid, nephrotic syndrome from, 300
Procarboxypeptidase, trypsin and, 149
Procarboxypeptidase A and B, in pancreas, 132
Proelastase, in pancreas, 132
Proelastomucase, in pancreas, 132
Progesterone
  and lower esophageal sphincter pressure, 120

Progesterone—*Continued*
  mechanism of action, 82
  in ovulation, 112, 113, 114
  in preeclampsia/eclampsia, 477
Proinsulin, insulin from, 106
Prolactin
  disorders of, 85, 86–87
  and ovarian failure, 113
  phenothiazines and, 86
  in preeclampsia/eclampsia, 479
  purpose of, 85
  release of, 85
  from tumors, 370
Proline, in bones, 313
Properdin (Factor P), in complement system, 221
Prophospholipase A, in pancreas, 132
Propranolol
  and asthma, 425
  for hyperthyroidism, 98, 100
  to lower renin secretion, 296
  and thyroid hormones, 96
Propylthiouracil, and thyroid hormones, 96, 98
Prostacyclin
  generation of, 177
  and platelet aggregation, 36, 176, 177
  and pulmonary vascular resistance, 450
Prostaglandins
  as allergic reaction mediators, 190–191
  in asthma, 195, 423
  and body temperature regulation, 240
  and hypercalcemia, 282
  and hypertension, 103
  as inflammation mediators, 233, 234
  and lower esophageal sphincter pressure, 120
  in lung, 449
  and pain nociceptors, 327
  in platelet aggregation, 36, 176, 177
  in preeclampsia/eclampsia, 477, 478
  and thromboemboli, 452
Prostaglandin E_1, and pulmonary vascular resistance, 450
Prostaglandin E_2
  in bone metastases, 369
  in mast cell degranulation, 424
  in tumor-induced hypercalcemia, 369
Prostaglandin F_2, and LES pressure, 120
Prostaglandin $F_{2\alpha}$, and pulmonary vascular resistance, 451
Prostheses, platelet disruption by, 177
Proteases
  abnormal, in cancer cells, 355
  deficiency of, 150
  in emphysema, 431
  gastric, 149
  and maldigestion, 150
  pancreatic, 149
  in rheumatoid arthritis, 207
Protein meal, and lower esophageal sphincter pressure, 120

Proteins
  clotting factors, 181
  contractile, 22
  and digestion, 125
  insulin and synthesis of, 106
  in interstitial fluid, 445
  maldigestion of, 150
  in malnutrition, 347–348
  in nephrotic syndrome, 299
  normal body store of, 464
  normal requirements for, 347, 463
  peptide hormones, 81
  post-trauma metabolism of, 466
  in pulmonary edema, 446
  serum, normal level of, 298–299
  in tumor cells, 355
Proteinuria
  with acute glomerulonephritis, 296
  Bence Jones, with multiple my-
    eloma, 381
  with chronic hypertension, 475
  from diabetes, 107
  nephrotic-range, clinical example,
    301–302
  in nephrotic syndrome, 298, 299
  with preeclampsia, 475, 477–478
Proteolysis, insulin and, 106
Proteolytic enzymes, in cancer cells,
  355
Prothrombin
  activation of, 183
  in clotting cascade, 181
  thrombin from, 181, 233
Protozoa, and immunodeficiency
  states, 225
Pseudocysts, with pancreatitis, 133,
  134
Pseudogout, 218
Pseudohyperkalemia, 264
Pseudohypoosmolality, 256
Pseudohyperparathyroidism, tumor
  induced, 369
Pseudohypoparathyroidism, hypocalcemia with, 283
Pseudomyasthenic syndrome, neuromuscular transmission in, 341,
  342
Psychogenic disorders, globus hystericus, 121
Psychosis
  chronic pain with, 330
  with renal failure, 309
Pulmonary alveolar-capillary membrane, lupus erythematosus in,
  204
Pulmonary aspiration, with achalasia,
  122
Pulmonary circulation, 59–60
Pulmonary congestion, and heart failure, 70
Pulmonary disease. See also Lung dis-
    ease
  chronic obstructive (COPD), 430–
    433
  diffusion impairment with, 401–403
  hypoventilation with, 398–399
  hypoxemia with, 398–404
  low ventilation-perfusion (V̇/Q̇)
    ratios with, 400–401
  shunt with, 398–399

Pulmonary edema, 442–448
  acute, with mitral regurgitation, 53
  acute, with ventricular pressure
    overload, 31
  with aortic regurgitation, 54
  chronic, interstitial lung disease
    from, 434
  clinical example, 71, 447–448
  dialysis effect on, 310–311
  from eclampsia, 479
  and heart failure, 70
  with heat illness, 243
  from left atrial pressure increase,
    68–69
  and lung fluid balance, 442, 443–
    445
  lymphatic drainage and, 445–446
  with mitral stenosis, 52
  with preeclampsia, 475
  with renal failure, 309
  shunt with, 399
  from surfactant deficiency, 411
  types of, 446
  vascular permeability and, 446–447
Pulmonary embolism
  respiratory alkalosis from, 414
  vascular disease and, 451
Pulmonary fibrosis
  with allergic alveolitis, 198
  from aspergillosis, 198
  idiopathic
    collagen in, 436
    and interstitial lung disease, 434,
      435
Pulmonary function, aging and, 7
Pulmonary gas exchange, 395–404
Pulmonary heart disease. See Cor pul-
    monale (pulmonary heart dis-
    ease)
Pulmonary hemosiderosis, idiopathic,
    and interstitial lung disease,
    435
Pulmonary neoplastic disease, 455–
    459. See also Cancer, lung
Pulmonary regurgitation, 55
Pulmonary stenosis, 55
Pulmonary system, airway described,
    194–195. See also Lung
Pulmonary vascular disease, 449–454
  clinical example of, 453
  cor pulmonale, 452–453
  primary pulmonary hypertension,
    451–452
  thromboemboli, 452
Pulmonary vascular resistance (PRV)
  in the fetus, 59, 61
  formula for, 450–451
  postnatal, 59–60
Pulmonary valve, sound of, 50
Pulmonary veno-occlusive disease,
    and interstitial lung disease, 435
Purified protein derivative (PPD), in
    malnutrition assessment, 350
Purine, metabolism and gout, 216
Purine nucleoside phosphorylase
    deficiency, 224
Purkinje network (fibers)
  and electrocardiogram, 17
  and excitation, 13, 14
  firing rates in, 16

Purpura
  in elderly, 4
  idiopathic autoimmune thrombocy-
    topenic, 176
  idiopathic thrombocytopenic, 203
  thrombocytopenic and thrombocy-
    topenia, 178
  thrombotic thrombocytopenic and
    platelet consumption, 177
Pyelonephritis, with multiple my-
    eloma, 381
Pyloric channel disease, ulcers with,
    127
Pylorus, in prepyloric ulcers, 127
Pyridoxine, deficiency in uremic syn-
    drome, 310
Pyrogen, endogenous and body tem-
    perature regulation, 241
Pyrosis, mechanisms and symptoms
    of, 121
Pyruvate, in glucose metabolism, 464,
    465
Pyuria, with hypokalemia, 263

QRS complex
  in electrocardiograms, 17
  in heart block, 19
  in Wolff-Parkinson-White syn-
    drome, 19
Quinidine, and platelet destruction,
    177

Radiation
  and interstitial lung disease, 435
  and lung cancer, 455
Radiation therapy
  and breast cancer, 386
  in Hodgkin's disease, 383
  for lung cancer, 458
Radioactive dye studies, anaphylaxis
    from dye, 192
Radiography, of lung cancer, 457
Radiotherapy, malnutrition and, 368
Radium, in bones, 313
Ranvier, nodes of, 333
Raynaud's phenomenon
  and pulmonary hypertension, 451
  with vasculitis, 203
Red cells
  overproduction of, 166
  production of, 160–161
Redox state of the body, in
    ketoacidosis, 108
Reed-Sternberg cell, in Hodgkin's dis-
    ease, 382
Reflux esophagitis
  described, 123–124
  mechanisms and symptoms of, 121
Refractory period, in myocardial exci-
    tation, 13, 14
Reifenstein's syndrome, 111–112
Reiter's syndrome, described, 208,
    209
Renal artery stenosis, and renal vascu-
    lar hypertension, 103
  polycythemia from, 166
Renal calculi, with hyperparathyroid-
    ism, 319
Renal cell carcinoma, 322–324

549

Renal cortex, vitamin D conversion in, 282

Renal disease. *See also specific diseases and manifestations*
and anemia, 161
chronic, and preeclampsia/eclampsia, 478
and chronic hypertension, 476
and hyperprolactinemia, 89
with nephrotic syndrome, 300
stages of, 308

Renal erythropoietic factor (REF), and erythrocyte production, 160

Renal failure. *See also* Renal insufficiency; Uremic syndrome
acute
azotemia, 303–307
clinical example of, 306–307
from hypercalcemia, 283
hyperkalemia with, 264
mechanisms and treatment of, 305–306
with pancreatitis, 133
with ventricular volume overload, 30–31
chemotaxis inhibition in, 172
chronic
adaptation to, 308–309
clinical example of, 311
hyperkalemia with, 264
hypocalcemia from, 284
osteodystrophy with, 318–319
platelet dysfunction in, 179
systemic effects of, 308, 309
with chronic hypokalemia, 263
defined, 308
early symptoms of, 311
from eclampsia, 479
from essential hypertension, 104
with heat stroke, 243
and hypocalcemia, 283
hyponatremia from, 256
metabolic acidosis from, 271
with multiple myeloma, 379, 380, 381
ulcers with, 127

Renal function, aging and, 6
Renal hypertension, 103–104
Renal hypoperfusion, from sodium depletion, 250
Renal insufficiency. *See also* Renal failure
chronic, gout with, 217
defined, 308
Renal medulla, glucose metabolism in, 464
Renal osteodystrophy, 318–319
Renal perfusion pressure, and renin release, 91
Renal plasma flow (RPF)
aging and, 5
in preeclampsia/eclampsia, 478
during pregnancy, 476
Renal reserve, diminished, 308
Renal stones, in Cushing's syndrome, 93
Renal tubular basement membrane, immune complex disease in, 202

Renal tubular defect, hypokalemia from, 262
Renal tubular proximal epithelial cell antigen, 201
Renin
in acute renal failure, 305
function of, 308
in hypertension, 103, 296
in nephrotic syndrome, 299
post-trauma secretion of, 466, 467
during pregnancy, 476
Renin-angiotensin-aldosterone system, in ascites formation, 145
Renin-angiotensin system, regulating aldosterone secretion, 91
Reproductive organs, endocrinology of, 111–115
Reserpine, and prolactin release, 88
Respiratory compensation, in acid-base disturbances, 270–274
Respiratory diseases. *See also* Lung diseases, *and Pulmonary entries*
allergic, 194–199
chronic nonspecific (CNSRD), 430
occupational, 197
Respiratory failure
acute, from hypophosphatemia, 285
cor pulmonale from, 411
with pancreatitis, 133
Reticulocytes
in anemia, 161
and erythrocyte production, 160, 163
Reticuloendothelial (RE) system
in erythrocyte removal, 160
and immune complex disease, 201
Retinopathy, from diabetes, 107
Reverse transcriptase, 356
Reversible obstructive airways disease. *See* Asthma
Rhabdomyolysis
with heat illness, 242–243
hyperkalemia from, 265
with hypokalemia, 263
from hypophosphatemia, 285
Rheumatic diseases
inflammatory noninfectious, 206–212
and neutropenia, 171
Rheumatic fever
etiology of, 206
pathophysiology of, 211
Rhinitis
allergic
with atopic dermatitis, 192
clinical aspects of, 196–197
clinical example of, 198–199
eosinophilic, 197
as hypersensitive disease, 189, 190
mechanisms of, 195
nonallergic eosinophilic, 189–190
Ribonucleic acid (RNA)
as antigen in immune complex diseases, 201
in carcinogenesis, 356
in cell cycle, 358
in tumor viruses, 356
Ribosomes, as antigens in immune complex diseases, 201

Rickets
nutritional, 283–284
vitamin D-dependent, 317
vitamin D-resistant, 317
x-linked hypophosphatemic, 285
RNA. *See* Ribonucleic acid (RNA)
Rokitansky, Karl Freiherr von, 35

Salicylates
hyperuricemia and, 217
intoxication and metabolic acidosis, 271
respiratory alkalosis from, 414
Salivary glands
amylase function, 149
in Sjögren's syndrome, 210
Salmonella flagellin, aging and immunity to, 7
Sarcoidosis
hypercalcemia with, 282
and interstitial lung disease, 434, 435
platelet pooling with, 177
secondary immunodeficiency from, 224
Sarcoma, Ewing's, doubling time in, 360
Sarcolemma, in ischemia, 42
Sarcomere
model of, 22
in myocardial contraction, 21
Satellitism, of platelets, 178
Schistocytes, in microangiopathic hemolytic anemia, 372
Schistosomiasis
with glomerulonephritis, 290
nephrotic syndrome from, 300
Scleroderma. *See* Sclerosis, progressive systemic (PSS)
Sclerosis
of bones in osteoarthritis, 214
focal
antiplatelet agents for, 295
with nephrotic syndrome, 300
progressive systemic (PSS), 209
antibodies in, 210
esophageal involvement, 122–123
and pulmonary hypertension, 451
with Sjögren's syndrome, 210
small vessel coronary disease with, 40
Scratch-itch cycle, with atopic dermatitis, 192
Secretin
and lower esophageal sphincter pressure, 120
in pancreas, 131–132, 149
from tumors, 370
Sedatives, and lower esophageal sphincter pressure, 120
Seizures
epileptic, 334
with hypocalcemia, 284
with renal failure, 309
with respiratory alkalosis, 414
Sellar tomography, 89
Senile dementia, 5
Senile plaques, 5

Sepsis
  clinical example of, 351–352
  with pancreatitis, 133
  shock from, 75–76
Septal defects, shunting with, 399
Septicemia, respiratory alkalosis from, 414
Serotonin
  in asthma, 423
  and body temperature, 240
  and glomerular injury, 294–295
  as inflammation mediator, 233, 234
  in lungs, 449
  in pain transmission, 327, 328
  and pulmonary vascular resistance, 451
Serratia, enzyme defects and defense against, 172
Sertoli-cell-only syndrome, 112
Set point, in body temperature regulation, 239, 240
Sexuality, hormones for, 111–115
Sézary syndrome, 378
Sheehan's syndrome, 113
Shigella, dysentery and Reiter's syndrome, 209
Shivering, as heat source, 238
Shock
  and acidemia, 272
  with anaphylaxis, 192
  cardiogenic, 42, 74–75
  clinical characteristics of, 73
  coronary, from myocardial infarction, 47
  distributive, 75–77
  hypovolemic, 73–74
  obstructive, 76
  from pancreatitis, 133
  with respiratory alkalosis, 414
  septic, 75–76
Short bowel syndrome
  malabsorption from, 151
  malnutrition with, 349
Shunts
  arteriovenous, heart failure with, 66
  in interstitial lung disease, 438
  intracardiac, 60–62
    congenital, 61–62
    left-to-right, 61
      clinical example of, 62–63
    right-to-left, 61
      clinical example of, 63–64
      oxygen saturation and pressures with, 64
  as mechanism of hypoxemia, 399–400
  normal, right-to-left, 395
Sick sinus syndrome, 16
Sickle cell anemia. See also Sickle cell disease
  and gallstones, 138
  and vasopressin, 88
Sickle cell disease. See also Sickle cell anemia
  hyperkalemia from, 265
  immune complex disease in, 201
  with splenic infarction and secondary immunodeficiency, 224
Silent zone, in lungs, 411

Sinoatrial (SA) node
  abnormal, 16
  excitation and the, 13, 14
Sjögren's syndrome, 210–211
  etiology of, 206
Skin
  aging and the, 3–4
  and heat regulation, 238, 240
  immune complex disease in, 202
  in malnutrition, 348
Skin tests, for asthma, 421
Skipper, Howard E., 359
Slow-reacting substance of anaphylaxis (SRS-A), in asthma, 423
Smoking. See also Nicotine
  and chronic bronchitis, 430
  and coronary artery disease, 33, 38
  and emphysema, 431
  and lung cancer, 455
  and platelet dysfunction, 179
  and polycythemia, 167
  and renal cell carcinoma, 322
Smooth muscle
  arteriolar, cortisol effect on, 102
  bronchial, influences on, 423–425
Smooth muscle cells (SMC), in atherosclerosis, 34, 36
Sodium
  and ascites formation, 145
  body fluid content of, 247, 248
  and body fluid osmolality, 247–248
  and body fluid volume, 248, 249
  in bones, 313
  cortisol effect on, 102
  depletion, 249–251
  in diabetic ketoacidosis, 108
  in essential hypertension, 104
  excess, 251, 252
  glucocorticoid's effect on, 93
  in heart failure, 65–66
  in heat illness, 243
  in hyperosmolality, 253
  in hypoosmolality, 256
  in myocardial excitation, 11, 12
  in neuron membrane potential, 333
  post-trauma balance of, 466, 467, 468, 469
  in preeclampsia/eclampsia, 477, 478
  regulation of balance of, 248–249
  in renal hypertension, 103–104
  and renin release, 91
  retention and blood volume, 101
Somatomedins
  in tumor-induced hypoglycemia, 370
  in uremic syndrome, 310
Somatostatin
  and growth hormone, 85
  and insulin, 106
  source of, 131
Spasm, coronary artery, 40–41
Spasticity, from disorders of upper motor neuron, 340
Spermatogenesis
  in hypogonadism, 111, 112
  process of, 111
  therapy for, 112
Sphincter of Oddi
  anatomy of, 137
  and gallstones, 139

Sphincteric smooth muscle, and lower esophageal sphincter pressure, 120
Spinal canal, stenosis of, with degenerative disks, 215
Spinal cord
  circuitry of, 328
  and herniated disk, 214–215
  in pain transmission, 330
Spine
  aging and changes of the, 3
  degenerative disks in, 213–214
Spirogram. See Spirometry
Spirometry
  in asthma, 425–426, 428
  in interstitial lung disease, 437
  to measure air flow, 408–409, 410
Spironolactone, for androgen excess, 114
Spleen
  and erythrocytes, 163
  granulocytes in, with leukemia, 173
  hypersplenism, 171
  platelet removal in, 175
Splenectomy
  secondary immunodeficiency from, 224
  thrombocytosis with, 179
Splenic vein occlusion, in pancreatitis, 134
Splenomegaly
  and erythrocyte phagocytosis, 163
  and leukocyte count, 174
  in Sjögren's syndrome, 210
Spondyloarthropathies, seronegative, 208–209
  etiology of, 206
Spondylosis, with degenerative disk disease, 215
Sputum cytology, for lung cancer, 458
Staphylococcus
  enzyme defects and defense against, 172
  in infectious arthritis, 206
  nephrotic syndrome from, 300
Starch, digestion of, 149
Starling forces
  in extracellular fluid volume, 251–252
  in pulmonary edema, 442–448
Starvation. See also Malnutrition
  physiologic response to, 463
  post-traumatic, 470
Status asthmaticus, 197
Steatorrhea
  with maldigestion and malabsorption, 150
  with pancreatic cancer, 155
  with pancreatitis, 134
Stem-cells (blood)
  committed, production of, 159
  disorders and erythrocyte production, 162
  in leukemia, 172, 173
  megakaryocyte-committed, 175
  and neutrophil production, 169, 171
  and platelet production, 176
  and thrombocytosis, 179
  totipotent, 159

Steroid hormones
  abnormal secretion of, 92–95
  characteristics of, 82
  normal secretion of, 90–92
Stomach
  anatomy and cell types of, 125
  cancer of, 154
  diseases of, 126–130
  function of, 149
  motility of, 126
  normal secretion in, 125–126
Storage pool disease, 179
Streptococcal infections
  Group A, and rheumatic fever, 211
  nephrotic syndrome from, 300
Streptococcus pneumoniae
  with multiple myeloma, 383–384
  pneumonia from, 8
Streptokinase-Streptodornase
    (SK-SD), in malnutrition assess-
    ment, 350
Stress
  and ACTH secretion, 91
  and atherosclerosis, 33, 34
  and chronic urticaria, 191
  and gastritis, 126
  hyponatremia from, 256, 257
  and pain perception, 329
  and preeclampsia/eclampsia, 478
  respiratory alkalosis from, 414
  and systemic lupus erythematosus,
    204
  ulcers from, 127
  and vasopressin release, 87
Stress erosions, in gastritis, 126
Stridor, with lung cancer, 457
Stroke
  from essential hypertension, 104
  pain from, 331
Stroke volume (cardiac)
  determination of, 25
  influences on, 101
  normal, 30
Strontium, in bones, 313
Subaortic muscular stenosis, and my-
    ocardial ischemia, 41
Substance P, in pain transmission, 327
Succinylcholine
  hyperkalemia from, 265
  and neuromuscular transmission,
    341–342
Sulfonamides, as antigens in immune
    complex diseases, 201
Superior vena cava, obstruction of,
    with lung cancer, 457
Superoxide dismutase (SD), in neu-
    trophil bacterial killing, 170,
    171
Supraoptic nuclei, in vasopressin os-
    molality, 87
Suppressor T cells
  and neutropenia, 171
  in rheumatic diseases, 207
  and systemic lupus erythematosus,
    204
Surfactant, alveolar, 411
Surgery
  convalescence from, 468–469
  energy requirements after, 463–
    464

Surgery—Continued
  metabolic response to, 463–471
  postoperative malnutrition, 368
Swallowing
  in dysphagia, 120–121
  mechanism of, 119
Synapses
  in cerebral physiology, 333
  dorsal, in pain transmission, 328
  of motor unit, 340
Syncope
  with aortic stenosis, 54
  with mitral stenosis, 52
Synovial membrane
  anatomy of, 213
  in rheumatoid arthritis, 207
Synoviocytes, 213
Synovium
  immune complex disease in, 202
  lupus erythematosus and, 204
Syphilis, nephrotic syndrome from,
    300
Systolic pressure, normal, 61–62

T_3 (3,5,3'-triiodothyronine)
  in hyperthyroidism, 96–98, 99–100
  in hypothyroidism, 98–99
  source of, 96
$_rT_3$ (3,3',5'-triiodothyronine), reverse
    T_3, 96
Tacharrhythmia. See Tachycardia
Tachycardia
  angina from, 47
  atrial, with hypokalemia, 263
  paroxysmal, with mitral stenosis, 52
  from reentrant arrhythmias, 15–16
  with shock, 73
  sinus, with high output heart fail-
    ure, 70
  supraventricular
    electrocardiographic diagnosis of,
      17
    mechanism of, 16
  ventricular
    clinical example of, 17–19
    electrocardiographic diagnosis of,
      17, 18
    with hypokalemia, 263
Tachypnea
  with interstitial lung disease, 438
  with shock, 73, 74
Taurine, in bile, 137
Temperature, body
  fever and, 240–242
  heat illnesses, 242–243
  homeostasis mechanisms for, 238–
    240
  hyperthermia, 240
  influences on, 239
  normal, 238
Temporal lobes, and auditory sensors,
    333
Tension-length relationship, in mus-
    cle contraction, 24
Terminal deoxynucleotidyl transfer-
    ase (TdT), in leukemia, 173–
    174, 377
Testes. See also Testosterone
  dysfunction of, 111–112
  and erythropoiesis, 160–161

Testes—Continued
  hormones and, 85
  normal function of, 111
Testicular feminization, clinical ex-
    ample of, 83
Testosterone
  excessive, in female, 113
  in hypogonadism, 112
  mechanism of, 82
  normal production of, 111
  in polycystic ovary syndrome, 114
  source of, 90
  therapy, 112, 115
Tetanus, serum as antigen in immune
    complex diseases, 201
Tetany
  with hypocalcemia, 284
  with pancreatitis, 133
  with respiratory alkalosis, 414
Tetracycline, in osteomalacia diag-
    nosis, 318
Tetraiodothyronine. See Thyroxine
Tetralogy of Fallot, pulmonic regurgi-
    tation after, 55
Tetrodotoxin (TTX), and electro-
    physiology, 11
Thalamus, in pain sensation, 331
Thalassemia, gout with, 217
Theophylline, and lower esophageal
    sphincter pressure, 120
Thiouracil, neutropenia from, 171
Thrombasthenin, in thrombus con-
    solidation, 176
Thrombin
  formation of, 181, 182, 233
  in hemostatic plug formation, 176
Thrombasthenia
  Glanzmann's, 179
  with renal failure, 309
Thrombocythemia, hemorrhagic, 179.
    See also Thrombocytosis
Thrombocytopenia. See also Platelets
  with anemia, 161
  bleeding with, 183
  cerebral hemorrhage with, 338
  with chronic lymphocytic leukemia,
    377
  classification of, 178
  clinical example, 179–180
  consequences of, 179
  with leukemia, 173
  mechanisms of, 176–178
  with multiple myeloma, 379, 380
  postperfusion, 178
  with preeclampsia, 475
  spurious, 178
  in systemic lupus erythematosus,
    204
  thrombopoiesis in, 175
  washout, 178
Thrombocytosis. See also Throm-
    bocythemia
  with cancer, 372–373
  hyperkalemia from, 265
  with polycythemia, 166
  primary and secondary, 179
  with renal cell carcinoma, 322
Thromboemboli, pulmonary, 452
  and pulmonary hypertension,
    451

Thrombophlebitis
  with lung cancer, 458
  with renal cell carcinoma, 323
Thrombopoiesis, 175. See also Platelets
  and thrombocytosis, 179
Thrombopoietin, and platelet production, 175
Thrombosis
  in coronary artery disease, 45–46
  lateral sinus, 338
  myocardial infarction from, 47
  with platelet hyperactivity, 179
  with preeclampsia/eclampsia, 477
  sagittal sinus, 338
  vasopressin and, 36
  venous, cerebral infarction from, 338
Thromboxane A_2
  and coronary spasm, 41
  generation of, 177
  in platelet aggregation, 176, 177
  with renal failure, 179
Thrombus, formation of, 176
Thymocytes, age and, 7
Thymomas, Cushing's syndrome with, 369
Thymosin, in tumor immunity, 364–365
Thymus
  aging and the, 7
  in inflammation, 235
  and T lymphocyte production, 220
Thymus-derived (T) cells, in type IV hypersensitivity, 200. See also Lymphocytes, T cells
Thyroglobulin
  as antigen in immune complex diseases, 201
  in thyroid, 96
Thyroid
  aging and the, 3
  and erythropoiesis, 160–161
  function of, 96
  in Graves' disease, 200
  hormones of, 82, 96–100
  hormones and bone metabolism, 319
  hormone therapy and surfactant production, 411
Thyroid acropachy, with Graves' disease, 97
Thyroid disease, autoimmune, hypothyroidism with, 98
Thyroiditis
  hyperthyroidism with, 97
  chronic lymphocytic (Hashimoto's), 97
    hypothyroidism with, 98
    type IV hypersensitivity in, 203
Thyroid-stimulating hormone (TSH)
  disorders of, 85
  function of, 85
  in Graves' disease, 97
  in hypothyroidism, 98–99
  regulation of thyroid by, 96
  release of, 85
  from tumors, 370
Thyrotoxicosis
  causing cardiac failure, 71
  hypercalcemia with, 282

Thyrotoxicosis—Continued
  and increased myocardial oxygen demand, 41
Thyrotropin-releasing hormone (TRH)
  as hormone stimulator, 85
  and TSH release, 96
Thyroxine (T_4)
  in hyperthyroidism, 96–98, 99–100
  deficiency, as cause of hyponatremia, 256
  in hypothyroidism, 98–99
  source of, 96
  synthetic, 99
L-thyroxine, 85
Tinnitus, with macroglobulinemia, 382
Tissue metabolic demand, increased, 66
Titratable acid (TA), hydrogen ion in, 272
Total peripheral resistance (TPR), and blood flow, 101
Totipotent stem cell, as blood cell precursor, 159
Tourniquet, pseudohyperkalemia with, 264
Toxins, in uremic syndrome, 310
Toxoplasmosis
  glomerulonephritis with, 290
  nephrotic syndrome from, 300
Trace elements, nutritional requirement for, 347
Tracheobronchial tree, 194–195
Transferrin
  in malnutrition assessment, 350
  in nephrotic syndrome, 299
Transfusions, blood
  neutrophil isoantibodies from, 171
  thrombocytopenia with, 178
Transient ischemic attacks (TIAs), cerebral, 337
Transplant rejection, and nephrotic syndrome, 301
Trauma
  clinical examples of, 470–471
  convalescence from, 468–469
  malnutrition with, 349
  metabolic response to, 463–471
Treponema pallidum, temperature and, 241
Triceps skin-fold thickness, to assess malnutrition, 349
Tricuspid incompetence. See Tricuspid regurgitation
Tricuspid regurgitation, 55
  jugular venous pulsation in, 52
Tricuspid stenosis, 55
Tricuspid valve, sound of, 50
Triglycerides
  digestion of, 150
  in nephrotic syndrome, 298, 299
Trihexyphenidyl, and sweating, 242
L-triiodothyronine, 85
Trophoblast antigen, with preeclampsia/eclampsia, 478
Tropical sprue, 150, 151

Trousseau's test, 284
Truncus arteriosus, 62
Trypanosomiasis, nephrotic syndrome from, 300
Trypsin
  in pancreatic secretion, 131, 132, 149
  in pancreatitis, 133
Trypsinogen
  enterokinase and, 149
  in pancreas, 132
Tubercules, and inflammation, 235
Tuberculosis
  age and, 7
  nephrotic syndrome from, 300
  secondary immunodeficiency from, 224
  syndrome of inappropriate ADH from, 88
d-Tubocurarine, and neuromuscular transmission, 341
Tubular basement membrane, lupus erythematosus and, 204
Tubular necrosis, acute. See Renal failure, acute
Tularemia, neutropenia with, 171
Tumors. See also Cancer and specific kinds of tumors
  adrenocortical, 92–93
  benign versus malignant, 356
  brain, syndrome of inappropriate ADH from, 88
  carcinoid, with Cushing's syndrome, 369
  diarrhea from, 151
  epilepsy from, 334
  erythropoietin and, 371
  gastrin-secreting, 128
  immunology
    antigens in, 362–363
    clinical example of, 365–366
    historical aspects of, 362
    mechanisms in, 363–364
    therapy, 364–365
  nephrotic syndrome from, 300
  of the pituitary, 85, 86, 88
  polycythemia from, 166
Tumor-specific transplantation antigens (TSTA), 362–363
Turbinates, nasal, 194
Turner's syndrome, 113
Typhoid, neutropenia with, 171

Ulcer, peptic
  defined, 126
  duodenal, 128–129
  gastric, 126–128, 129
  hydrochloric acid and, 127
  from hypercalcemia, 283
  jejunal, 128–129
  postbulbar, 128
  prepyloric, 127
Unidirectional block, in myocardial excitation, 15, 16
Upstroke, in cardiac electrophysiology, 11, 12, 14
Uranium, in bones, 313
Urate. See Uric acid
Uremia and uremic syndrome, 308–310. See also Renal failure

Uremia and uremic syndrome—
    Continued
  chronic, interstitial lung disease
    from, 435
  dialysis in, 310–311
  and potassium depletion, 262, 263
  with renal hypertension, 103
Ureterosigmoid anastomosis,
  metabolic acidosis from, 271
Urethritis, in Reiter's syndrome, 209
Uric acid
  crystallization of, 217–218
  excretion, 217
  and gout, 216–217
  nephropathy, with leukemia, 173
  renal lithiasis, with gout, 216
  supersaturation, levels of, 216
Uricase, and gout, 216
Urinary tract obstruction, postrenal
  azotemia with, 303, 304
Urine
  concentration and dilution, 252,
    253
  flow, and heart failure, 70
Urobilinogen, from bilirubin, 143
Uropathy, obstructive, differential
  diagnosis, 8
Urticaria (hives), 191–192
  as a hypersensitive disease, 189,
    190
  with vasculitis, 203

Valvular heart disease, 50–57
  aortic regurgitation (chronic), 54
  aortic stenosis, 53–54, 56
  clinical examples of, 55–56
  and coronary embolism, 41
  diagnosis of, 50
  mitral regurgitation, 53, 56
  mitral stenosis, 50, 52–53, 55–56
  pulmonary stenosis and regurgita-
    tion, 55
  tricuspid regurgitation, 55
  tricuspid stenosis, 55
Varicocele, from renal cell carcinoma,
  322
Vasa vasorum, 35
Vascular disease. *See* Cardiovascular
  disease *and specific diseases*
Vascular permeability
  through endothelium, 231–232
  and pulmonary edema, 446
  stimulation of, 233
Vascular resistance
  normal, 59–60, 62
  Ohm's law and, 60
  peripheral
    in hypertension, 103
    influences on, 101, 102
  with shunts, 62
Vasculitis
  as autoimmune disease, 203
  chronic pain with, 330
  from immune complex diseases,
    202–203
  and interstitial lung disease, 435
  necrotizing, with polyarteritis no-
    dosa, 209
  platelet consumption in, 177

Vasculitis—*Continued*
  and pulmonary vascular disease,
    451
  with renal parenchymal azotemia,
    305
  with rheumatoid arthritis, 208
  in Sjögren's syndrome, 210
  and thrombocytopenia, 178
  types of, 202
Vasoactive intestinal peptide (VIP)
  diarrhea from, 151
  and lower esophageal sphincter
    pressure, 120
  and pulmonary vascular resistance,
    250
  source of, 131
  from tumors, 370
Vasoconstriction
  afferent, in acute renal failure, 305
  in preeclampsia/eclampsia, 477
Vasodilation
  efferent, in acute renal failure,
    305–306
  for hypertension, 103
Vasopressin
  disorders with, 87–89
  normal secretion of, 87
  and plasminogen activator, 36
  and platelet aggregation, 36
  and post-trauma water balance,
    466, 467
  in preeclampsia/eclampsia, 479
Ventilation, alveolar, 413
  in emphysema and bronchitis, 415
  hypoventilation, 398–399
  in interstitial lung disease, 437–438
  measurements of, 425–426
Ventilation-perfusion ($\dot{V}/\dot{Q}$) ratios,
  low, 400–401
Ventricles
  diastolic function of, 27, 28
  myocardial infarction in right, 43
  myocardial ischemia in left, 42
  pressure overload, 30, 31–32
  systolic function of the, 27
  volume overload, 28–29, 30–31
Ventricular end-diastolic pressure
  (EDP), and preload, 25
Ventricular end-diastolic volume
  (EDV), and preload, 25
Ventricular fibrillation
  coronary death from, 48
  on electrocardiogram, 18
  from hyperkalemia, 264
  with hypokalemia, 263
Ventricular filling, constraint of, 66–
  67
Ventricular premature contractions,
  with hypokalemia, 263
Ventricular pressure-volume relationship, and cardiac contraction,
  24–25
Ventricular septal defect (VSD)
  clinical example of, 62–63
  oxygen saturations and pressures
    with, 63
Ventricular systolic ejection obstruction, 67
Ventriculogram, nuclear, and ventricular pressure overload, 31

Venule dilation, mediators of, 233
Vertebrae, aging and changes of, 3.
  See also Disks, intervertebral
Vertigo, with macroglobulinemia, 382
Vincristine, in tumor kill, 358, 361
Virchow, Rudolf, 35
Virilization, hormones causing, 113
Viruses
  kinds in immunodeficiencies, 225
  neutralized by complement system,
    222
  tumor, 356
Vision
  aging and, 4
  disorders in cerebral ischemia, 339
  sensors in brain, 333
Vitamin A
  and uremic syndrome, 310
  fat soluble, digestion of, 150
Vitamin B$_{12}$
  absorption of, 149
  deficiency of, 162
  deficiency and thrombocytopenia,
    178
  in enzyme/acid deficiency, 150
  and gastrectomy, 174
  in malabsorption, 151
Vitamin D
  and calcium homeostasis, 279, 280
  in calcium and phosphate regula-
    tion, 282
  fat soluble, digestion of, 150
  hypercalcemia from, 282
  and hypocalcemia, 283–284
  in osteomalacia, 317–318
  in renal osteodystrophy, 318
  in rickets, 317
  in uremic syndrome, 310
Vitamin E, fat soluble, digestion of,
  150
Vitamin K
  in blood clotting, 181, 182, 183, 185
  fat soluble, digestion of, 150
Vitamins, nutritional requirement for,
  347
Volume expansion, hypophosphatemia with, 285
Volume-pressure curves (lungs), normal versus interstitial disease,
  436
Vomiting, metabolic alkalosis from,
  276–277
von Willebrand's disease
  in atherosclerosis, 36
  factor VIII deficiency in, 177, 178–
    179, 184

Warfarin
  action of, 183, 184
  for glomerulonephritis, 295
Water
  absorption of, 150
  body content of, normal, 247, 248
  deficit estimation formula, 253–254
  excess, in body fluid, 256–257
  and fluid compartment osmolality,
    247–248, 249
  in hyperosmolality, 253–257
  in lung, 442, 443
  post-trauma metabolism of, 466–468

Water—*Continued*
    regulation of, normal, 252
    retention, with preeclampsia/
        eclampsia, 478
    and sodium in body fluid, 249, 250
Water brash, with reflux esophagitis, 124
West, John B., lung blood flow zones
        of, 449, 450

Willis, circle of, atherosclerosis in, 35
Wiskott-Aldrich syndrome, as
        immunodeficiency state, 224
Wolff-Parkinson-White syndrome
    clinical example of, 19
    reentrant arrhythmias in, 15
Wunderlich, Carl Reinhold August,
        238

X-rays, of gallstones, 138
Xerostomia, with Sjögren's syndrome,
        210

Zenker's diverticulum, 120
Zollinger-Ellison syndrome, from gas-
        trinoma, 128
Zymogen, clotting factors from, 181